Stephen M. Ansell, MD, PhD
Editor

Rare Hematological
Malignancies

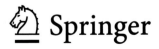 Springer

Stephen M. Ansell, MD, PhD
Associate Professor of Medicine
Mayo Clinic, College of Medicine
200 First Street SW
Rochester, Minnesota, USA

Series Editor:
Steven T. Rosen
Robert H. Lurie Comprehensive Cancer Center
Northwestern University
Chicago, IL
USA

ISBN-13: 978-0-387-73743-0   e-ISBN-13: 978-0-387-73744-7

Library of Congress Control Number: 2007932231

Contents

Contributors

Stephen M. Ansell
Mayo Clinic College of Medicine, Rochester, MN

Carlo Aul
St. Johannes Hospital, Duisburg, Germany

Milosav Beran
University of Texas M.D. Anderson Cancer Center, Houston TX

Peter Borchmann
University of Cologne, Cologne, Germany

Karen L. Chang
City of Hope National Medical Center, Duarte, CA

Angela Dispenzieri
Mayo Clinic College of Medicine, Rochester, MN

Michelle A. Fanale
University of Texas M.D. Anderson Cancer Center, Houston, TX

Paul T. Fanta
Scripps Clinic, La Jolla, CA

Guido Finazzi
Ospedali Riuniti, Bergamo, Italy

Aristoteles A.N. Giagounidis
St. Johannes Hospital, Duisburg, Germany

Lawrence E. Gibson
Mayo Clinic College of Medicine, Rochester, MN

Jason Gotlib
Stanford Cancer Center, Stanford, CA

Thomas M. Habermann
Mayo Clinic College of Medicine, Rochester, MN

Evdoxia Hatjiharissi
Dana Farber Cancer Institute, Boston, MA

Steven M. Horwitz
Memorial Sloan Kettering Cancer Center, New York, N Y

Ryan B. Lundell
Mayo Clinic College of Medicine, Rochester, MN

Giampaolo Merlini
Amyloidosis Center, Biotechnology Research Laboratories,
Fondazione IRCCS Policlinico San Matteo and Department of Biochemistry,
University of Pavia, Italy

Ana Maria Molina
Memorial Sloan Kettering Cancer Center, New York, NY

Kerry J. Savage
British Columbia Cancer Agency, Vancouver, Canada

Alan Saven
Scripps Clinic,. La Jolla, CA

Richard T. Silver
Weill Cornell Medical University, New York, NY

David S. Snyder
City of Hope National Medical Center, Duarte, CA

Ayalew Tefferi
Mayo Clinic College of Medicine, Rochester, MN

Xavier G. Thomas
Edouard Herriot Hospital, Lyon, France

Steven P. Treon
Dana Farber Cancer Institute, Boston, MA

Peter Valent
Medical University of Vienna, Vienna, Austria

Roger H. Weenig
Mayo Clinic College of Medicine, Rochester, MN

Anas Younes
University of Texas M.D. Anderson Cancer Center, Houston, TX

Chapter 1
Polycythemia Vera and Other Polycythemia Syndromes

Richard T. Silver

1.1 Introduction

Polycythemia vera (PV) is an acquired clonal hematopoietic stem cell disorder characterized by the overproduction of red and white blood cells and platelets in the absence of any appropriate stimulus for these events. For this reason, it is considered one of the four myeloproliferative diseases, which include essential thrombocythemia, primary myelofibrosis (PM), and chronic myeloid leukemia, all diseases which reflect varying degrees of erythroid, myeloid, and megakaryocytic marrow hyperplasia. Polycythemia, in general, can be defined as an increase in the volume of circulating red cells per kilogram of body weight or, equivalently, an increase in the red blood cell mass. Clinically, this is expressed as an absolute increase in the number of red cells, usually but not always accompanied by corresponding increases in the hemoglobin and hematocrit. Polycythemia might occur as a result of a primary disease of unknown cause, PV, or as a secondary manifestation of other illnesses. In the past, the diagnosis of PV was often an exclusionary diagnosis; now it is made more easily because of the $JAK2^{V617F}$ molecular abnormality (*vide infra*) found in this disease. Untreated PV leads to thrombohemorrhagic complications and eventually to progressive myelofibrosis, anemia, and splenomegaly.

1.2 Definitions

The terms "erythremia" and "erythrocytosis" are often used to refer to primary and secondary polycythemia, respectively. Others use erythremia as a classification for patients whose only abnormality is an increased red cell volume. The term "relative" polycythemia is a misnomer. A better term is "false" polycythemia, because it is not polycythemia since the red cell volume per kilogram of body weight is normal. In this instance, the increased hematocrit is related to a decrease in plasma volume. In PV, the plasma volume may be increased, normal, or decreased. Other terms referring to false or relative polycythemia include stress polycythemia, stress erythrocytosis, pseudopolycythemia, and benign polycythemia (1).

S.M. Ansell (ed.), *Rare Hematological Malignancies.*
© Springer 2008

The determination of red cell volume per kilogram of body weight separates both primary and secondary polycythemia from false polycythemia. PV is differentiated from secondary polycythemia by other means (to be described) but *not* by a red blood cell volume determination.

1.3   Presenting Signs and Symptoms

Polycythemia vera is twice as common in men as in women. It is usually a disease of middle age, but its range extends broadly from 20 to 60 or 70 years. Forty percent of our patients are under age 50 (1); rare cases of PV have been described in children (2). PV has been reported rarely in African Americans and is said to occur with increased frequency in Jews (3). Whether the latter observation is related to selection by virtue of specific hospital populations is not clear. The development of symptoms, which is often insidious, is related to increased red cell mass and whole-blood viscosity and an increased number of platelets. These symptoms include easy fatigue, weakness, shortness of breath, dizziness, tinnitus, bone pain, visual disturbances, headaches, erythromelalgia, pounding in the ears, and pruritus. The pruritus increases in intensity after a tub bath and less often after showering. It is worse when the temperature of the water is warm rather than cool. Burning or throbbing pain in the legs, feet, or hands might occur, which might be accompanied by a mottled redness.Abnormalities of coagulation are responsible for the hemorrhagic tendency and paradoxically contribute to thrombotic episodes. Either might be the presenting manifestation of PV, but thrombotic events predominate. Most often, these episodes result from qualitative and quantitative platelet abnormalities or to acquired abnormalities of Von Willebrand's factor (4), which resembles type II v WF disease.

The most common source of major hemorrhage is the upper gastrointestinal tract, where peptic ulcer has been reported in about 10% of patients (5). Thus, iron deficiency might distort the overall picture because of anemia, hypochromia, and microcytosis. Sometimes iron deficiency occurs in a previously polycythemic woman owing to menometrorrhagia producing the same distorted picture. In these instances, the nature of the underlying polycythemia is revealed when hemorrhage is controlled and the anemia has been treated with iron.

Patients referred because of small vessel thrombosis of the hands or feet may suffer from polycythemia. Erythromelalgia might be observed in PV, especially in those patients with significant thrombocythemia (6). Thrombosis of larger vessels may involve the arterial and venous circulations of the heart, brain, liver, spleen, gastrointestinal tract, and lung. Thrombophlebitis is common. Acute gouty attacks can accompany excess production of uric acid (7).

Particularly serious thrombotic events typically associated with PV include abdominal vein thrombosis (e.g., Budd-Chiari syndrome) and obstruction of the portal, mesenteric, and/or splenic system (8). In this case, red cell mass studies in addition to a *JAK2*^{V617F} determination can be extremely helpful because erythropoietin levels may be increased (9) and the presence of splenomegaly might not be diagnostically helpful. If the $JAK2^{V617F}$ abnormality is found and the red cell mass is increased, phlebotomy is usually required (10).

1.4   Physical Findings

In the early stage of PV, the conjunctivae are injected. The liver is palpable in about 50% of patients, and the spleen is palpable in about 60% of patients (1). The size of the spleen depends on the stage of the illness and ranges from barely palpable below the left costal margin to massive enlargement filling the left half of the abdomen. Extremely large spleens might herald the future development of myelofibrosis and myeloid metaplasia.

1.5   Hematologic Manifestations

Red cell counts of 7–10 million cells/μL, hematocrit values of 55–70%, and hemoglobin concentrations of 18–24 mg/dL have been observed (1). Often the hemoglobin is not increased as much as the red cell count; thus, the hematocrit might be slightly reduced in proportion to the erythrocyte count. If there has been hemorrhage, the hemoglobin content of the red blood cells is reduced more than their size, and the red cells appear hypochromic and microcytic. In general, however, the individual erythrocytes appear normocytic and normochromic. A rare normoblast may be found. The number of reticulocytes is usually normal except after hemorrhage.

In about half of the patients, there is a moderate increase in the peripheral leukocyte count, ranging from 10,000 to 30,000 cells/μL. Values greater than 50,000 cells/μL have been reported (11). Metamyelocytes may be seen in the peripheral blood smear. An increase in the absolute basophil count may be seen and might be related to certain features of PV, such as peptic ulcer and pruritus.

The number of blood platelets is increased above 400,000/μL in more than 80% of patients at the time of diagnosis and assumes diagnostic importance (12). In most of these patients, the platelet count ranges between 500,000 and 1 million/μL, but in some, the initial platelet count may be more than 1 million/μL. On occasion, the platelet count may increase after spontaneous bleeding or phlebotomy, although there has been no specific correlation between platelet count before phlebotomy and thrombosis.

The bone marrow in patients with PV is hypercellular, and marrow fat is reduced, findings particularly well appreciated in biopsy sections (13–15). Each of the three developmental series, erythroid cells, granulocytes and megakaryocytes, typically participate in the hyperplasia, although erythroid hyperplasia is paramount. (In contrast, the hyperplasia in *secondary* polycythemia is typically confined to the erythroid series.) There is no abnormality in erythroid maturation; orthochromic normoblasts predominate. There may be a slight shift to the left in the neutrophilic series. Eosinophils and basophils are prominent.

Bone marrow examination by itself cannot unequivocally distinguish primary and secondary polycythemia. However, a hyperplastic granulocyte series with evidence of cellular immaturity and an increase in megakaryocytes of variable size favor PV (16). Marrow iron stores are depleted more often in primary rather than in secondary polycythemia, a finding of diagnostic importance. However, because secondary iron deficiency is so common in women, the absence of marrow iron might not always be of significant differential diagnostic value in the female patient.

Normally, reticulin fibers, also known as type 3 collagen, extend throughout the marrow and provide a supporting stroma for hematopoietic cells. In disease states, two different patterns of the reticulin network can be recognized. The first consists of an increased prominence of the normal network, which probably occurs in response to an increase in functioning hematopoietic tissue. It is a nonspecific change, because it is found in many hematologic disorders (13–16). This second, or "fibroblastic," pattern, consisting of type 1 collagen, results in coarsening of the network, resulting from the formation of fibers that are thicker than normal. These thick fibers tend to form bundles or fascicles that follow a waving or swirling course. The fibroblastic pattern is seen in patients with PV and other myeloproliferative diseases (14–16).

1.6 Hyperuricemia

Hyperuricemia, a characteristic of all myeloproliferative diseases, occurs in many patients with PV. A good correlation between serum urate concentration and red and white cell counts has not been demonstrated. The incidence of gout in patients with PV has ranged from 5% to 10%. Although gout may precede the development of PV, it usually occurs 5–10 years after the onset of the disease (1).

Increased urate production and excretion may result in the precipitation of uric acid in the kidneys, causing stones or uric acid nephropathy. Renal colic is an unusual presenting manifestation of patients with PV, but it has been observed (1). Although serum uric acid may be increased in secondary polycythemia, it is rare to find the same high concentrations that occur in the primary disease.

1.7 Natural History

An appreciation of the natural history of PV is required because a patient might be observed during a stage when the disease is in transition. PV is an illness of reasonably long duration, usually ranging from 10 to 20 years. Although phlebotomy and other treatment modalities influence the course of the disease and its clinical manifestations, unsuccessful treatment and/or the natural history of the disease after a number of years is associated with a fall in hemoglobin concentration and the gradual development of anemia. The spleen (and sometimes the liver) progressively enlarges and may fill the entire abdomen. Splenic infarcts, causing mild to severe left upper quadrant pain, may mimic an acute abdominal crisis or renal colic. Rarely, the enormous spleen causes large bowel obstruction. Erythrocytes of variable size and shape, teardrop forms, nucleated red cells, and immature granulocytes appear in the peripheral blood. The white blood cell count, often normal or moderately increased throughout the early and middle phases of the illness, continues to rise. Blood platelets may increase or decrease in number. Bone marrow examination at this time reveals a prominent "fibroblastic" and reticulin network, myelofibrosis, and osteosclerosis. Although the degree of extramedullary hematopoiesis (myeloid metaplasia) generally is proportional to the duration of the disease, some patients display features of it early in the course of the illness and even relatively early during the polycythemic phase. Without an antecedent history of PV, it might appear that the patient is suffering from primary myelofibrosis (PM) with myeloid metaplasia. Sometimes the clinical and hematologic picture resembles chronic myeloid leukemia, which is readily excluded by examining the peripheral blood or marrow for the *BCR-ABL* gene rearrangement. Moreover, the Philadelphia chromosome, the hallmark of chronic myeloid leukemia, is never present in PV. Acute myeloid leukemia occurs as a terminal event in PV (17), indistinguishable from that which occurs in myelofibrosis with myeloid metaplasia or myeloid blast-phase chronic myeloid leukemia.

1.8   Diagnostic Tests

1.8.1   JAK2 [V617F]

Within the past few years, the finding of a specific mutation in the JAK-STAT signaling pathway in PV, essential thrombocythemia, and primary myelofibrosis with myeloid metaplasm has revolutionized our diagnostic abilities and our understanding of the pathophysiology of these disorders.

There are four members of the Janus kinase (JAK) family, Janus kinases 1, 2, and 3 and tyrosine kinase 2 (JAK1, JAK2, JAK3, and TYK2, respectively), with slightly different functions. Each has a kinase domain and a catalytically inactive pseudokinase domain, which has an important regulatory function. To some, the presence of these two similar domains in the protein, one active and the other inactive, suggested the Roman god of gates and passageways, Janus, who had the ability to look simultaneously in two directions (18).

The JAK proteins function as intermediates between membrane receptors and signaling molecules. When particular cytokines or growth factors bind to their receptors on JAK proteins, the kinases associated with the cytoplasmic regions of these receptors become phosphorylated and thereby activated. This activation causes docking sites for downstream molecules, notably those of the STAT system (signal transducers and activators of transcription), which become activated and enter the nucleus, where they function as transcription factors. JAK2, the third Janus kinase discovered, is activated particularly when receptors bind to hematopoietic growth factors, also known as type 1 cytokine receptors, such as erythropoietin, granulocyte-colony stimulating factor (G-CSF), granulocyte macrophage-colony stimulating factor (GM-CSF), and thrombopoietin (18, 19).

The $JAK2^{V617F}$ mutation lies within the negative regulatory domain of JAK2 known as the pseudokinase or Janus homology 2 (JH2) domain. In this mutation, phenylalanine is substituted for valine in codon 617 (V617F) of the JAK2 nucleotide 1849, which leads to independent activation of cellular pathways in erythropoietic receptor signaling and without need for erythropoietin. The mutation might be either heterozygous or homozygous. Homozygosity is thought to be related to more advanced disease (20) and to predict for major vascular events (21).

Our studies (22) and those of others (21–25) have shown that JAK2 is present in more than 95% of patients with the clinical phenotype of PV (19–23). It is also found in approximately 50% of patients with essential thrombocythemia (ET) or primary myelofibrosis, about 3% to 5% of patients with myelodysplasia, acute myeloid leukemia, systemic mastocytosis, and chronic neutrophilic leukemia, and 10–30% of normal individuals (20–25). Loss of the V617F gene has been observed in previously positive PV patients who develop acute myeloid leukemia (26).

The search for new mutations in members of the JAK family, particularly in those patients with V617F negative polycythemia has been the subject of intense scrutiny. New mutations, indeed, have been found in members of the JAK and STAT families in patients with V617F negative PV or idiopathic erythrocytosis. Four somatic gain of function mutations affecting JAK2 exon 12 have been described in 10 patients negative for $JAK2^{V617F}$ (27). These were found in marrow samples from patients who presented with an isolated erythrocytosis and distinctive bone marrow morphology. The platelet counts were less than $450,000/\mu L$ and the neutrophil counts were normal. Some also had reduced serum erythropoietin levels. Erythroid colonies could be grown from blood samples in the absence of exogenous erythropoietin. These erythroid colonies were heterozygous for the mutation, whereas colonies homozygous for the mutation occurred mostly in patients with V617F-positive PV. Three of the exon 12 mutations included a substitution of leucine for lysine at position 539 of JAK2.

The discovery of the JAK2 abnormality has broad implications for the present and the future both for diagnosis and treatment. There is now an intense search for new therapeutic agents that may affect JAK2 expression and might be effective in the treatment of PV and related disorders. The sensitivity of the techniques for detecting and measuring $JAK2^{V617F}$ or its variants will improve in the immediate future. Other mutations, similar to those described earlier, may soon be discovered. In the meantime, it is still important to review a recommended method for the diagnosis of PV in those patients with the phenotypic clinical and hematologic

Table 1.1 Clinical classification of polycythemia

Primary polycythemia (polycythemia vera)
  $JAK2^{V617F}$ – Positive   95+ % *(and variants)*
  JAK^{V617F} – Negative   < 5 %
Secondary polycythemia–$JAK2^{V617F}$ negative
  Related inadequate oxygen delivery to tissues with respect to need
    Due to increased arterial oxygen tension
      With physiologic or anatomic cardiopulmonary abnormalities
        Abnormalities of lungs, chest, bellows, or ventilator control mechanisms
        Right-to-left vascular shunts
      Without physiologic or anatomic cardiopulmonary abnormalities
        Impaired oxygen-carrying capacity of hemoglobin
        Normal oxygen-carrying capacity of hemoglobin
        Truncated erythropoietin receptor
        Congenital polycythemias (e.g., "Chubash")
      Due to increased blood flow-congestive heart failure
  Unrelated to inadequate oxygen delivery of need usually accompanied by increased serum levels
of erythropoietin and associated with benign or malignant lesions:
    Kidney—cysts, hydronephrosis, hypernephroma, sarcoma
    Cerebellum—hemangioblastoma
    Uterus— myoma
    Liver—hepatoma, hamartoma
    Other—adrenal (pheochromocytoma), lung

characteristics of PV in whom a $JAK2^{V617F}$ abnormality cannot be demonstrated. Until recently, the diagnosis of PV was essentially an exclusionary one, usually based on the criteria of the Polycythemia Vera Study Group (PVSG) or its many suggested modifications (28, 29). An alternative schema, which we have used and validated, is shown in Table 1.1.

1.8.2 Endogenous Erythroid Colonies

For many years, the measurement of endogenous erythroid colonies had been an important marker for diagnosing PV (30). However, this is a laborious test usually restricted to research laboratories, and from a diagnostic standpoint, this has fallen out of diagnostic favor because of the use of the JAK2 determination. However, it is described here because of its biologic importance.

In normal individuals, erythroid colonies grow only in culture media that are supplemented with erythropoietin (EPO). Erythroid progenitor cells obtained from blood or marrow from PV patients grow in semisolid serum-containing cultures in the absence of EPO (27, 31). This spontaneous growth of erythroid colonies, known as endogenous erythroid colony formation, is observed in some cases of essential thrombocythemia and idiopathic myelofibrosis but not in normal subjects. The formation of these cultures was first thought to be to the result of hypersensitivity of the cells to tiny amounts of EPO in the culture media and to sensitivity to other growth factors such as interleukin (IL)-3, stem cell factor, GM-CSF, and thrombopoietin, and GM-CSF insulin-like growth factor-1 (31,32). The augmented response of erythroid progenitors to growth factors suggested there was an abnormality in EPO signaling that controlled the process of proliferation, maturation, and cell death. However, subsequently, it became clear that growth of these colonies was truly independent of EPO because it was not blocked by anti-EPO neutralizing antibodies (31).

1.8.3   PRV-1 mRNA Overexpression

A molecular marker of interest in PV is the measurement of granulocyte levels of PRV-1 mRNA. Several studies suggested that overproduction of PRV-1 mRNA could be a marker of clonal hematopoiesis in PV (33–36). The frequency of finding this marker could be attributed to differences in sampling technique (37). Furthermore, elevations in granulocyte levels of PRV-1 mRNA are not specific for the chronic myeloproliferative diseases as initially believed. PRV-1 values, like the leukocyte alkaline phosphatase score, are higher in pregnancy, infection, and after G-CSF administration (36, 37). Thus, it appears to be a secondary phenomenon to myeloproliferation rather than a primary event, similar to high serum B_{12} levels and increased leukocyte alkaline phosphatase values (36–38).

1.8.4   Thrombopoietin Receptor (c-MPL)

Abnormalities of thrombopoietin receptor, c-MPL, have been involved in our understanding of the myeloproliferative diseases. Intuitively, one might think the expression of c-MPL would be increased in PV and ET; in fact its expression is reduced in ET and PV (39). This is related to impaired c-MPL glycoslation rather than c-MPL gene disruption or repression of transcription factors (40). Moreover, because c-MPL expression is also reduced in Idiopathic Myelofibrosis (IMF), it is not valuable as a diagnostic marker, notwithstanding its biologic interest.

1.8.5   Hematocrit

Polycythemia is first suspected most commonly because of abnormalities of hematocrit values. However, the extent of reliance on the hematocrit for the diagnosis of polycythemia is the source of much confusion both at the bedside and in published texts. Despite a reasonably good correlation between the hematocrit and the circulating total red cell volume over a wide range of hematocrit determinations, the value of a single hematocrit (HCT) measurement for predicting total red cell volume is poor (28) unless the hematocrit is more than 60% (41–44). At this level, there is excellent correlation between the hematocrit determination and actual red cell mass. For values of HCT ≤ 60%, the red cell mass must be measured with radioactive chromium (Cr^{51}) to ascertain whether it is increased. This is especially true for modest increases in HCT. To compare total red cell volume from one individual to another, it is best to express it in terms of corrected cubic centimeters per kilogram of body weight. Because fat tissue is relatively avascular, obese individuals might have a falsely low red cell mass. A satisfactory and widely used method for determining red cell volume is the direct tagging of red cells with Cr^{51}. The method is easy to perform and is reproducible with a coefficient of variation of 1.5% (28, 42–44). The red cell mass for a normal man is less than 36 cc/kg and for a woman is less than 32 cc/kg. Adjustments are made for obesity (42–44). A normal red blood cell mass might be found on occasion in patients with PV (e.g., after recent hemorrhage). In JAK2-negative patients with the phenotypic characteristics of PV, the diagnosis still relies upon the clinical criteria that has been discussed (*vide infra*).

The World Health Organization (WHO) recently revised its criteria for the diagnosis of PV (45) and recommended Cr^{51} red cell mass values as just described among other criteria for the diagnosis of polycythemia (45). However, it also allowed other surrogate markers for this test, including a hemoglobin value in men of 18.5 g/dL and a value of 16.5 g/dL or more in women, as published earlier (46). It is not clear how some of the hemoglobin values were selected (44). The use of a single hemoglobin value is no more reliable than the use of single hematocrit value, particularly in the lower ranges of presumed red blood cell mass increase (41). Moreover, hemoglobin values are often comparatively lower than hematocrit and red blood cell values because of iron deficiency. It is unfortunate that the use of these hemoglobin values has replaced the red cell mass in many reports and studies of PV (47) because it permits the addition of patients to studies who might not have had the disease. Moreover, the detection of endogenous erythroid colonies is a laborious process restricted to certain research laboratories. Thus, it is difficult to understand the reason why it was recently listed as a minor diagnostic criterion for PV by WHO, as its use will be so restricted.

1.8.6 *Erythropoietin*

Even in the JAK2 era, the easy availability of a relatively routine test for measuring serum erythropoietin remains important in the diagnosis of PV. Decreased arterial oxygen tension typically leads to increased red cell production, presumably mediated by erythropoietin. A major exception is in patients with emphysema who have diminished arterial oxygen tension but normal red cell mass (48). An increase in erythropoietin has, nevertheless, been demonstrated in some of these patients, implying that these patients are not polycythemic because of an inability to produce erythropoietin.

Polycythemia unrelated to tissue hypoxia might be due to autonomous erythropoietin production by benign or malignant tumors (49, 50). Biologically active erythropoietic substances, which have been demonstrated in plasma, urine, and tissue extracts from such patients, are not subject to physiologic control mechanisms and are independent of the red cell mass. The causal relationship between polycythemia and tumor is indicated by the fact that, in many patients, remission of polycythemia has occurred following removal of the tumor (51, 52). This type of polycythemia has been most frequently associated with renal abnormalities, especially neoplasms and benign cysts (51). From a diagnostic standpoint, it is important to stress that with polycythemia accompanying tumors, there might be increases in the platelet and white cell counts; even splenomegaly has been reported. To confound the situation even more, the coexistence of primary and secondary polycythemia (e.g., PV and chronic pulmonary disease) can occur. Therefore, a high level of diagnostic vigilance must be maintained.

In contrast to the observations in polycythemia secondary to anoxia and tumors, the polycythemia of PV is not oxygen dependent and is not usually associated with increased erythropoietin in plasma or urine. In fact, erythropoietin output is less than normal, because red cell production by the marrow is autonomous and erythropoietin output is suppressed by the increased red cell mass.

Despite the aforementioned, our data suggest that only low erythropoietin levels are of value in diagnosis. In analyzing our own data, we were surprised to find the number of normal or elevated EPO values in $JAK2^{V617F}$-positive patients at diagnosis; the cause for this is not clear (Table 1.2). The relation between erythropoietin and polycythemia can be summarized as follows:

1. Increased, but regulated, erythropoietin production is proportional to the stimulus in anemic but normal individuals and secondary hypoxemic polycythemia.
2. Autonomous erythropoietin production irrespective of red cell mass is observed in secondary polycythemia accompanying erythropoietic related tumors.
3. Autonomous erythropoiesis by the marrow, unrelated to erythropoietin production, and usually decreased levels of serum erythropoietin in PV.

Table 1.2 EPO levels determined in 77 PV patients at diagnosis at New York Presbyterian Hospital

EPO Level (mU/mL)	Number (%)
<5	39 (51%)
5–10	24 (31%)
10–15	7 (9%)
>15	7 (9%)

1.8.7 Arterial Oxygen Saturation

Causes of secondary polycythemia can be classified for clinical use as (1) those related to inadequate oxygen delivery that does not meet tissue needs and (2) those that are not related to oxygen delivery. Customarily, an arterial oxygen saturation of 92% or more has been considered characteristic of PV, whereas a lower saturation has been regarded as evidence of polycythemia related to hypoxemia. Recent studies have cast doubt on the usefulness of arterial oxygen saturation measurements in subtle cases in differentiating primary and secondary polycythemia, even when the latter is related to impaired arterial oxygen supply (48, 53). For example, some patients with pulmonary disease have respiratory alkalosis due to hyperventilation. This relates to the influence of pH on the oxyhemoglobin dissociation curve. Oxygen saturation in these patients might be normal even though arterial oxygen tension is significantly reduced. Of course, in primary PV, the JAK2 molecular abnormality is found, whereas in those cases of PV due to inadequate oxygenation the JAK2 test will be "negative."

1.8.8 Vitamin B and Its Binding Proteins

In PV and other myeloproliferative diseases, concentrations of serum vitamin B and vitamin B_{12} capacity are increased more than normal, paralleling the degree of leukocyte proliferation. Serum vitamin B_{12} levels tend to be modestly increased in PV and greatly increased in chronic myeloid leukemia (54). A similar, but more striking, increase occurs in the unbound B_{12} binding capacity (54). This test also had diagnostic value in days prior to JAK2.

1.8.9 Leukocyte Alkaline Phosphatase

Because of the ready availability of other tests to exclude chronic myeloid leukemia, including cytogenetics, fluorescent in situ hybridization tests, and analysis of the peripheral blood or marrow for the abnormal BCR-ABL gene by polymerase chain reaction (PCR), the LAP test is rarely used now. It is described briefly because of references to it in the older literature. The test was used as a diagnostic criterion of PV by the PVSG and to distinguish patients with PV from those with chronic myeloid leukemia (55). The principle of the LAP test is based on the amount and staining intensity of a dye precipitated at presumed sites of enzyme activity within mature and band neutrophils, which are the only granulocytes with significant LAP activity in the peripheral blood or bone marrow. Usually, peripheral blood is used and scored semiquantitatively; 100 neutrophils are graded 0 to 4+. The total score thus ranges from 0 to 400.

Abnormally low or absent LAP activity is observed in chronic myeloid leukemia and in some patients with myelofibrosis with myeloid metaplasia. A marked increase both in LAP activity and in the number of neutrophils showing such activity may be seen in PV, essential thrombocythemia, leukemoid reactions, and some patients with myelofibrosis with myeloid metaplasia (primary myelofibrosis).

The normal LAP score ranges from 25 to 50. In leukemoid reactions and in PV, it could rise to more than 200, whereas in chronic myeloid leukemia, it is usually less than 25 (55).

1.9   Differential Diagnosis of Polycythemia Vera

The JAK2 abnormality has made the diagnosis of PV much easier. As previously mentioned, it is found in 95% of patients with PV. However, because it is also found in approximately 50% of patients with ET and 50% of patients with PM, if the $JAK2^{V617F}$ abnormality is found, and if the HCT value is slightly elevated above normal median values, it is mandatory to perform a Cr^{51} red blood cell study to determine whether there is an increase in red cell mass. (In our institution we also routinely perform a radioactive iodinated albumin plasma volume study, which thus allows us to measure total blood volume.) This is especially important in patients with ET who have the $JAK2^{V617F}$ mutation for these patients have been reported to have a higher hemoglobin level than those without the mutation (56); it has been suggested these patients might evolve into PV. Of course, unless a red cell mass study is initially performed, it is impossible to unequivocally exclude PV at the onset of the illness, as the true red cell volume will not be known.

What is the approach for patients who are polycythemic but do not have the molecular JAK2 abnormality? As previously mentioned, the $JAK2^{V617F}$ mutation is found in approximately 95% of PV patients, a figure consistent with the findings in our own institution (Table 1.1). Among the 5% JAK2-negative PV patients, some carry the JAK2 exon 12 mutation. These patients have a different phenotype, because they do not have thrombocytosis or splenomegaly and the bone marrow shows only slight erythroid hyperplasia. However only one of our four $JAK2^{V617F}$-negative PV patients carried this mutation; therefore, other causes of polycythemia have to be considered.

In most patients with secondary polycythemia due to hypoxemia, the structural abnormalities of the heart and lung are sufficiently apparent to indicate the underlying cause of the polycythemia. In patients with familial high-affinity hemoglobin, the diagnosis is relatively easy because most, but not all, of these patients have a positive family history. The initial laboratory tests should, of course, include a hemoglobin electrophoresis and an oxygen tension at which hemoglobin is 50% saturated (P50). A low P50 suggests the presence of a high-affinity oxygen (57, 58) or bisphosphoglycerate (2,3-BPG) deficiency (59). High-affinity hemoglobins which include hemoglobin J Capetown, Yakima, Kemsey, Rainier, Ypsi, and Chesapeake may be found on electrophoresis (57). If the P50 is normal, mutations might involve the von Hippel-Lindau (VHL), tumor suppressive gene (60) or truncated EPO receptor (EPOR) (61). Another well-recognized cause of polycythemia is the so-called endemic Chubash polycythemia (62). Variations of these interesting polycythemias have been described and are detailed elsewhere (59–63).

1.10   Treatment of Polycythemia Vera

Considerable controversy surrounds the treatment of polycythemia vera ever since it was described 100 years ago. Current recommendations for its management are based upon a small number of randomized clinical trials, and a series of prospective and retrospective studies evaluating different treatment programs pertaining to different aspects of the disease. These include survival, reduction in phlebotomy requirements, thrombotic events, and evolution of the disease into myelofibrosis and acute leukemia.

1.10.1   Phlebotomy

Reduction of the red cell mass and maintaining it at a safe level by phlebotomy is the first principle of therapy in PV. Improperly treated, PV becomes a disease with serious consequences related to morbidity and mortality; this was recently emphasized by Marchioli et al, (64), who reported a death rate of 3.7 per 100 patients per year, far exceeding the normal. Important physiologic and pathologic components of the disease, which must be dealt with therapeutically, relate to the erythroid cell and the megakaryocyte, both of which play essential roles in causing complications of the disease. Hematologists agree that the mainstay in treatment is phlebotomy, with target levels of the hematocrit at <45% for men and <42% for women. Although a recent publication based on a retrospective review suggested higher red cell levels might be permissible (65). During pregnancy, the HCT should be <36%. Reduction of the red cell mass and maintaining it at a level close to normal will help to remove a major source of complications. A progressive increase in the incidence of vascular occlusive episodes at HCT levels >45% (66) has been shown as well as abnormal changes in blood viscosity above 45% (67). Iron replacement should not be used. Phlebotomy does not relieve pruritus. Repeated phlebotomy, overtime, causes severe iron deficiency. Venous access sites become exhausted. However, in a recent multivariate analysis of a large retrospective cohort of patients, a hematocrit in the evaluable range of 40–55% was not associated with the occurrence of an increased rate of thrombotic events or mortality (68). Although an appropriate controlled study to establish the real target range in PV is needed, it seems prudent to continue to recommend to the target of <45% (68) in men and <42% in women (69).

There is very little data in the literature pertaining to the frequency or the rate of phlebotomy which can be considered a manifestation of the aggressiveness of disease. In general, I believe that patients who have high phlebotomy requirements are those who might have a more aggressive form of the disease and should receive some form of myelosuppression prior to the development of splenomegaly and myelofibrosis. This is because a higher rate of phlebotomy may be associated not only with increased erythroid activity but also with more active megakaryocytic proliferation, leading to the earlier development of myelofibrosis (69).

Little quantifiable data exists, however, with respect to the phlebotomy requirements of patients with PV. It has been suggested that measurement of a Cr^{51} red cell mass provides an indication for the exact measurement of the blood to be removed (66). This statement, however, does not take into account that no study has correlated initial red blood cell mass with subsequent phlebotomy requirements. Additionally, as blood is removed by phlebotomy, it is replenished by the hyperactive bone marrow. Thus, each patient must provide sole source criteria on a measure of activity of the disease. In our series of 55 patients (71), the annual number of phlebotomies per year per patient ranged from 1 to 25, with a mean of 8 and a median of 9 phlebotomies per year. However, more than half the patients required 8–25 phlebotomies per year and thus became candidates for myelosuppressive therapy.

If the phlebotomy requirement is minimal (i.e., requiring 2 to 3 or even 4 units a year), a patient can be managed with phlebotomy only (PHO-O). All patients should receive low-dose aspirin (81– 100 mg daily). The use of acetylsalicylic acid (ASA) was originally discouraged because of the findings by the PVSG evaluating ASA 900 mg daily combined with dipyridamole (72). The trial was stopped because of an excess of major bleeding without preventing thrombotic events. The European Collaboration on Low-dose Aspirin in Polycythemia Study (ECLAP) provided compelling evidence for the efficacy and safety of low-dose ASA (for instance, 100 mg daily) in a double-blind, placebo-controlled, randomized clinical study (73). Five hundred eighteen patients without a clear indication or contraindications to ASA were enrolled. The median age was 61 years. Previous cardiovascular events were reported in only 10% of cases in this subgroup, so that the trial reflected an asymptomatic, low-risk population. Median follow-up was only 2.8 years. ASA significantly lowered the risk of a primary combined endpoint, including cardiovascular death, nonfatal myocardial infarction, nonfatal stroke, and major venous thromboembolism. Total and cardiovascular mortality were also reduced by 46% and 59%, respectively. Major bleeding was only slightly increased. The results of this trial eliminated the concerns raised by the PVSG about the risk:reward ratio with ASA. Different doses of ASA, mostly on the low side, have confirmed the value of this drug in treating microvascular symptoms such as erythromelalgia, transient ischemic attacks and other neurologic and ocular disturbances, dysarthria, scintillating scotoma, and so forth (74).

Should a patient have relatively frequent phlebotomies (more than six per year) and/or develop signs and symptoms of severe iron-deficiency anemia, progressive splenomegaly, or evidence of increasing marrow fibrosis or complain of the morbidity and discomfort of venesection in conjunction with frequent phlebotomy, myelosuppressive treatment should be considered (*vide infra*). Selection of the type of treatment for those patients who require some form of myelosuppression because of the frequency of phlebotomy and or its complications provides the basis for major discussion, confrontation, and disagreement since the days of the PVSG (72). For the most part, alkylating agents (including busulfan) are avoided because of the established risk of secondary leukemia, but these drugs and radioactive phosphorous (P^{32}) still play a role in treating the very elderly patient or those who have significant comorbid conditions. P^{32}, in particular, is associated with long periods of remission-free survival after 1 or 2 doses of 5 mCi intravenously (75).

The first systematic approach to myelosuppressive therapy of PV began with the PVSG in 1970 (72). Since then, a number of medications have been used for cytoreduction, including newer treatments such as recombinant interferon alpha (rIFN-α) and imatinib, which are therapeutically effective, have a biologic basis for their use and effect, and can modify JAK2 expression in some patients.

The first study of the PVSG (72), the 01 trial, included 431 patients who were randomized to receive either phlebotomy-only, phlebotomy plus radioactive phosphorous (P^{32}), or phlebotomy plus chlorambucil. The median survival of patients receiving phlebotomy-only (PHL-O), about 13.9 years, was superior to those receiving phlebotomy plus P^{32} (11.8 years) or phlebotomy plus chlorambucil (8.9 years). In the first 3 years of treatment, however, PHL-O was associated with an increased risk of thrombosis. Those in the second two groups experienced a higher rate of acute leukemia and other malignancies, which developed during the follow-up period. The frequency of myelofibrosis with myeloid metaplasia was essentially the same in all three groups.

Because treatment with chlorambucil predisposed patients to the development of acute myelogenous leukemia (AML), it is safe to presume other alkylating agents would do likewise. In general, such drugs should not be used in patients with PV. After the experience with chlorambucil, the PVSG tried to find a presumably nonmutagenic myelosuppressive drug. Hydroxyurea (HU) was selected (76); this agent is an antimetabolite affecting DNA synthesis by inhibiting the enzyme ribonucleotide reductase. In the first report by the PVSG, 51 patients were treated for a median of 8.6 years. The HU group showed a tendency for the development of acute leukemia in 5.8% of patients. This study was compared to the 134 patients treated with PHL-O in the PVSG 01 protocol. This noncontemporaneous, nonrandomized study is obviously statistically faulty, yet this information has been used to cite that HU is not leukemogenic (76). The limitations of the HU study of the PVSG include the fact that the patients were followed for a median of 8.6 years (maximum: 15.3 years) so that the true incidence of acute leukemia, which would increase by continuous exposure to HU, could not been determined (77, 78).

Few hematologists have followed serially and reported the treatment results of HU over the course of years; thus, the issues regarding potential leukemogenicity (69, 79, 80), although very suggestive, are not completely resolved. Likewise, it has also been presumed that HU is not leukemogenic because a recent study (64) indicated no increased risk of leukemia after HU; however, the median follow-up was only 2.8 years. Presumably, the development of leukemia in patients with PV occurs after more than 10 years of treatment (78). Others have observed acute leukemia developing in approximately 11.5% of PV patients after 10 years when HU was used as a myelosuppressive agent (79, 80). In another report, HU was not considered leukemogenic (69) because no increased leukemia risk was cited when compared with pipobroman, a drug not used in the United States. Although there was no difference in leukemia risk between the two drugs, there was a 10% frequency at the 13th year of follow-up in both, suggesting that both pipobroman and HU were associated with an increased risk of leukemia (78). Moreover, long-term maintenance therapy with HU was frequently ineffective, with complications appearing generally 5 years or more after initiation of treatment. These late occurrences explain why the frequency of complications is often underestimated. Indeed, the frequency of HU-induced leukemia was similar in that study to P^{32} in the PVSG studies!

Moreover, chromosomal abnormalities have been observed in cell cultures incubated with HU, in patients treated with HU for lung cancer (81), and in 36% of patients treated for PV with HU (82). Additional limitations of using HU in PV include an increased risk of squamous cell cancer, skin rash, and buccal aphthous ulcers, failure to control blood counts (high platelet count and macrocytic anemia), or leukopenia and thrombocytopenia in 15–30% of 109 patients reported by the PVSG; moreover, constitutional symptoms (night sweats and pruritus) persist and other toxicities of the drug (gastrointestinal, renal) were reported. Moreover, although PV customarily is thought of as a disease of older patients, the finding of this illness in patients under 50 years is noteworthy. In our series, the median age was 50 years and 23% were younger than 40 years (71). Obviously, selection of appropriate therapy for this younger group of patients is particularly important.

Further, HU, other than by general myelosuppressive does not affect abnormal megakaryocyte dysfunction, an abnormality leading to fibrosis as the disease evolves (70, 83). Unfortunately, clinical tradition has hardened into habit, and the therapeutic effects and the additional risk factors of therapy with HU have either been ignored or misinterpreted. The limitations of HU for treating PV have not received adequate attention. Even though the PVSG reported that only 61% of 51 patients treated with HU achieved long-term control (72, 76), the criteria for HU failure used by the PVSG allowed for the HCT to increase to more than 55% and permitted more than six phlebotomies in any consecutive 52-week period. This broad window for treatment failure would not be considered satisfactory in this era. Nevertheless, HU is considered by some to be very effective and should be considered the "drug of choice" in high-risk patients (69). An initial starting dose ranges between 500 and 1500 mg daily depending on the counts, with adjustment depending on response. In addition to its antiplatelet effect, HU might have additional mechanisms of activity, including myelosuppression, qualitative and quantitative changes in leukocytes, decreased expression of endothelial molecules, and increased nitric acid generation; all of which play a role in thrombosis in PV (83).

Hydroxyurea can be used with less reluctance for patients who require myelo-suppression, particularly with a high platelet count, and in older patients, especially for whom interferon is contraindicated.

1.10.2   Interferon

Since the initial studies of the use of recombinant interferon-α (rIFN-α) in treating patients with PV (85–88), many reports of its beneficial results have been published (89–91). Using rIFN-α avoids many of the problems and complications associated with PHL-O and/or chemotherapy and relieves pruritus and other constitutional symptoms. An update concerning long-term effects has recently been published (71).

The use of rIFN-α in PV is based on its broad effects on the hematopoietic system. Although PV, as noted, is a clonal stem cell disorder, there exist case reports of the resumption of polyclonal hematopoiesis after rIFN-α therapy (92, 93). rIFN-α inhibits erythroid progenitors and erythroid burst-forming units in vitro (94) and produces morphologic and biochemical changes in megakaryocytes (95), including a decrease in megakaryocyte density, size, and proliferation. rIFN-α inhibits megakaryocyte progenitor proliferation and reduces thrombopoietin-induced Mpl receptor signaling (96). The biochemical abnormalities of platelets in PV characterized by impaired conversion of exogenous arachidonic acid by platelet thromboxane B_2 and its correction by rIFN-α have been reported (97). rIFN-α also antagonizes platelet-derived growth factor (PDGF) (98). This is important because PDGF and other fibrogenic cytokines such as transforming growth factor β (TGF-β) and basic fibroblast growth factor play a major role in the pathogenesis of myelofibrosis (70, 84, 98). rIFN-α also inhibits the growth of marrow-derived fibroblasts (70, 84). rIFN-α, therefore, might retard the development of myelofibrosis because of its effect on megakaryocytes, thrombopoiesis, and various cytokines.

Recombinant IFN-α thus offers a physiologic basis for its use in PV. Compared with nonspecific myelosuppressive drugs or PHL-O, rIFN-α represents a treatment modality that could fundamentally alter the course of the disease and addresses the unmet therapeutic needs (64) of patients with PV.

Systematic studies in 55 patients with PV treated with rIFN-α have been reported recently (71); however, more than 70 patients have been treated in our clinic. In our studies, the criteria for the diagnosis and response to treatment were those of the PVSG (72). Response criteria were phlebotomy-free, HCT ≤ 45%, and platelets ≤ 600,000/μL. Our treatment program began with phlebotomy and rIFN-α 2b. Initially, we used doses of 3.0 MU/m² three times a week (tiw), but this was accompanied by frequent side effects over the long term. Beginning with low doses (1 MU tiw regardless of body surface area) and a gradual increase over the course of months, patient tolerance was enhanced. Then the dose was increased by 0.5 MU every 2–4 weeks until the target dose of 3 MU tiw was achieved, if necessary. Afterward, the dose was adjusted up or down depending on response until the patient remained phlebotomy-free at the target HCT. Supplemental antipyretics and analgesics were used liberally to treat side effects of rIFN-α. Aspirin, 81 mg daily, was given to all patients. Patients achieved partial response of their disease by 6 months and complete response by 1–2 years (phlebotomy free, HCT ≤ 45%, platelets 600,000/μL). Spleen size was reduced in 27 of 30 patients with prior splenomegaly. In our series (71), with a median disease duration of 7 years (range: 20 months to 20 years), the median disease-free survival was 11.9 years (range: 1.7–30 years). Strikingly, no thrombohemorrhagic events were observed.

The ubiquitous side effects of rIFN-α are described in detail elsewhere (99), and those that occurred in our patients are shown in Table 1.3. Although toxicity is acceptable for the majority of patients, 15–20% will not tolerate its long-term side effects, especially patients over the age of 65 years. Those patients who suffered influenzalike symptoms to a greater or lesser degree were in our early group of patients who had received higher initial doses of rIFN-α ($3.0 \, MU/m^2$ tiw). At lower doses (0.5–1.0 MU tiw), virtually no significant side effects were noted in many patients, but some degree of headache, fatigue, chills, and low-grade fever should be anticipated. Secondary hypothyroidism was common and easily treated. Hair loss and nail changes might occur. Neurological disorders such as demyelinating diseases or a history of seizures or other neuropsychiatric problems, including depression, are contraindications for rIFN-α (100).

A common error in treating PV patients with rIFN-α is to assume that it will replace the use of initial phlebotomy; it usually does not. rIFN-α suppresses the need for phlebotomy, once the target HCT values have been achieved by phlebotomy. The second major issue relates to the initial dose. In the majority of studies, the dose has been too high, modeling dosing used in the treatment of chronic myeloid leukemia. By way of contrast, the doses I advise suppresses the need for phlebotomy. I prefer nonpegylated forms of interferon, for this allows greater flexibility in dosing to avoid or reduce the frequency of side effects and to improve issues of quality of life.

Table 1.3 Toxicity of interferon seen in our patients with PV and an index of treatment continuation

Type of toxicity	Treatment Continued?	
	Yes	No
Initial influenzalike symptoms	√	
Liver function abnormalities	√	
Hypothyroidism	√	
Severe asthenia		√
Skin rash	√	
Complex seizures		√
Depression		√
Peripheral neuritis		√
Parkinson's syndrome		√
Bone pain	√	
Blurred vision		√

1.10.3 Imatinib Mesylate

Because of the side effects of interferon, alternative treatments are required and have been evaluated. Of interest, therefore, is the effect of imatinib mesylate (Gleevec®; Novartis Pharmaceuticals, Basel, Switzerland) in treating patients with PV. Reasons for using imatinib include inhibition of c-kit, which is involved in both normal and abnormal hematopoiesis (101, 102). Inhibition of c-kit reduces both erythroid and granulocyte/macrophage progenitor cells in patients with PV. Imatinib may also inhibit PDGF (101, 102), previously mentioned as involved in the production of marrow fibrosis. We initially reported that the erythrocytosis of PV was controlled with imatinib mesylate (101). We then reported treating an expanded cohort of 37 PV patients with imatinib in a multi-institutional phase II trial (103). All patients had an increased Cr^{51} red blood cell mass determined at diagnosis and fulfilled the other stipulated criteria for the diagnosis of PV. Men were initially phlebotomized to an HCT $\leq 45\%$ and women to $\leq 42\%$. Imatinib was started at 400 mg/day, escalating by 100 mg every 2 weeks to a maximum of 800 mg/day for those with persistent phlebotomy requirements or platelet counts greater than 600,000/μL. All patients received 81 mg/day of aspirin and prophylactic allopurinol. The study included 21 men and 16 women with a median age of 51 years (range: 29–83). Prior to imatinib, mean disease duration was 60.2 months; the patients had received a mean of nine phlebotomies per year (range: 0–23). After 1 year of imatinib, the mean phlebotomy requirement was only two per year, range: 0–9. There were 9 complete remissions (phlebotomy-free, platelet count <600,000/μL, no splenomegaly) and 10 partial remissions (phlebotomy and/or splenomegaly decreased by 50% of initial values, platelets less than 600,000/μL, or platelets more than 600,000/μL but no phlebotomy requirement or splenomegaly). There was one protocol violation. Thus, of 36 evaluable patients, 19 (53%) had a complete recovery (CR) or partial recovery (PR). Of the remaining 17, 10 showed disease progression: myelofibrosis (n = 2); platelets >1,000,000/μL, and/or persistent phlebotomy requirements or splenomegaly (n = 2) or increasing phlebotomy requirements (n = 2); progressive cytogenetic abnormalities (n = 1); increasing thrombocytosis (n = 1); and transient ischemic attacks (n = 2). Of these same 17, 7 developed toxicity: grade 3 dermatologic effects (n = 2); grade 3 diarrhea (n = 2); grade 3 bone pain (n = 1); liver toxicity (n = 1); and heart failure (n = 1). The median duration of response to date is 17.2 months. We concluded that imatinib is useful for treating erythrocytosis and controlling splenomegaly in a significant proportion of patients with PV, but it is less effective for controlling thrombocytosis or splenomegaly in others (101–103). These data suggest heterogeneity of hematopoietic stem cell proliferation in PV or patient variability with respect to imatinib metabolism. Dosage increases above 400 mg/day were usual and doses as high as 800 mg/day were associated with fluid retention, periorbital edema, and diarrhea. Clinical experience with imatinib facilitates its more effective use. The use of supplemental anagrelide could be considered, especially early in the course of treatment, particularly in those patients in whom HU had been used. Others have also reported the effectiveness of imatinib in the treatment of PV (104, 105). Continued investigation of this or related drugs would be of interest to explore the reason for heterogeneity of response, to determine the optimum dose and side effects, and the duration of response.

1.11   The Nature of the Response to rIFN-α and Imatinib

Despite these encouraging results with rIFN-α and imatinib, it is evident that for the most part, the results are quantitative and not qualitative in nature. Despite maintenance of a normal HCT and platelet count, marrows have remained hypercellular even in those patients who developed clinical and hematologic remission. Expression of c-kit by interval marrow immunohistochemistry tests was not reduced. Three patients with long-standing disease did develop progressive myelofibrosis after rIFN-α. (Whether earlier institution of rIFN-α treatment would have prevented this is moot.) rIFN-α has been reported to induce cytogenetic remission in a few patients with PV, with conversion of monoclonal to polyclonal hematopoiesis, as already mentioned. Such events have not yet been reported with imatinib treatment. Because only 20–30% of patients with PV present with a chromosomal abnormality, in general it has not been possible to gauge the depth of response to treatment (106). The recent finding of the $JAK2^{V617F}$ mutation in more than 95% of patients with PV suggests that this mutation might be exploited in order to measure the response to therapy in patients with PV (106). We examined change in gene expression in seven patients who received rIFN-α at an initial dose of 1 MU tiw increasing to 3 MU/day, with a median follow-up of 16 months (range: 13–132), and in 14 patients who received imatinib at initial doses of 400–800 mg/day, with a median follow-up of 17 months (range: 5–31). These patients were compared with 90 individuals who served as a control group; they had received phlebotomy only or HU, anagrelide, or both, or were untreated. We found that patients remained strongly positive for the $JAK2^{V617F}$ mutation after treatment, but there was significant reduction in the median percentage of mutant alleles, which correlated with hematologic response ($p = 0.001$). Furthermore, individuals who had achieved complete hematologic response had lower levels of $JAK2^{V617F}$ than those who did not. From a molecular standpoint, these results were modest, indeed. On the other hand, others have reported a more impressive molecular response to pegylated rIFN-α (107). These authors treated 40 patients, of whom 83% had a complete remission and 17% a partial remission, but judged after just 3 months of study. Three of the 40 patients were negative for JAK2 mutations at diagnosis (8%). Of 27 PV patients treated with pegylated IFN-α-2a, 24 (89%) had a mean decrease of 44% in the expression of mutated JAK2 allele by reverse transcription (RT)–PCR. There was no evidence of a plateau. In one patient, mutant JAK2 was not detected after 12 months. In three patients homozygous for the mutation, reappearance of 50% of wild-type allele was observed during treatment. Interferon has also been shown to preferentially target the malignant clone. These results suggest that rIFN-α-2a significantly decreased the proportion of circulating clonal cells in the majority of PV patients. Whether pegylated interferon results in a qualitative difference compared with nonpegylated interferon still remains to be determined.

In comparison with the myelosuppressive drugs that have been used in treating PV, why might rIFN-α be unique? Inhibition of erythroid progenitors has been discussed. Several observations suggest that the megakaryocytic and granulocytic myeloproliferations play a unique role in the production of cytokines, leading to secondary myelofibrosis (70, 84). The fact that the great majority of our patients, even those treated previously with HU, had increased platelet counts prior to the use of rIFN-α is significant. Hyperplasia and clustering of small to giant (pleomorphic) megakaryocytes in the bone marrow is a characteristic feature of PV (13–15). Although PDGF is involved in fibroblastic proliferation, it does not fully account for the complex production of myelofibrotic stroma.

Additional growth factors (cytokine storm) produced by megakaryocytic and granulocytic/monocyte precursor cells must be involved in the etiology of secondary myelofibrosis in Myeloproliferative Disorders (MPD), the most important of which is probably TGF-β (70, 98). How TGF-β, PDGF, other cell lineages, and cytokines interact to cause marrow fibrosis is unknown; after rIFN-α therapy, TGF-β values return to normal levels. Moreover, TGF-β has powerful angiogenic properties (70, 98). That rIFN-α has activities against erythropoiesis, megakaryocytopoiesis, PDGF, and TGF-β and is also antiangiogenic suggests that it might have a unique role in the treatment of the MPDs, particularly PV. The differentiation of erythroid-megakaryocyte precursor cells into one or another lineage might involve a balance between two related transcription factors, NF-E2 and BACH-1, which could conceivably be affected by rIFN-α (108). Finally, the effect of rIFN-α on JAK2 in patients with PV clearly requires further elucidation. rIFN-α might be the first drug that can alter the natural history of the disease.

1.12 Treatment of Other Aspects of PV

It is also my practice to treat all patients prophylactically with allopurinol or probenecid, particularly in patients with increased serum uric acid levels. Many patients take multivitamins containing relatively large amounts of vitamin C. By acidifying the urine, this agent might cause precipitation of uric acid crystals and result in renal colic. Of interest is the observation that acute gouty arthritis involving the right hallux can occur in patients who drive an automobile long distances. This is related to the right foot pressure, as the foot is applied repeatedly to the accelerator pedal. Except for fatigue associated with general metabolic symptoms and weight loss, leukocytosis does not require treatment *per se*. Blood cells of patients with polycythemia have normal phagocytic function; patients do not have an increased frequency of bacterial infection.

It is extremely important, as previously mentioned, to provide "total care" for the patient undergoing phlebotomy to reduce the risk of thrombosis. Thus, the use of birth control pills or estrogen supplementation is contraindicated. All cigarette smoking is forbidden. Obesity, hypertension, and diabetes should be treated in the usual fashion.

1.13 Summary

1. Evidence is presented indicating that rIFN-α effectively reduces phlebotomy requirements for thrombocythemia, splenomegaly, and thrombohemorrhagic events. It is an effective drug for treating PV with acceptable toxicity.
2. Because PV is a chronic disease and the use of rIFN-α is long term, the initial dose must be small. An initial dose of rIFN-α-2b 1 MU tiw subcutaneously is suggested. A dose that is too high should be avoided.
3. Treatment with rIFN-α cannot be expected to lower the HCT. Phlebotomies must be continued as necessary to maintain the HCT at target levels (men: HCT ≤ 45%; women: HCT ≤ 42%).
4. Attention to the side effects of rIFN-α must be addressed from the onset. Thus, it is best to give the injection of rIFN-α at night, with adequate coverage with nonsteroidal anti-inflammatory drugs.
5. Dose adjustments must be made; most patients will require an increased dose of total weekly rIFN-α during the first year of treatment. This is done initially by gradually increasing the frequency of the dose. In general, 9–10 MU/week is the usual target dose the first year. After the first year of treatment, the dose can be gradually decreased, so that the minimum dose is achieved to suppress erythropoiesis with minimum toxicity.
6. The platelet count should lower by the end of the first year of therapy to ≤600,000/μL.
7. All patients should receive aspirin, 80–100 mg/day.
8. Probenecid or allopurinol should be given to a patient with an elevated serum uric acid level. Liberal fluid intake is encouraged. (It is not necessary to routinely alkalinize the urine.)
9. For patients who are in the older age group or intolerant of rIFN-α, HU is the drug of choice for marrow suppression. Imatinib mesylate can be of value in selected patients.
10. For those in whom the leukemogenic potential is not an issue, such as significant comorbid illness, P32, busulfan, or other alkylating agents might be considered because they induce a smooth remission, which is associated with a very good quality of life. Of course, full informed consent must be obtained from such individuals prior to use. Anagrelide is of value in younger patients with platelet counts unresponsive to other agents which are considered to be clinically threatening.

11. Attention must be paid to other details of medical care such as the treatment of hypertension, diabetes, and obesity. Estrogen-containing compounds should be avoided.

1.14 Conclusion

These are exciting times for the study of PV and allied diseases. The discovery of $JAK2^{V617F}$ has lead to an enormous increase in activity in both understanding the pathobiology of this disease and attempting to find inhibitors which would affect the molecular abnormality. Hopefully, these advances will come soon.

References

1. Silver RT. Polycythemia. In: Barondess JA, editor. Diagnostic approaches to presenting syndromes (DAPS). Baltimore: Williams & Wilkins; 1971. p. 442–465.
2. Halbertsma T. Polycythemia in childhood. Am J Dis Child 1933;46:1356–1367.
3. Damon A, Holub DA. Host factors in polycythemia vera. Ann Intern Med 1958;49:43–60.
4. Mohri H. Acquired von Willebrand disease in patients with polycythemia rubra vera. Ann J Hematol 1987;25:135–46.
5. Videback A. Polycythemia vera. Course and prognosis. Acta Med Scand 1950;138:179.
6. Michiels JJ, Drenth JPH. Erythromelalgia: a review of clinical manifestations in pathophysiology. Am J Med 1991;91:416.
7. Talbott JH. Gout and blood dyscrasias. Medicine (Baltimore) 1959;38:173–205.
8. Lamy T, Devillers A, Bernard M, et al. Inapparent polycythemia vera: an unrecognized diagnosis. Am J Med 1997;102:14–20.
9. Thurmes PJ, Steensma DP. Elevated serum erythropoietin levels in patients with Budd-Chiari syndrome secondary to polycythemia vera: clinical implications for the role of JAK2 mutation analysis. Eur J Haemotol 2006;77:57–60.
10. Spivak JL, Silver RT, et al. The Budd-Chiari syndrome and V617F mutation in JAK2. New Engl J Med 2006;355:737–738.
11. Rosenthal N, Bassen FA. Course of polycythemia. Arch Intern Med 1938;62:903–917.
12. Silver RT, Jones AV, Feldman EJ, et al. Validation of JAK2 and new clinical criteria for the diagnosis of polycythemia vera (PV). Blood. Proceedings of the American Society of Hematology, Atlanta, GA. 2005 106:Abstract 4971.
13. Ellis J, Silver RT, Coleman M, et al. The bone marrow in polycythemia vera. Semin Hematol 1975;12:433–444.
14. Michiels JJ, Thiele J. Clinical and pathologic criteria for the diagnosis of essential thrombocythemia, polycythemia vera, and idiopathic myelofibrosis (agnogenic myeloid metaplasia). Int J Haematol 2002;76:133–145.
15. Thiele J., Kvaswicka HM. Clinicopathological criteria for the differential diagnosis of thrombocythemias in various myeloproliferative diseases. Semin Thromb Hemost 2006;32:219.
16. Thiele J, Kvasnicka HM, Zankovich R, et al. The value of bone marrow histology in differentiating between early stage polycythemia vera and secondary (reactive) polycythemias. Haematologica 2001;86:359–373.
17. Finazzi G, Caruso V, Marchioli R, et al. Acute leukemia in polycythemia vera: an analysis of 1638 patients enrolled in a prospective observational study. Curr Hematol Rep 2005;105:2664–2670.

18. Goldman JM. A unifying mutation in chronic myeloproliferative disorders. New Engl J Med 2005;352:1744–1746.
19. Bennett M, Stroncek DF. Recent advances in the bcr-abl negative chronic myeloproliferative diseases. J Transl Med 2006;4: 41.
20. Kralovics R, Passamonti F, Buser AS, et al. A gain-of-function mutation of JAK2 in myelo-proliferative disorders. New Engl J Med 2005;352:1779–1790.
21. Vannucchi AM, Antoniolim, E, Guglielmeli P, et al. Influence of the *JAK2^{V617F}* mutational load at diagnosis on major clinical aspects in patients with PV. Blood (ASH Annual Meeting Abstracts). 2006;108:5.
22. Jones AV, Kreil S, Zoi K, et al. Widespread occurrence of the *JAK2^{V617F}* mutation in chronic myeloproliferative disorders. Blood 2005;106:2162–2168.
23. Baxter EJ, Scott LM, Campbell PJ, et al. Acquired mutation of the tyrosine kinase JAK2 in human myeloproliferative disorders. Lancet. 2005;365:1054–1061.
24. James C, Ugo V, LeCouédic JP, et al. A unique clonal JAK2 mutation leading to constitutive signaling causes polycythemia vera. Nature 2005;434:1144–1148.
25. Levine RL, Wadleigh M, Cools J, et al. Activating mutation in the tyrosine kinase JAK2 in polycythemia vera, essential thrombocythemia, and myeloid metaplasia with myelofibrosis. Cancer Cell 2005;7:387–397.
26. Theocharides A, Boissinot M, Girodon F, et al. Leukemic blasts in transformed JAK2-V617F positive myeloproliferative disorders are frequently negative for the JAK2-V617F mutation. Blood 2007;110(1):375–379.
27. Scott LM, Tong W, Levine R, et al. JAK2 exon 12 mutations in polycythemia vera and idiopathic erythrocytosis. N Engl J Med 2007;356:459–468.
28. Berlin NI. Diagnosis of classification of the polycythemias. Sem Hematol 1975;12: 339–351.
29. Michiels JJ, Thiele J. Clinical and pathological criteria for the diagnosis of essential throm-bocythemia polycythemia vera and idiopathic myelofibrosis (agnogenic myeloid metapla-sia). Int J Hematol 2002; 76:133–145.
30. Prchal JF, Axelrad AA. Letter: Bone-marrow responses in polycythemia vera. N Engl J Med 1974;290:1382.
31. Dai CH, Krantz SB, Dessypris EN, et al. Polycythemia vera. II. Hypersensitivity of bone marrow erythroid, granulocyte-macrophage, and megakaryocyte progenitor cells to inter-leukin-3 and granulocyte-macrophage colony-stimulating factor. Blood 1992;80:891–899.
32. Correa PN, Eskinaz D, Axelrad AA. Circulating erythroid progenitors in polycythemia vera are hypersensitive to insulin-like growth factor-1 in vitro: studies in an improved serum-free medium. Blood 1994;83:99–112.
33. Kralovics R, Buser AS, Teo SS, et al. Comparison of molecular markers in a cohort of patients with chronic myeloproliferative diseases. Blood 2003;102:1869.
34. Liu E, Jelinek J, Pastore YD, et al., Discrimination of polycythemias and thrombocytoses by novel, simple, accurate clonality assays and comparison with PRV-1 expression and BFU-E response to erythropoietin. Blood 2003;101:3294.
35. Rickstein A, Palmquist L, Wasllavikc, et al. High PRV-1 mRNA expression, the diagnostic marker for polycythemia vera (Abstract). Blood 2002;100:3156A.
36. Bench AJ, Pa HL. Chromosomal abnormalities and molecular markers in myeloproliferative disorders. Semin Hematol 2005;42:196.
37. Caruccio L, Bettinotti M, Director-Myska AE, et al. The gene over expressed in poly-cythemia rubra vera, PRV-1 and the gene encoding a neutrophil alloantigen, MBI are alle-les of the single gene, CD177 in chromosome ban 19Q13.31. Transfusion 2006;46:441.
38. Stroncek DF, Caruccio L, Bettinotti M. CD177: a member of the LY-6 gene super family involved with neutrophil proliferation and polycythemia vera. J Transl Med 2004;2:8.
39. Moliterno AR, Hankins WD, Spivak JL. Impaired expression of the thrombopoietin receptor by platelets in patients with polycythemia vera. New Engl J Med 1998;338:572.
40. Moliterno AR, Spivak JL. Post translational processing of the thrombopoietin receptor is impaired in polycythemia vera. Blood 1999;94:2555.

41. Pearson TC, Weatherley-Mein G. Vascular occlusive episodes and venous haematocrit in primary proliferative polycythaemia. Lancet 1978;2:1219–1221.
42. Pearson TC, Botterill CA, Glass UH, et al. Interpretation of measured red cell mass and plasma volume in males with elevated venous PCV values. Scand J Haematol 1984;33: 68–74.
43. Pearson TC, Guthrie DL, Simpson J, et al. Interpretation of measured red cell mass and plasma volume in adults: Expert panel on radionuclides of the International Council for Standardization in Haemotology. Br J Haematol 1995;89:748–756.
44. McMullin MF, Bareford D, Campbell P, et al. Guidelines for the diagnosis, investigation and management of polycythaemia/erythrocytosis. Br J Haematol 2005;130:174–195.
45. Tefferi A, Thile J, Orazi A, et al. Proposals and rationale for revision of the World Health Organization diagnostic criteria for Polycythemia vera, Essential Thrombocythemia, and idiopathic Myelofibrosis. Blood 2007;110(4):1092–1097.
46. Pierre R, Imbert M, Thiele I, et al. Polycythaemia vera. In: Jaffe E, Harris N, Stein H, et al., editors. WHO pathology and genetics of tumours of the haemopoietic and lymphoid tissues. Lyon: IARC Press; 2001. p. 32–34.
47. Johansson PL, Safai-Kutti S, Kutti J. An elevated venous haemoglobin concentration cannot be used as a surrogate marker for absolute erythrocytosis: a study of patients with polycythaemia vera and apparent polycythaemia. Br J Haematol 2005;129:701–705.
48. Murray JF. Arterial studies in primary and secondary polycythemic disorders. Am Rev Resp Dis 1965;92:435–449.
49. Murray JF. Classification of polycythemic disorders. Ann Intern Med 1966;64:892.
50. Stohlman F. Pathogenesis of erythrocytosis. Semin Hematol 1966;3:181–192.
51. Brandt PW, Dacie JV, Steiner RE, et al. Incidence of renal lesions in polycythemia. Br Med. J 1963;2:468–472.
52. Hertko E. Polycythemia (erythrocytosis) associated with uterine fibroids and apparent surgical cure. Amer J Med 1963;34:228–294.
53. Cassels DE, Morse M. The arterial blood gases, the oxygen dissociation curve and the acid base balance in polycythemia vera. J Clin Invest 1953;32:52.
54. Herbert V. Diagnostic and prognostic values of measurement of serum b^{12}- binding proteins. Blood 1968;32:305.
55. Block JB., Carbone PP, Oppenheim JJ, et al. The effect of treatment in patients with chronic myelogenous leukemia. Ann Int J Med 1963;59:629–636.
56. Campbell PJ, Green AR. The myeloproliferative disorders. New Engl J Med 2006;355: 2452–2466.
57. Weatherall DJ. Polycythemia resulting from abnormal hemoglobins. New Engl J Med. 1969;280:6004.
58. Charache S. Weatherall DJ. Polycythemia associated with a hemoglobinopathy. J Clin Invest 1966;45:813.
59. Hoyer JD, Allen SL, Beutler E, et al. Erythrocytosis due to bisphosphal glycerate mutates deficiency with concurrent gluco-6 phosphate dehydrogenate (G6PD deficiency). Am J Hematol 2004;75:205–208.
60. Carlo H, Schwarz, Jorch N, et al. Mutations in the von Hippel-Lindau (VHL) tumor suppressor gene and VHL-haplotype analysis in patients with presumable congenital erythrocytosis. Haematologica 2005;90:19–24.
61. De la Chapelle A. Truncated erythropoietin receptor causes dominantly inherited benign human erythrocytosis. Proc Natl Acad Sci USA 1993;90:4495–4499.
62. Ang SO, Chen H, Hirota K, et al. Disruption of oxygen homeostasis underlies congenital Chubash polycythemia. Nat Genet 2002;32:614–621.
63. Bento MC, Chang KT, Guan Y, et al. Congenital polycythemia with homozygous and heterozygous mutations of von Hippel-Lindau gene: five new Caucasian patients. Haematologica 2005;90:128–129.
64. Marchioli R, Finazzi G, Landolfi R. Vascular and neoplastic risk in a large cohort of patients with polycythemia vera. J Clin Oncol 2005;23(10) 2224–2232.

65. Pearson TC, Wetherley-Mein G. Vascular occlusive episodes and venous haematocrit in primary proliferative polycythaemia. Lancet 1978;2:1219–1222.
66. Spivak JL. Polycythemia vera: myths, mechanisms and management. Blood 2002;100:4272–4290.
67. Pearson TC. Rheology of the absolute polycythemias. Baillieres Clin Hematol 1987;1: 637–664.
68. DiNisio M, Barbui T, Di Gennaro L, et al. The haematocrit and platelet target in polycythemia vera. Br J Haematol. 2007; 136:249–259.
69. Finazzi G, Barbui T. How we treat patients with polycythemia vera. Blood 2007. doi: 10.1182/blood-2006-12-038968.
70. Martyre MC. TGF-β and megakaryocytes in the pathogenesis of myelofibrosis in myeloproliferative disorders. Leuk Lymphoma 1995;20: 39–44.
71. Silver RT. Long-term results in the treatment of polycythemia vera with recombinant interferon-α. Cancer 2006;27:451–448.
72. Berk PD, Wasserman LR, Fruchtman SM. Treatment of polycythemia vera: a summary of clinical trials conducted by the Polycythemia Vera Study Group In: Wasserman LR, Berk PD, Berlin N, editors. Polycythemia vera and the myeloproliferative disorders. Philadelphia: WB Saunders; 1995. p. 166–194.
73. Landolfi R, Marchioli R, Kutti J. Efficacy and safety of low-dose aspirin in polycythemia vera. N Engl J Med 2004;350(2):114–124.
74. Michiels JJ, Berneman Z, Schroyens W, et al. Platelet-mediated thrombotic complications in patients with ET: reversal by aspirin, platelet reduction, and not by coumadin. Blood Cells Mol Dis 2006;36:199–205.
75. Silver RT. Treatment of polycythemia vera. Semin Thromb 2006;32-437–442.
76. Kaplan ME, Mack K, Goldberg JB. Long-term management of polycythemia vera with hydroxyurea: a progress report. Semin Hematol 1986;23:167–171.
77. Najean Y, Dresch C, Rain JD. The very-long-term course of polycythaemia: a complement to the previously published data of the Polycythaemia Vera Study Group. Br J Haematol 1994;86:233–235.
78. Najean Y, Rain JD. Treatment of polycythemia vera: the use of hydroxyurea and pipobroman in 292 patients under the age of 65 years. Blood 1997;90: 3370–3377.
79. Nand S, Messmore H, Fisher SG. Leukemia transformation in polycythemia vera: analysis of risk factors. Am J Hematol 1990;34:32–36.
80. Weinfeld A, Swolin B, Westin J. Acute leukemia after hydroxyurea therapy in polycythemia vera and allied disorders: prospective study of efficacy and leukemogenicity with therapeutic implications. Eur J Haematol 1994;52:134–139.
81. Kaung DT, Swartzendruber AA. Effect of chemotherapeutic agents on chromosomes of patients with lung cancer. Dis Chest 1969;55:98–100.
82. Landaw SA. Acute leukemia in polycythemia vera In: Wasserman LR, Berk PD, Berlin N, editors. Polycythemia vera and the myeloproliferative disorders. Philadelphia: WB Saunders; 1995. p. 154–165.
83. Falanga A, Marchetti M, Vignoli A, et al. Leukocyte-platelet interaction in patients with essential thrombocythemia and polycythemia vera. Exp Hematol 2005;33:523–530.
84. Le Bousse-Kerdiles MC, Martyre MC. Involvement of the fibrogenic cytokines, TGF-β and bFGF, in the pathogenesis of idiopathic myelofibrosis. Pathol Biol (Paris) 2001;49:153–157.
85. Silver RT. Recombinant interferon-alpha for treatment of polycythemia vera. Lancet 1988;2:403.
86. Silver RT. A new treatment for polycythemia vera: recombinant interferon alpha. Blood 1990;76:664–665.
87. Silver RT. Interferon-α 2b: a new treatment for polycythemia vera. Ann Intern Med 1993;119:1091–1092.
88. Silver RT. Interferon alpha: effects of long-term treatment for polycythemia vera. Semin Hematol 1997; 34: 40–50.

89. Lengfelder E, Berger U, Hehlmann R. Interferon in the treatment of polycythemia vera. Ann Hematol 2000;79:103–109.
90. Sacchi S, Leoni P, Liberati M. A respective comparison between treatment with phlebotomy alone and with interferon alpha in patients with polycythemia vera. Ann Hematol 1994;68:247–250.
91. Taylor PC, Dolan G, Ng JP. Efficacy of recombinant interferon-alpha (rIFN-α) in polycythemia vera: a study of 17 patients and an analysis of published data. Br J Haematol 1996;92:55–59.
92. Hino M, Futami E, Okuno S. Possible selective effects of interferon α-2b on a malignant clone in a case of polycythemia vera. Ann Hematol 1993;66:161–162.
93. Messora C, Be Qsi L, Vecchi A. Cytogenetic conversion in a case of polycythemia vera treated with interferon-alpha. Br J Haematol 1994;86:402–404.
94. Means RT, Krantz SB. Inhibition of human erythroid colony-forming units can be corrected by recombinant human erythropoietin. Blood 1991;78:2564–2567.
95. Chott A, Gisslinger H, Thiele J. Interferon-alpha induced morphological changes of megakaryocytes: a histomorphological study on bone marrow biopsies in chronic myeloproliferative disorders with excess thrombocytosis. Br J Haematol 1990;74:10–16.
96. Wang O, Miyakawa Y, Fox N. Interferon-α directly represses megakaryopoiesis by inhibiting thrombopoietin-induced signaling through induction of SOCS-1. Blood 2000;96:2093–2099.
97. Sinzinger H, Linkesch W, Ludwig H. Impaired conversion of exogenous arachidonic and by platelets to thromboxane b2 and correction of that deficiency by interferon-alpha. Prostaglandins 1990;40:351–360.
98. Martyre MC, Magdelenat H, Calvo F. Interferon gamma in vivo reverses the increased platelet levels of platelet-derived growth factors in transforming growth factor-13 in patients with myelofibrosis with myeloid metaplasia. Br J Haematol 1991;77:431–435.
99. Silver RT, Woolf SH, Hehlmann R. An evidence-based analysis of the effect of busulfan, hydroxyurea, interferon and allogeneic bone marrow transplantation in treating the chronic phase of chronic myeloid leukemia: developed for the American Society of Hematology. Blood 1999;94:1515–1516.
100. Hensley ML, Peterson B, Silver RT, et al. Risk factors for severe neuropsychiatric toxicity in patients receiving interferon alfa-2b and low-dose cytarabine for chronic myelogenous leukemia: analysis of Cancer and Leukemia Group B 9013. J Clin Oncol 2000;18:1301–1308.
101. Silver RT. Imatinib mesylate (Gleevec™) reduces phlebotomy requirements in polycythemia vera. Leukemia 2003;17:1186–1187.
102. Silver RT, Fruchtman S, Feldman E, et al. Imatinib mesylate (Gleevec™) is effective in the treatment of polycythemia vera: a multi-institutional clinical trial (Abstract). Blood (ASH Annual Meeting Abstracts). 2004;104:Abstract 656.
103. Feldman EJ, Spivak JL, Lee S, et al. Imatinib mesylate is effective in the treatment of polycythemia vera: a multi-institutional clinical trial (Abstract). J Clin Oncol (ASCO Annual Meeting Proceedings). 2006;24:6532.
104. Jones CM, Dickinson TM: Polycythemia vera responds to imatinib mesylate. Am J Med Sci 2003;325:149–152.
105. Hasselbalch H: Imatinib mesylate in polycythemia vera. A heterogeneous response pattern but a consistent reduction in phlebotomy requirements (Abstract). Blood (ASH Annual Meeting Abstracts). 2004;104:Abstract 4747.
106. Jones A, Silver RT, Waghorn K. Minimal molecular response in polycythemia vera patents treated with Imatinib or interferon alpha. Blood 2006;107:3339–3341.
107. Kiladjian JJ, Cassinat B, Turlure P, et al: High molecular response rate of polycythemia vera patients treated with pegylated interferon α-2a. Blood 2006;108:2037–2040.
108. Poncz M. BACH and the megakaryocyte symphony. Blood 2005;105:3001–3002.

Chapter 2
Primary Myelofibrosis

Ayalew Tefferi

2.1 Introduction

Myelofibrosis (MF) in the context of a myeloproliferative disorder is a clinicopatho-logically defined entity characterized by anemia, marked splenomegaly, constitutional symptoms, leukoerythroblastosis (i.e., the presence of immature granulocytes and nucleated red blood cells), dacryocytosis (i.e., presence of teardrop-shaped red blood cells), and a bone marrow that displays dysplastic megakaryocyte hyperplasia, granulocyte proliferation, and reticulin and/or collagen fibrosis (1). Disease presentation could be either *de novo* (primary MF; PMF) or preceded by either polycythemia vera (post-PV MF) or essential thrombocythemia (post-ET MF). PMF is also known by many other names (Table 2.1), including chronic idiopathic myelofibrosis (CIMF), the term used by the World Health Organization (WHO) system for classification of myeloid neoplasms (2). However, the use of the term "PMF" was recently endorsed by the International Working Group for Myelofibrosis Research and Treatment (IWG-MRT) (3).

2.2 Historical Perspective and Disease Classification

The first description of PMF is credited to Heuck (1879) (4). He described two cases, which he referred to at the time as "splenic-medullary leukemia" and "pure splenic leukemia" (4). The term "osteosclerosis," which refers to the new bone formation that often accompanies bone marrow fibrosis in PMF, was first introduced by Assman in 1907 (5). Post-PV MF was recognized as early as 1935 by Hirsch-. (6). Similarly, the typical histological characteristics of the disease, including hepatosplenic extramedullary hematopoiesis (1908) (7, 8), bone marrow fibrosis (8), and leukoerythroblastosis (1939) (9), were all recognized in the first half of the 20th century. PMF was referred to as agnogenic myeloid metaplasia of the spleen (AMM), a term first used in 1940 (10) and later endorsed by Dameshek in 1951 (11).

Dameshek classified PMF as a myeloproliferative disorder (MPD), along with chronic myeloid leukemia (CML), ET, and PV (11). In 1960, Nowell and

Table 2.1 Terms used to refer to primary myelofibrosis

Agnogenic myeloid metaplasia
Atypical myeloid leukemia
Atypical myelosis
Aleukemic myelosis with osteosclerosis
Chronic idiopathic myelofibrosis
Chronic nonleukemic myelosis
Chronic erythroblastosis
Chronic megakaryocytic leukemia
Chronic megakaryocytic-granulocytic myelosis
Heuck–Assman disease
Idiopathic myelofibrosis
Idiopathic myeloid metaplasia
Leukoerythroblastic anemia
Leukanemia
Megakaryocytic myelosis with osteosclerosis
Megakaryocytic splenomegaly
Myelosis
Myelofibrosis with myeloid metaplasia
Myeloid metaplasia with myelofibrosis
Megakaryocytic myelosis
Myelosclerosis
Osteosclerotic pseudoleukemia
Osteomyeloreticulosis
Osteomyelosclerosis
Osteosclerotic anemia
Osteomyelofibrosis
Primary myelofibrosis

Hungerford described the Philadelphia chromosome in CML (12),which was later shown to harbor first the t(9;22)(q32;q13) (13) and subsequently the *BCR-ABL* disease-causing mutation (14). Accordingly, modern classification systems list PMF, PV, and ET as *BCR-ABL*-negative classic MPDs (15). In 1978, G6PD-based clonality studies established PMF as a stem-cell-derived clonal myeloproliferation (16). In 2005, a novel gain-of-function (GOF) mutation involving the JAK2 tyrosine kinase (*JAK2*V617F) was described in approximately 50% of PMF patients but also in the majority of those with PV as well as ET (17). In 2006, another GOF mutation involving MPL (*MPL*W515L/K) was described in approximately 5% of patients with PMF (18).

In 1967, an International Polycythemia Vera Study Group (PVSG) was created under the auspices of the National Cancer Institute and the group provided, for the first time, formal criteria for the diagnosis of each one of the *BCR-ABL*-negative classic MPDs, including PMF (19). Subsequently, a WHO-sponsored committee on the classification of hematological malignancies revised the PVSG diagnostic criteria for PMF and reorganized the overall classification system for myeloid neoplasms (2). The WHO system considers two broad categories of myeloid malignancies: acute myeloid leukemia (AML) and chronic myeloid disorders (CMDs) (20). AML is defined by the presence of 20% or more "blasts" in either the bone marrow or blood and/or certain recurring cytogenetic abnormalities including t(8;21)(q22;q22), t(15;17)(q22;q12), inv(16)(p13;q22), and t(16;16)(p13;q22) (20). Table 2.2 presents the current WHO classification scheme for CMD. Most recently, a semimolecular classification system has been proposed (Table 2.3) (21).

2.3   Epidemiology

The prevalence of PMF is similar in men and women (M:F = 1.6:1) and overall reported incidence figures range from 0.4 to 1.5/100,000 (22–26). A higher incidence has been suggested in persons of Jewish ancestry (27). Median age at diagnosis is estimated between 55 and 60 years and approximately 2%, 10%, and 30% of patients are diagnosed before age 30, 40, and 50 years, respectively (28). In one study of 323 patients, 9 (2.8%; 6 females) were age 30 years or younger (range: 17–30). The clinical course in these nine young patients was more indolent compared to that seen in older adults and more like that seen in children, where disease occurrence is very rare (29, 30). In general, there is little evidence that links PMF to environmental toxins. However, the possibility of some association with exposure to benzene, other industrial solvents, thorotrast injections, and radiation accidents has been suggested in the past (31–35).

Table 2.2   The World health Organization classification system for chronic myeloid disorders

Major categories	Subcategories
1. Myelodysplastic syndrome (MDS)	
2. Myeloproliferative disorder (MPD)	i. Chronic myeloid leukemia (CML)
	ii. Polycythemia vera
	iii. Essential thrombocythemia
	iv. Primary myelofibrosis
	v. Chronic neutrophilic leukemia
	vi. Chronic eosinophilic leukemia
	viii. Hypereosinophilic syndrome
	ix. Unclassified MPD
3. MDS/MPD	i. Chronic myelomonocytic leukemia
	ii. Juvenile myelomonocytic leukemia
	iii. Atypical CML
4. Systemic mastocytosis (SM)	

Table 2.3 A semimolecular classification of chronic myeloid disorders

Main categories	Clinicopathologic subcategories	Molecular subcategories
I. Myelodysplastic syndrome	*According to WHO classification system*	
II. Classic myeloproliferative disorders	**1. Chronic myeloid leukemia**	*100% BCR-ABL*[(+)]
	2. Polycythemia vera	*~100% JAK2V617F*[(+)]
	3. Essential thrombocythemia	*~50% JAK2V617F*[(+)]
		~1% MPLW515L/K[(+)]
	4. Primary Myelofibrosis	*~50% JAK2V617F*[(+)]
		~5% MPLW515L/K[(+)]
III. Atypical myeloproliferative disorders	**1. Chronic myelomonocytic leukemia**	*~3% JAK2V617F*[(+)]
	2. Juvenile myelomonocytic leukemia	*~30% PTPN11 mutation*[(+)]
		~15% NF1 mutation[(+)]
		~15% RAS mutation[(+)]
	3. Chronic neutrophilic leukemia	*~20% JAK2V617F*[(+)]
	4. Chronic eosinophilic leukemia/eosinophilic MPD	**A. *PDGFRA*-rearranged**
		B. *PDGFRB*-rearranged
		C. *FGFR1*-rearranged
		D. Molecularly undefined
	5. Hypereosinophilic syndrome	
	6. Chronic basophilic leukemia	
	7. Systemic mastocytosis	**A. *KIT*D816V**[(+)]
		B. Other *KIT* mutation
		C. *FIP1L1-PDGFRA*[(+)]
		D. Molecularly undefined
	8. Unclassified MPD	*~20% JAK2V617F*[(+)]
	i. Mixed/overlap MDS/MPD	
	ii. CML-like but *BCR-ABL*[(−)]	

2.4   Pathogenesis

The central pathogenetic process in PMF is stem-cell-derived clonal myeloproliferation (16, 36). Unlike the case with CML and *BCR-ABL*, the primary oncogenic event in PMF has not been characterized. However, activating mutations of the JAK2 tyrosine kinase (*JAK2*V617F) and thrombopoietin receptor (*MPL*W515L/K) have recently been reported in approximately 50% and 5% of patients, respectively (17, 18). *JAK2*V617F is an exon 14 *JAK2* mutation at nucleotide position 1849 representing a G to T somatic point mutation. The mutation results in the substitution of valine to phenylalanine at codon 617. *MPL*W515L mutation represents a G to T transition at nucleotide 1544, resulting in a tryptophan to leucine substitution at codon 515 of the transmembrane region of the MPL receptor (18). *JAK2*V617F has also been described in ET at a similar mutational frequency and in PV, where almost all patients carry the mutation (17, 37–39). Similarly, *MPL*W515L/K also occurs in approximately 1% of ET patients (40). Both mutations induce an MPD phenotype in mice, the former a PV-like disease (17, 41, 42) and the latter a PMF-like disease (43). Regardless, about half of the patients with PMF do not display either mutation and the precise pathogenetic role of these mutations, when they are present, remains to be clarified.

The bone marrow stromal reaction in PMF, including reticulin/collagen fibrosis, osteosclerosis, and angiogenesis is currently believed to be reactive in nature and cytokine mediated. In mice, for example, PMF-associated bone marrow stromal changes have been induced by either systemic overexpression of thrombopoietin (TPO^{high} mice) or by megakaryocyte lineage restricted underexpression of the transcription factor GATA-1 (GATA-1^{low} mice). In both instances, the megakaryocytes display abnormal distribution of P-selectin that is believed to promote a pathologic interaction between megakaryocytes and neutrophils (emperipolesis), resulting in the release of both fibrogenic and

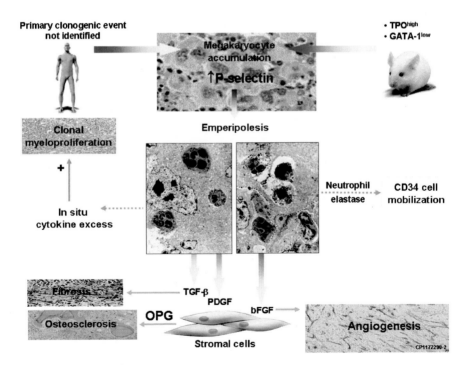

Figure 2.1 Pathogenesis of primary myelofibrosis. TPO, thrombopoietin; TGF, transforming growth factor; PDGF, platelet-derived growth factor; FGF, fibroblast growth factor; OPG, osteoprotegerin. (From Ref. 51; published with permission)

angiogenic cytokines, including transforming growth factor-β1 (TGF-β), platelet-derived growth factor (PDGF), basic fibroblast growth factor (bFGF), vascular endothelial growth factor (VEGF), tissue inhibitors of matrix metalloproteinases, and neutrophil-derived elastase and other proteases (44, 45). Among the latter, megakaryocyte-derived TGF-β1 might be the most important in the pathogenesis of the stromal reaction in PMF (46–48). Peripheral blood expansion of both CD34-positive myeloid progenitors and endothelial cells provide additional evidence for aberrant bone microenvironment in PMF (49, 50). Figure 2.1 summarizes the current speculation regarding the mechanisms of stromal reaction in PMF (51, 52).

2.5   Clinical Features and Diagnosis

Most, but not all, patients with PMF are symptomatic at diagnosis. The typical presentation includes anemia, marked splenomegaly, and profound constitu tional symptoms, including fatigue and night sweats. Other manifestations, either at diagnosis or during the course of the disease, include left upper quadrant discomfort, including recurrent pain from splenic infarcts (may be referred to the left shoulder), early satiety and change in bowel habits, pruritus, easy bruising, peripheral edema, lymphadenopathy, ascites, bleeding, and thrombosis (53–55). The spleen is palpably enlarged in approximately 80% of patients at diagnosis (marked splenomegaly in half of the cases) and the liver in 50% (56). Organomegaly in PMF is secondary to extramedullary hematopoiesis (EMH) that might also involve other organs: lymph nodes (lymphadenopathy), pleura (effusion), peritoneum (ascites), lung (interstitial process), and the paraspinal and epidural spaces (spinal cord and nerve root compression) (57–60).

The peripheral blood smear in PMF often shows leukoerythroblastosis (presence of nucleated red blood cells and immature granulocytes) and teardrop-shaped red blood cells (Figure 2.2). Anemia is present at diagnosis in the majority of the patients and approximately 20% might be red blood cell transfusion-dependent at presentation (59, 61–63). Other laboratory abnormalities at diagnosis include leukocytosis (41–49% incidence), leukopenia (7–22%), thrombocytosis (13–31%), thrombocytopenia (21–37%), presence of circulating blasts (33–53%), increased serum levels of lactate dehydrogenase (LDH; 83%), and low cholesterol levels (32%) (59, 60, 62, 63).

Bone marrow examination reveals both "cellular phase" and "overtly fibrotic" stages of the disease (Figure 2.3) (64). In cellular-phase disease, reticulin fibrosis, might be absent (i.e., prefibrotic stage). Therefore, the most helpful diagnostic feature in the bone marrow is the presence of dense megakaryocyte clusters with atypical megakaryocyte morphology (cloudlike nuclear morphology) that is accompanied by increased granulocyte proliferation and reduced erythropoiesis (64). Additional histological features of advanced disease include osteosclerosis, dilated sinuses, and intrasinusoidal hematopoiesis (Figure 2.4).

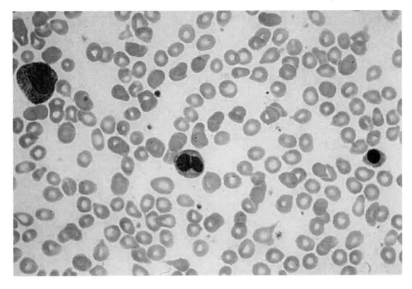

Figure 2.2 Peripheral blood smear in primary myelofibrosis showing myelophthisis; presence of nucleated red blood cells, immature granulocytes, and dacryocytes

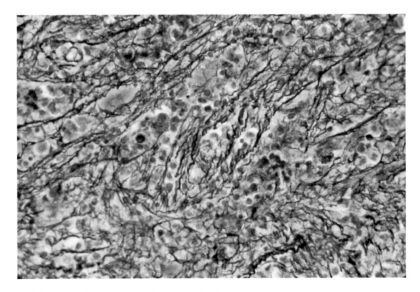

Figure 2.3 Reticulin fibrosis in primary myelofibrosis

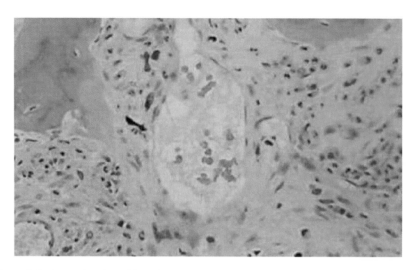

Figure 2.4 Osteosclerosis and intrasinusoidal hematopoiesis in primary myelofibrosis

2.6 Differential Diagnosis

Neither leukoerythroblastosis nor bone marrow fibrosis is specific to PMF. Bone marrow fibrosis might accompany a number of hematologic and nonhematologic conditions, as listed in Table 2.4. In most situations, mutation screening for *BCR-ABL* (to exclude the diagnostic possibility of CML) and *JAK2*V617F (to exclude the possibility of bone marrow fibrosis associated with nonmalignant condition, lymphoid disorder, or metastatic cancer) is highly recommended. It should be noted, however, that *JAK2*V617F cannot distinguish PMF from other myeloid disorders such as MDS, ET, PV, or atypical MPD. Therefore, accurate diagnosis requires careful morphological evaluation of the bone marrow.

Primary MF is typically characterized by the presence of morphologically abnormal megakaryocytes (bulbous and hyperchromatic nuclei) in dense clusters. MDS is characterized by the presence of erythroid and/or granulocytic dysplasia. As mentioned earlier, reticulin fibrosis can be absent in cellular-phase PMF and it is thus possible to confuse cellular-phase PMF with ET. Unlike ET, however, bone marrow in PMF is markedly hypercellular with both granulocytic and megakaryocytic proliferation in PMF as opposed to often normocellular bone marrow with only megakaryocytic hyperplasia in ET (65). Other distinguishing features between cellular-phase PMF and ET include the presence of myelophthisis and/or increased LDH in the former but not the latter.

Acute myelofibrosis, considered a variant of AML, can sometimes be confused with PMF. In general, patients with acute myelofibrosis usually present with severe constitutional symptoms, pancytopenia, mild or no splenomegaly, and circulating blasts. Both immunohistochemistry and cytogenetic studies are helpful in

Table 2.4 Causes of bone marrow fibrosis

Hematologic disorders		Nonhematologic disorders
Myeloid disorders	Lymphoid disorders	
• Primary myelofibrosis (1)	• Hairy cell leukemia (122)	• Metastatic cancer (126)
• Chronic myeloid leukemia (112)	• Hodgkin's lymphoma (123)	• Autoimmune myelofibrosis (127)
• Myelodysplastic syndrome (113)	• Non-Hodgkin's lymphoma (124)	• Systemic lupus erythematosus (128)
• Chronic myelomonocytic leukemia (114)		• Kala-Azar (leishmaniasis) (129)
	• Multiple myeloma (125)	• Tuberculosis (130)
• Chronic eosinophilic leukemia (115)		• Paget's disease (131)
• Systemic mastocytosis (116)		• HIV infection (132)
• Acute megakaryocytic leukemia (117)		• Vitamin D-deficient rickets (133)
• Other acute myeloid leukemias (118)		• Renal osteodystrophy (134)
• Acute lymphocytic leukemia (119)		• Hyperparathyroidism (135)
• Acute myelofibrosis (120)		• Gray platelet
• Malignant histiocytosis (121)		• Familial infantile myelofibrosis (137)
		• Idiopathic pulmonary hypertension (138)

distinguishing PMF from both acute myelofibrosis and MDS with fibrosis. For example, CD34 and CD61 immunoperoxidase staining provides a better estimate of the marrow blast and megakaryocyte content, respectively. Similarly, although cytogenetic abnormalities that occur in approximately half of the patients with PMF are mostly not specific to the disease [e.g., del(20)(q11;q13), del(13)(q12;q22), trisomy 8, trisomy 9, del(12)(p11;p13), monosomy or long arm deletions involving chromosome 7, and partial trisomy 1q] (66). the presence of either del(13)(q12;q22) or der(6)t(1;6)(q21–23;p21–23) is strongly suggestive of PMF diagnosis (67).

2.7 Clinical Course and Prognosis

Primary MF displays a progressive course in the majority of cases, and disease complications include cachexia, peripheral edema, severe fatigue, excessive night sweats, low-grade fever, symptomatic portal hypertension, variceal bleeding, ascites, debilitating diffuse and/or extremity bone pain, and "idiopathic" pulmonary hypertension (68). Causes of death includes development of blast-phase PMF, which occurs in approximately 10% of patients during the first decade of their disease (60, 63, 69, 70), infections (26–29%), bleeding (11–22%), heart failure (7–15%), liver failure (3–8%), solid tumor (3%), respiratory failure (3%), and portal hypertension (6%) (63, 69).

Survival in PMF is estimated by the use of one of several prognostic scoring systems (PSSs) that rely on the presence or absence of well-established adverse prognostic features (Table 2.5) (62, 63, 69, 71). Among the latter, the Mayo Clinic PSS has been reported to be superior, compared to other PSSs, in delineating both low-risk and intermediate-risk disease categories. According to the Mayo PSS (Table 2.5), median survival for low-risk young patients (age < 60 years) approaches 15 years compared to approximately 5 years in intermediate-risk patients and less than 3 years in high-risk patients. Additional risk factors for inferior survival, in addition to those listed in Table 2.5, include circulating immature granulocytes of ≥ 10% (59), circulating blast count of ≥ 3% (69), advanced age (61, 69, 72), male sex (69), and cytogenetic abnormalities other than 13q- or 20q- (66, 73, 74).

2.8   Management

Unfortunately, current therapy for PMF is inadequate and often palliative at best. Among the several treatment modalities that are currently employed, allogeneic stem cell transplantation (ASCT) is the only one with a potential for prolonging survival. However, ASCT is associated with substantial mortality and morbidity and is currently utilized in a select group of patients with high-risk disease. Drug therapy in PMF is used to alleviate symptomatic cytopenias, organomegaly, or marked thrombocytosis and/or leukocytosis. Other treatment modalities are also palliative and include involved field radiation, splenectomy, and blood component transfusions. Therefore, in the asymptomatic patient with low-risk PMF, it is currently reasonable to defer therapy (i.e., watchful waiting), regardless of age. In the presence of symptoms, either conventional or experimental drug therapy is advised in older patients as well as in younger low-risk patients. The risk associated with ASCT might be justified in young patients with high-risk disease and in some with intermediate-risk disease (Table 2.6). The choice between myeloablative versus reduced intensity conditioning (RIC) ASCT is made taking age and the presence of other comorbid conditions into consideration (Table 2.6).

2.8.1   Drug Therapy

The primary reason for using drug therapy in PMF is the presence of either anemia or splenomegaly that is symptomatic. Drug options for the former include subcutaneous (SC) erythropoietin (Epo) or oral drugs, including androgen preparations, corticosteroids, danazol, thalidomide, and lenalidomide. The starting dose for SC

Table 2.5 Prognostic models in primary myelofibrosis

Prognostic scoring system	Risk category	Score sum	Median survival (months)	Score for Hgb < 10 g/dL	Score for WBC < 4 or > 30 × 10⁹/L	Score for Plt < 100 × 10⁹/L	Score for AMC ≥ 1 × 10⁹/L	Score for symptoms*	Score for circulating blasts ≥ 1%
Elliott et al. (139) (n = 129) (ages < 60 years; median: 52) (Mayo prognostic model)	Low	0	173	1	1	1	1	N/A	N/A
	Intermediate	1	61						
	High	≥2	26						
Dingli et al. (71) (n = 160) (ages < 60 years; median: 52)	Low	0	155	1	1	1	N/A	N/A	N/A
	Intermediate	1	69						
	High	≥2	24						
Cervantes et al. (140) (n = 116) (ages ≤ 55 years; median: 46)	Low	0 or 1	176	1	N/A	N/A	N/A	1	1
	High	≥2	33						
Cervantes et al.63 (n = 106) (all ages; median: 64 years)	Low	0 or 1	99	1	N/A	N/A	N/A	1	1
	High	≥2	21						
Dupriez et al.62 (n = 195) (all ages; median: 65 years)	Low	0	93	1	1	N/A	N/A	N/A	N/A
	Intermediate	1	26						
	High	2	13						

Hgb, hemoglobin; WBC, white blood cell count; Plt, platelet count; AMC, absolute monocyte count.

Table 2.6 Suggested treatment algorithm in primary myelofibrosis

Risk stratification	Age <45 years	Age 45–60 years	Age >60 years
Low risk (no risk factors)[a]	Watchful waiting or Experimental drug therapy	Watchful waiting or Experimental drug therapy	Watchful waiting or Experimental drug therapy
Intermediate risk (one risk factor)	Experimental drug therapy or RIC ASCT	Experimental drug therapy	Experimental drug therapy
High risk (≥2 risk factors)	Myeloablative ASCT	RIC ASCT	Experimental drug therapy

RIC, reduced-intensity conditioning; ASCT, allogeneic stem cell transplant.

[a]According to Mayo prognostic scoring system; hemoglobin <10 g/dL, platelet count < 100×10^9/L, monocyte count ≥ 1×10^9/L, leukocyte count > 30×10^9/L or < 4×10^9.

Epo injection is 40,000 units weekly and such therapy is most appropriate in the presence of an endogenous serum Epo level below 100 U/L, where an approximately 50% response rate is expected (75). Some patients under Epo therapy experience further enlargement of their spleen. Several androgen preparations, including testosterone enanthate (400–600 mg IM weekly) and oral fluoxymesterone (10 mg TID) have been shown to improve anemia in a third of treated patients (76). The response rate from androgen therapy is improved by the concomitant use of corticosteroids (e.g., prednisone 30 mg/day) and compromised by the presence of cytogenetic abnormalities (76, 77). Danazol (600 mg/day) is a synthetically modified testosterone and produces response rates in PMF that is similar to that seen with other androgen preparations (78).

Thalidomide and lenalidomide have recently been shown to have therapeutic activity in PMF (79, 80). The mechanism of action for both drugs is not clearly understood but believed to be related to their anticytokine and immunomodulatory properties. The anticytokine treatment approach in PMF is based on both circumstantial evidence from affected patients and experimental myelofibrosis in mice. Thalidomide displays both antiangiogenic (81) and anti-tumor necrosis factor (TNF)-α (82) activity. There are currently two classes of thalidomide analogs: the selective cytokine inhibitory drugs (SelCIDs) and the immunomodulatory drugs (ImiDs) (83). Like thalidomide, both drug classes have anti-TNF-α, antiangiogenic, and anti-inflammatory activity (84). The activity of SelCIDs is mostly tied to phosphodiesterase 4 inhibition. The ImiDs, including CC-5013 (lenalidomide™) and CC-4047 (actimid™), do not inhibit phosphodiesterase 4 and have a broader cytokine inhibitory activity [inhibit TNF-α, interleukin (IL)-1β, IL-6, and IL-12]. In addition, they costimulate T-cells with upregulation of IL-2 and interferon (IFN)-γ production by T helper-1 cells and IL-5 and IL-10 production by T helper-2 cells (85). Lenalidomide (CC-5013) is the lead compound among the ImiDs and its ex vivo antiangiogenic as well as anti-TNF property is estimated to be at least 50-fold higher than that of thalidomide (83, 84). In PMF, thalidomide works best at low doses (50 mg/day) and in combination with corticosteroids (prednisone 15–30 mg/day) (86) and lenalidomide in the presence of del(5)(q31) (80). Single-agent therapy in unselected patients with either thalidomide or lenalidomide produces 15% and 20% response rates in anemia, respectively. The addition of corticosteroids doubles the response rate with thalidomide and the presence of del(5)(q31) is associated with complete hematologic remission in the majority of patients treated with lenalidomide. In addition, both drugs have been shown to improve thrombocytopenia (approximately 50% response rates) and splenomegaly (approximately 30% response rate) (79, 80).

The drug of choice for symptomatic splenomegaly in PMF is hydroxyurea (starting dose 500 mg TID). The drug is also used for controlling symptomatic thrombocytosis and/or leukocytosis. Hydroxyurea-refractory cases are sometimes managed by the use of alternative myelosuppressive agents, including intravenous cladribine (5 mg/m²/day in a 2-h infusion for 5 consecutive days to be repeated monthly for four to six cycles) (87), oral melphalan (2.5 mg three times a week) (88), and oral busulfan (2–6 mg/day with close monitoring of blood counts) (89, 90). In contrast, interferon-α therapy is poorly tolerated and has limited efficacy in the treatment of PMF (91–96).

It is expected that all clinicians disclose the side effects of the above-mentioned drugs before prescribing them. In addition, one must always look out for the presence of contraindications to the use of these drugs. For example, androgen use requires monitoring of serum prostate-specific antigen in men, liver function tests in both men and women, and underscoring the possibility of masculinizing side effects in women. Similarly, the use of thalidomide requires strict supervision and any possibility of pregnancy during its use must be prevented. Other side effects of thalidomide include somnolence, constipation, rash, and neuropathy. Lenalidomide is myelosuppressive and can result in neutropenic fever and sepsis. Therefore, one has to follow CBC closely and intervene with myeloid growth factors if the absolute neutrophil count drops to below 1×10^9/L. Other notable side effects of drugs used in PMF include mucocutaneous ulcers and skin/nail pigmentations associated with hydroxyurea use and the usual complications of corticosteroid use.

2.8.2 Splenectomy

Splenectomy is a strictly palliative treatment modality in PMF and does not alter the natural history of the disease. The procedure is associated with approximately 10% mortality and a higher incidence of morbidity that includes thrombosis, bleeding, postsplenectomy enlargement of the liver, and exacerbation of thrombocytosis/leukocytosis. Current indications for splenectomy in PMF include complications of portal hypertension, including ascites and variceal bleeding, drug-refractory symptomatic splenomegaly, or very frequent red blood cell transfusions (97). Severe thrombocytopenia in PMF is a marker of impending leukemic transformation and overall outcome in its presence might not be favorably affected with splenectomy.

In preparation for splenectomy, prophylactic therapy with hydroxyurea is advised in patients with leukocyte count of $>5 \times 10^9/L$ and/or platelet count $>150 \times 10^9/L$ in order to prevent postsplenectomy thrombocytosis and/or leukocytosis that might facilitate thrombotic complications (97). In addition, there is some evidence that suggests an increased incidence of bleeding in patients displaying laboratory evidence of DIC (i.e., presence of markedly increased d-dimer). Anecdotal evidence supports the use of low-dose prednisone (20 mg/day) in preparation for surgery. In addition, short-term (4–8 weeks) systemic anticoagulation, once hemostasis is secured after surgery, might reduce the risk of postoperative thrombotic complications.

2.8.3   Radiation Therapy

Involved field radiotherapy provides transient (median response duration of 3–6 months) relief of mechanical discomfort from hepatosplenomegaly (98, 99). However, such therapy is often complicated by protracted pancytopenia and drug therapy is instead preferred. In contrast, irradiation therapy is very useful in patients with nonhepatosplenic EMH; most frequent sites include vertebral column, lungs, pleura, and peritoneum. When symptomatic, nonhepatosplenic EMH is effectively treated with low-dose radiation therapy (0.1–1 Gy in 5–10 fractions) (58). Sometimes, occult pulmonary EMH presents with "idiopathic" pulmonary hypertension and a technetium 99m sulfur colloid scintigraphy is recommended if such an occurrence is suspected and treatment with single-fraction (0.1 Gy) whole-lung irradiation has been shown to be effective (68, 100).

2.8.4   Allogeneic Stem Cell Transplant

An increasing amount of information is being gathered regarding the use of ASCT in PMF, in the context of both myeloablative (101–104) and RIC (105, 106) transplant. Early engraftment rate is acceptable in both instances regardless of whether a related or matched unrelated donor is used. The experience so far with myeloablative ASCT is encouraging in very young patients (age <45 years), but posttransplant long-term survival in older patients is less than 20% (103, 104). Furthermore, the majority of survivors after ASCT experience reduced quality of life because of chronic graft versus host disease (GVHD) (101). A recent multi-variable analysis involving 320 patients with PMF registered to an international transplant database identified young age, HLA-matched sibling transplant, excellent performance status, absence of circulating blasts, and more recent transplant date as independent indicators of favorable transplant outcome (107). To date, the advantage of RIC transplant over myeloablative ASCT has not been examined in a controlled setting, although single-cohort studies suggest better outcome in terms of both 1-year mortality (0–33%) and morbidity (0–50% rate of acute GVHD) (108).

2.9   Conclusions

Over the last two decades, many drugs have been investigated for their therapeutic value in PMF. Negative studies have included drugs such as IFN-α, anagrelide, suramin, pirfenidone, imatinib mesylate, farnesyl transferase inhibitors such as R115777, and certain VEGF receptor inhibitors, including PTK-787 and SU5416 (109). In contrast, promising results were obtained with cladribine (87), etanercept (110), thalidomide (111), and lenalidomide (80). Despite such progress, treatment in PMF remains suboptimal in terms of both survival and quality of life. At present, it is reasonable to consider all high-risk patients for either ASCT (if transplant-eligible) or experimental drug therapy. It is equally reasonable to undertake a "watchful waiting" approach in low-risk patients. Management in intermediate-risk patients should be individualized and is often dictated by age, performance status, and patient preference. In all patients, the presence of del(5)(q31–32) warrants a therapeutic trial with lenalidomide. The recent discovery of PMF-associated activating mutations involving *JAK2* and *MPL* has raised the prospect of small molecule drug therapy that targets JAK2.

References

1. Tefferi A. Myelofibrosis with myeloid metaplasia. N Engl J Med 2000;342:1255–1265.
2. Thiele J, Vardiman JW, Pierre R, et al. Chronic idiopathic myelofibrosis. In: Jaffe ES, Harris NL, Stein H, et al., editors. World Health Organization classification of tumors: Tumours of the haematopoietic and lymphoid tissues. Lyon: International Agency for Research on Cancer (IARC) Press; 2001. p. 35–38.
3. Mesa R, Verstovsek S, Cervantes F, et al. Primary myelofibrosis (PMF), post polycythemia vera myelofibrosis (post-PV MF), post essential thrombocythemia myelofibrosis (post-ET MF), blast phase PMF (PMF-BP): Consensus on terminology by the International Working Group for Myelofibrosis Research and Treatment (IWG-MRT). Leuk Res 2007; in press.
4. Heuck G. Zwei Falle von Leukamie mit eigenthumlichem Blut- resp. Knochenmarksbefund [Two cases of leukemia with peculiar blood and bone marrow findings, respectively]. Arch Pathol Anat Physiol Virchows 1879;78:475–496.
5. Assmann H. Beitrage zur osteosklerotischen anamie. Beitr Pathol Anat Allgemeinen Pathol (Jena) 1907;41:565–595.
6. Hirsch R. Generalized osteosclerosis with chronic polycythemia vera. Arch Pathol 1935;19:91–97.
7. Donhauser J. The human spleen as an haematoplastic organ, as exemplified in a case of splenomegaly with sclerosis of the bone-marrow. J Exp Med 1908;10:559–574.
8. Askanazy M. Ueber extrauterine Bildung von Blutzellen in der Leber. Verh Dtsch Pathol Ges 1904;7:58–65.
9. Vaughan JM HC. Leuco-erythrobalstic anaemia and myelosclerosis. J Pathol Bacteriol 1939;48:339–352.
10. Jackson H Jr, PFJ, Lemon HM. Agnogenic myeloid metaplasia of the spleen: a syndrome simulating other more definite hematological disorders. N Engl J Med 1940;222:985–994.
11. Dameshek W. Some speculations on the myeloproliferative syndromes. Blood 1951;6:372–375.
12. Nowell PC, Hungerford DA. A minute chromosome in human chronic granulocytic leukemia. J Nat Cancer Inst 1960;25:85.

13. Rowley JD. Letter: A new consistent chromosomal abnormality in chronic myelogenous leukae-mia identified by quinacrine fluorescence and Giemsa staining. Nature 1973;243:290–293.
14. Daley GQ, Van Etten RA, Baltimore D. Induction of chronic myelogenous leukemia in mice by the P210bcr/abl gene of the Philadelphia chromosome. Science 1990;247:824–830.
15. Tefferi A, Gilliland DG. Classification of myeloproliferative disorders: From Dameshek towards a semi-molecular system. Best Pract Res Clin Haematol 2005; in press.
16. Jacobson RJ, Salo A, Fialkow PJ. Agnogenic myeloid metaplasia: a clonal proliferation of hematopoietic stem cells with secondary myelofibrosis. Blood 1978;51:189–194.
17. James C, Ugo V, Le Couedic JP, et al. A unique clonal JAK2 mutation leading to constitutive signalling causes polycythaemia vera. Nature 2005;434:1144–1148.
18. Pikman Y, Lee BH, Mercher T, et al. MPLW515L is a novel somatic activating mutation in myelofibrosis with myeloid metaplasia. PLoS Med 2006;3:e270.
19. Wasserman LR. The treatment of polycythemia. A panel discussion. Blood 1968;32:483–487.
20. Vardiman JW, Harris NL, Brunning RD. The World Health Organization (WHO) classifica-tion of the myeloid neoplasms. Blood 2002;100:2292–2302.
21. Tefferi A, Gilliland DG. Classification of myeloproliferative disorders: From Dameshek towards a semi-molecular system. Best Pract Res Clin Haematol 2006;19:361–364.
22. Mesa RA, Silverstein MN, Jacobsen SJ, et al. Population-based incidence and survival fig-ures in essential thrombocythemia and agnogenic myeloid metaplasia: An Olmsted County study, 1976–1995. Am J Hematol 1999;61:10–15.
23. Ridell B, Carneskog J, Wedel H, et al. Incidence of chronic myeloproliferative disorders in the city of Goteborg, Sweden 1983–1992. Eur J Haematol 2000;65:267–271.
24. Woodliff HJ, Dougan L. Myelofibrosis in Western Australia: an epidemiological study of 29 cases. Med J Aust 1976;1:523–525.
25. Heudes D, Carli PM, Bailly F, et al.. Myeloproliferative disorders in the department of Cote d'Or between 1980 and 1986. Nouv Rev Francaise Hematol 1989;31:375–378.
26. McNally RJ, Rowland D, Roman E, et al. Age and sex distributions of hematological malig-nancies in the U.K. Hematol Oncol 1997;15:173–189.
27. Chaiter Y, Brenner B, Aghai E, et al. High incidence of myeloproliferative disorders in Ashkenazi Jews in northern Israel. Leuk Lymphoma 1992;7:251–255.
28. Cervantes F, Barosi G, Hernandez-Boluda JC, et al. Myelofibrosis with myeloid metaplasia in adult individuals 30 years old or younger: presenting features, evolution and survival. Eur J Haematol 2001;66:324–327.
29. Sekhar M, Prentice HG, Popat U, et al. Idiopathic myelofibrosis in children. Br J Haematol 1996;93:394–397.
30. Altura RA, Head DR, Wang WC. Long-term survival of infants with idiopathic myelofibro-sis. Br J Haematol 2000;109:459–462.
31. Tondel M, Persson B, Carstensen J. Myelofibrosis and benzene exposure. Occup Med (Lond) 1995;45:51–52.
32. Honda Y, Delzell E, Cole P. An updated study of mortality among workers at a petroleum manufacturing plant. J Occup Environ Med 1995;37:194–200.
33. Mueller K. [Panmyelopathy and myelofibrosis after therapy with thorium X (peteosthor)]. Med Monatsschr 1960;14:241–243.
34. Bastrup-Madsen P, Jensen BN. Myelofibrosis with myeloid metaplasia and pancytopenia after thorotrast injection. Acta Med Scand 1971;189:355–358.
35. Anderson RE, Hoshino T, Yamamoto T. Myelofibrosis with myeloid metaplasia in survivors of the atomic bomb in Hiroshima. Ann Intern Med 1964;60:1–18.
36. Reeder TL, Bailey RJ, Dewald GW, et al. Both B and T lymphocytes may be clonally involved in myelofibrosis with myeloid metaplasia. Blood 2003;101:1981–1983.
37. Baxter EJ, Scott LM, Campbell PJ, et al. Acquired mutation of the tyrosine kinase JAK2 in human myeloproliferative disorders. Lancet 2005;365:1054–1061.
38. Levine RL, Wadleigh M, Cools J, et al. Activating mutation in the tyrosine kinase JAK2 in polycythemia vera, essential thrombocythemia, and myeloid metaplasia with myelofibrosis. Cancer Cell 2005;7:387–397.

39. Kralovics R, Passamonti F, Buser AS, et al. A gain of function mutation in Jak2 is frequently found in patients with myeloproliferative disorders. New Engl J Med 2005;352:1779–1790.
40. Pardanani AD, Levine RL, Lasho T, et al. MPL515 mutations in myeloproliferative and other myeloid disorders: a study of 1182 patients. Blood First Edition Paper, prepublished online July 25, 2006; doi 101182/blood-2006-04-018879. 2006.
41. Wernig G, Mercher T, Okabe R, Levine RL, Lee BH, Gilliland DG. Expression of Jak2V617F causes a polycythemia vera-like disease with associated myelofibrosis in a murine bone marrow transplant model. Blood. 2006;107:4274–4281.
42. Lacout C, Pisani DF, Tulliez M, et al. JAK2V617F expression in murine hematopoietic cells leads to MPD mimicking human PV with secondary myelofibrosis. Blood First Edition Paper, prepublished online May 2, 2006; doi 101182/blood-2006-02-002030. 2006.
43. Pikman Y, Lee BH, Mercher T, et al. MPLW515L is a novel somatic activating mutation in myelofibrosis with myeloid metaplasia. PLoS. 2006; in press.
44. Schmitt A, Jouault H, Guichard J, et al. Pathologic interaction between megakaryocytes and polymorphonuclear leukocytes in myelofibrosis. Blood 2000;96:1342–1347.
45. Xu M, Bruno E, Chao J, et al. Constitutive mobilization of CD34+ cells into the peripheral blood in idiopathic myelofibrosis may be due to the action of a number of proteases. Blood 2005;105:4508–4515.
46. Chagraoui H, Komura E, Tulliez M, et al. Prominent role of TGF-beta 1 in thrombopoietin-induced myelofibrosis in mice. Blood 2002;100:3495–3503.
47. Chagraoui H, Tulliez M, Smayra T, et al. Stimulation of osteoprotegerin production is responsible for osteosclerosis in mice overexpressing TPO. Blood 2003;101:2983–2989.
48. Vannucchi AM, Bianchi L, Cellai C, et al. Development of myelofibrosis in mice genetically impaired for GATA-1 expression (GATA-1(low) mice). Blood 2002;100:1123–1132.
49. Massa M, Rosti V, Ramajoli I, et al. Circulating CD34+, CD133+, and vascular endothelial growth factor receptor 2-positive endothelial progenitor cells in myelofibrosis with myeloid metaplasia. J Clin Oncol 2005;23:5688–5695.
50. Barosi G, Viarengo G, Pecci A, et al. Diagnostic and clinical relevance of the number of circulating CD34(+) cells in myelofibrosis with myeloid metaplasia. Blood 2001;98:3249–3255.
51. Tefferi A. New insights into the pathogenesis and drug treatment of myelofibrosis. Curr Opin Hematol 2006;13:87–92.
52. Tefferi A. Pathogenesis of myelofibrosis with myeloid metaplasia. J Clin Oncol. 2005;23:8520–8530.
53. Ward HP, Block MH. The natural history of agnogenic myeloid metaplasia (AMM) and a critical evaluation of its relationship with the myeloproliferative syndrome. Medicine 1971;50:357–420.
54. Cervantes F, Alvarez-Larran A, Arellano-Rodrigo E, et al. Frequency and risk factors for thrombosis in idiopathic myelofibrosis: analysis in a series of 155 patients from a single institution. Leukemia 2006;20:55–60.
55. Jaroch MT, Broughan TA, Hermann RE. The natural history of splenic infarction. Surgery 1986;100:743–750.
56. Cervantes F, Pereira A, Esteve J, et al. The changing profile of idiopathic myelofibrosis: a comparison of the presenting features of patients diagnosed in two different decades. European Journal of Haematology 1998;60:101–105.
57. Mesa RA, Li CY, Schroeder G, et al. Clinical correlates of splenic histopathology and splenic karyotype in myelofibrosis with myeloid metaplasia. Blood 2001;97:3665–3667.
58. Koch CA, Li CY, Mesa RA, et al. Nonhepatosplenic extramedullary hematopoiesis: associated diseases, pathology, clinical course, and treatment. Mayo Clinic Proc 2003;78: 1223–1233.
59. Visani G, Finelli C, Castelli U, et al. Myelofibrosis with myeloid metaplasia: clinical and haematological parameters predicting survival in a series of 133 patients. Br J Haematol 1990;75:4–9.
60. Rupoli S, Da Lio L, Sisti S, et al. Primary myelofibrosis: a detailed statistical analysis of the clinicopathological variables influencing survival. Ann Hematol 1994;68:205–212.

61. Strasser-Weippl K, Steurer M, Kees M, et al. Age and hemoglobin level emerge as most important clinical prognostic parameters in patients with osteomyelofibrosis: introduction of a simplified prognostic score. Leuk Lymphoma 2006;47:441–450.
62. Dupriez B, Morel P, Demory JL, et al. Prognostic factors in agnogenic myeloid metaplasia: a report on 195 cases with a new scoring system. Blood 1996;88:1013–1018.
63. Cervantes F, Pereira A, Esteve J, et al. Identification of 'short-lived' and 'long-lived' patients at presentation of idiopathic myelofibrosis. Br J Haematol 1997;97:635–640.
64. Thiele J, Kvasnicka HM. Hematopathologic findings in chronic idiopathic myelofibrosis. Semin Oncol 2005;32:380–394.
65. Thiele J, Kvasnicka HM. A critical reappraisal of the WHO classification of the chronic myeloproliferative disorders. Leuk Lymphoma 2006;47:381–396.
66. Tefferi A, Mesa RA, Schroeder G, et al. Cytogenetic findings and their clinical relevance in myelofibrosis with myeloid metaplasia. Br J Haematol 2001;113:763–771.
67. Dingli D, Grand FH, Mahaffey V, et al. Der(6)t(1;6)(q21–23;p21.3): a specific cytogenetic abnormality in myelofibrosis with myeloid metaplasia. Br J Haematol 2005;130:229–232.
68. Dingli D, Utz JP, Krowka MJ, et al. Unexplained pulmonary hypertension in chronic myeloproliferative disorders. Chest 2001;120:801–808.
69. Okamura T, Kinukawa N, Niho Y, et al. Primary chronic myelofibrosis: clinical and prognostic evaluation in 336 Japanese patients. Int J Hematol 2001;73:194–198.
70. Mesa RA, Tefferi A. Survival and outcomes to therapy in leukemic transformation of myelofibrosis with myeloid metaplasia; a single institution experience with 91 patients. Blood 2003;102:917a–918a.
71. Dingli D, Schwager SM, Mesa RA, et al. Prognosis in transplant-eligible patients with agnogenic myeloid metaplasia: A simple CBC-based scoring system. Cancer 2005;in press.,
72. Kvasnicka HM, Thiele J, Werden C, et al. Prognostic factors in idiopathic (primary) osteomyelofibrosis. Cancer 1997;80:708–719.
73. Reilly JT, Snowden JA, Spearing RL, et al. Cytogenetic abnormalities and their prognostic significance in idiopathic myelofibrosis: a study of 106 cases. Br J Haematol 1997;98:96–102.
74. Tefferi A, Dingli D, Li CY, et al. Prognostic diversity among cytogenetic abnormalities in myelofibrosis with myeloid metaplasia. Cancer 2005;104:1656–1660.
75. Cervantes F, Alvarez-Larran A, Hernandez-Boluda JC, et al.. Erythropoietin treatment of the anaemia of myelofibrosis with myeloid metaplasia: results in 20 patients and review of the literature. Br J Haematol 2004;127:399–403.
76. Silverstein MN. Agnogenic myeloid metaplasia. Acton, MA Publishing Science Group; 1975, p. 126.
77. Besa EC, Nowell PC, Geller NL, et al. Analysis of the androgen response of 23 patients with agnogenic myeloid metaplasia: the value of chromosomal studies in predicting response and survival. Cancer 1982;49:308–313.
78. Cervantes F, Alvarez-Larran A, Domingo A, et al. Efficacy and tolerability of danazol as a treatment for the anaemia of myelofibrosis with myeloid metaplasia: long-term results in 30 patients. Br J Haematol 2005;129:771–775.
79. Elliott MA, Mesa RA, Li CY, et al. Thalidomide treatment in myelofibrosis with myeloid metaplasia. Br J Haematol 2002;117:288–296.
80. Tefferi A, Cortes J, Verstovsek S, et al. Lenalidomide therapy in myelofibrosis with myeloid metaplasia. Blood 2006;108:1158–1164.
81. D'Amato RJ, Loughnan MS, Flynn E, et al. Thalidomide is an inhibitor of angiogenesis. Proc Natl Acad Sci USA 1994;91:4082–4085.
82. Moreira AL, Sampaio EP, Zmuidzinas A, et al. Thalidomide exerts its inhibitory action on tumor necrosis factor alpha by enhancing mRNA degradation. J Exp Med 1993;177: 1675–1680.
83. Corral LG, Haslett PA, Muller GW, et al. Differential cytokine modulation and T cell activation by two distinct classes of thalidomide analogues that are potent inhibitors of TNF- alpha. J Immunol 1999;163:380–386.

84. Dredge K, Marriott JB, Macdonald CD, et al. Novel thalidomide analogues display anti-angiogenic activity independently of immunomodulatory effects. Br J Cancer 2002;87: 1166–1172.
85. Schafer PH, Gandhi AK, Loveland MA, et al. Enhancement of cytokine production and AP-1 transcriptional activity in T cells by thalidomide-related immunomodulatory drugs. J Pharmacol Exp Ther 2003;20:20.
86. Mesa RA, Steensma DP, Pardanani A, et al. A phase 2 trial of combination low-dose thalidomide and prednisone for the treatment of myelofibrosis with myeloid metaplasia. Blood 2003;101:2534–2541.
87. Tefferi A, Silverstein MN, Li CY. 2-Chlorodeoxyadenosine treatment after splenectomy in patients who have myelofibrosis with myeloid metaplasia. Br J Haematol 1997;99: 352–357.
88. Petti MC, Latagliata R, Spadea T, et al. Melphalan treatment in patients with myelofibrosis with myeloid metaplasia. Br J Haematol 2002;116:576–581.
89. Shojania AM. Reversion of post polycythemia vera (PV) myelofibrosis (MF) to PV following busulfan therapy. Blood 2002;100:343b–343b.
90. Naqvi T, Baumann MA. Myelofibrosis: response to busulfan after hydroxyurea failure. Int J Clin Pract 2002;56:312–313.
91. Parmeggiani L, Ferrant A, Rodhain J, et al. Alpha interferon in the treatment of symptomatic myelofibrosis with myeloid metaplasia. Eur J Haematol 1987;39:228–232.
92. Seewann HL, Gastl G, Lang A, et al. Interferon-alpha-2 in the treatment of idiopathic myelofibrosis. Blut 1988;56:161–163.
93. Barosi G, Liberato LN, Costa A, et al. Cytoreductive effect of recombinant alpha interferon in patients with myelofibrosis with myeloid metaplasia. Blut 1989;58:271–274.
94. Barosi G, Liberato LN, Costa A, et al. Induction and maintenance alpha-interferon therapy in myelofibrosis with myeloid metaplasia. Eur J Haematol 1990;52(Suppl):12–14.
95. Gilbert HS. Long term treatment of myeloproliferative disease with interferon-alpha-2b - feasibility and efficacy. Cancer 1998;83:1205–1213.
96. Tefferi A, Elliot MA, Yoon SY, et al. Clinical and bone marrow effects of interferon alfa therapy in myelofibrosis with myeloid metaplasia. Blood 2001;97:1896.
97. Tefferi A, Mesa RA, Nagorney DM, et al. Splenectomy in myelofibrosis with myeloid metaplasia: a single-institution experience with 223 patients. Blood 2000;95:2226–2233.
98. Elliott MA, Chen MG, Silverstein MN, et al. Splenic irradiation for symptomatic splenomegaly associated with myelofibrosis with myeloid metaplasia. Br J Haematol. 1998;103: 505–511.
99. Tefferi A, Jimenez T, Gray LA, et al. Radiation therapy for symptomatic hepatomegaly in myelofibrosis with myeloid metaplasia. Eur J Haematol 2001;66:37–42.
100. Steensma DP, Hook CC, Stafford SL, et al. Low-dose, single-fraction, whole-lung radiotherapy for pulmonary hypertension associated with myelofibrosis with myeloid metaplasia. Br J Haematol 2002;118:813–816.
101. Deeg HJ, Gooley TA, Flowers ME, et al. Allogeneic hematopoietic stem cell transplantation for myelofibrosis. Blood 2003;102:3912–3918.
102. Ditschkowski M, Beelen DW, Trenschel R, et al. Outcome of allogeneic stem cell transplantation in patients with myelofibrosis. Bone Marrow Transplant 2004;34:807–813.
103. Daly A, Song K, Nevill T, et al. Stem cell transplantation for myelofibrosis: a report from two Canadian centers. Bone Marrow Transplant 2003;32:35–40.
104. Guardiola P, Anderson JE, Gluckman E. Myelofibrosis with myeloid metaplasia. N Engl J Med 2000;343:659; discussion 659–660.
105. Kroger N, Zabelina T, Schieder H, et al. Pilot study of reduced-intensity conditioning followed by allogeneic stem cell transplantation from related and unrelated donors in patients with myelofibrosis. Br J Haematol 2005;128:690–697.
106. Rondelli D, Barosi G, Bacigalupo A, et al. Allogeneic hematopoietic stem-cell transplantation with reduced-intensity conditioning in intermediate- or high-risk patients with myelofibrosis with myeloid metaplasia. Blood 2005;105:4115–4119.

107. Ballen K, Sobocinski KA, Zhang MJ, et al. Outcome of bone marrow transplantation for myelofibrosis. Blood 2005;106:53a–53a.
108. Arana-Yi C, Quintas-Cardama A, Giles F, et al. Advances in the therapy of chronic idiopathic myelofibrosis. Oncologist 2006;11:929–943.
109. Hennessy BT, Thomas DA, Giles FJ, et al. New approaches in the treatment of myelofibrosis. Cancer 2005;103:32–43.
110. Steensma DP, Mesa RA, Li CY, et al. Etanercept, a soluble tumor necrosis factor receptor, palliates constitutional symptoms in patients with myelofibrosis with myeloid metaplasia: results of a pilot study. Blood 2002;99:2252–2254.
111. Tefferi A, Elliot MA. Serious myeloproliferative reactions associated with the use of thalidomide in myelofibrosis with myeloid metaplasia. Blood 2000;96:4007.
112. Buesche G, Georgii A, Duensing A, et al. Evaluating the volume ratio of bone marrow affected by fibrosis: a parameter crucial for the prognostic significance of marrow fibrosis in chronic myeloid leukemia. Hum Pathol 2003;34:391–401.
113. Steensma DP, Hanson CA, et al. Myelodysplasia with fibrosis: a distinct entity? Leuk Res 2001;25:829–838.
114. Tefferi A, Hoagland HC, Therneau TM, et al. Chronic myelomonocytic leukemia: natural history and prognostic determinants. Mayo Clin Proc 1989;64:1246–1254.
115. Michel G, Thuret I, Capodano AM, et al. Myelofibrosis in a child suffering from a hypereosinophilic syndrome with trisomy 8: response to corticotherapy. Med Pediatr Oncol 1991;19:62–65.
116. Baek JY, Li CY, Pardanani A, et al. Bone marrow angiogenesis in systemic mast cell disease. J Hematother Stem Cell Res 2002;11:139–146.
117. Ruiz-Arguelles GJ, Marin-Lopez A, Lobato-Mendizabal E, et al. Acute megakaryoblastic leukaemia: a prospective study of its identification and treatment. Br J Haematol 1986;62:55–63.
118. Mori A, Wada H, Okada M, et al. Acute promyelocytic leukemia with marrow fibrosis at initial presentation: possible involvement of transforming growth factor-beta(1). Acta Haematol 2000;103:220–223.
119. Wallis JP, Reid MM. Bone marrow fibrosis in childhood acute lymphoblastic leukaemia. J Clin Pathol 1989;42:1253–1254.
120. Thiele J, Krech R, Vykoupil KF, Georgii A. Malignant (acute) myelosclerosis: a clinical and pathological study in 6 patients. Scand J Haematol 1984;33:95–109.
121. Hasselbalch H. Idiopathic myelofibrosis: a clinical study of 80 patients. Am J Hematol 1990;34:291–300.
122. Shehata M, Schwarzmeier JD, Hilgarth M, et al. TGF-beta1 induces bone marrow reticulin fibrosis in hairy cell leukemia. J Clin Invest 2004;113:676–685.
123. Meadows LM, Rosse WR, Moore JO, et al. Hodgkin's disease presenting as myelofibrosis. Cancer 1989;64:1720–1726.
124. Matsunaga T, Takemoto N, Miyajima N, et al. Splenic marginal zone lymphoma presenting as myelofibrosis associated with bone marrow involvement of lymphoma cells which secrete a large amount of TGF-beta. Ann Hematol 2004;83:322–325.
125. Meerkin D, Ashkenazi Y, Gottschalk-Sabag S, et al. Plasma cell dyscrasia with marrow fibrosis. A reversible syndrome mimicking agnogenic myeloid metaplasia. Cancer 1994;73:625–628.
126. Kiely JM, Silverstein MN. Metastatic carcinoma simulating agnogenic myeloid metaplasia and myelofibrosis. Cancer 1969;24:1041–1044.
127. Paquette RL, Meshkinpour A, Rosen PJ. Autoimmune myelofibrosis. A steroid-responsive cause of bone marrow fibrosis associated with systemic lupus erythematosus. Medicine 1994;73:145–152.
128. Inoue Y, Matsubara A, Okuya S, et al. Myelofibrosis and systemic lupus erythematosus: reversal of fibrosis with high-dose corticosteroid therapy. Acta Haematol. 1992;88:32–36.
129. Rocha Filho FD, Ferreira FV, Mendes FdO, et al. Bone marrow fibrosis (pseudo-myelofibrosis) in human kala-azar. Rev Soc Bras Med Trop 2000;33:363–366.

130. Viallard JF, Parrens M, Boiron JM, et al. Reversible myelofibrosis induced by tuberculosis. Clin Infect Dis 2002;34:1641–1643.
131. Murrin RJ, Harrison P. Abnormal osteoclasts and bone marrow fibrosis in Paget's disease of the bone. Br J Haematol 2004;124:3.
132. Sitalakshmi S, Srikrishna A, Damodar P. Haematological changes in HIV infection. Indian J Pathol Microbiol 2003;46:180–183.
133. Stephan JL, Galambrun C, Dutour A, et al. Myelofibrosis: an unusual presentation of vitamin D-deficient rickets. Eur J Pediatr 1999;158:828–829.
134. Nomura S, Ogawa Y, Osawa G, et al. Myelofibrosis secondary to renal osteodystrophy. Nephron 1996;72:683–687.
135. Kumbasar B, Taylan I, Kazancioglu R, et al. Myelofibrosis secondary to hyperparathyroidism. Exp Clin Endocrinol Diabetes 2004;112:127–130.
136. Falik-Zaccai TC, Anikster Y, Rivera CE, et al. A new genetic isolate of gray platelet syndrome (GPS): clinical, cellular, and hematologic characteristics. Mol Genet Metab 2001;74: 303–313.
137. Sheikha A. Fatal familial infantile myelofibrosis. J Pediatr Hematol Oncol 2004;26:164–168.
138. Popat U, Frost A, Liu E, et al. New onset of myelofibrosis in association with pulmonary arterial hypertension. Ann Intern Med 2005;143:466–467.
139. Elliott M, Dingli D, Schwager S, et al. Absolute monocyte count is an independent prognostic factor for survival in agnogenic myeloid metaplasia. Blood 2006: Abstract.
140. Cervantes F, Barosi G, Demory JL, et al. Myelofibrosis with myeloid metaplasia in young individuals: disease characteristics, prognostic factors and identification of risk groups. Br J Haematol 1998;102:684–690.

Chapter 3
Essential Thrombocythemia

Guido Finazzi

3.1 Introduction

Essential thrombocythemia (ET) is currently classified as a myeloproliferative disorder (MPD), which is a heterogeneous category of clonal stem cell diseases that also includes polycythemia vera (PV), myelofibrosis with myeloid metaplasia (MMM), chronic myeloid leukemia (CML), and atypical MPDs (1). A major advance in our understanding of the pathogenesis of MPDs was made with the recent identification of the V617F JAK2 mutation in a substantial proportion of patients, especially with PV (2–7). This discovery has had a major impact on disease classification, diagnostic approach, and in addressing research strategies in these disorders.

Among the classic MPDs (1), ET shows a longer median survival as well as lower transformation rates into acute myelogenous leukemia (AML). However, the clinical course of ET is complicated by thrombotic and hemorrhagic episodes that occur more frequently in older patients and those with previous vascular events. There is an ongoing debate as to whether the evolution to AML is part of the natural history of the disease or is related to the use of cytoreductive agents given to control the myeloproliferation and avoid vascular complications. Hence, the best strategy is to limit the use of cytotoxic therapy by stratifying patients on the basis of their risk for developing vascular events.

This chapter reviews recent progress in the management of ET with particular emphasis on four key areas: pathogenesis, diagnostic criteria, clinical course, and risk-adapted therapy.

3.2 Pathogenesis

Essential thrombocythemia is thought to result from transformation of a multipotent hematopoietic progenitor. This concept was originally proposed by Fialkow and colleagues, who demonstrated a clonal pattern of X inactivation in multiple myeloid lineages but not in lymphoid cells (8). Subsequent studies in ET have demonstrated that a significant proportion of ET patients do not appear to have clonal hematopoie-sis (9, 10). This observation, however, might reflect the limited ability of current techniques to detect a small proportion of clonally derived cells in a background of polyclonal hematopoesis since a recent study has demonstrated the presence of JAK2 V617F in the majority of patients with "polyclonal" ET (11).

Cytogenetic studies have not been helpful. Almost 95% of ET patients have normal cytogenetics and, when present, karyotypic abnormalities are highly varia-ble (12). A clue to the nature of the underlying defect came from the realization that as in PV, hematopoietic progenitors from many patients with ET are hypersensitive to cytokines such as thrombopoietin or erythropoietin (13–15). These observations focused attention on cytokine signal transduction pathways.

In 2005, an identical acquired mutation of JAK2 has been found in the vast majority of patients with PV, as well as approximately half those with ET and MMM (2–7). The mutation (V617F) is located in the negative regulatory JH2 domain and replaces a highly conserved valine with a bulky phenylalanine. As predicted by previous structural and biochemical studies, the consequence of this mutation is increased tyrosine kinase acytivity of JAK2. JAK2 plays a central role in signal transduction from multiple growth factors, and so its activation is consistent with the growth-factor-independent phenotype. Sequence analysis of peripheral blood granulocytes detected the mutation in 12–40% of patients with ET (2–5), but over 50% were positive by allele-specific polymerase chain reaction (PCR) (3). These results demonstrate that ET can be divided into JAK2-positive and JAK2-negative subgroups. The molecular basis for JAK-2-negative ET remains obscure. It is also unclear how the same mutation can give rise to PV, ET, MMM, and other atypical MPDs. Potential explanations include differences between individuals with respect to genetic background, additional acquired mutations, or the target cell for transformation (16).

3.3 Diagnostic Criteria

Also in the current JAK2 V617F era, there is no single clinical or laboratory finding that permits a diagnosis of ET. Thus, the diagnosis must be reached by a mix of positive criteria in conjunction with the exclusion of other myeloproliferative or myelodysplastic disorders as well as conditions that are associated with a reactive thrombocytosis. This principle was used in the diagnostic criteria developed by the World Health Organization (WHO) (17) (Table 3.1).

3.3.1 Platelet Count

The current criteria for ET require a persistent platelet count of $>600 \times 10^9$/L. However, it has been suggested that the platelet count criterion should be reduced to $>400 \times 10^9$/L because, in long-term follow-up studies, the clinical course of

Table 3.1 WHO diagnostic criteria for essential thrombocythemia

Positive criteria

1. Sustained platelet count $>600 \times 10^9$/L
2. Bone marrow biopsy specimen showing proliferation mainly of the megakaryocytic lineage with increased number of enlarged, mature megakayocytes

Criteria of exclusion

No evidence of PV

- Normal red cell mass or Hb < 18.5 g/dL in men, 16.5 g/dL in women
- Stainable iron in bone marrow, normal serum ferritin, or normal MCV
- If the former condition is not met, failure of iron trial to increase red cell mass or Hb levels to the PV range.

2. No evidence of CML

- No Philadelphia chromosome and no BCR/ABL fusion gene

3. No evidence of myelodysplastic syndrome

- No del(5q), t(3;3)(q21;q26), inv(3)(q21q26)
- No significant granulocytic dysplasia, few if any micromegakaryocytes

4. No evidence that thrombocytosis is reactive due to:

- Underlying inflammation or infection
- Underlying neoplasm
- Prior splenectomy

MCV: Mean cell volume. Source: Adapted from Ref. 17.

patients with platelet counts between 400 10^9/L and 600×10^9/L was found to be indistinguishable from that of patients with a clearly diagnosed ET (18, 19). The major problem with this approach is that lowering the threshold of platelet count will improve the sensitivity but reduce the specificity of ET diagnosis. Therefore, the selection of a cutoff of 600×10^9/L is probably the most appropriate for the selection of ET patients to be put in therapeutic trials. In the current clinical practice, a lower platelet count can be taken for an initial screening, but this should be supported by other clinical and laboratory ET features.

3.3.2 JAK2 Mutation

The V617F JAK2 mutation is detectable in 40–60% of ET patients ([2–7) and the technology required to detect it is very simple, being generally PCR based (20). Hence, for those patients presenting with an isolated thrombocytosis, or with clinical findings suspicious for a MPD [e.g., patients presenting with Budd Chiari syndrome (21)], a positive screen for V617F JAK2 will confirm the diagnosis as a MPD. The traditional difficulty in making a diagnosis of ET has been excluding a reactive thrombocytosis in those patients with other comorbidities. This distinction will be simpler in patients with detectable V617F JAK2 but does not, of course, preclude careful clinical history and examination. For V617F JAK2-negative patients, the diagnosis will rely on the WHO criteria (17). A proposed diagnostic scheme including JAK2 mutation screening is reported in Table 3.2 (22).

3.3.3 Bone Marrow Biopsy

It has been suggested that ET can be positively diagnosed by careful, quantitative examination of the bone marrow biopsy (23): this forms the basis of a positive marker for ET in the WHO diagnostic criteria (17). Typical clustering of enlarged megakaryocytes with multilobated nuclei has been advocated to represent the hallmark feature of the disease. The background hematopoiesis in ET is characterized by a discrete pattern of minimal or no hyperplastic erythropoiesis, no change in granulopoiesis, almost no fibrosis, and a reduction of stainable iron. A detailed evaluation of bone marrow features might also help to distinguish "true" ET from the initial stages of MMM, PV, or myelodysplasia. "Early" myelofibrosis is characterized by increasing cellularity with prominent neutrophil granulopoiesis,

Table 3.2 Proposed diagnostic criteria for essential thrombocythemia including JAK2 V617F mutation

A

1. Platelet count $>600 \times 10^9$/L for >2 months
2. Presence of JAK2 V617F mutation

B

1. No cause for a reactive thrombocytosis
2. No evidence of iron deficiency
3. No evidence of PV
   - Normal red cell mass or haematocrit $<40\%$
4. No evidence of myelofibrosis
   - Collagen fibrosis of the bone marrow absent or less than one-third of the biopsy area without both marked splenomegaly and a leukoerythroblastic blood film
5. No evidence of CML
   - No Philadelphia chromosome and no BCR/ABL fusion gene
6. No evidence of myelodysplastic syndrome
   - No del(5q), t(3;3)(q21;q26), inv(3)(q21q26)
   - No significant granulocytic dysplasia, few if any micromegakaryocytes

Note: Diagnosis of ET requires either A1, A2 and B3-6 or A1 and B1-6.
Source: Adapted from Ref. 22.

borderline to slight reticulin fibrosis, and pronounced abnormalities of megakaryo-cyte differentiation, including hyperchromasia and marked nuclear-cytoplasmatic deviation. Notably, patients with these morphological features frequently develop an overt myelofibrosis and have a significantly worse life expectancy. However, an experienced observer and a well-standardized procedure are required to diagnose ET by examination of the bone marrow biopsy.

3.3.4 Other Criteria

Some authors have shown that endogenous erythroid colonies or culture examining CFU-Mk (megakaryocytic colony-forming unit) growth might be reliable markers of the disease (13, 24). However, these investigations are not widely available, are expensive, and are technically demanding and, therefore, might be suitable for research purposes or in the occasional patient but not for general use.

Nonstimulated metaphases obtained from marrow aspirates should be examined for cytogenetic abnormalities. This is primarily important in order to exclude the presence of the Philadelphia (Ph) chromosome, the genotypic hallmark of CML, particularly in those patients with very high platelet counts (25). Karyotypic abnormalities generally arise upon transformation of ET to acute leukemia when deletions or elongations of the short arm of chromosomes 1, 2, 5, 17, 20, and 21 are the most frequent defects (12).

3.4 Clinical Course

3.4.1 Frequency

According to population-based epidemiological studies (26, 27), the incidence rates of ET range from 15 to 25 cases per million inhabitants annually. These figures are in agreement with a recent systematic screening for erythrocytosis and thrombocy-tosis in 10,000 consecutive persons living in the city of Vicenza, Italy (28). This cross-sectional study of healthy people led to the identification of four cases of ET (platelet count $\geq 600 \times 10^9$/L) with an estimated prevalence of 400 cases per million inhabitants (95% confidence interval 109–1020/million). Interestingly, no throm-botic or hemorrhagic complications occurred over 5 years of follow-up in these incidentally discovered ET patients.

The disorder appears to affect primarily middle-aged people, with an average age at diagnosis of about 55 years (29). There is a higher prevalence of females (26, 29), mainly due to a second peak frequency at around 30 years of age for women. This predisposition of young women to develop ET is relevant for the issue of pregnancy discussed below.

3.4.2   Incidence and Type of Major Thrombotic and Hemorrhagic Complications

Thrombosis and hemorrhage are the most frequent clinical complications observed in ET patients (30). In uncontrolled studies, reported cumulative rates for thrombosis and hemorrhage during follow-up ranged from 7% to 17% and 8% to 14%, respectively (31). In one study that also evaluated a control population (32), the incidence of thrombotic episodes was 6.6% per patient-year in ET versus 1.2% in control subjects and the rate of major hemorrhagic complications was 0.33% per patient-year in ET versus 0% in controls.

The most frequent types of major thrombosis include stroke, transient ischemic attack, myocardial infarction, peripheral arterial thrombosis, and deep venous thrombosis often occurring in unusual sites, such as hepatic (Budd-Chiari syndrome), portal, and mesenteric veins. In addition to large-vessel occlusions, ET patients might suffer from microcirculatory symptoms, including vascular headaches, dizziness, visual disturbances, distal paresthesia, and acrocyanosis. The most characteristic of these disturbances is erythromelalgia, consisting of congestion, redness, and burning pain to ischemia and gangrene of distal portions of toes and fingers (33). The most frequent bleeding events are hemorrhages from the gastrointestinal tract, followed by hematuria and other mucocutaneous hemorrhages. Hemarthrosis and large muscle hematomas are uncommon.

3.4.3   Risk Factors

Age over 60 and a previous thrombotic event were identified as major risk factors for thrombosis in a controlled study (32) and in an uncontrolled series of patients (34, 35). Additional risk factors have been also recognized: clonal disease, impaired expression of c-*Mpl* in bone marrow megakaryocytes, overexpression of PRV-1, presence of factor V Leiden, and antiphospholipid antibodies were associated with a higher incidence of vascular complications (reviewed in Ref. 31). The risk is increased by the concomitant presence of hypertension, hypercholesterolemia, and smoking, but it should be recognized that these associations are not consistently found in all studies.

Recently, a prognostic role for leukocytosis in MPDs has been advocated. Three large cohort studies have demonstrated that an increased leukocyte count is a novel independent risk factor for both thrombosis and inferior survival in ET (29, 36) and for thrombosis in PV (37). In one study, a correlation between leukocytosis and the V617F JAK2 mutation was reported (36). In ET and PV, in vivo leukocyte activation has been shown to occur and to be associated with signs of activation of both platelets and endothelial cells (38). Platelet activation is increased in ET patients carrying the V617F JAK2 mutation (39). Thus, leukocyte and platelet activation might play a role in the generation of the prethrombotic state that characterizes ET and PV.

The presence of the V617F JAK2 mutation in about 50% of patients with ET raises the question of whether mutated and nonmutated patients differ in terms of thrombotic risk. The largest relevant study on 806 patients suggested that JAK2 mutation was associated with venous but not arterial events (40). An increased risk of thrombosis in JAK2-mutated patients with essential thrombocythemia was also reported by other investigators (41, 42). However, the rate of vascular complications was not affected by the presence of the mutation in two other relatively large studies, including 150 and 130 patients, respectively (11, 43). It is possible that the higher age distribution and hematocrit and leukocyte levels consistently found in mutation-positive patients (11, 40–43) contributed to the apparent association between JAK2 V617F and thrombosis reported in some studies.

Paradoxically, a very high platelet count ($>1500 \times 10^9$/L) was found to be a major predictor of bleeding rather than thrombosis (44). The explanation of this comes from the well-documented impairment of von Willebrand factor (vWF) multimers found both in patients with ET and those with reactive thrombocytosis (30, 44). Large vWF multimers have been found to be decreased in parallel with the degree of thrombocythemia. Moreover, normalization of the platelet count was accompanied by restoration of a normal plasma vWF multimeric distribution and correction of bleeding tendency. However, in a retrospective study of 99 consecutive young patients (aged <60 years) who presented with extreme thrombocytosis (platelet count $\geq 1000 \times 10^9$/L) and without a previous history of thrombohemorrhagic complications, the incidences of major thrombosis and hemorrhage during the follow-up were similar between those who were treated with prophylactic cytoreductive therapy and those who did not receive such therapy (45). This clinical observation challenges the role of extreme thrombocytosis as a major risk factor for vascular events in otherwise low-risk patients with ET.

3.4.4 Progression of the Disease

Essential thrombocythemia might transform to MMM or acute leukemia (AL) as part of the natural history. In a series of 195 patients followed for a median of 7.2 years (range: 1.9–24), conversion to MMM was observed in 13 cases, with an actuarial probability of 2.7% at 5 years, 8.3% at 10 years, and 15.3% at 15 years (46). In a long-term cohort study of 322 consecutive patients followed for a median of 13.6 years life expectancy, survival was similar to that of the control population in the first decade of disease [risk ratio: 0.72; 95% confidence interval (CI): 0.50–0.99) but became significantly worse thereafter (risk ratio: 2.21; 95% CI: 1.74–2.76)]. Multivariable analysis identified age at diagnosis of 60 years or older, leukocytosis, tobacco use, and diabetes mellitus as indendent predictors of poor survival. The risk of leukemic or any myeloid disease transformation was low in the first 10 years (1.4% and 9.1%, respectively) but increased substantially in the second (8.1% and 28.3%, respectively) and third (24.0% and 58.5%, respectively) decades of the disease (43).

3.5   Risk-Adapted Therapy

Before deciding whether to start platelet-lowering treatment, ET patients should be evaluated for history of thrombotic or hemorrhagic events and the presence of cardiovascular risk factors (i.e., smoking, hypertension, hypercholesterolemia, and diabetes). Then they should be stratified according to their probability of developing major bleeding or thrombosis (Table 3.3)(1, 47).

3.5.1   Low Risk

Avoiding cytoreduction is an option for low-risk ET patients. The natural history of such patients left untreated was prospectively evaluated in a controlled study that compared 65 low-risk patients with 65 age- and sex-matched normal controls (48). After a median follow-up of 4.1 years, the incidence of thrombosis was not significantly higher in patients than in controls (1.91% vs. 1.5% per patient-year; age- and sex-adjusted risk ratio: 1.43; 95% CI: 0.37–5.4). No major bleeding was observed. Thrombotic deaths seem very rare in low-risk ET subjects, and there are no data indicating that fatalities can be prevented by starting cytoreductive drugs early. Therefore, withholding chemotherapy might be justifiable in young, asymptomatic ET patients with a platelet count below $1,500 \times 10^9$/L. This policy is based on the low risk of complications and the potential leukemogenicity of cytotoxic drugs. However, the strength of these recommendations is based on studies with small number of patients, and further data from large clinical trials are needed.

Aspirin at different doses (30–500 mg/day) has been found to control microvascular symptoms, such as erythromelalgia, and transient neurological and ocular disturbances (TIAs), including dysarthria, hemiparesis, scintillating scotomas, amaurosis fugax, migraines, and seizures (33). The efficacy and safety of aspirin, 100 mg daily, in preventing major thrombotic events has been formally assessed in a randomized clinical trial in PV (49). Aspirin lowered significantly the risk of a primary combined

Table 3.3 Classification of essential thrombocythemia based on thrombotic and hemorrhagic risk

Low risk	Age < 60 years, and
	No history of thrombosis or major bleeding, and
	Platelet count < 1500 x 10^9/L
Intermediate risk	Neither low risk nor high risk
High risk	Age > 60 years, or
	A previous history of thrombosis or major bleeding

Note: Correction of cardiovascular risk factors (smoking, hypertension, hypercolesterolemia, diabetes) is recommended in all patients; their contribution to thrombotic risk classification is controversial (see text).

Source: Adapted from Ref. 1.

endpoint, including cardiovascular death, nonfatal myocardial infarction, nonfatal stroke, and major venous thromboembolism (relative risk: 0.4; 95% CI: 0.18–0.91, $p = 0.0277$) without increasing major bleeding (relative risk: 1.6; 95% CI: 0.27–9.71). Based on these findings, an antithrombotic preventive strategy with low-dose aspirin is recommended in all PV patients. Translating evidence from this study to ET can be considered, but formal clinical trials have not hitherto been produced.

3.5.2 Intermediate Risk

Whether some patients might be classified as at "intermediate risk" of thrombosis is more contentious. The rationale for assigning this risk category is the increase in incidence of thrombotic events in the age range 40–60 years compared to less than 40 years (32) and the uncertainty over the weighting that might be ascribed to weaker or more controversial risk factors. The Italian Consensus Criteria define "intermediate risk" as age 40–60 years, platelets less than $1000 \times 10^9/L$, and either vascular risk factors or familial thrombophilia with no consensus on treatment (31). In a recent review, Elliott and Tefferi suggested that those aged 60 years, with no history of thrombosis and either a platelet count $1500 \times 10^9/L$ or cardiovascular risk factors (e.g., smoking, diabetes) are of intermediate risk and should be treated with aspirin, but they concluded there was no consensus on cytoreductive therapy (30). Finally, in the United Kingdom, intermediate-risk patients, aged 40–60 years with all of the following: platelets less than $1500 \times 10^9/L$, no prior thrombosis or hemorrhage, no hypertension or diabetes, are entering into an ongoing randomized study comparing HU plus aspirin or aspirin alone (50).

3.5.3 High Risk

3.5.3.1 Hydroxyurea

Hydroxyurea (HU) has emerged as the treatment of choice in high-risk patients with ET (Table 3.3) because of its efficacy in preventing thrombosis (see Section 3.5.3.4) and rare acute toxicity. Hematopoietic impairment, leading to neutropenia and macrocytic anemia, is the main short-term toxic effect of HU. Other less frequent side effects include oral and leg ulcers and skin lesions.

The leukemogenicity of this agent is still debated. Some long-term studies found that a proportion of ET patients treated with HU developed acute leukemia (51, 52). In other studies, however, this drug was rarely associated with secondary malignancies when used alone (53–56). In an analysis of 25 ET patients younger than 50 years and treated with HU for a high risk of thrombosis, no leukemic or neoplastic transformation occurred after a median follow-up of 8 years (range: 5–14) (53). In 1638 patients with PV enrolled in a prospective study, HU alone did not enhance the risk of leukemia in comparison with patients treated with phlebotomy only (hazard ratio: 0.86; 95% CI: 0.26–2.88; $p = 0.8$), whereas this risk was significantly increased by any other cytoreductive drug, namely radiophosphorus, busulphan, or pipobroman, either used alone or in combination (hazard ratio: 5.46; 95% CI: 1.84–16.25; $p = 0.002$) (54). The incidence of acute leukemic transformation is higher in patients with ET treated with HU if they have cytogenetic abnormalities (51, 52) or have received other cytotoxic drugs with different mechanisms of action (51, 54–56).

3.5.3.2 Anagrelide

Anagrelide, an imidazo quinazinoline derivative, has been shown to reduce the platelet count in a species-specific manner (57, 58). The mechanism by which anagrelide induces thrombocytopenia is unclear, but current attention is focused on inhibition of megakaryocytes differentiation and maturation (58). Major side effects of the drug include palpitations, headaches, noncardiac edema, and congestive cardiac failure (58). In one report, patients treated with anagrelide developed cardiomyopathy (59).

There is extensive experience with the use of this drug, which is licensed in United States as a first-line agent by the Food and Drug Administration for control of thrombocytosis associated with any myeloproliferative disorders. In Europe, the drug has been granted a license only for ET patients refractory to or intolerant of first-line therapy. The criteria for defining resistance or intolerance to HU have been recently established by an International Working Group (60). They include the following: platelet count greater than $600 \times 10^9/L$ after 3 months of at least 2 g/day of HU (2.5 g/day in patients with a body weight over 80 kg); platelet count greater than $400 \times 10^9/L$, and white blood count (WBC) less than $2.5 \times 10^9/L$ or Hb less than 10 g/dL at any dose of HU; presence of leg ulcers or other unacceptable mucocutaneous manifestations at any dose of HU; and HU-related fever.

Until recently, studies of anagrelide in ET were nonrandomized, lacked a control arm, and had relatively limited follow-up. The largest study to date evaluated 934 ET patients for efficacy and 2251 for safety and had a maximum follow-up of 7 years; there was no evidence that anagrelide increased conversion to AL and no mention was made of myelofibrosis (61). A study of 35 consecutive young ET patients treated with anagrelide, with a median follow-up of 10.7 years, demonstrated that 20% had thrombotic complications and a similar proportion had major hemorrhagic complications, raising a question about the efficacy of anagrelide (62). These events occurred when the platelet count was above $400 \times 10^9/L$ suggesting that control of the platelet count to below $400 \times 10^9/L$ might reduce this risk. A second major finding from this study was the development of a significant anemia of more than 3 g/dL in a quarter of patients.

3.5.3.3 Interferon-alpha

Interferon (IFN)-α has been evaluated in several cohorts of ET patients (reviewed in Ref. 63). Platelet count was reduced to below $600 \times 10^9/L$ in about 90% of cases after about 3 months, with an average dose of 3 million international units (IU) daily. The time and degree of platelet reduction during the induction phase were dose dependent. The IFN-α dose can be tapered during maintenance, but after its discontinuation, the platelet count rebounds in the majority of patients. IFN-α is not known to be teratogenic and does not cross the placenta. Thus, it has been used successfully throughout pregnancy in some ET patients with no adverse fetal or maternal effects.

Side effects are a major problem with this drug. In addition to flulike symptoms observed in the early treatment phase, signs of chronic toxicity include weakness, myalgia, weight and hair loss, gastrointestinal toxicity, and depression. In a series of 273 ET patients (63), IFN-α therapy was terminated in 25% (67 cases) before completion of the treatment. The rate of withdrawal ranged between 0% and 66% in the different studies. This wide range might be partly explained by the difference in observation times that ranged from 1 month to 4 years. So far, no leukemogenic effects have been reported.

Recently, semisynthetic pegylated forms of interferon-α (peg-IFN-α) have been used to treat ET, which in a limited number of studies (reviewed in Ref. 64) have been shown to be superior to unmodified IFN as related to its adverse event profile and efficacy. Interestingly, the use of peg-IFN-α-2a in 27 patients with PV was able to decrease the percentage of mutated JAK2 allele in 24 cases (89%), from a mean of 49% to a mean of 27% (65). However, a more limited effect on JAK2 mutational status of another form of peg-IFN-α (peg-IFN-α-2b) in patients with PV and ET has been reported (66). Despite its high cost and toxicity, IFN remains a useful agent in cytoreductive treatment of ET, especially in very young patients and pregnant women.

3.5.3.4 Clinical Trials

Two randomized clinical trials assessing benefits and risks of myelosuppressive therapy in ET patients at high risk of thrombosis have been carried out so far. The first was performed about 10 years ago in Italy and evaluated HU versus untreated controls (67): 114 ET patients were randomized to HU or no cytoreductive treatment. During a median follow-up of 27 months, 2 thromboses were recorded in the HU-treated group (1.6%/patient-year) compared with 14 in the control group (10.7%/patient-year; p = 0.003). This study provided the basis for considering HU as the standard therapy for high-risk ET patients and the reference arm for other randomized trials.

The second trial was carried out in United Kingdom and compared HU plus aspirin with anagrelide plus aspirin in 809 high-risk ET patients analyzed with a median follow-up of 39 months (68). Overall, patients randomized to anagrelide and aspirin were more likely to reach the composite primary endpoint of major thrombosis (arterial or venous), major hemorrhage, or death from a vascular cause ($p = 0.03$). When individual endpoints were assessed, arterial thrombosis, major hemorrhage, and myelofibrosis were all significantly more frequent for patients treated with anagrelide ($p = 0.004$, 0.008, and 0.01 respectively). However anagrelide and aspirin seems to offer at least partial protection from thrombosis, as the prevalence of thrombotic events was significantly lower than the control arm of the Italian study (67) (actuarial rate of first thrombosis 8% versus 26% at 2 years, respectively), whereas the HU arms were approximately equivalent (actuarial rate of first thrombosis 4% at 2 years in both trials). The success of HU is likely to reflect the importance of additional factors such as the hematocrit, leukocyte count, or subtle effects on the endothelium in the pathogenesis of thrombosis. Intriguingly, venous thrombosis was, however, less frequent in patients treated with anagrelide ($p = 0.006$).

Major hemorrhage was increased for anagrelide plus aspirin treatment ($p = 0.008$). The most frequent of these endpoints were gastrointestinal hemorrhages. Hemorrhagic events might result from some subtle effect on platelet function, possibly accentuated by aspirin or in relation to combined gastric toxicity.

Myelofibrotic transformation was seen in 16 patients treated with anagrelide in comparison with 5 with HU. It seems logical that anagrelide might be less effective than HU at suppressing the natural evolution of ET to myelofibrosis, as the number of megakaryocytes remains elevated in ET patients treated with anagrelide compared to those given HU. There is also evidence that despite control of the platelet count, levels of tranforming growth factor-β remain elevated in patients treated with anagrelide (69). The incidence of myelofibrosis in the anagrelide arm (3.95%) at median follow-up of 39 months is approximately in accordance with what has previously reported (0.9% per annum) (46), supporting the view that HU might be more effectively suppressing myelofibrosis.

3.5.4 Pregnancy

Essential thrombocythemia is unique among the other Philadelphia negative MPDs, as it is relatively common among women of child-bearing age (70). In a recent systematic review of the literature, outcome data from 461 pregnancies reported by retrospective and prospective cohort studies were evaluated (31). The rate of spontaneous abortions was 44%, which is about threefold higher than in the general population. Placental infarction was reported in 18 cases: these were often responsible for intrauterine fetal growth retardation (11 cases). Abruptio placentae was reported in nine cases (3.6%), a rate that is higher than in the general population (1%). Maternal complications are relatively rare with no fatalities, but postpartum thrombotic episodes were reported in 13 patients (5.2% of the pregnancies) emphasizing the need for postpartum thrombo-prophylaxis.

The average platelet count at the beginning of pregnancy in patients with successful pregnancies was $1010 \times 10^9/L$, whereas it was $977 \times 10^9/L$ among those with an unsuccessful outcome (31); thus, the baseline platelet count did not predict pregnancy outcome. During the second trimester, a spontaneous decline was registered to a nadir of $599 \times 10^9/L$. In the postpartum period, the platelet counts rose back up to their earlier levels and rebound thrombocytosis occured in some patients.

The apparent low risk of maternal complications must be considered in context, as the majority of these patients are "low-risk" ET. Most pregnant ET patients not in the high-risk category should be treated with aspirin and postpartum prophylaxis with heparin and closely monitored for complications. For those patients with previous pregnancy or disease–related complications (>3 first-trimester or 1 second- or third-trimester loss, severe Intrauterine Growth Retardation (IUGR), preeclampsia, significant hemorrhage or thrombotic event, and/or extreme thrombocytosis) therapeutic options include aspirin, low-molecular-weight heparin, and IFN-α (30,70) (Table 3.4). However, only limited literature to support optimal management strategies is available and there is a need for international collaboration to address these issues and define best care (71).

3.6 Personal Approach to Therapy

My first step in deciding the treatment of a patient with ET is to assess his/her risk of major thrombotic or bleeding complications (Table 3.3). I do not treat patients clearly classifiable as "low risk," but I give low-dose aspirin (100 mg daily) if they present with microvascular symptoms, such as erythromelalgia, paresthesiae or atypical visual disturbances or associated cardiovascular risk factors (Figure 3.1). The management of patients with extreme thrombocytosis ($>1500 \times 10^9$/L) and otherwise low-risk ET is more contentious (45). I favor patient's age and symptoms over platelet count, avoiding cytoreductive therapy in very young (<40 years),

Table 3.4 Risk-adapted management of ET in pregnancy

1. Risk stratification.
   At least one of the following defines high-risk pregnancy:

   - Previous major thrombotic or bleeding complication
   - Previous severe pregnancy complications*
   - Platelet count $>1500 \times 10^9$/L

2. Therapy

   a) Low-risk pregnancy

   - Aspirin 100 mg/day
   - LMWH 4000 U/day after delivery until 6 weeks postpartum

   b) High-risk pregnancy
      As above, plus

   - If previous major thrombosis or severe pregnancy complications: LMWH throughout pregnancy (stop aspirin if bleeding complications)
   - If platelet count $>1500 \times 10^9$/L: consider IFN-α
   - If previous major bleeding: avoid aspirin and consider IFN-α to reduce thrombocytosis

*Note: Severe pregnancy complications: ≥3 first-trimester or ≥1 second- or third-trimester losses, birth weight <5th centile of gestation, preeclampsia, intrauterine death or stillbirth.
LMWH: Low molecular weight heparin.
Source: Adapted from Ref. 70.

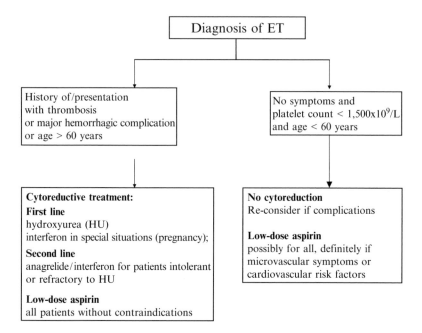

Figure 3.1 An algorithm of risk-adapted treatment recommendations in patients with ET. Classification of intermediate risk is controversial: A randomized study comparing aspirin versus aspirin plus HU in intermediate risk patients is ongoing (see text)

completely asymptomatic patients with stable platelet count also in the range of $(1600-1800) \times 10^9/L$. However, I start therapy in the presence of rapidly increasing platelet counts and/or minor bleeding or vascular disturbances. In patients younger than 40 years of age, my first choice is IFN-α. If the drug is ineffective or not tolerated, I use HU. In patients over 40 years of age with more than $1500 \times 10^9/L$ platelets and in those with definitely "high-risk" ET, the therapy of choice is HU plus low-dose aspirin (47). I consider anagrelide as second-line treatment in high-risk patients intolerant or refractory to HU (60), provided they have a normal cardiac function. I assess JAK2 V617F in all patients with ET, but, for the time being, I do not use the mutation status to decide therapy. It is hoped that molecularly targeted treatment will be available in the near future, as promising JAK2-targeted small molecule drugs are already on the horizon.

References

1. Tefferi A, Barbui T. *bcr/abl* negative, classic myeloproliferative disorders: diagnosis and treatment. Mayo Clin Proc 2005;80:1220–1232.
2. James C, Ugo V, Le Couedic JP, et al. A unique clonal JAK2 mutation leading to constitutive signalling causes polycythaemia vera. Nature 2005;434:1144–1148.

3. Baxter EJ, Scott LM, Campbell PJ, et al. Acquired mutation of the tyrosine kinase JAK2 in human myeloproliferative disorders. Lancet 2005;365:1054–1061.
4. Levine RL, Wadleigh M, Cools J, et al. Activating mutation in the tyrosine kinase JAK2 in polycythemia vera, essential thrombocythemia, and myeloid metaplasia with myelofibrosis. Cancer Cell 2005;4:387.
5. Kralovics R, Passamonti F, Buser AS, et al. A gain-of-function mutation of JAK2 in myelo-proliferative disorders. N Engl J Med 2005;352: 1779–1790.
6. Zhao R, Xing S, Li Z, et al. Identification of an acquired JAK2 mutation in polycythemia vera. J Biol Chem 2005;280:22,788–22,792.
7. Jones AV, Kreil S, Zoi K, et al. Widespread occurrence of the JAK2 V617 mutation in chronic myeloproliferative disorders. Blood 2005;106:2162–2168.
8. Fialkow PJ, Faguet GB, Jacobson RJ, et al. Evidence that essential thrombocythemia is a clonal disorder with origin in a multipotent stem cell. Blood 1981;58:916–919.
9. el-Kassar N, Hetet G, Briere J, et al. Clonality analysis of hematopoiesis in essential thrombo-cythemia: advantages of studying T lymphocytes and platelets. Blood 1997;89:128–134.
10. Harrison CN, Gale RE, Machin SJ, et al. A large proportion of patients with a diagnosis of essential thrombocythemia do not have a clonal disorder and may be at lower risk of throm-botic complications. Blood 1999;93:417–424.
11. Antonioli E, Guglielmelli P, Pancrazzi A, et al. Clinical implications of the JAK2 V617F mutation in essential thrombocythemia. Leukemia 2005;19:1847–1849.
12. Steensma DP, Tefferi A. Cytogenetic and molecular genetic aspects of essential thrombo-cythemia. Acta Haematol 2002;108:55–65.
13. Axelrad AA, Eskinazi D, Correa PN, et al. Hypersensitivity of circulating progenitor cells to megakaryocyte growth and development factor (PEG-rHu MGDF) in essential thrombo-cythemia. Blood 2000;96:3310–3321.
14. Kawasaki H, Nakano T, Kohdera U, et al. Hypersensitivity of megakaryocyte progenitors to thrombopoietin in essential thrombocythemia. Am J Hematol 2001;68:194–197.
15. Li Y, Hetet G, Maurer AM, et al. Spontaneous megakaryocyte colony formation in myelopro-liferative disorders is not neutralizable by antibodies against IL3, IL6 and GM-CSF. Br J Haematol 1994;87:471–476.
16. Schafer AI. Molecular basis of the diagnosis and treatment of polycythemia vera and essential thrombocythemia. Blood 2006;107:4214–4122.
17. Imbert M, Pierre R, Thiele J, et al. Essential thrombocythemia. In: Jaffe ES, Harris NL, Stein H, et al., editors. Pathology and genetics of tumours of hematopoietic and lymphoid tissues. Lyon: IARC Press; 2001. p. 39–41.
18. Lengfelder E, Hochhaus A, Kronawitter U, et al. Should a platelet limit of $600 \times 10^9/l$ be used as a diagnostic criterion in essential thrombocythemia? An analysis of the natural course including early stages. Br J Haematol 1998;100:15:23.
19. Sacchi S, Vinci G, Gugliotta L, et al. Diagnosis of essential thrombocythemia at platelet counts between 400 and $600 \times 10^9/l$. Haematologica 2000;85:492–495.
20. Campbell PJ, Scott LM, Baxter EJ, et al. Methods for the detection of the JAK2 V617F muta-tion in human myeloproliferative disorders. Methods Mol Med 2006;125:253–264.
21. Patel RK, Lea NC, Heneghan MA, et al. Prevalence of the activating JAK2 tyrosine kinase mutation V617F in the Budd-Chiari syndrome. Gastroenterology 2006;130:2031–2038.
22. Harrison CN, Green AR. Essential thrombocythemia. Best Pract Res Clin Haematol 2006;19:439–453.
23. Thiele J, Kvasnicka HM, Zankovich R, et al. Relevance of bone marrow features in the dif-ferential diagnosis between essential thrombocythemia and early stage idiopathic myelofibro-sis. Haematologica 2000;85:1126–1134.
24. Westwood NB, Pearson TC. Diagnostic applications of hemopoietic progenitor culture tech-niques in polycythaemias and thrombocythaemias. Leuk Lymphoma 1996;22(SUppl):95–103.
25. Tefferi A. Ultra high platelet count might be a characteristic feature of chronic myeloid leukemia rather than essential thrombocyhthemia. Leuk Res 2006;Sep 27 [Epub ahead of print].

26. Mesa RA, Silverstein MN, Jacobsen SJ, et al. Population-based incidence and survival figures in essential thrombocythemia and agnogenic myeloid metaplasia: an Olmsted County study, 1976–1995. Am J Hematol 1999;61:10–15.
27. Johansson P, Kutti J, Andreasson B, et al. Trends in the incidence of chronic Philadelphia chromosome negative (Ph-) myeloproliferative disorders in the city of Goteborg, Sweden, during 1983–99. J Intern Med 2004;256:161–165.
28. Ruggeri M, Tosetto A, Frezzato M, et al. The rate of progression to polycythemia vera or essential thrombocythemia in patients with erythrocytosis or thrombocytosis. Ann Intern Med 2003;139:470–475.
29. Wolanskyj AP, Schwager SM, McClure RF, et al. Essential thrombocythemia beyond the first decade: life expectancy, long-term complication rates, and prognostic factors. Mayo Clin Proc 2006;81:159–166.
30. Elliott MA, Tefferi A. Thrombosis and haemorrhage in polycythemia vera and essential thrombocythaemia. Br J Haematol 2005;128:275–290.
31. Barbui T, Barosi G, Grossi A, et al. Evidence- and consensus-based practice guidelines for the therapy of essential thrombocythemia. A statement from the Italian Society of Hematology. Haematologica 2004;89:215–232.
32. Cortelazzo S, Viero P, Finazzi G, et al. Incidence and risk factors for thrombotic complications in a historical cohort of 100 patients with essential thrombocythemia. J Clin Oncol 1990;8:556–562.
33. van Genderen PJ, Michiels JJ. Erythromelalgic, thrombotic and hemorrhagic manifestations of thrombocythaemia. Presse Med 1994;23:73–77.
34. Tefferi A, Fonseca R, Pereira D, et al. A long-term retrospective study of young women with essential thrombocythemia. Mayo Clin Proc 2001;76:22–28.
35. Besses C, Cervantes F, Pereira A, et al. Major vascular complications in essential thrombocythemia: a study of the predictive factors in a series of 148 patients. Leukemia 1999;13:150–154.
36. Carobbio A, Finazzi G, Guerini V, et al. Leukocytosis is a risk factor for thrombosis in essential thrombocythemia: intercation with tratement, standard risk factors and JAK2 mutation status. Blood 2007;109:2310–2313.
37. Landolfi R, Di Coennazo L, Barbui T, et al. Leukocytosis as a major thrombotic risk factor in patients with polycythemia vera. Blood 2007;109:2446–2452.
38. Falanga A, Marchetti M, Barbui T, et al. Pathogenesis of thrombosis in essential thrombocythemia and polycythemia vera: the role of neutrophils. Semin Hematol 2005;42:239–247.
39. Arellano-Rodrigo E, Alvarez-Larran A, Reverter JC, et al. Increased platelet and leukocyte activation as contributing mechanisms for thrombosis in essential thrombocythemia and correlation with the JAK2 mutation status. Haematologica 2006;91:169–175.
40. Campbell PJ, Scott LM, Buck G, et al. Definition of subtypes of essential thrombocythaemia and relation to polycythaemia vera based on JAK2 V617F mutation status: a prospective study. Lancet 2005;366:1945–1953.
41. Cheung B, Radia D, Pantedelis P, et al. The presence of the JAK2 V617F mutation is associated with higher haemoglobin and increased risk of thrombosis in essential thrombocythaemia. Br J Haematol 2005;132:244–250.
42. Finazzi G, Rambaldi A, Guerini V, et al. Risk of thrombosis in patients with essential thrombocythemia and polycythemia vera according to JAK2 V617F status. Haematologica 2007; 92:135–136.
43. Wolanskyj AP, Lasho TL, Schwager SM, et al. JAK2 V617F mutation in essential thrombocythaemia: clinical associations and long-term prognostic relevance. Br J Haematol 2005;131:208–213.
44. van Genderen PJ, Budde U, Michiels JJ, et al. The reduction of large vonWillebrand multimers in plasma in essential thrombocythemia is related to the platelet count. Br J Haematol 1996; 93:962–965.
45. Tefferi A, Gangat N, Wolanskyj AP. Management of extreme thrombocytosis in otherwise low-risk essential thrombocythemia: does number matter? Blood 2006;108:2493–2494.

46. Cervantes F, Alvarez-Larran A, Talarn C, et al. Myelofibrosis with myeloid metaplasia following essential thrombocythemia: actuarial probability, presenting characteristics and evolution in a series of 195 patients. Br J Haematol 2002; 118:786–790.
47. Barbui T, Finazzi G. When and how to treat essential thrombocythemia. N Engl J Med 2005;85–86.
48. Ruggeri M, Finazzi G, Tosetto A, et al. No treatment for low-risk essential thrombocythemia: results from a prospective study. Br J Haematol 1998;103:772–777.
49. Landolfi R, Marchioli R, Kutti J, et al. Efficacy and safety of low-dose aspirin in polycythemia vera. N Engl J Med 2004;350:114–124.
50. Harrison CN, Green AR. Essential thrombocythemia. Hematol Oncol Clin North Am 2003;17:1175–1190.
51. Sterkers Y, Preudhomme C, Lai J-L, et al. Acute myeloid leukemia and myelodyslastic syndromes following essential thrombocythemia treated with hydroxyurea: high proportion of cases with 17p deletion. Blood 1998;91:616–622.
52. Lofvenberg E, Nordenson I, Walhlin A. Cytogenetic abnormalities and leukemic transformation in hydroxyurea-treated patients with Philadelphia chromosome negative chronic myeloproliferative disease. Cancer Genet Cytogenet 1990;49:57–67.
53. Finazzi G, Ruggeri M, Rodeghiero F, et al. Efficacy and safety of long-term use of hydroxyurea in young patients with essential thrombocythemia and a high risk of thrombosis. Blood 2003;101:3749.
54. Finazzi G, Caruso V, Marchioli R, et al. Acute leukemia in polycythemia vera. An analysis of 1638 patients enrolled in a prospective observational study. Blood 2005;105:2664–2670.
55. Finazzi G, Ruggeri M, Rodeghiero F, et al. Second malignancies in patients with essential thrombocythemia treated with busulphan and hydroxyurea: long-term follow-up of a randomized clinical trial. Br J Haematol 2000;110:577–583.
56. Murphy S, Peterson P, Iland H, et al. Experience of the Polycythemia Vera Study Group with essential thrombocythemia: a final report on diagnostic criteria, survival and leukemic transition by treatment. Semin Hematol 1997;34:29–39.
57. Anagrelide study group. Anagrelide, a therapy for thrombocythemic states: experience in 577 patients. Anagrelide Study Group. Am J Med 1992;92:69–76.
58. Wagstaff AJ, Keating GM. Anagrelide. A review of its use in the management of essential thrombocythaemia. Drugs 2006;66:111–131.
59. Jurgens DJ, Moreno-Aspitia A, Tefferi A. Anagrelide-associated cardiomyopathy in polycythemia vera and essential thrombocythemia. Haematologica 2004;89:1394–1395.
60. Barosi G, Besses C, Birgegard G, et al. A unified definition of clinical resistance/intolerance to hydroxyuea in essential thrombocythemia: results of a consensus process by an international working group. Leukemia 2007;24:277–280.
61. Fruchtman SM, Petitt RM, Gilbert HS, et al. Anagrelide: analysis of long term safety and leukemogenic potential in myeloproliferative disorders Leuk Res 2005;29:481–491.
62. Storen EC, Tefferi A Long-term use of anagrelide in young patients with essential thrombocythemia. Blood 2001; 97:863–866.
63. Lengfelder E, Griesshammer M, Hehlmann R. Interferon-alpha in the treatment of essential thrombocythemia. Leuk Lymphoma 1996;22(Suppl 1):135–142.
64. Quintas-Cardama A, Kantarjian HM, Giles F, et al. Pegylated interferon therapy for patients with Philadelphia chromosome–negative myeloproliferative disorders. Semin Thromb Hemost 2006;32:409–416.
65. Kiladjian JJ, Cassinat B, Turlure P, et al. High molecular response rate of polycythemia vera patients treated with pegylated interferon α-2a. Blood 2006;108: 2037–2040
66. Samuelsson J, Mutschler M, Birgegard G, et al. Limited effects on JAK2 mutational status after pegylated interferon α-2b therapy in polycythemia vera and essential thrombocythemia. Haematologica 2006;91:1281–1282.
67. Cortelazzo S, Finazzi G, Ruggeri M, et al. Hydroxyurea in the treatment of patients with essential thrombocythemia at high risk of thrombosis: a prospective randomized trial. N Engl J Med 1995;332:1132–1136.

68. Harrison CN, Campbell P, Buck G, et al. Hydroxyurea compared with anagrelide in high-risk essential thrombocythemia. N Engl J Med 2005;353:33–45.
69. Lev PR, Salim JP, Kornblihtt LI, et al. PDGF-A, PDGF-B, TGFbeta, and bFGF mRNA levels in patients with essential thrombocythemia treated with anagrelide. Am J Hematol 2005;78:155–157.
70. Harrison C. Pregnancy and its management in the Philadelphia negative myeloproliferative diseases. Br J Haematol 2005;129:293–306.
71. Griesshammer M, Struve S, Harrison C. Essential thrombocythemia/polycythemia vera: the need for a observational study in Europe. Semin Thromb Haemost 2006;32:422–429.

Chapter 4
Chronic Eosinophilic Leukemia/ Hypereosinophilic Syndrome

Jason Gotlib

4.1 Introduction

The eosinophil was histopathologically characterized in 1879 by Paul Ehrlich who mastered the use of aniline dyes to distinguish cell types (1). The term "eosinophil" was thus borne from the observation that the acidic dye eosin reacted strongly with the abundance of highly basic proteins found within the granules of these cells. Eosinophils serve a central function in the host defense against helminth infections and undergo recruitment and activation in allergic and inflammatory responses. However, as part of the immune system's effort to maintain normal homeostasis, the potential for collateral tissue damage by eosinophils exists. This chapter focuses on the relatively rare but fascinating hematologic diseases: chronic eosinophilic leukemia (CEL) and hypereosinophilic syndrome (HES). These entities share a common theme of abnormal persistent elevation of the eosinophil count and the potential for substantial morbidity and mortality from organ complications. The study of pathologic hypereosinophilia was originally rooted in descriptive and morphologic investigations; however, with an increasingly sophisticated understanding of the cellular and molecular bases of these eosinophilic disorders, new biologically oriented classification schemes have emerged that carry therapeutic implications.

4.2 Definition of Eosinophilia

The upper limit of normal for the range of % eosinophils in the peripheral blood is 3–5%, with a corresponding absolute eosinophil count (AEC) of 350–500/mm^3 (2, 3). The severity of eosinophilia has been arbitrarily divided into mild (AEC from the upper limit of normal to 1500/mm^3), moderate (AEC 1500–5000/mm^3), and severe (AEC >5000/mm^3) (3, 4). For subsets of certain eosinophilic diseases, the degree of peripheral eosinophilia might help narrow the differential diagnosis. For example, among the pulmonary eosinophilic syndromes, peripheral eosinophilia tends to be relatively mild in drug-induced and idiopathic eosinophilia pneumonia (IEP); in contrast, chronic IEP and tropical pulmonary eosinophilia are usually characterized by more severe elevations in the AEC (4).

S.M. Ansell (ed.), *Rare Hematological Malignancies.*
© Springer 2008

4.3   Eosinophil Biology

The T-cell-derived eosinophilopoietic cytokines interleukin-3 (IL-3), granulocyte macrophage colony-stimulating factor (GM-CSF), and interleukin-5 (IL-5) are primarily responsible for the commitment, proliferation, and differentiation of multipotent hematopoietic progenitors into the eosinophilic lineage (3). These cytokines also contribute to the priming, activation, and recruitment of eosinophils within specific tissue compartments. Type 1 (Th1) and type 2 (Th2) T-helper cells produce IL-3 and GM-CSF, whereas IL-5 is predominantly produced by Th2 cells and mast cells (3, 5). IL-5 is a more eosinophil-specific cytokine critical for the terminal differentiation and proliferation of eosinophils (6).

Migration of eosinophils from the circulation to tissues is mediated by their interaction with endothelial cells. Rolling of eosinophils along the endothelium is facilitated by adhesion molecules such as P-selectin (7). Eosinophil adherence to endothelium is promoted by interactions between intercellular adhesion molecule 1 (ICAM-1) on endothelial cells and β2 integrins (e.g., CD18) on eosinophils; similar interactions also occur between endothelium vascular cell adhesion molecule 1 (VCAM1) and β1 integrins (e.g. very late antigen-4 (VLA-4) (3, 5, 8). Migratory responses of eosinophils are enhanced by numerous potent eosinophil chemoattractants, including, but not limited to, complement fragment 5a, leukotriene β_4, platelet activating factor, various interleukins, RANTES, and specific eotaxins that are ligands for the CCR3 receptor expressed on eosinophils (3, 5, 9–11).

The pro-inflammatory effects of eosinophils are related to the release of mediators from well-characterized intracellular granule compartments. The relatively large-sized specific granules contain an electron-dense crystalloid core containing preformed major basic protein, surrounded by a matrix consisting of eosinophil cationic protein, eosinophil-derived neurotoxin, and eosinophil peroxidase (5). Small granules contain hydrolytic enzymes such as acid phosphatase, arylsulfatase, and catalase. Newly synthesized mediators, including oxidative products (e.g., hydrogen peroxide), lipid mediators (e.g., leukotriene C_4), inflammatory/hematopoietic cytokines, and chemokines, instigate the tissue damage and fibrosis that characterize the pathologic eosinophilia of CEL and HES (3, 5).

4.4   Nomenclature

"Reactive" or "secondary" eosinophilia refers to identifiable conditions that mediate cytokine-driven eosinophilia. "Primary" eosinophilia is typically used to denote eosinophilia related to an underlying bone marrow disease. Among the marrow-related primary eosinophilias, a clonal marker can be found in a subset of patients, consistent with an underlying acute or chronic myeloid or lymphoid disorder. In such cases, the presence of a cytogenetic or molecular abnormality does not necessarily imply that the eosinophil population is derived from the malignant clone, as eosinophilia can be a reactive phenomenon accompanying both solid and hematologic malignancies (see below).

Historically, the term "idiopathic hypereosinophilic syndrome" (HES) or simply "hypereosinophilic syndrome" has been applied to patients for whom a persistent primary or secondary cause of acquired eosinophilia has not be ascertained. Hardy and Anderson inaugurated the term "hypereosinophilic syndrome" for such patients in 1968 (12), the first of several modern clinico-pathologic landmarks in the study of hypereosinophilic syndromes (Table 4.1). Chusid and colleagues established its diagnostic criteria in 1975: (1) persistent eosinophilia of 1500/mm^3 or greater for longer than 6 months; (2) lack of evidence for parasitic, allergic, or other known reactive causes of eosinophilia (Table 4.2); and (3) signs and symptoms of organ involvement (13). In the last 15 years, the pool of classically defined HES patients has diminished in size due to an increasing proportion of cases that have been molecularly/cytogenetically reassigned as chronic eosinophilic leukemia (Figure 4.1). The HES pool has also decreased in size with the recognition of

Table 4.1 Modern landmarks in the classification, diagnosis, and treatment of hypereosinophilic syndrome/eosinophilic disorders

Year	Authors	Event
1968	Hardy and Anderson	Term "hypereosinophilic syndrome" coined
1975	Chusid et al.	Diagnostic criteria for idiopathic HES established
1994	Golub et al.	Characterization of the PDGFRB-related rearrangement, t(5;12)(q31-q33;p13), the first molecular abnormality to become associated with eosinophilia
1998	Popovic et al., Reiter et al., Smedley et al., Xiao et al.	Identification of rearrangement of the FGFR1 gene (ZNF198-FGFR1) as a molecular basis for the 8p11 myeloproliferative syndrome
2001	Bain et al.	World Health Organization diagnostic criteria for idiopathic HES and CEL published
2001	Schaller and Burkland	Successful empiric treatment of an HES patient with imatinib
2002	Apperley et al.	Imatinib responsiveness in patients with chronic myeloproliferative disorders associated with eosinophilia and rearrangements of PDGFRB
2002	Baxter et al.	Characterization of the first PDGFRA rearrangement (BCR-PDGFRA), t(4;22)(q12;q11), in two patients with atypical CML with eosinophilia
2003	Trempat et al.	Successful imatinib treatment of a patient with the BCR-PDGFRA fusion
2003	Cools et al.	Identification of the FIP1L1-PDGFRA fusion as the basis for therapeutic response to imatinib in HES/CEL
2003	Pardanani	Identification of the FIP1L1-PDGFRA fusion (using FISH for the CHIC2 deletion) in patients with systemic mastocytosis with eosinophilia

HES: hypereosinophilic syndrome; CEL: chronic eosinophilic leukemia; PDGFRA: platelet-derived growth factor receptor alpha; PDGFRB: platelet derived growth factor receptor beta; FGFR1: fibroblast growth factor receptor 1.

Source: Gotlib et al. (60), with permission from Elsevier.

Table 4.2 Reactive causes of eosinophilia

Allergic/hypersensitivity diseases

 Asthma, rhinitis, drug reactions, allergic bronchopulmonary aspergillosis,
 allergic gastroenteritis

Infections

 Parasitic

  Strongyloidiasis, *Toxocara canis, Trichinella spiralis*, visceral larva migrans,
  filariasis, Schistosomiasis, *Ancylostoma duodenale, Fasciola hepatica,*
  Echinococcus, Toxoplasma, other parasitic diseases

 Bacterial/mycobacterial

 Fungal (coccidioidomycosis, cryptococcus)

 Viral (HIV, HSV, HTLV-II)

 Rickettsial

Connective tissue diseases

 Churg-Strauss syndrome, Wegener's granulomatosis, rheumatoid arthritis,
 polyarteritis nodosa, systemic lupus erythematosus, scleroderma,
 eosinophilic fasciitis / myositis

Pulmonary diseases

 Bronchiectasis, cystic fibrosis, Loeffler's syndrome,
 eosinophilic granuloma of the lung

Cardiac diseases

 Tropical endocardial fibrosis, eosinophilic endomyocardial fibrosis or myocarditis

Skin diseases

 Atopic dermatitis, urticaria, eczema, bullous pemphigoid, dermatitis herpetiformis,
 episodic angioedema with eosinophilia (Gleich syndrome)

Gastrointestinal diseases

 Eosinophilic gastroenteritis, celiac disease

Malignancies

 Hodgkin's and non-Hodgkin's lymphoma, acute lymphoblastic leukemia,
 Langerhans cell histiocytosis, angiolymphoid hyperplasia with eosinophilia
 (Kimura's disease), angioimmunoblastic lymphadenopathy, solid tumors
 (e.g., renal, lung, breast, vascular neoplasms, female tract cancers)

Immune system diseases/abnormalities

 Wiskott-Aldrich syndrome, hyper-IgE (Job's) syndrome, hyper-IgM syndrome,
 IgA deficiency

Metabolic abnormalities

 Adrenal insufficiency

Other

 IL-2 therapy, L-tryptophan ingestion, toxic oil syndrome, renal graft rejection

Source: Gotlib et al. (79).

a pathologically distinct, lymphocyte-mediated form of hypereosinophilia, characterized by a T-cell population with an aberrant immunophenotype and/ or abnormal eosinophilopoietic cytokine production (e.g., elevated levels of serum interleukin-5) (14, 15).

In 2001, the World Health Organization established criteria that distinguished HES from chronic eosinophilic leukemia (CEL) and lymphocyte-variant

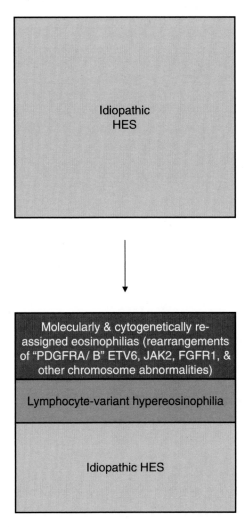

Figure 4.1 The schematic illustrates the shrinking pool of patients with hypereosinophilic syndrome. The relative frequency of patients with idiopathic hypereosinophilia is decreasing due to an increasing number of patients who are diagnosed with either a previously unrecognized molecularly defined myeloproliferative variant or lymphocyte-variant of hypereosinophilia

hypereosinophilia (Table 4.3) (15). In the absence of increased peripheral blood or marrow blasts or cytogenetic/molecular evidence of clonality, a diagnosis of CEL is also suggested by additional clinical or laboratory features: hepato/splenomegaly, dysplasia in eosinophils or other cell lineages, myeloid immaturity, bone marrow fibrosis, or an elevated serum cobalamin and/or serum tryptase level (Figure 4.2). Because these supporting clinical and laboratory features are

Table 4.3 WHO classification of chronic eosinophilic leukemia and hypereosinophilic syndrome

1. Exclude all causes of reactive eosinophilia secondary to:
   - Allergy
   - Parasitic disease
   - Infectious disease
   - Pulmonary diseases (hypersensitivity pneumonitis, Loeffler's, etc.)
2. Exclude all neoplastic disorders with secondary, reactive eosinophilia:
   - T-Cell lymphomas, including mycosis fungoides, Sezary syndrome
   - Hodgkin lymphoma
   - Acute lymphoblastic leukemia/lymphoma
   - Mastocytosis
3. Exclude other neoplastic disorders in which eosinophils are part of the neoplastic clone:
   - CML (Ph chromosome or BCR-ABL-positive)
   - AML including those with inv(16), t(16;16) (p13;q22)
   - Other myeloproliferative diseases (PV, ET, AMM)
   - Myelodysplastic syndromes
4. Exclude T-cell population with aberrant phenotype and abnormal cytokine population
5. If there is no demonstrable disease that could cause eosinophilia, no abnormal T-cell population, and no evidence of a clonal myeloid disorder, diagnose HES.
6. If requirements 1–4 have been met and if the myeloid demonstrates a clonal cytogenetic abnormality or clonality is shown by other means, or if blasts are present in the peripheral blood (>2%) or marrow (>5% but less than 19%), diagnose CEL.

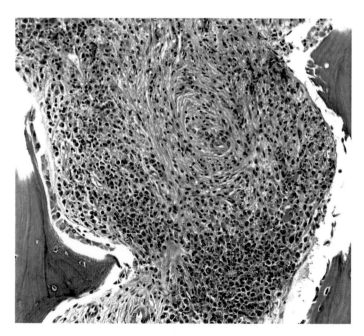

Figure 4.2 Histopathologic features suggestive of chronic eosinophilic leukemia in this bone marrow core biopsy from a 28-year-old man include marked hypercellularity (100%), panmyelosis, and increased focal fibrosis (2+ on reticulin stain), in addition to the increased numbers of eosinophils. In addition, the serum tryptase and vitamin B_{12} levels were elevated. Interphase FISH for the CHIC2 deletion, a surrogate test for the FIP1L1-PDGFRA rearrangement, was positive in 37% of 200 cells analyzed. (Photo courtesy of Dr. Tracy George and Dr. Bruno Medeiros, Stanford University School of Medicine)

common to chronic myelogenous leukemia (CML) and related classic myeloproliferative disorders, these cases of CEL have also been broadly categorized as "myeloproliferative variants" of hypereosinophilia (16). In addition to the aforementioned laboratory features of lymphocyte-mediated hypereosinophilia, this variant is clinically characterized primarily by skin disease and usually a benign course (16).

4.5 Epidemiology

Hypereosinophilic syndrome is a rare disease, and although the precise incidence is unknown, it is estimated at 0.5–1.0 cases per 100,000 persons per year. HES exhibits a marked gender bias, with men ninefold more frequently affected than women. Although usually diagnosed between the ages of 20 and 50 (17), idiopathic hypereosinophilia or CEL might arise at the extremes of age, with infrequent cases being described in infants and children (18–21).

4.6 Laboratory and Morphology Assessment of Hypereosinophilia

In addition to increased peripheral blood or bone marrow blasts, demonstration of clonality can be used to establish a diagnosis of CEL versus HES. A clonal process can be identified by widely available techniques such as conventional cytogenetics or fluorescent *in situ* hybridization (22) or more research-based assays such as cytogenetic analysis of purified eosinophils (23) and X-chromosome inactivation analysis in females (24, 25). The latter method has limited utility in the heavily male-biased population of idiopathic hypereosinophilia patients.

Attempts have also been made to use eosinophil morphology to distinguish HES from CEL. However, several studies have highlighted the difficulty in using this approach because abnormal eosinophil morphology (e.g., cytoplasmic hypogranularity or vacuolization, abnormal lobation, ring nuclei) might be present in both conditions (26–28).

4.7 Clinico-Pathologic Manifestations

In one large series, eosinophilia was an incidental finding in 12% of HES patients (17). The most common presenting signs and symptoms were weakness and fatigue (26%), cough (24%), dyspnea (16%), myalgias or angioedema (14%), rash or fever

(12%), and rhinitis (10%) (17). Table 4.4 shows the cumulative frequency of organ involvement in 105 patients previously compiled from three series (17, 28–31).

4.7.1 Hematologic Findings

Persistent eosinophilia without a clinically identifiable cause forms the basis of HES. Elevation of the leukocyte count (e.g., 20,000–30,000/mm^3) with peripheral eosinophilia in the range of 30–70% is a common finding (13), but higher leukocyte

Table 4.4 Organ Involvement in Hypereosinophilic Syndrome

Organ System	Cumulative Frequency from 3 studies (%)[17,29,30]	Examples of Organ-Specific Manifestations
Hematologic	100	Leukocytosis with eosinophilia; neutrophilia, basophilia, myeloid immaturity, immature and/or dysplastic eosinophils; anemia, thrombocytopenia or thrombocytosis, increased marrow blasts, myelofibrosis
Cardiovascular	58	Cardiomyopathy, constrictive pericarditis, endomyocarditis, mural thrombi, valvular dysfunction, endomyocardial fibrosis, myocardial infarction
Dermatologic	56	Angioedema, urticaria, papules/nodules, plaques, aquagenic pruritis, erythroderma, cellulitis, mucosal ulcers, vesico-bullous lesions, microthrombi, vasculitis, Well's syndrome
Neurologic	54	Thromboembolism, peripheral neuropathy, encephalopathy, dementia, epilepsy, cerebellar disease, eosinophilic meningitis
Pulmonary	49	Pulmonary infiltrates, effusions,' fibrosis, emboli, nodules/focal ground glass attentuation, acute respiratory distress syndrome (ARDS)
Splenic	43	Hypersplenism, infarct
Liver/gallbladder	30	Hepatomegaly, focal or diffuse hepatic lesions on imaging, chronic active hepatitis, hepatic necrosis, Budd-Chiari syndrome, sclerosing cholangitis, cholecystitis, cholestasis
Ocular	23	Microthrombi, choroidal infarcts, retinal arteritis, episcleritis, keratoconjunctivitis sicca, Adie's syndrome (pupillotonia)
Gastrointestinal	23	Ascites, diarrhea, gastritis, colitis, pancreatitis
Musculoskeletal	N/A	Arthritis, effusions, bursitis, synovitis, Raynaud's phenomena, digital necrosis, polymyositis/myopathy
Renal	N/A	Acute renal failure with Charcot-Leyden crystalluria, nephrotic syndrome, immunotactoid glomerulopathy, crescentic glomerulonephritis

Modified from Weller PF and Bubley GJ. *Blood.* 1994;83:2760, and Brito-Babapulle F. *Blood Reviews.* 1997;11:139. N/A: not available
Source: Gotlib et al. (79).

counts have also been reported (29, 30). Other hematologic findings include peripheral blood or bone marrow neutrophilia, basophilia, myeloid immaturity, and both mature and immature eosinophils with varying degrees of dysplasia (29, 32). In one series, anemia was present in 53% of patients, thrombocytopenia was more common than thrombocytosis (31% vs. 16%), and bone marrow eosinophilia ranged from 7% to 57% (mean: 33%) (32). Marrow findings of Charcot-Leyden crystals, and sometimes increased blasts and myelofibrosis, are also observed (32).

4.7.2 Cardiac Disease

Although all organ systens might be susceptible to the effects of sustained eosinophilia, the eosinophil count does not necessarily predict the development or extent of organ damage. Given the potential for significant cardiac-related morbidity and mortality, the effects of eosinophilia on this organ merit review. Cardiac injury involves a multistep pathophysiological process involving eosinophil infiltration of cardiac tissue and release of toxic mediators from eosinophils (reviewed in Refs. 17 and 31). In the initial necrotic stage, cardiac disease is initiated by eosinophil damage to the endocardium, with local platelet thrombus leading to mural thrombi that have the potential to embolize (thrombotic stage). The contents of eosinophil granules, including major basic protein and eosinophilic cationic protein, might promote endothelial damage and hypercoagulablity, enhancing the thromboembolic risk (33, 34). In the later fibrotic stage, organization of thrombus can lead to fibrous thickening of the endocardial lining and a restrictive cardiomyopathy (17, 31). Valvular insufficiency is related to mural endocardial thrombosis and fibrosis involving leaflets of the mitral or tricuspid valves (35–37). The diversity of hypereosinophilia-related organ findings in addition to hematologic and cardiac manifestations are shown in Table 4.4.

4.8 Prognosis

Historically, the lives of patients with HES were overshadowed by early cardiac death. A review of 57 HES cases published through 1973 reported a median survival of 9 months and the 3-year survival was only 12% (13). Patients usually presented with advanced disease, with congestive heart failure accounting for 65% of deaths at autopsy. In addition to cardiac disease, peripheral blood blasts or a white blood cell (WBC) count greater than 100,000/mm^3 were poor prognostic factors (13). A later report of 40 HES patients cited a 5-year survival rate of 80%, decreasing to 42% at 15 years (30). In this cohort, factors predictive of a worse outcome included the presence of a concurrent myeloproliferative syndrome, corticosteroid-refractory hypereosinophilia, cardiac disease, male sex, and the height of eosinophilia (30). Improved diagnostic methods (e.g., echocardiography), better medical treatment and surgery for cardiovascular sequelae, and now the availability of effective targeted therapy for molecularly defined cases of hypereosinophilia probably contribute to improved survival in the modern era.

4.9   Reactive and Clonal Eosinophilia Associated with Hematologic Malignancies

Numerous nonrecurrent chromosomal abnormalities have been published in literature-described reports of CEL or HES. These cases have been cataloged and updated in recent reviews (4, 38, 39). The overwhelming majority of patients with HES exhibit a normal karyotype; however, among patients with abnormal cytogenetics, trisomy 8 is most commonly observed (40–44). However, trisomy 8 is not specific to eosinophilic disorders, as it is commonly found in other myeloid leukemias. Very few of the reciprocal translocations, additions, or deletions in eosinophilic disorders have been molecularly characterized.

Although eosinophilia accompanies solid and hematologic malignancies, eosinophils are not always derived from the neoplastic clone. Instead, reactive eosinophilia might result from the production of cytokines such as IL-3, IL-5, and GM-CSF, which promote eosinophil differentiation and survival. These cytokines are elaborated from malignant cells in T-cell lymphomas (5), Hodgkin's disease (46), and acute lymphoblastic leukemias (47, 48). Tumor-associated eosinophilia might signify worse outcomes in particular disease types. For example, in a multivariate analysis of 158 patients with adult T-cell leukemia/lymphoma (ATLL), peripheral blood eosinophilia was a significant adverse prognostic factor that was independent of other variables, including lactate dehydogenase (LDH) (49).

In several myeloid malignancies associated with eosinophilia, eosinophils are in fact part of the malignant clone. Examples include systemic mastocytosis (e.g., FIP1L1-PDGFRA-associated) (50), BCR-ABL-positive chronic myelogenous leukemia, and chronic myeloproliferative disorders associated with rearrangements of PDGFRA and PDGFRB. As classified by the French-American-British classification, M2 (inv(16)(p13q22) or t(16;16)(p13;q22)) (51) and M4Eo (t(8;21)(q22;q22)) (52) are well-defined subtypes of acute myeloid leukemia (AML) with associated clonal eosinophila. In cases of eosinophilic myelodysplastic syndrome (MDS) with t(1;7) or dic(1;7) karyotypes (22, 53), the eosinophils have also been shown to be clonal. In a case of eosinophilia-associated chronic myelomonocytic leukemia characterized by t(5;12)(q31;p13) with t(1;7)(q10;p10), clonality of eosinophils was demonstrated using fluorescence in situ hybridization (FISH) probes for chromosome 1 (54).

4.10   Molecularly Characterized Bone Marrow Eosinophilic Disorders: PDGFRA- and PDGFRB-Rearranged

In the current era, in which molecular discrimination of eosinophilic disorders is becoming increasingly available, rearrangements involving the tyrosine kinases PDGFRα and PDGFRβ have emerged as a common theme, specifically among eosinophilia-associated chronic myeloproliferative sisorders (MPDs). These proteins belong to the family of class III receptor tyrosine kinases, which also include c-KIT, FLT3, KDR, and c-FMS (reviewed in Ref. 55). In the normal state, the ligand PDGF binds to its receptor, resulting in dimerization and subsequent autophosphorylation of tyrosine residues located in intracellular portions of the molecule. Activation of tyrosine kinase activity leads to a cascade of signaling via downstream effectors such as Src and STAT5 and the phosphatidylinositol-3(PI-3)-kinase and Ras/mitogen-activated (MAP) protein kinase pathways (56–59).

Rearrangements involving the *PDGFRA* and *PDGFRB* genes lead to deregulated kinase activity and abrogates the requirement for normal ligand-induced receptor stimulation. Several structural and functional relationships are shared among the different *PDGFRB* rearrangements [reviewed in Refs. 39 and 60]. *PDGFRB* fusions are in-frame, and only rarely are reciprocal fusion transcripts detected. Another structural theme is that the PDGFRβ tyrosine kinase domain is preserved and fused to an N-terminal protein in all of the chimeric oncoproteins. The amino-terminal partner protein always contains dimerization/oligomerization motif(s) that can mimic receptor dimerization and activation without ligand. In vitro and in vivo transforming activity has been demonstrated for most of these fusions and depends both on the presence of a catalytic domain of PDGFRβ and the dimerization motif(s) of the partner protein. Other regions of the N-terminal protein might also modulate the transforming capacity of the fusion, as exemplified by studies of the PDGFRβ fusion partners H4 and HIP1 (61, 62).

4.10.1   PDGFRA-Rearranged

In 2002, Baxter and colleagues described two patients with atypical CML with peripheral blood eosinophilia and a t(4;22)(q12;q11) reciprocal translocation (63). In both cases, molecular analysis revealed an in-frame *BCR-PDGFRA* fusion mRNA, with either *BCR* exon 7 or 12 (followed by short BCR-intronic sequences) fused to exon 12 of *PDGFRA*. Similar to FIP1L1-PDGFRα or structural rearrangements involving PDGFRβ, the BCR-PDGFRα fusion would be expected to have properties of a deregulated tyrosine kinase with transforming properties in vitro. In 2003, Trempat and colleagues described a third patient with the *BCR-PDGFRA* fusion in the setting of acute pre-B-cell ALL (64). In this case, the mRNA breakpoint involved fusion of *BCR* exon 1 with *PDGFRA* exon 13. A fourth case of t(4;22)(q12;q11.2) was reported in a patient with secondary atypical CML with eosinophilia arising after treatment for diffuse large-B-cell lymphoma (65). Sequence analysis of the mRNA revealed the breakpoint in *BCR* exon 17 and *PDGFRA* exon 12. In 2006, two novel PDGFRA chimeric oncoproteins were described in patients with chronic eosinophilic leukemia: one with ins(9;4)(q33;q12;q25), molecularly defined as a CDK5RAP2-PDGFRA (66), and a patient with a KIF5B-PDGFRA fusion, which joined KIF5B on 10p11 to PDGFRA on 4q12 as part of a complex karyotype involving chromosomes 3, 4, and 10 (67). In all six cases, breakpoints clustered in the juxtamembrane domain of *PDGFRA*. Disruption of this negative regulatory domain contributes to deregulation of the protein's tyrosine kinase activity, similar to the mechanism of oncogenesis attributed to the FIP1L1-PDGFRα fusion (see below). Treatment with imatinib in the latter four patients resulted in hematologic remissions in all cases (64–67). FISH was used to identify additional novel translocation partners involving PDGFRA and chromosomal segments 1q44, 3q25, and 17q23, but the molecular fusions were not described (68).

4.10.2   A Recurrent PDGFRA Rearrangement in Eosinophilic Disorders: FIP1L1-PDGFRA

Because of some overlapping phenotypic clinical and laboratory features with CML, imatinib was empirically investigated in HES. In 2001, Schaller and Burkland published the initial case of HES treated with imatinib (69). The patient was resistant or intolerant to prior therapies, including corticosteroids, hydroxyurea, and interferon-α. A low imatinib dose of 100 mg daily resulted in a rapid and complete hematologic remission. This initial description heralded several case reports or series of imatinib's use in HES in 2002 and 2003: Among 24 total patients treated among 6 reports (69–74), 14 complete and 2 partial hematologic remissions were observed. These reports reenforced the observation that imatinib could elicit rapid (e.g., within 1–4 weeks) and complete hematologic responses, including normalization of eosinophilia, in the majority of HES patients. These data also recapitulated the successful experience with imatinib in BCR-ABL-positive leukemias and strongly implicated a constitutively activated tyrosine kinase involving one of its known targets.

A benchtop-to-bedside collaborative trial deciphered the molecular basis for the response to imatinib in HES (75). Of the16 HES/CEL patients enrolled, 11 were treated with imatinib. Nine of the treated patients had normal karyotypes. Hematologic responses were observed in 10 of 11 HES patients treated with imatinib doses of 100–400 mg daily. The median time to response was 4 weeks (range: 1–12 weeks). Nine of 10 patients demonstrated a durable hematologic response (lasting ≥ 3 months), with a median duration of 7 months at the time of publication (range: 3–15 months).

In responding patients, the molecular basis for response was found to be imatinib's inhibition of a novel fusion tyrosine kinase, FIP1L1-PDGFRα (75). The *FIP1L1* gene encodes a 520-amino-acid protein that is homologous to a previously characterized *Saccharomyces cerevisiae* protein, Fip1, a component of its mRNA polyadenylation machinery (76). *FIP1L1-PDGFRA* was present in 9/16 (56%) HES patients (75). All five patients with the *FIP1L1-PDGFRA* fusion responded to imatinib. Imatinib's mechanism of action in four additional responding patients who lacked *FIP1L1-PDGFRA* is unknown but might involve cryptic fusions involving one of imatinib's known targets.

FIP1L1-PDGFRα was independently discovered by Griffin and colleagues in the cell line EOL-1, derived from a patient with acute eosinophilic leukemia, which transformed from HES (77). Imatinib and additional PDGFRα inhibitors reduced the viability of EOL-1 cells and a prominent 110-kDa phosphoprotein, ultimately identified as FIP1L1-PDGFRα. EOL-1 cell line growth was also inhibited by the tyrosine kinase inhibitors PKC412 and SU5614, which was due to induction of apoptosis and inhibition of phoshorylation of FIP1L1-PDGFRα and STAT5 (78).

The FIP1L1-PDGFRA fusion frequency of 56% in the cohort of HES patients described by Cools and colleagues likely overestimates its actual prevalence in patients with idiopathic hypereosinophilia. The median frequency of the fusion among 7 reports enrolling at least 10 patients is 23% (range: 0–56%) (reviewed in Ref. 39). Differences in the prevalence of *FIP1L1-PDGFRA*-positive patients in these studies reflect some degree of selection bias, the specialty clinics in which the patients were evaluated, assay sensitivity in detecting the fusion, and the proportion of individuals with lymphocyte versus myeloproliferative variants of the disease, with the fusion segregating with the latter group.

4.10.3   *Molecular Biology of the FIP1L1-PDGFRA Fusion*

The *FIP1L1-PDGFRA* fusion gene is a cryptic molecular abnormality that is generated by an 800-kb interstitial deletion on chromosome 4q12, not by reciprocal translocation, which is the molecular basis for most constitutively activated fusion tyrosine kinases in myeloproliferative disorders (75). The deletion is not visible using standard cytogenetic banding techniques and thus accounts for the normal karyotype observed in most HES patients.

The deletion that disrupts the *FIP1L1* and *PDGFRA* genes fuses the 5' part of *FIP1L1* to the 3' part of *PDGFRA* (75). In each patient, the breakpoints in *FIP1L1* and *PDGFRA* are different. Most cases might have multiple *FIP1L1-PDGFRA* fusions, many of which are out of frame, but an in-frame fusion can be identified in each case (75, 79). The breakpoints in *FIP1L1* are scattered over introns 7–10, whereas the breakpoints in *PDGFRA* are restricted exclusively to *PDGFRA* exon 12.

Walz and colleagues characterized the molecular breakpoints of the *FIP1L1-PDGFRA* rearrangement in an additional 43 patients with CEL or systemic mastocytosis with eosinophilia (80). Because of the variability of breakpoints within *FIP1L1*, insertion of additional sequences derived from *FIP1L1* introns or exons (or from a complex chromosomal rearrangement in one case), reverse transcription–polymerase chain reaction (RT-PCR) assays to detect the fusion and monitor response to therapy need to consider this molecular heterogeneity of the *FIP1L1-PDGFRA* fusion.

The protein product of FIP1L1-PDGFRA has properties a deregulated tyrosine kinase. Expression of FIP1L1-PDGFRα in the Ba/F3 hematopoietic cell line results in constitutive tyrosine phosphorylation, and transformation to IL-3-independent growth (75). In addition, FIP1L1-PDGFRα phosphorylates STAT5, but in contrast with the native PDGFRα, it does not activate the MAP kinase pathway (58, 75, 81, 82). The difference in MAP kinase signaling might be explained by the difference in subcellular localization, as PDGFRα is a transmembrane protein with access to farnesylated RAS (upstream in the MAPK pathway), whereas FIP1L1-PDGFRα is predicted to have a cytosolic location.

The mechanism of constitutive activation of FIP1L1-PDGFRα tyrosine kinase activity is independent of the N-terminal partner FIP1L1 (83). Instead, it relates to the disruption of the PDGFRA exon 12-encoded juxtamembrane domain, the recurrent breakpoint site in all PDGFRA fusions described to date. This region of the kinase serves an autoinhibitory function in PDGFFRA and related tyrosine kinases. For example, juxtamembrane internal tandem duplications in *FLT3* result in its constitutive activation in approximately 25% of cases of AML (84). Mutations of the juxtamembrane domain of both *KIT* and PDGFRA result in tyrosine kinase activation in the majority of cases of gastrointestinal stromal cell tumors (85, 86).

Assays have been developed to detect the presence of *FIP1L1-PDGFRA* in patients with newly diagnosed hypereosinophilia and to monitor response during imatinib treatment. Commercially available FISH probes that detect the deletion region between the FIP1L1 and PDGFRA genes (e.g., "FISH for the CHIC2 deletion") are now commonly used for these purposes (Figure 4.3). Sensitive RT-PCR-based assays are also used to gauge molecular response. Molecular remissions were first reported by PCR testing of the peripheral blood in five of six FIP1L1-PDGFRA-positive patients after 1–12 months of imatinib therapy (87). Numerous reports have since described molecular remissions in imatinib-treated patients with FIP1L1-PDGFRA-positive disease (41, 88–94 or after bone marrow transplantation (95).

The basis for the apparent lineage predilection of FIP1L1-PDGFRα for eosinophils is not well understood. The *FIP1L1-PDGFRA* fusion has been detected in enriched eosinophils, neutrophils, and mononuclear cells by FISH and RT-PCR in a patient with a diagnosis of systemic mast cell disease and eosinophilia (96). Using a combination of Taqman quantitative PCR, nested PCR, and FISH, the *FIP1L1-PDGFRA* fusion was identified in purified populations of eosinophils, neutrophils, mast cells, T-cells, B-cells and monocytes (97). Taken together, these findings are consistent with the notion that FIP1L1-PDGFRα-mediated disease probably arises from a pluripotent hematopoietic progenitor. It is possible that it is present in all myeloid lineages but that eosinophils are particularly sensitive to the FIP1L1-PDGFRα proliferative signal.

4.10.4 Clinical Correlates of the **FIP1L1-PDGFRA** *Fusion*

The *FIP1L1-PDGFRA* genotype segregates with a clinical phenotype including myeloproliferative-like HES (HES-MPD), tissue fibrosis, and increased serum tryptase levels (87, 98). *FIP1L1-PDGFRA* might also be related to the pathogenesis of eosinophilic subsets of systemic mastocytosis (SM). Deletion of the CHIC2 locus, a surrogate for the *FIP1L1-PDGFRA* fusion, was detected in imatinib-responsive patients diagnosed with systemic mastocytosis (SM) and eosinophilia, but not in two other patients with SM and the KIT Asp816 to Val (D816V) mutation who exhibited no response to imatinib (99).

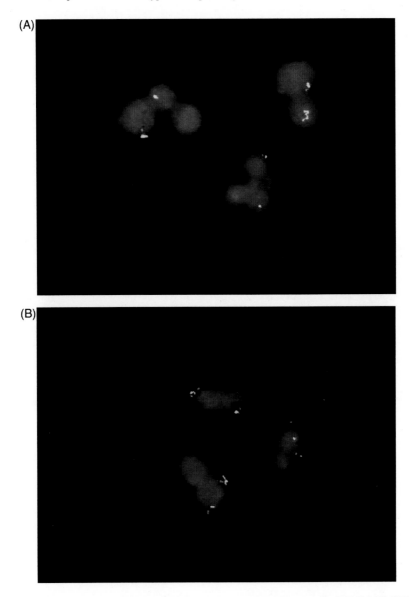

Figure 4.3 FISH for the CHIC2 deletion is used as a diagnostic test for FIP1L1-PDGFRA-positive CEL. (**A**) Three cells are shown with deleted CHIC2 (1 red/ 2 aqua signals); (**B**) three normal cells are shown (2 red/ 2 aqua signals). The CHIC2 probe is red, and a CEP4 probe (Vysis) is shown in aqua. CEP4 is a centromeric probe for chromosome 4, an identifier to indicate that chromosome 4 is present, and is deleted for CHIC2 as opposed to monosomy 4. These FISH photographs are from a 51-year-old man with FIP1L1-PDGFRA-positive CEL in whom 74% of cells were positive for the fusion. Treatment with imatinib mesylate resulted in a complete normalization of the FISH pattern. (Photos courtesy of Dr. Susan Olson, Oregon Health and Science University)

The ability of imatinib to reverse eosinophil-related organ damage is now emerging in several reports. Among three HES-MPD patients with endomyocardial fibrosis and congestive heart failure, there was no improvement in cardiac disease despite complete hematologic responses to imatinib (87). However, significant improvement of respiratory symptoms associated with clearing of interstitial infiltrates on chest computed tomography (CT))70, 87) and normalization of pulmonary function testing has been reported (87). We and others have demonstrated reversal of myelofibrosis (79, 87). Improvements in skin disease, hepato/splenomegaly, and both peripheral and central nervous system findings have also been reported in *FIP1L1-PDGFRA*-positive CEL (reviewed in Ref.100).

The natural history of imatinib-treated FIP1L1-PDGFRA-positive chronic eosinophilic leukemia was recently reported by an Italian study that prospectively followed 21 patients (all male) for a median follow-up period of 28 months (range: 13–67 months) (101). Patients were initiated on imatinib 400 mg daily, resulting in a complete hematologic response in less than 1 month in all cases. The longest follow-ups recorded were 42, 46, and 67 months; in these 3 patients, both hematologic and PCR remissions were maintained. Imatinib was well tolerated with minimal side effects, with dose reduction to 100–300 mg undertaken in several individuals.

A European study prospectively assessed the natural history of molecular responses to imatinib 100–400 mg daily in HES patients, Of 376 patients with hypereosinophilia, 40 (11%) were found to have the *FIP1L1-PDGFRA* fusion by quantitative PCR. Although fusion-positive patients exhibited higher absolute and % eosinophil counts than other patients, there was no correlation between the load of *FIP1L1-PDGFRA* expression and variables such as the WBC count, absolute or % eosinophil count, or % cells with the CHIC2 deletion by interphase FISH. Interestingly, there was a variability up to 3 logs in the *FIP1L1-PDGFRA* transcript load before treatment. Among 11 patients with high pretreatment transcript levels, all achieved a 3-log reduction in transcripts from baseline by 12 months of therapy and 9/11 patients achieved a molecular remission. Withrawal of imaitnib resulted in a rapid rise in transcript levels. These data confirm the considerable sensitivity of the FIP1L1-PDGFRA fusion to imatinib and the drug's capacity to elicit in-depth molecular responses in the majority of patients tested.

4.10.5   Molecular Basis for Resistance to Imatinib in FIP1L1-PDGFRα-Mediated Disease

In in vitro experiments, the concentration of imatinib required to inhibit FIP1L1-PDGFRα-transformed Ba/F3 cell growth by 50% (IC_{50}) was 3 nM.[75] This IC_{50} was at least 100-fold lower than for BCR-ABL-transformed cell growth (582 nM), consistent with the clinical observation that lower doses of imatinib are effective in CEL (100 mg daily) compared to BCR-ABL-positive CML (300–400 mg daily).

In the study by Cools et al., one patient with AML arising from CEL who harbored *FIP1L1-PDGFRA* and a complex karyotype obtained a complete hematologic remission with imatinib (75). After 5 months, he relapsed back into AML and was found to have a new mutation in the ATP-binding region of PDGFRα. The T674I mutation is in an analogous position to the T315I mutation that confers resistance to imatinib in CML. When Ba/F3 cells were transformed with this FIP1L1-PDGFRα T674I mutant, there was more than 1000-fold resistance to imatinib inhibition, compelling evidence that FIP1L1-PDGFRα is the target of imatinib in CEL (75). The FIP1L1-PDGFRα T674I mutation was subsequently described in a second patient at the time of relapse into myeloid blast crisis (102) and, more recently, in a third patient whose Langerhans cell histiocytosis evolved into CEL after chemotherapy (103). To date, primary resistance to imatinib in FIP1L1-PDGFRα-mediated disease has not been observed.

Although clinical use of alternative small molecular inhibitors was not described in the three relapsed patients with the FIP1L1-PDGFRα T674I mutation, second-generation tyrosine kinase inhibitors have been assessed against the T674I mutant in preclinical in vitro and in vivo models. For example, the alternative PDGFRα inhibitor PKC412 effectively inhibited the FIP1L1-PDGFRα T674I mutant in vitro and in an in vivo murine model of myeloproliferative disease (104). These in vivo experiments provided the first proof that one strategy to preclude or overcome tyrosine kinase resistance mutations is the use of structurally varied tyrosine kinase inhibitors. More recently, it was found that sorafenib could inhibit the FIP1L1-PDGFRα T674I mutation in vitro at nanomolar concentrations (105), whereas conflicting data exist regarding the efficacy of nilotinib in this context (106, 107).

4.10.6   PDGFRβ Rearrangements in Eosinophilic Disorders

In 1987, four patients were described in whom eosinophilia and abnormalities involving the short arm of chromosome 12p13 were shared features (108); in two of these cases, there were coexisting abnormalities of chromosome segment 5q3. In 1994, the t(5;12)(q31-q33;p13) translocation found in a small subset of patients with chronic myelomonocytic leukemia (CMML) was molecularly characterized as a fusion joining the tyrosine kinase domain of the platelet-derived growth factor receptor-beta (*PDGFRB*) on chromosome 5q33 to *TEL* (now named *ETV6*) on chromosome 12p13 (109). In addition to male predominance and splenomegaly, the hematologic picture of these patients is characterized by monocytosis, peripheral blood/marrow eosinophilia, and evolution to AML in some patients.

In addition to ETV6, 14 additional rearrangements of PDGFRB associated with 5q31-q33 translocations have been molecularly characterized to date (Table 4.5): *CEV14, HIP1, H4(D10S170), Rapabtin (RAB5), PDE4DIP (Myomegalin), HCMOGT, NIN, TP53BP1, KIAA1509*, TPM3, WDR48, and GOLGA4, and more recently, GIT2 and GPIAP1 (110–123). These fusions were identified in patients with diagnoses of CMML and juvenile myelomonocytic leukemia (JMML), and in patients alternatively described as having a BCR-ABL-negative chronic myeloproliferative disorder, atypical CML, or an overlap MPD/MDS syndrome. The

Table 4.5 Cytogenetic abnormalities and corresponding rearrangements of *PDGFRB* in eosinophilic disorders

Year	Authors	[Ref.]	Cytogenetics	Molecular abnormality	Clinical disease
1994	Golub et al.	[109]	t(5;12)(q33;p13)	*TEL(ETV6)-PDGFRB*	CMML
1997	Abe et al.	[110]	t(5;14)(q33;q32)	*CEV14-PDGFRB*	AML after clonal evolution
1998	Ross et al.	[111]	t(5;7)(q33;q11.2)	*HIP1-PDGFRB*	CMML
2000	Schwaller et al.	[112]	t(5;10)(q33;q21-22)	*H4 (D10S170)-PDGFRB*	Atypical CML
2001	Kulkarni et al.	[113]	t(5;10)(q33;q21-22)	*H4 (D10S170)-PDGFRB*	Atypical CML
2001	Magnusson et al.	[114]	t(5;17)(q33;p13)	*RAB5-PDGFRB*	CMML
2003	Baxter et al.	[115]	t(1;5)(q21;q33)[a]	Not characterized	Atypical CML
			t(1;5)(q22;q31)[a]	Not characterized	CMPD
			t(1;3;5)(p36;p21;q33)[a]	Not characterized	CMPD
			t(2;12;5)(q37;q22;q33)[a]	Not characterized	MDS
			t(3;5)(p21;q31)[a]	Not characterized	Atypical CML
			t(5;14)(q33;q24)[a]	*NIN-PDGFRB*[b]	Atypical CML
2003	Wilkinson et al.	[116]	t(1;5)(q23;q33)	*PDE4DIP-PDGFRB*	Atypical CML
2004	Morerio et al.	[117]	t(5;17)(q33;p11.2)	*HCMOGT-1-PDGFRB*	JMML
2004	Vizmanos et al.	[118]	t(5;14)(q33;q24)	*NIN-PDGFRB*	Atypical CML
2004	Grand et al.	[119]	t(5;15)(q33;q22)	*TP53BP1-PDGFRB*	Atypical CML
2004	Ketterling et al.	[124]	t(1;5)(q21;q33)[a]	Not characterized	N/A
			t(5;14)(q33;q32)[a]	Not characterized	N/A
			t(5;16)(q33;16p13.1)[a]	Not characterized	N/A
2005	Levine et al.	[120]	t(5;14)(q33;q32)	*KIAA1509-PDGFRB*	CMPD
2005	Curtis et al.	[121]	t(1;3;5)(p36;p21;q33)	*WD48-PDGFRB*	CEL
			t(3;5)(p21-25;q31-35)	*GOLGA4-PDGFRB*	CEL
2006	Rosati et al.	[122]	t(1;5)(q21;q33)	TMP53-PDGFRB	CEL
2006	Walz et al.	[123]	t(5;12)(q31;q24)	*GIT2-PDGFRB*	Eos-CMPD
			t(1;5;11)(?;q33;p13)	*GPIAP1-PDGFRB*	Eos-CMPD

CMML: chronic myelomonocytic leukemia; JMML: juvenile myelomonocytic leukemia; CML: chronic myelogenous leukemia; EosCMPD: eosinophilic chronic myeloproliferative disorder; MDS: myelodysplastic syndrome; CEL: chronic eosinophilic leukemia; Y: yes; N: no; ND: not determined; N/A: not available.

[a]*PDGFRB* rearranged by FISH analysis.

[b]Although not characterized in this report, this case was later molecularly defined by Vizmanos et al. as a *NIN-PDGFRB* fusion.

molecular breakpoints and partner genes of several reciprocal chromosomal translocations involving 5q31-5q33 in which FISH analysis has confirmed involvement of *PDGFRB* have not yet been identified (Table 4.5) (124, 125). These *PDGFRB* gene fusions invariably result in constitutively activated tyrosine kinases, and imatinib therapy has been successful in eliciting both hematologic and cytogenetic remissions in almost all cases tested (reviewed in Ref. 60).

The t(5;12) translocation is rare among cytogenetically categorized myeloid diseases. In their 2002 review, Steer and Cross found 34 cases of t(5;12) (q31-q33;p12-p13) in the literature, including 8 patients who had a documented rearrangement of either *ETV-6* or *PDGFRB* by FISH or RT-PCR (126). Among 56,709 cytogenetically defined cases at the Mayo Clinic, 25 (0.04%) exhibited the t(5;12) breakpoint (127). The classic variant t(5;12)(q33;p13) was present in only four of these cases.

Because several genes encoding cytokines involved in proliferation and differentiation of eosinophils reside in the 5q31-33 region, it was suspected that myeloid disorders with hypereosinophilia and non-PDGFRB rearrangements involving this region would involve these eosinophilopoietic factors (128–130). However, with the exception of IL-3 (chromosome 5q31) being fused to the immunoglobulin heavy-chain gene (chromosome 14q32) in a subset of eosinophilia-associated B-cell acute lymphoblastic leukemias (131), none of these genes (e.g., GM-CSF, IL-4, IL-5, and IL-13) has been implicated. In three cases of MDS/AML with associated eosinophilia and a t(5;12)(q31;p13) translocation, an *ETV6-ACS2* gene fusion was identified, the pathogenic relevance of which is unclear (132).

4.11 Eosinophilia Associated with Rearrangements of ETV6 at 12p13

Eosinophilia is also a feature of acute and chronic hematologic malignancies with rearrangements involving transcription factor ETV6 on chromosome 12p13. In addition to the aforementioned *ETV6-PDGFRB* fusion, examples include the ETV6-ABL fusion in t(9;12)(q34;p13) cases of atypical CML (133) or AML associated with eosinophilia (134). Interphase FISH has been used to prove that eosinophils are part of the neoplastic clone in *ETV6-ABL*-positive AML (134). In a patient with M4Eo AML, and the CBFb/MYH11 rearrangement, an additional rearrangement was found, t(1;12)(q25;p13), characterized by fusion of *ETV6* to the Abelson-related gene (*ARG*) (135). In addition to the ETV6-ASC2 fusion noted earlier in three MDS/AML cases with eosinophilia, an *ETV6-SYK* rearrangement has been reported in a case of MDS with eosinophilia and a t(9;12)(q22;p12) translocation (136). In 2006, an *ETV6-FLT3* fusion gene was identified in a patient with an eosinophilic myeloproliferative disorder and a t(12;13)(p13;q12) translocation (137).

4.12 Eosinophilia Associated with Rearrangements of JAK2 at 9p24

In 2005, the t(8;9)(p22;p24) translocation was reported in seven patients with chronic and acute leukemias (138). One patient had a diagnosis of CEL, and two patients exhibited mild eosinophilia. The rearrangement was subsequently identified in patients with atypical CML, acute erythroid leukemia, and T-cell lymphoma (139–141). In all cases, the human autoantigen pericentriolar material (*PCM1*) gene on 8p22 is fused to the gene encoding the *JAK2* tyrosine kinase on 9p24 (138–141). The protein fuses the coiled-coil domains of PCM1 and the tyrosine kinase domain of JAK2. The development of JAK2 inhibitors for chronic myeloproliferative disorders with the *JAK2* V617F mutation might have crossover applicability to hematologic malignancies with the constitutively activated PCM1-JAK2 fusion.

4.13 Fibroblast Growth Factor Receptor 1 (FGFR1) Fusions

In the 8p11 myeloproliferative syndrome (EMS, or stem cell leukemia/lymphoma syndrome), mutation in a pluripotent hematopoietic progenitor results in a spectrum of diseases including T-cell (less commonly B-cell) lymphoblastic lymphoma, bone marrow myeloid hyperplasia, and eosinophilia (reviewed in Ref. 142). These poor-prognosis disorders frequently transform to acute myeloid leukemia within 1–2 years after diagnosis. Early, intensive therapy with allogeneic transplantation remains the only potential curative option.

The 8p11 myeloproliferative syndrome is related to recurrent breakpoints on chromosome 8p11 (found in both myeloid and lymphoid cells) that involve translocation of the fibroblast growth factor receptor 1 (*FGFR1*) gene to several identified partner loci: *FIM/ZNF198* at 13q12 (143–146), *FOP* at 6q27 (147), *CEP110* at 9q33 (148), *BCR* at 22q11 (149, 150), and the human endogenous retrovirus gene (*HERV-K*) at 19q13 (Table 4.6) (151). More recently, the cytogenetic abnormality ins(12;8)(p11;p11p22) was described in a patient with T-cell lymphoblastic lymphoma and mild eosinophilia that progressed rapidly to AML (152). A chimeric gene was identified, resulting from the fusion of FGFR1, to part of a sixth novel partner gene, *FGFR1OP2* (*FGFR1* oncogenic partner 2), derived from chromosome 12p11. The FOP-FGFR1 fusion kinase localizes to the centrosome, activates signaling pathways within this compartment, and sustains cell cycle entry by overcoming G1 arrest. In 2005, two more fusions were characterized, *TIF1-FGFR1*153 and *MYO18A-FGFR1* (154), representing the translocations t(7;8)(q34;p11) and t(8;17)(p11;q25), respectively. All *FGFR1* fusions characterized to date have involved an mRNA junction in exon 9 of the *FGFR1* gene, and, thus, all chimeric proteins include the entire FGFR1 tyrosine kinase domain (155).

Table 4.6 Rearrangements of fibroblast growth factor receptor 1 (FGFR1) in EMS and other hematologic malignancies

Cytogenetics	Molecular abnormality	Clinical disease	Author (year)	[Ref.]
t(8;13)(p12;q12)	ZNF198-FGFR1	EMS	Popovici et al. (1998)	[143]
			Reiter et al. (1998)	[144]
			Smedley et al. (1998)	[145]
			Xiao et al. (1998)	[146]
t(6;8)(q27;p12)	FOP-FGFR1	EMS	Popovici et al. (1999)	[147]
t(8;9)(p12;q33)	CEP110-FGFR1	EMS	Guasch et al. (2000)	[148]
t(8;22)(p11;q11)	BCR-FGFR1	EMS	Demiroglu et al. (2001)	[149]
			Fioretes et al. (2001)	[150]
t(8;17)(p11;q25)	?-FGFR1[a]	SM	Sohal et al. (2001)	[155]
	MYO18A-FGFR1	EMS	Walz et al. (2005)	[154]
t(8;19)(p12;q13.3)	HERVK-FGFR1	EMS	Guasch et al. (2003)	[151]
ins(12;8)(p11;p11p22)	FGFR1OP2-FGFR1	EMS	Grand et al. (2004)	[152]
t(7;8)(q34;p11)	TIF1-FGFR1	EMS	Belloni et al. (2005)	[153]

AML: acute myeloid leukemia; SM: systemic mastocytosis.

[a]Material not available to determine the molecular breakpoint.

Similar to *PDGFRB* rearrangements, FGFR fusions exhibit aberrant tyrosine kinase activity, related to the dimerization motif(s) provided by the amino-terminal partner protein (156, 157). However, the specific partner protein might modify the disease phenotype. Using a mouse retroviral bone marrow transplant model, Roumiantsev and colleagues demonstrated that the *ZNF198-FGFR1* fusion induced MPD and T-cell lymphoma, whereas the *BCR-FGFR1* fusion induced a CML-like disease without lymphoma (158). These murine diseases recapitulated the distinct leukemia variants associated with these two deregulated fusion tyrosine kinases in human 8p11 syndrome. These murine models also provide a platform for evaluating targeted therapies against dysregulated FGFR1 oncoproteins. For example, the tyrosine kinase inhibitor PKC412 demonstrated activity in a both a murine model and a patient with EMS with the *ZNF198-FGFR1* fusion tyrosine kinase (159).

4.14 T-Cell-Mediated (Lymphocyte-Variant) Hypereosinophilia

In the healthy state, the cytokines GM-CSF, IL-3, and IL-5 direct the proliferation, survival, and differentiation of eosinophils. IL-5 is a specific eosinophil differentiation factor that is overproduced (primarily from CD4+ T-cells) as part of the immune response leading to the hypereosinophilia observed in parasitoses and atopy/allergic disorders (16).

Some patients might exhibit expansion of abnormal lymphocyte populations without any other recognized cause of their hypereosinophilia (16). These patients typically have cutaneous signs and symptoms as the primary disease manifestation.

The immunophenotypic profile of these lymphocytes include double-negative, immature T-cells (e.g., CD3$^+$CD4$^-$CD8$^-$) or the absence of CD3 (e.g., CD3$^-$CD4$^+$), a normal component of the T-cell receptor complex (160–162). Additional immunophenotypic abnormalities include elevated CD5 expression on CD3$^-$CD4$^+$ cells and loss of surface CD7 and/or expression of CD27 (16). In patients with T-cell-mediated hypereosinophilia with elevated IgE levels, lymphocyte production of IL-5, and in some cases IL-4 and IL-13, suggests that these T-cells have a Th2 cytokine profile (16, 160, 162–164). In a study of 60 patients recruited primarily from dermatology clinics, 16 had a unique population of circulating T-cells with an abnormal immunophenotype (165). Clonal rearrangement of T-cell receptor genes was demonstrated in half of these individuals (8/60 total patients). The abnormal T-cells secreted high levels of IL-5 in vitro and displayed an activated immunophenotype (e.g. CD25 and/or HLA-DR expression). Four of these patients were ultimately diagnosed with either T-cell lymphoma or Sézary syndrome, indicating that lymphocyte-variant hypereosinophilia can exhibit malignant potential. The factors that contribute to neoplastic transformation are not well characterized. In some cases, accumulation of cytogenetic changes (e.g., partial 6q and 10p deletions, trisomy 7) in T-cells, and proliferation of lymphocytes with the CD3$^-$CD4$^+$ phenotype have been observed (164, 166–168). In patients with the CD3$^-$CD4+ T-cell phenotype, loss of CD3gamma gene transcripts was found to be responsible for the defect in CD3 surface expression. In the abnormal T-cells, increased NFATc2 overexpression and binding to NFAT motifs in the CD3gamma gene promoter negatively regulate its activity, resulting in loss of CD3 (169).

Large panels of monoclonal antibodies with a wider repertoire to the variable domains (Vβ) to the T-cell receptor might increase the potential for detecting clonal T-cells as a cause for idiopathic hypereosinophilia (170). Elevation of serum thymus and activation-regulated chemokine (TARC) levels has been found in patients with T-cell-mediated hypereosinophilia versus other HES patients and controls (171). Further studies will need to assess its validity as a diagnostic marker of this variant and its relevance to the clinical course of these patients.

4.15   Treatment

In patients with eosinophilia-related organ damage (e.g., heart, lungs, gastrointestinal, central nervous system, skin), therapy should be directed to the underlying reactive or clonal disorder. Inadequate data exist to support initiation of therapy based on a specific eosinophil count in the absence of organ disease, although an absolute eosinophil count of 1500–2000/mm^3 has been recommended by some as the threshold for starting treatment (5). Treatment algorithms have incorporated serial monitoring of eosinophil counts, evaluation of clonality (e.g., T-cell receptor gene rearrangement, immunophenotyping), bone marrow aspiration and biopsy with cytogenetics, and directed organ assessment (e,g., echocardiography, pulmonary function testing) in order to identify occult organ disease and alternative causes of eosinophilia that might slowly emerge after an initial diagnosis of hyper-eosinophilia (26, 31). In patients with HES, prednisone (1 mg/kg/day) is indicated for organ involvement and is effective in producing rapid reductions in the eosinophil count (31, 172, 173). Lack of steroid responsiveness warrants considera-tion of cytotoxic therapy. Hydroxyurea is an effective first-line chemotherapeutic for HES that could be used in conjunction with corticosteroids or in steroid nonresponders (21, 172, 173). Case reports have also cited benefit from second-line agents, including vincristine (174–176), pulsed chlorambucil (31), cyclophospha-mide (177), and etoposide (178, 179). Responses to cyclosporin-A (180, 181) and 2-chlorodeoxyadenosine have also been reported in HES (182). The cumulative experience with imatinib treatment of eosinophilic disorders with rearrangements of *PDGRB* and *PDGFRA* (including *FIP1L1-PDGFRA*-positive disease) was discussed earlier.

Interferon-α (IFN-α) can elicit sustained hematologic and cytogenetic remissions in HES and CEL patients refractory to other therapies, including prednisone and hydroxyurea (44, 183–188). Some have advocated its use as initial therapy for these diseases (187). Remissions have been associated with improvement in clinical symptoms and organ disease, including hepatosplenom-egaly (183, 187), cardiac and thromboembolic complications (44, 184), mucosal ulcers (186), and skin involvement (188). The benefits of IFN-α derive from pleiotropic activities, including inhibition of eosinophil proliferation and differentiation (189). Inhibition of IL-5 synthesis from CD4+ helper T-cells mighr be relevant to its mechanism of action in lymphocyte-mediated hypere-osinophilia (190). IFN-α might also act more directly via IFN-α receptors on eosinophils, suppressing the release of IL-5 and mediators of tissue injury, such as cationic protein and neurotoxin (191).

Anti-IL-5 antibody approaches (e.g., mepolizumab, SCH55700) have been undertaken in HES based on the cytokine's role as a differentiation, activation, and survival factor for eosinophils. Mepolizumab is a fully humanized monoclonal IgG antibody that inhibits binding of IL-5 to the α-chain of the IL-5 receptor expressed on eosinophils (192). Treatment with mepolimuzab or SCH55700 could elicit rapid reductions in the periperhal blood eosinophil count within 48 h and/or decreases in serum levels of eosinophil mediators (e.g., cationic protein, eotaxin, TARC) (193–195). Clinical benefit has included regression of constitutional symptoms, dermatologic lesions (including decreases in skin/tissue-infiltrating eosinophils), and improvements in FEV_1 measurements in patients with pulmonary disease (193–195).

Clinical and/or hematologic improvements have been observed for 30 days after a single dose of SCH55700 (195) and for 12 weeks after 3 monthly doses of mepolizumab (194). Among the few patients studied, response has not been predicted by pretreatment serum IL-5 levels or the presence of the *FIP1L1-PDGFRA* fusion. Rebound eosinophilia, accompanied by increases in serum IL-5 levels, has been noted in some cases, and tachyphylaxis has been observed with repeated doses, not linked to the development of neutralizing antibodies to the recombinant antibody (195).

In phase I studies, anti-IL-5 therapy has been well tolerated except for mild infusional side effects (193–195). In the largest study of HES patients to date, the safety and steroid-sparing effects of mepolizumab was evaluated in a multicenter, randomized, double-blind, placebo-controlled trial of 85 FIP1L1-PDGFRα-negative patients (196, 197). Blood eosinophil levels were stabilized at <1000 cells/μL on 20–60 mg/day prednisone during a run-in period of up to 6 weeks. Patients were subsequently randomized to intravenous mepolizumab 750 mg or placebo every 4 weeks for 36 weeks. No adverse events were significantly more frequent with mepolizumab compared to placebo. A significantly higher proportion of mepolizumab-treated HES patients versus placebo were able to achieve the primary efficacy endpoint of a daily prednisone dose of ≤10 mg daily for at least 8 consecutive weeks.

Case reports have described the effective use of alemtuzumab (anti-CD52 monoclonal antibody) in refractory HES based on expression of the CD52 antigen on eosinophils (198, 199). In one patient with an abnormal T-cell population and an elevated serum IL-5 level of 280 pg/mol (normal < 10 pg/mol), a dose of 30 mg sc weekly resulted in resolution of fever, improvement in painful skin lesions and left ventricular function, and normalization of the serum IL-5 level (198). In another HES patient who exhibited progressive disease despite a nonmyeloablative peripheral blood stem cell transplant, use of alemtuzumab 20 mg weekly provided marked improvement in skin, joint, and cardiac complications, with striking eosinopenia (albeit transient) after infusions of the drug (199). Durable control (6 months to 2.5 years) was achieved in both cases with a maintenance regimen of 30 mg every 3 weeks.

Bone marrow/peripheral blood stem cell allogeneic transplantation has been attempted in patients with aggressive disease. Disease-free survival ranging from 8 months to 5 years has been reported (200–204) with one patient relapsing at 40 months (205). Allogeneic transplantation using nonmyeloablative conditioning regimens have been reported in three patients, with remission duration of 3–12 months at the time of last reported follow-up (206, 207). In one patient who underwent an allogeneic stem cell transplantation from an HLA-matched sibling, the patient was disease-free at 3 years, and there was no evidence of the FIP1L1-PDGFRA fusion that was present at diagnosis (95). Despite success in selected cases, the role of transplantation in HES is not well established. Transplant-related complications, including acute and chronic graft-versus-host disease as well as serious infections, have been frequently observed (208, 209).

Advances in cardiac surgery have extended the life of patients with late-stage heart disease manifested by endomyocardial fibrosis, mural thrombosis, and valvular insufficiency (3, 172). Mitral and/or tricuspid valve repair or replacement (210–214) and endomyocardectomy for late-stage fibrotic heart disease (211, 215) can improve cardiac function. Bioprosthetic devices are preferred over their mechanical counterparts because of the reduced frequency of valve thrombosis.

Leukapheresis can elicit transient reductions in high eosinophil counts, but it is not an effective maintenance therapy (216–218). Similar to other myeloproliferative disorders, splenectomy has been performed for hypersplenism-related abdominal pain and splenic infarction, but it is not considered a mainstay of treatment (219, 220). Anticoagulants and antiplatelet agents have shown variable success in preventing recurrent thromboembolism (72, 219, 221, 222).

The development of severe left ventricular dysfunction during the 7–10 days of imatinib treatment of HES is a previously unrecognized safety concern that has now been reported in a few patients (70, 223) All three patients experienced clinical recovery and improvement in LV function with high-dose corticosteroids. Although not extensively studied, a 10–14-day course of corticosteroids in conjunction with imatinib is advised in patients with echocardiogram abnormalities and/or elevated serum troponin T levels.

4.16   A Diagnostic, Classification, and Treatment Algorithm for Hypereosinophilia

The discovery of targetable molecular lesions in patients with hypereosinophilia facilitates the development of diagnostic and treatment algorithms for specific subsets of patients. In patients whose workup is negative for secondary causes of eosinophilia, screening for the *FIP1L1-PDGFRA* gene fusion (RT-PCR or interphase/metaphase FISH) is potentially the next most useful diagnostic maneuver. In cases where FIP1L1-PDGFRA screening is not available, testing for elevation of the serum tryptase might be useful as a surrogate marker for FIP1L1-PDGFRA-positive disease because it segregates with this molecular finding and the myeloproliferative variant of hypereosinophilia. Fusion-positive patients (with <20% marrow blasts) would be classified into the clonal category of ***FIP1L1-PDGFRA*-positive clonal eosinophilia, consisting of either chronic eosinophilic leukemia** or ***FIP1L1-PDGFRA*–positive systemic mast cell disease with eosinophilia**, depending on additional clinicopathological findings. Patients without reactive eosinophilia and a negative screen for *FIP1L1-PDGFRA* would be categorized into one of three possible diagnostic groups (Figure 4.4). *FIP1L1-PDGFRA*-negative patients with a nonspecific clonal cytogenetic abnormality, clonal eosinophils, or increased marrow blasts (5–19%) would be categorized as **CEL, unclassified**. This grouping would exclude well-characterized recurrent molecular abnormalities such as rearrangements involving *PDGFRA, PDGFRB, FGFR1*, and *ETV6*. *FIP1L1-PDGFRA*-negative patients without any of these clonal features or without increased marrow blasts would be assigned to the diagnostic group ***HES***. A third group, designated **T-cell associated hypereosinophilia**, would consist of patients with hypereosinophilia in whom an abnormal T-cell population is demonstrated. Such diagnostic groups might not be mutually exclusive in all cases; for example, some patients have been described with both nonspecific cytogenetic abnormalities and either the *FIP1L1-PDGFRA* fusion or a clonal T-cell expansion.

These categorizations of hypereosinophilia have implications for treatment (Figure 4.4B). Patients with *FIP1L1-PDGFRA*-positive disease as well as

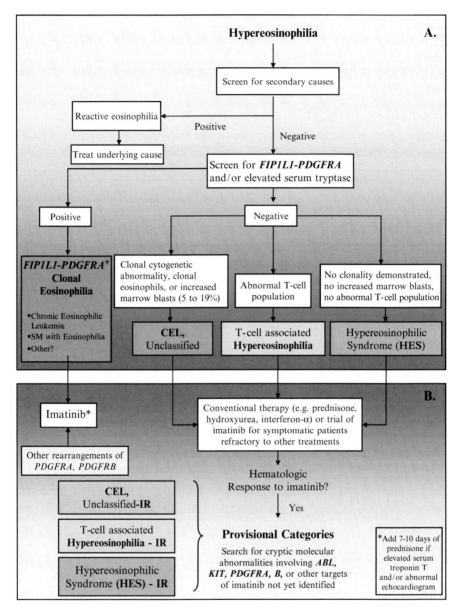

Figure 4.4 Diagnostic, classification, and treatment algorithm for hypereosinophilia. See text for details. (Originally published in Gotlib et al. (79), with permission from Churchill Livingstone for adapted figure by Ackerman and Buttefield in Ref. 5)

rearrangements involving *PDGFRA or PDGFRB* are expected to be imatinib-responsive, and treatment at doses of 100–400 mg daily should be considered first-line treatment. In *FIP1L1-PDGFRA* -negative patients, conventional therapeutic approaches (e.g., prednisone, hydroxyurea) should be undertaken. However, a trial of imatinib could be considered in some of these symptomatic *FIP1L1-PDGFRA*-negative patients (e.g., **CEL, unclassified** or **HES**) who demonstrate refractory or relapsed disease, because responses to imatinib might occur in some individuals. It might be useful to provisionally categorize *FIP1L1-PDGFRA*-negative patients with hematologic responses to imatinib as **imatinib-responsive (IR)**. Imatinib-responsiveness is likely indicative of alternate molecular targets of imatinib that contribute to the pathogenesis of these eosinophilic diseases. The utility of imatinib in a cytokine-driven disease such as **T-cell associated hypereosinophilia** has not yet been described. In cases where abnormal production of IL-5 is relevant to the hypereosinophilia, anti-IL-5 antibody therapy merits consideration.

4.17 Summary

Although HES and CEL are indeed rare clinical entities, interest in these disorders has been reborn due to a renaissance in uncovering the biologic basis of previously idiopathic cases. Unmasking the molecular basis for such cases has, in turn, led to the development of semimolecular classification schemes for categorizing patients based on recurrent genetic alterations, usually related to constitutively activated tyrosine kinases. In turn, increasing sophistication in unmasking the molecular underpinnings of eosinophilia in patients heretofore classified as idiopathic HES now permits the rationale use biologically targeted therapies such as imatinib mesylate and recombinant anti-IL-5 antibody. The WHO convenes in 2007 to review prior diagnostic criteria for both HES and CEL. It will be of interest to see how the new genetic information becomes integrated with traditional histopathologic criteria in establishing a practical road map for clinicians who treat these diseases.

References

1. Perkins WH. Beitrage zur Kenntnis der granulirten Bindewebzellen und der eosinophilen Leukocythen. Achiv Anat Physiol Physiol Abteil (Leipzi) 1879;166–169.
2. Brigden M, Graydon C. Eosinophilia detected by automated blood cell counting in ambulatory North American outpatients. Incidence and clinical significance. Arch Pathol Lab Med 1997;121:963–967.
3. Rothenberg ME. Eosinophilia. New Engl J Med 1998;338:1592–1600.
4. Pardanani A, Patnaik MM, Tefferi A. Eosinophilia: secondary, clonal and idiopathic. Br J Haematol 2006;133:468–492.
5. Ackerman SJ, Butterfield JH. Eosinophilia, eosinophil-associated diseases, chronic eosinophilic leukemia, and the hypereosinophilic syndromes. In: Hoffman R, Benz E Jr., Shattil SJ, et al., editors. Hematology, 4th ed. Philadelphia: Churchill Livingstone: 2005. p. 763–786.
6. Sanderson CJ. Interleukin-5, eosinophils, and disease. Blood 1992;79:3101–3109.
7. Wein M, Sterbinsky SA, Bickel CA, Schleimer RP, Bochner BS. Comparison of human eosinophil and neutrophil ligands for P-selectin: ligands for P-selecton differ from those for E-selectin. Am J Respir Cell Mol Biol. 1995; 12:315–319.
8. Schleimer RP, Sterbinsky SA, Kaiser J, et al. IL-4 induces adherence of human eosinophils and basophils but not neutrophils to endolthelium: association with expression of VCAM-1. J Immunol 1992;148:1086–1092.

9. Wardlaw AJ, Moqbel R, Cromwell O, et al. Platelet-activating factor: a potent chemotactic and chemokinetic factor for human eosinophils. J Clin Invest 1986;78:1701–1706.
10. Forssman U, Uguccioni M, Loetscher P, et al. Eotaxin-2, a novel CC chemokine that is selective for the chemokine receptor CCR3, and acts like eotaxin on human eosinophil and basophil leukocytes. J Exp Med 1997;185:2171–2176.
11. Kameyoshi Y, Dorschner A, Mallet AI, et al. Cytokine RANTES released by thrombin-stimulated platelets is a potent attractant for human eosinophils. J Exp Med 1992;176:587–592.
12. Hardy WR, Anderson RE. The hypereosinophilic syndromes. Ann Intern Med 1968;68:1220–1229.
13. Chusid MJ, Dale DC, West BC, et al. The hypereosinophilic syndrome. Analysis of fourteen cases with review of the literature. Medicine 1975;54:1–27.
14. Simon HU, Plotz SG, Dummer R, et al. Abnormal clones of T cells producing interleukin-5 in idiopathic hypereosinophilia. N Eng J Med 1999;341:1112–1120.
15. Bain B, Pierre R, Imbert M, et al. Chronic eosinophilic leukaemia and the hypereosinophilic syndrome. In: Jaffe ES, Harris NL, Stein H, et al., editors. World Health Organization of tumours: tumours of haematopoietic and lymphoid tissues. Lyon: IARC Press; 2001. p. 29–31.
16. Roufosse F, Cogan E, Goldman M. Recent advances in pathogenesis and management of hypereosinophilic syndromes. Allergy. 2004;59:673–689.
17. Fauci AS, Harley JB, Roberts WC, et al. NIH conference. The idiopathic hypereosinophilic syndrome. Clinical, pathophysiologic, and therapeutic considerations. Ann Intern Med 1982;97:78–92.
18. Alfaham MA, Ferguson SD, Sihra B, et al. The idiopathic hypereosinophilic syndrome. Arch Dis Child 1987;62:601–613.
19. Wynn SR, Sachs MI, Keating MU, et al. Idiopathic hypereosinophilic syndrome in a 5 ½-month-old infant. J Pediatr 1987;111:94–97.
20. Bakhshi S, Hamre M, Mohamed AM, et al. t(5;9)(q11;q34): a novel familial translocation involving Abelson oncogene and association with hypereosinophilia. J Pediatr Hematol Oncol 2003;25:82–84.
21. Rives S, Alcorta I, Toll T, et al. Idiopathic hypereosinophilic syndrome in children: report of a 7-year-old boy with FIP1L1-PDGFRA rearrangement. J Pediatr Hematol Oncol 2005;27:663–665.
22. Forrest DL, Horsman DE, Jensen CL, et al. Myelodysplastic syndrome with hypereosinophilia and a nonrandom chromosomal abnormality dic(1;7): confirmation of eosinophil clonal involvement by fluorescence in situ hybridization. Cancer Genet Cytogenet 1998;107:65–68.
23. Goldman JM, Najfeld V, Th'ng. KH. Agar culture and chromosome analysis of eosinophilic leukaemia. J Clin Pathol 1975;28:956–961.
24. Chang HW, Leong KH, Koh DR, et al. Clonality of isolated eosinophils in the hypereosinophilic syndrome. Blood 1999;93:1651–1657.
25. Luppi M, Marasca R, Morselli M, et al. Clonal nature of hypereosinophilic syndrome. Blood 1994;84:349–350.
26. Brito-Babapulle F. The eosinophilias, including the idiopathic hypereosinophilic syndrome. Br J Haematol 2003; 121:203–223.
27. Bain BJ. Eosinophilic leukaemias and the idiopathic hypereosinophilic syndrome. Br J Haematol 1996;95:2–9.
28. Brito-Babapulle F. Clonal eosinophilic disorders and the hypereosinophilic syndrome. Blood Rev 1997;11:129–145.
29. Spry CJ, Davies J, Tai PC, et al. Clinical features of fifteen patients with the hypereosinophilic syndrome. Q J Med 1983;52:1–22.
30. Lefebvre C, Bletry O, Degoulet P, et al. Prognostic factors of hypereosinophilic syndrome. Study of 40 cases. Ann Med Intern (Paris) 1989;140:253–257.
31. Weller PF, Bubley GJ. The idiopathic hypereosinophilic syndrome. Blood 1994;83:2759–2779.

32. Flaum MA, Schooley RT, Fauci AS, et al. A clinicopathologic correlation of the idiopathic hypereosinophilic syndrome. Blood 1981;58:1012–1020.
33. Tai PC, Ackerman SJ, Spry CJ, et al. Deposits of eosinophil granule proteins in cardiac tissues of patients with eosinophilic endomyocardial disease. Lancet 1987;1:643–647.
34. Venge P, Dahl R, Hallgren R, et al. Cationic proteins of human eosinophils and their role in the inflammatory reaction. In: Mahmoud AAF, Austen KF, editors. The eosinophil in health and disease. New York; Grune and Stratton; 1980. p. 131–144.
35. Tanino M, Kitamura K, Ohta G, et al. Hypereosinophilic syndrome with extensive myocardial involvement and mitral valve thrombus instead of mural thrombi. Acta Pathol Jpn 1983;33:1233–1242.
36. Radford DJ, Garlick RB, Pohlner PG. Multiple valvar replacement for hypereosinophilic syndrome. Cardiol Young 2002;12:67–70.
37. Ommen SR, Seward JB, Tajik AJ. Clinical and echocardiographic features of hypereosinophilic syndromes. Am J Cardiol 2000;86:110–113.
38. Bain BJ. Cytogenetic and molecular genetic aspects of eosinophilic leukaemias. Br J Haematol 2003;122:173–179.
39. Gotlib J. Molecular classification and pathogenesis of eosinophilic disorders: 2005 update. Acta Haematol. 2005; 114:7–25.
40. Schoch C, Reiter A, Bursch S, et al. Chromosome banding analysis, FISH and RT-PCR performed in parallel in hypereosinophilic syndrome establishes the diagnosis of chronic eosinophilic leukemia in 22% of cases: a study on 40 patients (Abstract). Blood 2004;104:671a.
41. Vandenberghe P, Wlodarska I, Michaux L, et al. Clinical and molecular features of FIP1L1-PDGFRA (+) chronic eosinophilic leukemias. Leukemia 2004;18:734–742.
42. Maubach PA, Bauchinger M, Emmerich B, et al. Trisomy 7 and 8 in Ph-negative chronic eosinophilic leukemia. Cancer Genet Cytogenet 1985;17:159–164.
43. Guitard AM, Horschowski N, Mozziconacci MJ, et al. Hypereosinophilic syndrome in childhood: trisomy 8 and transformation to mixed acute leukaemia. Nouv Rev Fr Hematol 1994;35:555–559.
44. Quiquandon I, Claisse JF, Capiod JC, et al. Alpha-interferon and hypereosinophilic syndrome with trisomy 8: karyotypic remission. Blood 1995;85:2284–2285.
45. Kawasaki A, Mizushima Y, Matsui S, et al. A case of T-cell lymphoma accompanying marked eosinophilia, chronic eosinophilic pneumonia and eosinophilic pleural effusion. A case report. Tumori 1991;77:527–530.
46. Endo M, Usuki K, Kitazume K, et al. Hypereosinophilic syndrome in Hodgkin's disease with increased granulocyte-macrophage colony-stimulating factor. Ann Hematol 1995;71:313–314.
47. Catovksy D, Bernasconi C, Verdonck PJ, et al. The association of eosinophilia with lymphoblastic leukaemia or lymphoma: a study of seven patients. Br J Haematol 1980;45:523–534.
48. Takai K, Sanada M. Hypereosinophilic syndrome evolving to acute lymphoblastic leukemia. Int J Hematol 1991;54:231–239.
49. Utsunomiya A, Ishida T, Inagaki A, et al. Clinical significance of a blood eosinophilia in adult T-cell leukemia/lymphoma: a blood eosinophilia is a significant unfavorable prognostic factor. Leukemia Res 2007;31:915–920.
50. Pardanani A, Reeder T, Li CY, et al. Eosinophils are derived from the neoplastic clone in patients with systemic mastocytosis and eosinophilia. Leuk Res 2003;27:883–885.
51. Le Beau MM, Larson RA, Bitter MA, et al. Association of inversion 16 with abnormal marrow eosinophils in acute myelomonocytic leukemia. N Eng J Med 1983;309:630–636.
52. Swirsky DM, Li YS, Matthews JG, et al. 8;21 translocation in acute granulocytic leukemia: cytological, cytochemical, and clinical features. Br J Haematol 1984;56:199–213.
53. Matsushima T, Murakami H, Kim K, et al. Steroid-responsive pulmonary disorders associated with myelodysplastic syndromes with der(1q;7p) chromosomal abnormality. Am J Hematol 1995;50:110–115.

54. Kim M, Lim J, Lee A, et al. A case of chronic myelomonocytic leukemia with severe eosinophilia having t(5;12)(q31;p13) with t(1;7)(q10;p10). Acta Haematol 2005;114:104–107.
55. Reilly JT. Class III receptor tyrosine kinases: role in leukaemogenesis. Br J Haematol 2002;116:744–757.
56. Claesson-Welsh L. Platelet-derived growth factor receptor signals. J Biol Chem 1994;269:32,023–32,026.
57. Heldin CH, Ostman A, Ronnstrand L. Signal transduction via platelet-derived growth factor receptors. Biochim Biophys Acta 1998;1378:F79–F113.
58. Valgeirsdottir S, Paukku K, Silvennoinen O, et al. Activation of Stat5 by platelet-derived growth factor (PDGF) is dependent on phosphorylation sites in PDGF beta-receptor juxtamembrane and kinase insert domains. Oncogene 1998;16:505–515.
59. Sachsenmaier C, Sadowski HB, Cooper JA. STAT activation by the PDGF receptor requires juxtamembrane phosphorylation sites but not Src tyrosine kinase activation. Oncogene 1999;18:3583–3592.
60. Gotlib J, Cross NC, Gilliland DG. Eosinophilic disorders: molecular pathogenesis, new classification, and modern therapy. Best Pract Res Clin Haematol 2006;19:535–569.
61. Schwaller J, Anastasiadou E, Cain D, et al. H4/D10S170, a gene frequently rearranged in papillary thyroid carcinoma, is fused to the platelet-derived growth factor receptor beta gene in atypical chronic myeloid leukemia with t(5;10)(q33;q22). Blood 2001;97:3910–3918.
62. Ross TS, Gilliland DG. Transforming properties of the Huntingtin interacting protein 1 platelet-derived growth factor beta receptor fusion protein. J Biol Chem 1999;274:22,328–22,336.
63. Baxter EJ, Hochhaus A, Bolufer P, et al. The t(4;22)(q12;q11) in atypical chronic myeloid leukaemia fuses BCR to PDGFRA. Hum Mol Genet 2002;11:1391–1397.
64. Trempat P, Villalva C, Laurent G, et al. Chronic myeloproliferative disorders with rearrangement of the platelet-derived growth factor alpha receptor: a new clinical target for STI571/Glivec. Oncogene 2003;22:5702–5706.
65. Safley AM, Sebastian S, Collins TS, et al. Molecular and cytogenetic characterization of a novel translocation t(4;22) involving the breakpoint cluster region and platelet-derived growth factor receptor-alpha genes in a patient with atypical chronic myeloid leukemia. Genes Chromosomes Cancer 2004;40:44–50.
66. Walz C, Curtis C, Schnittger S, et al. Transient response to imatinib in a chronic eosinophilic leukemia associated with ins(9;4)(q33;q12q25) and a CDK5RAP2-PDGFRA fusion gene. Genes Chromosomes Cancer 2006; 45:950–956.
67. Score J, Curtis C, Waghorn K, et al. Identification of a novel imatinib responsive KIF5B-PDGFRA fusion gene following screening for PDGFRA overexpression in patients with hypereosinophilia. Leukemia 2006; 20:827–832.
68. Ketterling RP, Knudson RA, Gilmer HCF. Discovery of 6 novel translocations involving the imatinib responsive genes PDGFRA and PDGFRB from screening 29,047 abnormal bone marrow specimens (Abstract). Blood 2004;104:793a.
69. Schaller JL, Burkland GA. Case report: rapid and complete control of idiopathic hypereosinophilia with imatinib mesylate. Med Gen Med. 2001;3:9.
70. Pardanani A, Reeder T, Porrata L, et al. Imatinib therapy for hypereosinophilic syndrome and other eosinophilic disorders. Blood 2003;101:3391–3397.
71. Gleich GJ, Leiferman KM, Pardanani A, et al. Treatment of hypereosinophilic syndrome with imatinib mesilate. Lancet 2002;359:1577–1578.
72. Ault P, Cortes J, Koller C, et al. Response of idiopathic hypereosinophilic syndrome to treatment with imatinib mesylate. Leuk Res 2002;26:881–884.
73. Nolasco I, Carvalho S, Parreira A. Rapid and complete response to imatinib mesylate (STI-571) in a patient with idiopathic hypereosinophilia (Abstract). Blood 2002;100:346b.
74. Cortes J, Ault P, Koller C, et al. Efficacy of imatinib mesylate in the treatment of idiopathic hypereosinophilic syndrome. Blood 2003;101:4714–4716.

75. Cools J, DeAngelo DJ, Gotlib J, et al. A tyrosine kinase created by fusion of the PDGFRA and FIP1L1 genes as a therapeutic target of imatinib in idiopathic hypereosinophilic syndrome.N Engl J Med 2003;348:1201–1214.

76. Preker PJ, Lingner J, Minvielle-Sebastia L, et al. The FIP1 gene encodes a component of a yeast pre-mRNA polyadenylation factor that directly interacts with poly(A) polymerase. Cell 1995;81:379–389.

77. Griffin JH, Leung J, Bruner RJ, et al. Discovery of a fusion kinase in EOL-1 cells and idiopathic hypereosinophilic syndrome. Proc Natl Acad Sci USA 2003;100:7830–7835.

78. Cools J, Quentmeier H, Huntly BJP, et al. The EOL-1 cell line as an in vitro model for the study of FIP1L1-PDGFRA-positive chronic eosinophilic leukemia. Blood 2004;103:2802–2805.

79. Gotlib J, Cools J, Malone JM, et al. The FIP1L1-PDGFRα fusion tyrosine kinase in hypereosinophilic syndrome and chronic eosinophilic leukemia: implications for diagnosis, classification, and management. Blood 2004;103:2879–2891.

80. Walz C, Cilloni D, Soverini S, et al. Molecular heterogeneity of the *FIP1L1-PDGFRA* fusion gene in chronic eosinophilic leukemia (CEL) and systemic mastocytosis with eosinophilia (SME): a study of 43 cases (Abstract). Blood 2004;104:667a.

81. Zhang GS, Li B, Pei MF, et al. Identification of FIP1L1-PDGFRA fusion, and expression of signal transducer and activator of transcription 5 in hypereosinophilic syndrome. Zhonghua Yi Xue Za Zhi 2004; 84:1541–1544.

82. Yu J, Deuel TF, Kim HR. Platelet-derived growth factor (PDGF) receptor-alpha activates c-Jun NH2-terminal kinase-1 and antagonizes PDGF receptor-beta -induced phenotypic transformation. J Biol Chem 2000;275:19,076–19,082.

83. Stover EH, Chen J, Folens C, et al. Activation of FIP1L1-PDGFRalpha requires disruption of the juxtamembrane domain of PDGFRalpha and is FIP1L1-independent. Proc Natl Acad Sci USA 2006;103:8078–8083.

84. Gilliland DG, Griffin JD. The roles of FLT3 in hematopoiesis and leukemia. Blood 2002;100:1532–1542.

85. Hirota S, Isozaki K, Moriyama Y, et al. Gain-of-function mutations in c-kit in human gastrointestinal tumors. Science 1998;279:577–580.

86. Heinrich MC, Corless CL, Duensing A, et al. PDGFRA activating mutations in gastrointestinal stromal tumors. Science 2003; 299:708–710.

87. Klion AD, Robyn J, Akin C, et al. Molecular remission and reversal of myelofibrosis in response to imatinib mesylate treatment in patients with the myeloproliferative variant of hypereosinophilic syndrome. Blood 2004;103:473–478.

88. Martinelli G, Cilloni D, Ottaviani E, et al. Idiopathic hypereosinophilic syndrome (HES) with FIP1L1-PDGFRA rearrangement can be effectively treated with imatinib (Abstract). Blood 2004;104:421a.

89. Rose C, Dupire S, Roche-Lestienne C, et al. Sustained molecular response with imatinib in a leukemic form of idiopathic hypereosinophilic syndrome in relapse after allograft. Leukemia 2004;18:354–355.

90. Frickhofen N, Marker-Hermann E, Reiter A, et al. Complete molecular remission of chronic eosinophilic leukemia complicated by CNS disease after targeted therapy with imatinib. Ann Hematol 2004;83:477–480.

91. Martinelli G, Malagola M, Ottaviani E, et al. Imatinib mesylate can induce complete molecular remission in FIP1L1-PDGFRα–positive hypereosinophilic syndrome. Haematologica 2004;89:236–237.

92. Rotoli B, Catalano L, Galderisi M, et al. Rapid reversion of Loeffler's endocarditis by imatinib in early stage clonal hypereosinophilic syndrome. Leuk Lymphoma 2004;45:2503–2507.

93. Malagola M, Martinelli G, Rondoni M, et al. Soft tissue and skeletal involvement in FIP1L1-PDGFR-alpha positive chronic eosinophilic leukemia: imatinib mesylate may induce complete molecular and imaging remission. Haematologica 2004; 89:ECR25.

94. Jovanovic JV, Score J, Waghorn K, et al. Low-dose imatinib mesylate leads to rapid induction of major molecular responses and achievement of complete molecular remission in FIP1L1-PDGFRA positive chronic eosinophilic leukemia. Blood 2007;109:4635–4640.

95. Halaburda K, Prejzner W, Szatkowski D, et al. Allogeneic bone marrow transplantation for hypereosinophilic syndrome: long-term follow-up with eradication of FIP1L1-PDGFRA fusion transcript. Bone Marrow Transplant 2006;38:319–320.

96. Tefferi A, Lasho TL, Brockman SR, et al. FIP1L1-PDGFRA and c-kit D816V mutation-based clonality studies in systemic mast cell disease associated with eosinophilia. Haematologica 2004;89:871–873.

97. Robyn J, Lemery S, McCoy JP, et al. Multilineage involvement of the fusion gene in patients with FIP1L1/PDGFRA-positive hypereosinophilic syndrome. Br J Haematol 2006;132:286–292.

98. Klion AD, Noel P, Akin C, et al. Elevated serum tryptase levels identify a subset of patients with a myeloproliferative variant of idiopathic hypereosinophilic syndrome associated with tissue fibrosis, poor prognosis, and imatinib responsiveness. Blood 2003;101:4660–4666.

99. Pardanani A, Ketterling RP, Brockman SR, et al. CHIC2 deletion, a surrogate for *FIP1L1-PDGFRA* fusion, occurs in systemic mastocytosis associated with eosinophilia and predicts response to imatinib therapy. Blood 2003;102:3093–3096.

100. Muller AMS, Martens UM, Hofmann SC, et al. Imatinib mesylate as a novel treatment option for hypereosinophilic syndrome: two case reports and a comprehensive review of the literature. Ann Hematol 2006; 85:1–16.

101. Rondoni M, Ottaviani E, Paolo P, et al. FIP1L1-PDGFRalpha positive hypereosinophilic syndrome (HES). The response to imatinib (IM) is durable. A report of 21 patients with a follow-up of 12 to 67 months (Abstract). Blood 2006;108:763a.

102. Von Bubnoff N, Sandherr M, Schlimok G, et al. Myeloid blast crisis evolving during imatinib treatment of an FIP1L1-PDGFRalpha-positive chronic myeloproliferative disease with prominent eosinophilia. Leukemia 2004;19:286–287.

103. Ohnishi H, Kandabashi K, Maeda Y, et al. Chronic eosinophilic leukaemia with FIP1L1-PDGFRA fusion and T674I mutation that evolved from Langerhans cell histiocytosis with eosinophilia after chemotherapy. Br J Haematol 2006;134:547–549.

104. Cools J, Stover EH, Boulton CL, et al. PKC412 overcomes resistance to imatinib in a murine model of FIP1L1-PDGFRA-induced myeloproliferative disease. Cancer Cell 2003;3:459–469.

105. Lierman E, Folens C, Stover EH, et al. Sorafenib is a potent inhibitor of FIP1L1-PDGFRalpha and the imatinib-resistant FIP1L1-PDGFRalpha T674I mutant. Blood 2006;108:1374–1376.

106. von Bubnoff N, Gorantla SP, Thone S, et al. The FIP1L1-PDGFRA T674I mutation can be inhibited by the tyrosine kinase inhibitor AMN107 (nilotinib). Blood 2006;107:4970–4971.

107. Stover EH, Chen J, Lee BH, et al. The small molecule tyrosine kinase inhibitor AMN107 inhibits TEL-PDGFRbeta and FIP1L1-PDGFRalpha in vitro and in vivo. Blood 2005;106:3206–3213.

108. Keene P, Mendelow B, Pinto MR, et al. Abnormalities of chromosome 12p13 and malignant proliferation of eosinophils: a non-random association. Br J Haematol 1987;67:25–31.

109. Golub TR, Barker GF, Lovett M, et al. Fusion of PDGF receptor beta to a novel ets-like gene, tel, in chronic myelomonocytic leukemia with t(5;12) chromosomal translocation. Cell 1994;77:307–316.

110. Abe A, Emi N, Tanimoto M, et al. Fusion of the platelet-derived growth factor beta receptor to a novel gene CEV14 in acute myelogenous leukemia after clonal evolution. Blood 1997;90:4271–4277.

111. Ross TS, Bernard OA, Berger R, et al. Fusion of Huntington interacting protein 1 to platelet-derived growth factor beta receptor (PDGFbetaR) in chronic myelomonocytic leukemia with t(5;7)(q33;q11.2). Blood 1998;91:4419–4426.

112. Schwaller J, Anastasiadou E, Cain D, et al. H4/D10S170, a gene frequently rearranged in papillary thyroid carcinoma, is fused to the platelet-derived growth factor receptor beta gene in atypical chronic myeloid leukemia with t(5;10)(q33;q22). Blood 2001;97:3910–3918.

113. Kulkarni S, Heath C, Parker S, et al. Fusion of H4/D10S170 to the platelet-derived growth factor receptor beta in BCR-ABL negative myeloproliferative disorders with a t(5;10)(q33;q21). Cancer Res 2000;60:3592–3598.

114. Magnusson MK, Meade KE, Brown KE, et al. Rabaptin-5 is a novel fusion partner to platelet-derived growth factor receptor beta in chronic myelomonocytic leukemia. Blood 2001;98:2518–2525.

115. Baxter EJ, Kulkarni S, Vizmanos JL, et al. Novel translocations that disrupt the platelet-derived growth factor receptor beta (PDGFRB) gene in BCR-ABL-negative chronic myeloproliferative disorders. Br J Haematol 2003; 120:251–256.

116. Wilkinson K, Velloso ER, Lopez LF, et al. Cloning of the t(1;5)(q23;q33) in a myeloproliferative disorder associated with eosinophilia: involvement of PDGFRB and response to imatinib. Blood 2003;102:4187–4190.

117. Morerio C, Acquila M, Rosanda C, et al. HCMOGT-1 is a novel fusion partner to PDGFRB in juvenile myelomonocytic leukemia with t(5;17)(q33;p11.2). Cancer Res 2004;64:2649–2651.

118. Vizmanos JL, Novo FJ, Roman JP, et al. NIN, a gene encoding a CEP110-like centrosomal protein, is fused to PDGFRB in a patient with a t(5;14)(q33;q24) and an imatinib-responseive myeloproliferative disorder. Cancer Res 2004;64:2673–2676.

119. Grand FH, Burgstaller S, Kuhr T, et al. P53-binding protein 1 is fused to the platelet-derived growth factor receptor beta in a patient with a t(5;15)(q33;q22) and an imatinib-responsive eosinophilic myeloproliferative disorder. Cancer Res 2004;64:7216–7219.

120. Levine RL, Wadleigh M, Sternberg DW, et al. KIAA1509 is a novel PDGFRB fusion partner in imatinib-responsive myeloproliferative disease associated with a t(5;14)(q33;q32). Leukemia 2005;19:27–30.

121. Curtis C, Apperley J, Dang R, et al. The platelet-derived growth factor receptor beta fuses to two distinct loci at 3p21 in imatinib responsive chronic eosinophilic leukemia (Abstract). Blood 2005;106:909a

122. Rosati R, La Starza R, Luciano L, et al. TPM3/PDGFRB fusion transcript and its reciprocal in chronic eosinophilic leukemia. Leukemia 2006;20:1623–1624.

123. Walz C, Metzgeroth G, Claudia Schoch C, et al. Characterization of two new imatinib-responsive fusion genes generated by disruption of *PDGFRB* in eosinophilia-associated chronic myeloproliferative disorders (Abstract). Blood 2006;108:200a

124. Ketterling RP, Knudson RA, Gilmer HCF. Discovery of 6 novel translocations involving the imatinib responsive genes PDGFRA and PDGFRB from screening 29,047 abnormal bone marrow specimens (Abstract). Blood 2004;104:793a.

125. Baxter EJ, Kulkarni S, Vizmanos JL, et al. Novel translocations that disrupt the platelet-derived growth factor receptor beta (PDGFRB) gene in BCR-ABL-negative chronic myeloproliferative disorders. Br J Haematol 2003; 120:251–256.

126. Steer EJ, Cross NC. Myeloproliferative disorders with translocations of chromosome 5q31-5q35: role of the platelet-derived growth factor receptor beta. Acta Haematol 2002;107:113–122.

127. Greipp PT, Dewald GW, Tefferi A. Prevalence, breakpoint distribution, and clinical correlates of t(5;12). Cancer Genet Cytogenet 2004;153:170–172.

128. Sato H, Danbara M, Tamura M, et al. Eosinophilic leukemia with a t(2;5)(p23;q35) translocation. Br J Haematol 1994;87:404–406.

129. Darbyshire PJ, Shortland D, Swansbury GJ, et al. A myeloproliferative disease in two infants associated with eosinophilia and chromosome t(1;5) translocation. Br J Haematol 1987;66:483–486.

130. Jani K, Kempski HM, Reeves BR. A case of myelodysplasia with eosinophilia having a translocation t(5;12)(q31;q13) restricted to myeloid cells but not involving eosinophils. Br J Haematol 1994;87:57–60.

131. Meeker TC, Hardy D, Willman C, et al. Activation of the interleukin-3 gene by chromosome translocation in acute lymphoblastic leukemia with eosinophilia. Blood 1990;76:285–289.

132. Yagasaki F, Jinnai I, Yoshida S, et al. Fusion of TEL/ETV6 to a novel ACS2 in myelodys-plastic syndrome and acute myelogenous leukemia with t(5;12)(q31;p13). Genes Chromosomes Cancer 1999;26:192–202.

133. Keung YK, Beaty M, Steward W, et al. Chronic myelocytic leukemia with eosinophilia, t(9;12)(q34;p13) and ETV6-ABL gene rearrangement: case report and review of the litera-ture. Cancer Genet Cytogenet 2002;138:139–142.

134. La Starza R, Trubia M, Testoni N, et al. Clonal eosinophils are a morphologic hallmark of ETV6/ABL1 positive acute myeloid leukemia. Haematologica 2002;87:789–794.

135. Cazzaniga G, Tosi S, Aloisi A, et al. The tyrosine kinase abl-related gene ARG is fused to ETV6 in an AML-M4Eo with a t(1;12)(q25;p13): molecular cloning of both reciprocal tran-scripts. Blood 1999;94:4370–4373.

136. Kuno Y, Abe A, Emi N, et al. Constitutive kinase activation of the TEL-Syk fusion gene in myelodysplastic syndrome with t(9;12)(q22;p12). Blood 2001;97:1050–1055.

137. Vu HA, Xinh PT, Masusa M, et al. FLT3 is fused to ETV6 in a myeloproliferative disorder with hypereosinophilia and a t(12;13)(p13;q12) translocation. Leukemia 2006;20:1414–1421.

138. Reiter A, Walz C, Watmore A, et al. The t(8;9)(p22;p24) is a recurrent abnormality in chronic and acute leukemia that fuses PCM1 to JAK2. Cancer Res 2005;65:2662–2667

139. Murati A, Gelsi-Boyer V, Adelaide J, et al. PCM1-JAK2 fusion in myeloproliferative disorders and acute erythroid leukemia with t(8;9) translocation. Leukemia 2005;19(9):1692–1696.

140. Bousquet M, Quelen C, De Mas V, et al. The t(8;9)(p22;p24) translocation in atypical chronic myeloid leukaemia yields a new PCM1-JAK2 fusion gene. Oncogene 2005;24:7248–7252.

141. Adelaide J, Perot C, Gelsi-Boyer V, et al. A t(8;9) translocation with PCM1-JAK2 fusion in a patient with T-cell lymphoma. Leukemia 2006:536–537.

142. Macdonald D, Reiter A, Cross NCP. The 8p11 myeloproliferative syndrome: a distinct clini-cal entity caused by constitutive activation of *FGFR1*. Acta Haematol 2002;107:101–107.

143. Popovici C, Adelaide J, Ollendorff V, et al. Fibroblast growth factor receptor 1 is fused to FIM in stem-cell myeloproliferative disorder with t(8;13). Proc Natl Acad Sci USA 1998;95:5712–5717.

144. Reiter A, Sohal J, Kulkarni S, et al. Consistent fusion of ZNF198 to the fibroblast growth factor receptor 1 in the t(8;13)(p11;q12) myeloproliferative syndrome. Blood 1998;92:1735–1742.

145. Smedley D, Hamoudi R, Clark J, et al. The t(8;13)(p11;q11-12) rearrangement associated with an atypical myeloproliferative disorder fuses the fibroblast growth factor receptor 1 gene to a novel gene RAMP. Hum Mol Genet 1998;7:637–642.

146. Xiao S, Nalabolu SR, Aster JC, et al. FGFR1 is fused with a novel zinc-finger gene, ZNF198, in the t(8;13) leukaemia/lymphoma syndrome. Nat Genet 1998;18:84–87.

147. Popovici C, Zhang B, Gregoire MJ, et al. The t(6;8)(q27;p11) translocation in a stem cell myeloproliferative disorder fuses a novel gene, FOP, to fibroblast growth factor receptor 1. Blood 1999;93:1381–1389.

148. Guasch G, Mack GJ, Popovici C, et al. FGFR1 is fused to the centrosome-associated protein CEP110 in the 8p12 stem cell myeloproliferative disorder with t(8;9)(p12;q33). Blood 2000;95:1788–1796.

149. Demiroglu A, Steer EJ, Heath C, et al. The t(8;22) in chronic myeloid leukemia fuses BCR to FGFR1: transforming activity and specific inhibition of FGFR1 fusion proteins. Blood 2001;98:3778–3783.

150. Fioretos T, Panagopoulos I, Lassen C, et al. Fusion of the BCR and the fibroblast growth factor receptor-1 (FGFR1) genes as a result of t(8;22)(p11;q11) in a myeloproliferative disorder: the first fusion gene involving BCR but not ABL. Genes Chromosomes Cancer 2001;32:302–310.

151. Guasch G, Popovici C, Mugneret F, et al. Endogenous retroviral sequence is fused to FGFR1 kinase in the 8p12 stem-cell myeloproliferative disorder with t(8;19)(p12;q13.3). Blood 2003;101:286–288.

152. Grand EK, Grand FH, Chase AJ, et al. Identification of a novel gene, FGFR1OP2, fused to FGFR1 in 8p11 myeloproliferative syndrome. Genes Chromomosomes Cancer 2004;40:78–83.

153. Belloni E, Trubia M, Gasparini P, et al. 8p11 myeloproliferative syndrome with a novel t(7;8) translocation leading to fusion of the FGFR1 and TIF1 genes. Genes Chromosomes Cancer 2005;42:320–325.
154. Walz C, Chase A., Weisser A., et al. The t(8;17)(p11;q25) in the 8p11 myeloproliferative syndrome fuses MYO18A to FGFR1. Leukemia 2005;19:1005–1009.
155. Sohal J, Chase A, Mould S, et al. Identification of four new translocations involving FGFR1 in myeloid disorders. Genes Chromosomes Cancer 2001;32:155–163.
156. Ollendorff V, Guasch G, Isnardon D, et al. Characterization of FIM-FGFR1, the fusion product of the myeloproliferative disorder-associated t(8;13) translocation. J Biol Chem 1999;274:26,922–26,930.
157. Smedley D, Demiroglu A, Abdul-Rauf M, et al. ZNF198-FGFR1 transforms Ba/F3 cells to growth factor independence and results in high level tyrosine phosphorylation of STATs 1 and 5. Neoplasia 1999;1:349–355.
158. Roumiantsev S, Krause DS, Neumann CA, et al. Distinct stem cell myeloproliferative/T lymphoma syndromes induced by ZNF198-FGFR1 and BCR-FGFR1 fusion genes from 8p11 translocations. Cancer Cell 2004;5:287–298.
159. Chen J, DeAngelo DJ, Kutok JL, et al. PKC412 inhibits the zinc finger 198-fibroblast growth factor receptor 1 fusion tyrosine kinase and is active in treatment of stem cell myeloproliferative disorder. Proc Natl Acad Sci USA 2004;101:14,479–14,484.
160. Cogan E, Schandene L, Crusiaux A, et al. Brief report: clonal proliferation of type 2 helper T cells in a man with the hypereosinophilic syndrome. N Engl J Med 1994;330: 535–538.
161. Simon HU, Yousefi S, Dommann-Scherrer CC, et al. Expansion of cytokine-producing CD4-CD8- T cells associated with abnormal Fas expression and hypereosinophilia. J Exp Med 1996;183:1071–1082.
162. Brugnoni D, Airo P, Rossi G, et al. CD4+ T-cell population able to secrete large amounts of interleukin-5. Blood 1996;87:1416–1422.
163. Roufosse F, Schandene L, Sibille C, et al. T-cell receptor-independent activation of clonal Th2 cells associated with chronic hypereosinophilia. Blood 1999;94:994–1002.
164. Bank I, Amariglio N, Reshef, A, et al. The hypereosinophilic syndrome associated with CD4+CD3- helper type 2 (Th2) lymphocytes. Leuk Lymphoma 2001;42:123–133.
165. Simon HU, Plotz SG, Dummer R, et al. Abnormal clones of T cells producing interleukin-5 in idiopathic hypereosinophilia. N Eng J Med 1999;341:1112–1120.
166. Brugnoni D, Airo P, Tosoni C, et al. CD3-CD4+ cells with a Th2-like pattern of cytokine production in the peripheral blood of a patient with cutaneous T cell lymphoma. Leukemia 1997;11:1983–1985.
167. Roufosse F, Schandene L, Sibille C, et al. Clonal Th2 lymphocytes in patients with the idiopathic hypereosinophilic syndrome. Br J Haematol 2000;109:540–548.
168. Kitano K, Ichikawa N, Shimodaira S, et al. Eosinophilia associated with clonal T-cell proliferation. Leuk Lymphoma 1997;27:335–342.
169. Willard-Gallo KE, Badran BM, Ravoet M, et al. Defective CD3gamma gene transcription is associated with NFATc2 overexpression in the lymphocytic variant of hypereosinophilic syndrome. Exp. Hematol. 2005;33:1147–1159.
170. Bassan R, Locatelli G, Borleri G, et al. Immunophenotypic evaluation of circulating T-cell clones in hypereosinophilic syndromes with or without abnormal CD3 and CD4 lymphocytes. Haematologica 2004;89:238–239.
171. DeLavareille A, Roufosse F, Schmid-Grendelmeier P, et al. High serum thymus and activation-regulated chemokine levels in the lymphocytic variant of the hypereosinophilic syndrome. J Allergy Clin Immunol 2002;110:476–479.
172. Fauci AS, Harley JB, Roberts WC, et al. NIH conference. The idiopathic hypereosinophilic syndrome. Clinical, pathophysiologic, and therapeutic considerations. Ann Intern Med 1982;97:78–92.
173. Parrillo JE, Fauci AS, Wolff SM. Therapy of the hypereosinophilic syndrome. Ann Intern Med 1978;89:167–172.

174. Chusid MJ, Dale DC. Eosinophilic leukemia. Remission with vincristine and hydroxyurea. Am J Med 1975;59:297–300.
175. Cofrancesco E, Cortellaro M, Pogliani E, et al. Response to vincristine treatment in a case of idiopathic hypereosinophilic syndrome with multiple clinical manifestations. Acta Haematol 1984;72:21–25.
176. Sakamoto K, Erdreich-Epstein A, deClerck Y, et al. Prolonged clinical response to vincristine treatment in two patients with hypereosinophilic syndrome. Am J Pediatr Hematol Oncol 1992;14:348–351.
177. Lee JH, Lee JW, Jang CS, et al. Successful cyclophosphamide therapy in recurrent eosinophilic colitis associated with hypereosinophilic syndrome. Yonsei Med J 2002;43:267–270.
178. Smit AJ, van Essen LH, de Vries EG. Successful long-term control of idiopathic hypereosinophilic syndrome with etoposide. Cancer 1991;67:2826–2827.
179. Bourrat E, Lebbe C, Calvo F. Etoposide for treating the hypereosinophilic syndrome. Ann Intern Med 1994;121:899–900.
180. Zabel P, Schlaak M. Cyclosporin for hypereosinophilic syndrome. Ann Hematol 1991;62:230–231.
181. Nadarajah S, Krafchik B, Roifman C, et al. Treatment of hypereosinophilic syndrome in a child using cyclosporine: implication for a primary T-cell abnormality. Pediatrics 1997;99:630–633.
182. Ueno NT, Zhao S, Robertson LE, et al. 2-chlorodeoxyadenosine therapy for idiopathic hypereosinophilic syndrome. Leukemia 1997;11:1386–1390.
183. Luciano L, Catalano L, Sarrantonio C, et al. αIFN–induced hematologic and cytogenetic remission in chronic eosinophilic leukemia with t(1;5). Haematologica 1999;84:651–653.
184. Yamada O, Kitahara K, Imamura K, et al. Clinical and cytogenetic remission induced by interferon-α in a patient with chronic eosinophilic leukemia associated with a unique t(3;9;5) translocation. Am J Hematol 1998;58:137–141.
185. Malbrain ML, Van den Bergh H, Zachee P. Further evidence for the clonal nature of the idiopathic hypereosinophilic syndrome: complete haematological and cytogenetic remission induced by interferon-alpha in a case with a unique chromosomal abnormality. Br J Haematol 1996;92:176–183.
186. Butterfield JH, Gleich GJ. Response of six patients with idiopathic hypereosinophilic syndrome to interferon alpha. J Allergy Clin Immunol 1994;94:1318–1326.
187. Ceretelli S, Capochiani E, Petrini M. Interferon-alpha in the idiopathic hypereosinophilic syndrome: consideration of five cases. Ann Hematol 1998;77:161–164.
188. Yoon TY, Ahn GB, Chang SH. Complete remission of hypereosinophilic syndrome after interferon-alpha therapy: report of a case and literature review. J Dermatol 2000;27:110–115.
189. Broxmeyer HE, Lu L, Platzer E, et al. Comparative analysis of the influences of human gamma, alpha and beta interferons on human multipotential (CFU-GEMM), erythroid (BFU-E), and granulocyte-macrophage (CFU-GM) progenitor cells. J Immunol 1983;131:1300–1305.
190. Schandene L, Del Prete GF, Cogan E, et al. Recombinant interferon-alpha selectively inhibits the production of interleukin-5 by human CD4+ T cells. J Clin Invest 1996;97:309–315.
191. Aldebert D, Lamkhioued B, Desaint C, et al. Eosinophils express a functional receptor for interferon alpha: inhibitory role of interferon alpha on the release of mediators. Blood 1996;87:2354–2360.
192. Hart TK, Cook RM, Zia-Amirhosseini P, et al. Preclinical efficacy and safety of mepolizumab (SB—240563), a humanized monoclonal antibody to IL-5, in cynomolgus monkeys. J Allergy Clin Immunol 2001;108:250–257.
193. Plotz SG, Simon HU, Darsow U, et al. Use of an anti-interleukin-5 antibody in the hypereosinophilic syndrome with eosinophilic dermatitis. N Engl J Med 2003;349:2334–2339.
194. Garrett JK, Jameson SC, Thomson B, et al. Anti-interleukin-5 (mepolizumab) therapy for hypereosinophilic syndrome. J Allergy Clin Immunol 2004;113:115–119.

195. Klion AD, Law MA, Noel P, et al. Safety and efficacy of the monoclonal anti-interleukin-5 antibody SCH55700 in the treatment of patients with hypereosinophilic syndrome. Blood 2004;103:2939–2941.
196. Klion AD, Rothenberg ME, Murray JJ, et al. Safety and tolerability of anti-IL-5 monoclonal antibody (Mepolizumab) therapy in patients with HES: A multicenter, randomized, double-blind, placebo-controlled trial (Abstract). Blood 2006;108:762a.
197. Rothenberg ME, Gleich GJ, Roufosse FE, et al. Steroid-sparing effects of anti-IL-5 monoclonal antibody (Mepolizumab) therapy in patients with HES: A multicenter, randomized, double-blind, placebo-controlled trial (Abstract). Blood 2006;115a.
198. Pitini V, Teti D, Arrigo C, Righi M, et al. Alemtuzumab therapy for refractory idiopathic hypereosinophilic syndrome. Br J Haematol 2004;127:477.
199. Sefcick, A, Sowter D, DasGupta E, et al. Alemtuzumab therapy for refractory idiopathic hypereosinophilic syndrome. Br J Haematol 2004;124:558–559.
200. Vazquez L, Caballero D, Canizo CD, et al. Allogeneic peripheral blood cell transplantation for hypereosinophilic syndrome with myelofibrosis. Bone Marrow Transplant 2000;25:217–218.
201. Chockalingam A, Jalil A, Shadduck RK, et al. Allogeneic peripheral blood stem cell transplantation for hypereosinophilic syndrome with severe cardiac dysfunction. Bone Marrow Transplant 1999;23:1093–1094.
202. Basara N, Markova J, Schmetzer B, et al. Chronic eosinophilic leukemia: successful treatment with an unrelated bone marrow transplantation. Leuk Lymphoma 1998;32:189–193.
203. Sigmund DA, Flessa HC. Hypereosinophilic syndrome: successful allogeneic bone marrow transplantation. Bone Marrow Transplant 1995;15:647–648.
204. Esteva-Lorenzo FJ, Meehan KR, Spitzer TR, et al. Allogeneic bone marrow transplantation in a patient with hypereosinophilic syndrome. Am J Hematol 1996;51:164–165.
205. Sadoun A, Lacotte L, Delwail V, et al. Allogeneic bone marrow transplantation for hypereosinophilic syndrome with advanced myelofibrosis. Bone Marrow Transplant 1997;19:741–743.
206. Juvonen E, Volin L, Kopenen A, et al. Allogeneic blood stem cell transplantation following non-myeloablative conditioning for hypereosinophilic syndrome. Bone Marrow Transplant 2002;29:457–458.
207. Ueno NT, Anagnostopoulos A, Rondon G, et al. Successful non-myeloablative allogeneic transplantation for treatment of idiopathic hypereosinophilic syndrome. Br J Haematol 2002;119:131–134.
208. Archimbaud E, Guyotat D, Guillaume C, et al. Hypereosinophilic syndrome with multiple organ dysfunction treated by allogeneic bone marrow transplantation. Am J Hematol 1988;27:302–303.
209. Fukushima T, Kuriyama K, Ito H, et al. Successful bone marrow transplantation for idiopathic hypereosinophilic syndrome. Br J Haematol 1995;90:213–215.
210. Radford DJ, Garlick RB, Pohlner PG. Multiple valvar replacement for hypereosinophilic syndrome. Cardiol Young 2002;12:67–70.
211. Harley JB, McIntosh XL, Kirklin JJ, et al. Atrioventricular valve replacement in the idiopathic hypereosinophilic syndrome. Am J Med 1982;73:77–81.
212. Hendren WG, Jones EL, Smith MD. Aortic and mitral valve replacement in idiopathic hypereosinophilic syndrome. Ann Thorac Surg 1988;46:570–571.
213. Cameron J, Radford DJ, Howell J, et al. Hypereosinophilic heart disease. Med J Aust 1985;143:408–410.
214. Weyman AE, Rankin R, King H. Loeffler's endocarditis presenting as mitral and trucuspid stenosis. Am J Cardiol 1977;40:438–444.
215. Chandra M, Pettigrew RI, Eley JW, et al. Cine-MRI-aided endomyocardectomy in idiopathic hypereosinophilic syndrome. Ann Thorac Surg 1996;62:1856–1858.
216. Blacklock HA, Cleland, JF, Tan P, et al. The hypereosinophilic syndrome and leukapheresis. Ann Intern Med 1979;91:650–651.
217. Davies J, Spry C. Plasma exchange or leukapheresis in the hypereosinophilic syndrome. Ann Intern Med 1982;96:791.

218. Chambers LA, Leonard SS, Whatmough AE, et al. Management of hypereosinophilic syndrome with chronic plasma- and leukapheresis. Prog Clin Biol Res 1990;337:83–85.
219. Spry CJ, Davies J, Tai PC, et al. Clinical features of fifteen patients with the hypereosinophilic syndrome. Q J Med 1983;52:1–22.
220. Narayan S, Ezughah F, Standen GR, et al. Idiopathic hypereosinophilic syndrome associated with cutaneous infarction and deep venous thrombosis. Br J Dermatol 1993;148:817–820.
221. Moore PM, Harley JB, Fauci AS. Neurologic dysfunction in the idiopathic hypereosinophilic syndrome. Ann Intern Med 1985;102:109–114.
222. Johnston AM, Woodcock BE. Acute aortic thrombosis despite anticoagulant therapy in idiopathic hypereosinophilic syndrome. J R Soc Med 1998;91:492–493.
223. Pitini V, Arrigo C, Azzarello D, et al. Serum concentration of cardiac troponin T in patients with hypereosinophilic syndrome treated with imatinib is predictive of adverse outcomes. Blood 2003;102:3456–3457.

Chapter 5
Chronic Myelomonocytic Leukemia

Miloslav Beran

5.1 Definition and Classification

Owing to its variable pathologic features and clinical course, chronic myelo-monocytic leukemia (CMML) is both a diagnostic and a therapeutic challenge. The French-American-British (FAB) classification system included CMML as one of the five categories of myelodysplastic syndrome (1), and its definition of CMML as a disease characterized by absolute monocytosis is still used today (Table 5.1). The FAB classification includes a wide spectrum of patients with cytopenias and ineffective hematopoiesis reminiscent of myelodysplastic syndromes (MDS) and those with leukocytosis and organ involvement typical of myeloproliferative disorders, suggesting differences in pathology. Based on expert opinion, the FAB group proposed the use of a white blood cell (WBC) count of 13×10^9/L as an arbitrary cutoff point to separate CMML into "dysplastic" and "proliferative" varieties (2). The International Working Group followed the FAB recommendation (3) and excluded CMML patients with WBC >12 × 10^9/L from the risk-oriented International Prognostic Scoring System for MDS (IPSS) (3), limiting its usefulness for assessing the expected outcomes of CMML patients (4, 5). The World Health Organization (WHO) included CMML in a category of mixed myelodysplastic/myeloproliferative disorders (MDS/MPD) (6). The prognostic significance of bone marrow and circulating blasts and eosinophilia led to the creation of further subcategories (Table 5.1).

The major contribution of the FAB classification was the creation of a defined category of CMML. The unintended consequence of including CMML in the MDS group was that in reporting the results of clinical trials, data from patients with CMML were often combined with those from patients with high-risk MDS, which made it difficult to assess the impact specifically on CMML. The WHO classification, which further highlights distinct features of CMML, should encourage research and stimulate the initiation of clinical trials focusing specifically on CMML.

Table 5.1 Diagnostic criteria for CMML according to (A) French-American-British (FAB) and (B) World Health Organization (WHO) criteria

A. FAB Classification (adapted from Bennett et al. 1982) (1)

- Persistant blood monocytosis $\geq 1 \times 109/L$
- Bone marrow blasts <20% associated with dysplasia in either erythroid, granulocytic, or megakaryocytic lineages
- Circulating blasts below 5%
- Absence of Auer rods in myeloid cells

B. WHO Criteria (adapted from Vardiman et al. 2002) (6)

- Persistent blood monocytosis $\geq 1 \times 10^9/L$
- Absence of Philadelphia chromosome or BCR-ABL rearrangement
- Bone marrow or peripheral blood blasts <20%
- Dysplasia in one or more myeloid lineages. In the absence of dysplasia, all other criteria are met along with the following: presence of cytogenetic abnormality, or persistent monocytosis of unknown origin for ≥ 3 months.

Subcategories:

- CMML-1. Blasts <10% in bone marrow and <5% in peripheral blood
- CMML2: Blasts 10–20% in bone marrow, 5–19% in peripheral blood, or Auer rods are present and blasts <20% in peripheral blood or bone marrow.
- CMML-1 or CMML-2 with eosinophilia (eosinophils in blood >$1.5 \times 10^9/L$).

5.2   Ethiology and Epidemiology

The causes of CMML are largely unknown, as is the molecular basis. At present, it is not clear to what extent environmental factors—exposure to carcinogens, ionizing radiation, or DNA-damaging drugs—are involved in the development of the disease. CMML is infrequently reported as therapy related (7). In a series of 213 patients, one-fifth had a prior malignancy (4). Only in those treated with DNA-damaging agents should CMML be considered a treatment-related, secondary malignancy, more frequently seen in dysplastic CMML, and like in secondary MDS, it appears more frequently associated with chromosomal abnormalities, particularly monosomy 7 or a complex karyotype (Beran, unpublished observation). In others, however, CMML arose as a second, unrelated malignancy. The potential involvement of growth-regulatory genes is supported by the detection of abnormal fusion tyrosine kinases (TKs) in some patients (see below). The incidence and prevalence of CMML are largely unknown. Population studies estimate that CMML constitutes approximately 10–15% of MDS cases. The reported median age varies between 65 years and 75 years, and there is an approximately 2:1 male predominance (4, 5, 8, 9).

5.3   Clinical Features

Chronic myelomonocytic leukemia patients might remain asymptomatic for years, ultimately developing anemia, thrombocytopenia, and neutropenia. Weight loss, night sweats, and a catabolic state are more often observed in patients with proliferative disease. Splenomegaly is observed in one-third (4, 5, 8) and hepatomegaly is observed in 15–20% of patients (4, 8). The involvement of other organs, seen particularly in patients with severe monocytosis, includes the skin and serous membranes of the pericardium, pleura, or peritoneum. Renal excretion of lysozyme, produced by monocytic cells, might cause tubular damage, which, along with monocytic infiltration of the kidneys, is a common cause of abnormal renal function. Skin rashes like pruritus are thought to be related to the activated state of monocytes (10) or to represent a paramalignant condition.

5.4   Laboratory Features and Differential Diagnosis

Absolute monocytosis is the only objective feature characteristic of CMML and is required for diagnosis. The pathological process behind monocytosis is not understood. A formal analysis of its significance in patients with MDS/MPD documented a significant negative association between monocytosis and survival (11). Monocytosis could also be seen as a nonspecific reactive phenomenon in patients with inflammatory disorders and might represent a component in other malignant disorders, such as systemic mastocytosis (12). The elevation of serum lysozyme levels might be helpful in assessing the tumor load, particularly in cases with organ involvement. The remaining laboratory features are nonspecific and shared with MDSs or with typical and atypical MPDs. The laboratory findings and their variability (8) are shown in Table 5.2. Eosinophilia might be relevant to the pathology of the disease being frequently associated with abnormalities in the PDGFRβ gene (*vide infra*).

Bone marrow morphology is, *per se*, not diagnostic of CMML and the guidelines provided to distinguish CMML from atypical chronic myelogenous leukemia (aCML) (2, 13) still retain a degree of subjectivity. The percentage of monocytic cells is often, but not always, elevated. The upper limit of blast cells defining the disease has been arbitrarily set by the FAB (1) and WHO (6) classifications. Reticulin fibrosis might be seen, although collagen fibrosis is uncommon. The current diagnosis and classification of CMML is the result of a temporary consensus. Ultimately, knowledge of the pathogenetic mechanisms involved in the initiation and evolution of the disease or empirical identification, by clinical trials, of subpopulations of patients responsive to clinical treatment will provide a more meaningful and treatment-oriented classification.

The present categorization of CMML as dysplastic or proliferative (2) remains controversial (14–18), although it bears some consequences for management. The

Table 5.2 Laboratory characteristics of patients with CMML[a]

Variable	Proliferative WBC > 13000			Dysplastic WBC ≤ 13000			p-Value
	Number	Mean	SD	Number	Mean	SD	
Age	184	64.8	10.7	120	64.5	12.5	0.963
Blood:							
Neutrophils (%)	176	50.3	17.9	118	38.3	17.8	0.000
Neutrophils (× 10⁹/L)	177	24.1	25.3	119	3.2	2.2	0.000
Monocytes (%)	182	24.4	16.8	120	29.2	13.2	0.000
Monocytes (× 10⁹/L)	182	11.5	16.2	120	2.2	1.1	0.000
Lymphocytes (%)	177	12.2	7.9	119	26.6	12.4	0.000
Lymphocytes (× 10⁹/L)	177	4.6	4.3	119	2.0	1.0	0.000
IMC	168	9.2	9.0	117	3.0	3.9	0.000
Hemoglobin (g/dL)	184	10.3	2.1	120	10.3	2.0	0.819
Platelets (× 10⁹/L)	180	146.1	144.3	120	110.0	121.2	0.033
B2M (mg/L)	84	5.9	3.7	59	4.0	2.4	0.000
LDH (U/L)	175	1170.1	1034.3	116	663.5	334.9	0.000
Bone Marrow:							
Blood (%)	181	5.5	4.9	117	5.7	4.9	0.790
Neutrophils (%)	175	22.4	12.2	115	16.0	9.8	0.000
Monocytes (%)	156	15.9	12.1	116	11.4	9.3	0.000
Normoblasts (%)	171	13.0	10.5	112	22.3	14.0	0.000
Lymphocytes (%)	170	5.8	4.6	110	8.8	6.7	0.000
Basophils (%)	62	0.8	2.1	9	0.1	0.3	0.087
M:E Ratio	171	11.3	20.2	112	5.5	9.5	0.000
Cellularity (%)	165	83.0	18.5	111	64.3	26.1	0.000

[a]M.D. Anderson Cancer Center data registry.
Source: Beran et al. unpublished data.

categories might represent pathogenetically diverse disorders or various stages of a disease initiated by the same event and evolving as a consequence of new genetic or epigenetic alterations. Serial laboratory evaluation of patients presenting with dysplastic CMML documented increasing leukocytosis and transition into disease with proliferative features (16, 17). The transition from proliferative to dysplastic CMML has not been reported, however. There might even be a dynamic disease continuum from patients with MDS and relative monocytosis (>8–10% of monocytes but < 10⁹/L) who seem to have a prognosis close to that of CMML (19), some of whom will progress to CMML, to patients who have a high absolute monocyte count >1 × 10⁹ /L due to leukocytosis but who do not have relative monocytosis; these patients would likely be classified as having aCML (2) or atypical MPD (6, 12). In proliferative CMML, aCML, or aMPD, the predominant underlying molecular abnormalities might involve the products of genes regulating lineage–favoring proliferation (e.g., receptor tyrosine kinases) and/or antiapoptotic pathways, whereas genes regulating differentiation and favoring apoptosis might be more important in dysplastic CMML and MDS.

5.5   Pathophysiology and Biology

5.5.1   Progenitor Cells and Sensitivity to Hematopoetic Growth Factors

Clonality studies support the involvement of myeloid but not lymphoid cells in the CMML (20, 21). With the initiating event likely confined to progenitor cells committed to myeloid/monocytic lineage, these might display abnormal behavior. In vitro cultures of bone marrow or blood cells have shown abnormalities in the frequency and properties of such leukemic clonogenic, granulocyte-macrophage colony-forming cells (GM-CFCs) (22–28). The small colonies, composed predominantly of macrophagelike cells (25), are the consequence of abnormalities in both the growth rate and differentiation of GM-CFC progeny. In CMML patients, the frequency of GM-CFCs in the bone marrow or blood varies from increased to normal or decreased, and in some instances, no GM-CFCs are detectable, suggesting heterogeneity and variable degree of growth and maturation defect(s). With limited data available, the frequency of circulating GM-CFCs appears to be higher in cases of CMML with proliferative features. Definite correlations with other characteristics, particularly degree of leukocytosis or prognostic significance have yet to be reported.

These results are of interest when compared to those in other MPDs. In the chronic phase of BCR-ABL-positive CML, the number of circulating GM-CFCs is invariably elevated. Their growth and differentiation appears normal and is strictly dependent on the presence of exogenous hematopoietic growth factors (HGFs) but changes during the evolution into accelerated and blastic-phase CML. In polycythemia vera (PV), the requirement of progenitor cells for erythropoietin is decreased (29). Similarly, GM-CFCs in juvenile myelomonocytic leukemia (JMML) display an increased sensitivity to GM-CSF (30). This finding is particularly interesting, as it is potentially linked to abnormalities in the Ras pathway (31, 32). In CMML, the evidence of an increased sensitivity to GM-CSF is less compelling. A "spontaneous," or exogenous, GM-CSF-independent colony formation in CMML (22–28) might be due to the paracrine production of such factor(s) by accessory cells. Removal of adherent cells is invariably associated with a decrease in the clonogenic growth (26, 27, Beran, unpublished). The addition of HGF-specific antibodies to CMML cell cultures reduces spontaneous colony formation (27, 33, 34). An increased sensitivity to GM-CSF reminiscent of that in JMML (30) was seen in adherent cell-depleted blood GM-CFCs from a minority of patients with CMML, whereas in others, the GM-CFC growth was entirely dependent on exogenous growth factors (Beran, unpublished). Whether the spontaneous clonogenic growth is due to autocrine production of growth factors by progenitor cells or to paracrine mechanisms is unresolved. Colony formation by purified CD34-positive CMML-derived cells is, however, strictly dependent on the addition of exogenous GM-CSF or the reconstitution of the cultures with autologous adherent cells, themselves devoid of colony-forming ability (Beran, unpublished).

The clinical significance of these findings and relationship to other pathophysiological and molecular features of the disease remain to be determined.

5.5.2   Genetic Alterations and Abnormalities in Signaling Pathways

5.5.2.1   Karyotype

There are no CMML-specific chromosomal or molecular abnormalities. Because of the similarity between proliferative CMML and typical CML, it is mandatory to exclude the presence of Ph+ by karyotype or fluorescence *in situ* hybridization (FISH) probing or BCR-ABL by polymerase chain reaction (PCR) and specific primers. Similarly, CMML patients with inv(16) or t(8; 21) karyotype are considered to have evolving acute myeloid leukemia (AML) (6) and should be treated accordingly. Balanced translocations involving chromosome 5 (q31–33) [e.g., t(5;12)] have been described in patients with MDS/MPD, including those with CMML (35–37), with the underlying pathogenetic event identified as TEL-PDGFRβ fusion TK, in which fusion of the Tel oligomerization domain to the PDGFRβ catalytic domain results in dimerization and subsequent constitutive activation of the receptor (38). Subsequently, additional fusion partners of PDGFRβ were identified in CMML and aCML, all resulting in the activation of a resulting fusion TKs and dysregulated growth ([39–9). In CMML-like MPD, activation of PDGFRα tyrosine kinase was reported in BCR-PDGFRα fusion (50), and JAK2 tyrosine kinase was activated after JAK2 fusion with ETV6 in t(9;12) (51) or with PCM1 in t(8;9) (52). Early identification of such abnormalities is important for choice of treatment. Karyotype analysis will identify the majority of such patients. Negative results in patients displaying features associated with rearranged PDGFRβ, such as eosinophilia (35, 44, 48), might justify further workup using either FISH probing or PCR. Because of its rarity (4), routine screening of CMML patients for PDGFRβ rearrangements with PCR is probably not indicated.

An abnormal karyotype is found in about 30% of patients (4, 8, 9, 11, 16, 53–55). The striking finding in studies comparing CMML, MDS, and aCML is the low frequency of a complex karyotype in CMML and aCML . The most frequent single chromosomal abnormality in both CMML and aCML is trisomy 8, followed by monosomy 7 in CMML but not in BCR-ABL-negative aCML (58, 59) (Table 5.3). Contrary to initial reports suggesting the association of t(5; 12) with CMML (35–38), the abnormality is rare in both CMML and aCML. The same is true for other cytogenetic abnormalities involving PDGFRβ rearrangement (35–490. In cohorts of consecutive patients with CMML, t(5;12) was identified in 0/213 (4) and 1/27 (57) cases, respectively. It was found in 2/219 consecutive cases of Ph-negative, aCML (58) (Table 5.3).

Table 5.3 Comparison of cytogenetic abnormalities for CMML (*n* = 228), Ph- CML (*n* = 219), BCR- CML (82), and MDS (*n* = 1284)[a]

Abnormality	CMML No. (%)	Ph- CML No. (%)	BCR/ABL- CML[b] No. (%)	MDS No. (%)
Not available	10 (4.4)	29 (13.2)	5 (6.1)	167 (13.0)
Available	218 (95.6)	190 (86.8)	77 (94.0)	1117 (88.2)
Diploid	142 (65.1)	136 (71.6)	56 (72.7)	451 (40.4)
−5	2 (0.9)	0 (0.0)	0 (0.0)	20 (1.8)
−7	16 (7.3)	0 (0.0)	0 (0.0)	41 (3.7)
−5, −7	3 (1.4)	0 (0.0)	0 (0.0)	15 (1.3)
−7 and other single abnormality (but −5)	0 (0.0)	0 (0.0)	0 (0.0)	69 (6.2)
7q- (+/− other single abnormality)	0 (0.0)	1 (0.5)	1 (1.3)	16 (1.4)
+8	13 (6.0)	10 (5.3)	5 (6.5)	64 (5.7)
+8 and other single abnormality	2 (0.9)	2 (1.1)	6 (7.8)	83 (7.4)
+21	3 (1.4)	0 (0.0)	0 (0.0)	10 (0.9)
5q- (± other single abnormailty)	1 (0.5)	2 (1.1)	0 (0.0)	36 (3.2)
20q- (± other single abnormality)	4 (1.8)	4 (2.1)	3 (3.9)	34 (3.0)
−Y	2 (0.9)	1 (0.5)	0 (0.0)	21 (1.9)
12p-	2 (0.9)	0 (0.0)	0 (0.0)	9 (0.8)
Iso17	2 (0.9)	1 (0.5)	1 (1.3)	4 (0.4)
13q-	0 (0.0)	3 (1.6)	2 (2.6)	4 (0.4)
Inv 16	0 (0.0)	0 (0.0)	0 (0.0)	9 (0.8)
t(8;21)	0 (0.0)	0 (0.0)	0 (0.0)	10 (0.9)
Complex (without −5 or −7)[c]	8 (3.7)	5 (2.6)	2 (2.6)	81 (7.3)
Complex (included −5 or −7)	13 (6.0)	7 (3.7)	2 (2.6)	252 (22.6)
Other CMML abnormality[d]	13 (6.0)[e]	16 (8.4)[e]	7 (9.1)	135 (12.1)

[a]M.D. Anderson data registry and modified from Onida et al. (58).

[b]Subset of Ph- CML examined with PCR for BCR/ABL transcripts.

[c]Complex = ≥3 abnormalities.

[d]Other CMML abnormalities [number of patients]: Inv Y [1], +10 [1], +14 [1], +19 [1], +X [1], 11q- [1], 12q- [1], add 4(q35) [1], t(11;22) [1], t(11;16) [1], t(4;15) [1], t(7;10) [1], t(9;21) [1]. Other Ph- CML abnormalities [Ph- number, BCR- number]: Inv 5 [1,1], Inv 9 [1,0], 12q- [1,0], +14 [2,1], add 17p [1,1], add 15p, +frag [1,0], Ins (X;4) [1,1], t(5;12) [2,0], t(8;9) [2,0], t(9;14) [1,1], t(1;13) [1,1].

[e]All single abnormality.

5.5.2.2. Ras Pathway

Mutation of the N-*ras* or K-*ras* oncogene results in the activation of the ras pathway in hematological malignancies (60), including myeloproliferative, myelodysplastic, and MDS/MPD disorders (61–67), particularly in high-risk MDS (63), CMML (61, 62, 65–67), and JMML (31). *Ras* mutations are virtually absent in BCR-ABL-positive

CML (62, 64, 65) and are relatively rare in aCML (59, 65). They are present in approximately one-third of CMML patients (4, 8) (Table 5.4), although the frequency has been reported as high as 60% in smaller studies (65), likely reflecting selection of patients with proliferative CMML (65). The frequency of *ras* mutation in proliferative CMML is double that in dysplastic CMML (43% vs.. 22%, respectively) (8, 16, 66, 67). *Ras* mutation has been reported to be associated with the progression of MDS to AML (68) and transition of dysplastic into proliferative CMML (69), but a causative relationship between the acquisition of ras mutation and disease progression has not yet been established. *Ras* mutation was not a significant independent variable associated with survival (67), although in the most recent update in an extended patient cohort, the presence of *ras* mutation was significantly associated with a shorter median survival (9.9 months vs. 15.5 months, $p = 0.02$) (8; Beran, unpublished) (Figure 5.1A).

Other molecular abnormalities associated with activation of the Ras pathway, studied in JMML, have received less attention in CMML. Several lines of evidence support the role of hyperactive Ras in JMML. The frequent loss of the normal *NF1* allele in JMML indicates the role of *NF1* as a tumor suppressor gene and a negative regulator of Ras activation (70). Such a role is further supported by the development of JMML-like disease in mice with somatic inactivation of the *NF1* gene (71). Involvement of *NF1* has not been reported in CMML, although abnormal levels of neurofibromin were found in bone marrow (72). Mutation of the *PTPN11* gene, leading to disregulation of SHP-2 phosphatase activity and increased *ras* downstream signaling, observed in 43% of JMML patients (73, 74), is rare in adult CMML. It was found in only 1 of 84 (75) and in 0 of 35 (76) patients with CMML. The molecular profile of adult CMML thus differs noticeably from that of JMML, where alternative and perhaps mutually exclusive molecular events activate Ras via mutations of *RAS*, *NF1*, or *PTPN11*.

5.5.2.3   JAK/STAT

Activation of JAK/STAT signaling via specific mutations of the *JAK2* gene (JAKV617F) in PV (77, 78), essential thrombocytemia, and myeloid metaplasia with myelofibrosis (78) is less frequent in CMML, varying from 3% to 10% (78–80). Unlike in PV, where JAK2V617F is believed to confer hypersensitivity to

Table 5.4 Frequence of *ras* mutation in CMML[a]

Category, given either intravenously of subcutaneously,	*n*	*ras* mutation %	Distribution of mutations by codon (%)		
			N-ras	K-ras	Unknown
All CMML	242	29	38	10	52
"Proliferative" (WBC > 12 × 10⁹/L)	147	36			
"Dysplastic" (WBC ≤ 12 × 10⁹/L)	95	19			

[a]MD Anderson Cancer Center Data Registry.

Source: Beran, unpublished.

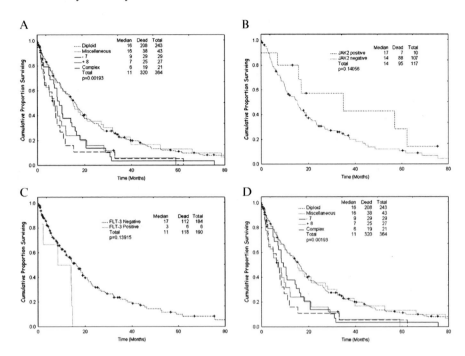

Figure 5.1 Survival of patients with CMML as a function of ras mutation (**A**), JAK2 mutation (**B**), FLT-3 mutation (**C**), and karyotype (**D**). Kaplan-Meier plots

erythropoietin, its role in CMML is unknown. Finding both *RAS* and *JAK2* mutations in two patients with CMML suggests that both the JAK-STAT and RAS-MAPK pathways can be activated and contribute to the disease phenotype (78). In 10 CMML patients, JAK2V617F mutation was associated with proliferative features such as leukocytosis in 8 with splenomegaly in 7 (4 with and 3 without hepatomegaly) but had no apparent effect on survival (Beran, unpublished) (Figure 5.1B). Although experimental evidence supports a nonredundant role of JAK2 in the function of specific cytokine receptors, including interleukin (IL)-3 and GM-CSF (81), the molecular mechanism by which JAK2V617F operates in CMML is not known.

5.5.2.4 FLT3 Mutation

Internal tandem duplication (ITD) or mutation within the kinase domain (D835) of the FLT3 receptor gene results in ligand-independent dimerization and activation of the receptor, with subsequent constitutive activation of the tyrosine kinase and signaling through the RAS, MAPK, and STAT5 pathways (82). It is associated with an unfavorable prognosis of AML, both previously untreated (83–87) and in first relapse (Beran, unpublished)]. FLT3 mutation is frequent in patients with monocytic or myelomonocytic AML (83, 88, 89). Because 20–30% of patients with CMML will develop AML, FLT3 mutations might be involved in the leukemic transformation. FLT3 mutations are rare in CMML; screening of 163 consecutive patients for the presence of ITD or D835 mutations documented only five (3%) with ITD. Four of the five patients had a diploid karyotype and none had *ras* mutations. All patients had features of proliferative disease, and four had an enlarged liver, spleen, or both. Survival was shorter than expected by prognostic scoring (4, 8) (Beran, unpublished) (Figure 5.1) and all patients succumbed to progressive disease or AML. Therefore, it appears that FLT3 mutation in CMML is associated with proliferative disease, organ involvement, and poor prognosis (Beran, unpublished).

5.5.3   Epigenetic Abnormalities

The methylation of gene promoters, resulting in gene inactivation, is an alternative mechanism regulating cellular proliferation and differentiation (90, 91). Although there has been long-standing interest in abnormalities in gene methylation in MDS in the context of prognosis and changes during therapy (92–95), information specific to CMML is limited (96), with cases of CMML often being included in MDS studies (94, 95). Methylation of the promoter of the cell-cycle–regulating gene p15^{INK4b} was found in 58% of 33 CMML patients and was correlated with reduced mRNA and protein expression and with increased expression of DNA methyltransferase (DNMT) 3A (96). The methylation of RASSFA1 and Ship1 promoter are rare in CMML (94). The data on SOCS1 are conflicting, with promoter methylation being virtually absent in 26/27 CMML patients (94), yet hypermethylation of exon 2 of SOCS1 was detected in the bone marrow of 10/25 patients. Statistical analysis of the whole MDS group, including CMML, found that SOCS1 methylation was associated with a higher frequency of N-*ras* mutations, poor prognosis, and a higher cumulative risk of leukemic transformation but had no independent effect on survival (94).

5.6   Natural History and Risk Assessment/ Stratification

Chronic myelomonocytic leukemia is a heterogeneous disease and the overall survival has been reported to vary between 7 and 60 months (4, 5, 8, 52). Some differences in survival might be accounted for by delayed referral to a hematologist-oncologist or a tertiary referral center to establish the diagnosis (Figure 5.2). Repeated multivariate analyses in large cohorts of patients have failed to document any treatment modality as significantly and independently associated with survival (4, 8), thus justifying the inclusion of treated patients into prognostic modeling. Numerous studies have reported a large number of variables that are significantly associated with survival. These served as the basis of risk-oriented prognostic scoring systems aimed at stratifying patients according to expected survival (reviewed in Refs.4 and 5). Of those specifically

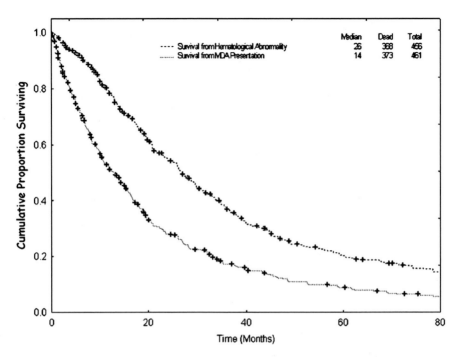

Figure 5.2 Survival of CMML patients from the first detection of hematological abnormality and from referral to and diagnosis of CMML at M.D. Anderson Cancer Center

developed for CMML, the Bornemouth system used bone marrow blast, platelet, hemoglobin, and neutrophil counts to stratify patients according to expected survival of 32 or 9 months (97), whereas the Dusseldorf system used bone marrow blast, lactate dehydrogenase (LDH), hemoglobin, and platelet levels (5, 98, 99). The M. D. Anderson Prognostic Score (MDAPS) identified hemoglobin and bone marrow blast levels, the presence of circulating immature myeloid cells, and absolute lymphocyte count as significant independent prognostic variables, stratifying patients into four survival categories (4). The unique prognostic significance of lymphocytes was subsequently independently verified (100). The MDAPS was recently prospectively validated in an independent group of patients with CMML at the same institution (8). Abnormal karyotype, although negatively associated with survival (4, 8), was never formally documented to be an independent prognostic variable in multivariate analysis in described CMML risk models. Recent follow-up of 320 patients demonstrated significant negative association of +8, −7, and complex karyotypes with survival (8) (Figure 5.1D). There is currently no evidence for the superiority of any of these models, as would be expected due to limitations inherent in any prognostic scoring (101). With expansion of cohort size by additional patients, the significance of variables selected by multiple regression models might change, affecting the final model and stratification, as was indeed documented (8). With the exception of IPSS, which proved unsuitable for CMML (4, 5), all of the above-mentioned models recognize CMML as a separate entity and could be used to stratify patients for prognostic purposes, for assignment to clinical trials, and for alternative evaluation of response according to expected survival. Although age is not considered in any of the models, it is important that it is taken into account for treatment selection. In patients with low-risk disease, supportive care might be appropriate for the elderly, whereas allogeneic stem cell transplantation (SCT), with or without prior chemotherapy, might be considered in low-risk patients younger than 50–60 years.

5.7 Management and Treatment Options

Traditionally, the management of patients with CMML has been centered on supportive care and the control of disease-associated symptoms, with the main aim of improving quality of life. The identification of activated PDGFRβ fusion tyrosine kinases as molecular targets for imatinib mesylate and the introduction and approval of hypomethylating agents 5-azacytidine and decitabine for the treatment of CMML in the United States, offers new treatment options. A reduced-intensity SCT, developed as an alternative to standard myeloablative allogeneic SCT, is another addition to the management of CMML. Finally, a better understanding of prognostic risk models might allow improved risk assessment and assignment to treatment modalities.

5.7.1 Risk Assessment and Choice of Therapy

With an increasing number of therapeutic options available, it is becoming important to consider major disease- and patient-associated variables using one of the published prognostic scores (4, 5, 8, 97, 98). In patients with rearrangement of the PDGFRβ gene, imatinib is the initial treatment of choice. Patients potentially eligible for allogeneic SCT and their siblings should be HLA typed. In selected cases, discussion of an unrelated matched donor SCT might be initiated. It is important to provide patients and their families with detailed information about treatment options, the potential advantages of investigational agents, and the importance of using them in the context of supervised clinical trials. Finally, the patient's personal wishes and quality of life expectations should be respected.

5.7.2 General Supportive Care

Pending the final selection of treatment, it is appropriate to initiate supportive care tailored to the patient's clinical symptoms and the activity of the disease. Many patients are completely asymptomatic, and in these cases, observation might be prudent to assess the stability of the disease. Anemia is initially managed by red blood cell transfusions, with frequency ideally based on the degree of anemia tolerated by the individual patient. A trial of erythropoietin might benefit some patients (102). Platelet transfusions are indicated in severely thrombocytopenic patients with clinical signs of bleeding; prophylactic transfusions based on low platelet counts in asymptomatic patients are less likely beneficial and might lead to rapid allo-sensitization. Single-donor platelets are preferable. For cytomegalovirus (CMV)-negative patients who are candidates for allogeneic SCT, blood products from CMV-negative donors are recommended. The use of blood products from the potential stem cell donor should be avoided. The benefit of prophylactic use of G-CSF or GM-CSF has not been documented. In febrile patients with severe neutropenia not responding to antibiotics, G-CSF can be considered. Excessive leukocytosis and monocytosis are occasionally seen in response to G-CSF therapy, suggesting cautious use of long-acting preparations.

5.7.3   Single-Agent Therapy

Several oral agents such as hydroxyurea, 6-mercaptourine, busulphan, and etoposide were used in CMML. Of those, hydroxyurea is the most commonly used agent for initial cytoreductive treatment in patients with leukocytosis, organomeg-aly, and constitutional symptoms. Its superior activity over etoposide was documented in a randomized trial involving mostly CMML patients with prolifera-tive features (103). Although hydroxyurea treatment might achieve a rapid reduction in WBCs in most patients, improvement of anemia and platelet counts are infrequent. The impact on the bone marrow is less evident, and reduction of organomegaly, if achieved, is often partial and transient.

   Of investigational agents, topoisomerase I inhibitors, topotecan given either intravenously (104) or orally (105), and orally administered 9-nitro20-(S)-campthothecin (106) demonstrated activity in CMML, including complete responses. Their oral formulation might facilitate drug delivery, but additional investigations would be necessary to define an optimal treament schedule and prolong response duration. It is not known whether they are superior to hydroxyurea. Antiangiogenic and immunomedulatory properties of thalidomide prompted treatment of few CMML patients (107). No responses were observed. Thalidomide analog, lenalinomide (Revlimid), is currently being investigated in MPDs.

5.7.4   Hypomethylating Agents

Azacytidine and decitabine are believed to have a dual effect on treated cells. At higher doses, they mainly inhibit DNA synthesis and are cytotoxic; at low doses, they modulate the activity of genes associated with the growth and differen-tiation, presumably due to hypomethylation. Thus, from the early stages of drug development, the importance of dose intensity was apparent. The activity of 5-azacytidine (5-aza; Vidaza®) in MDS was first demonstrated in two phase II studies of patients with high-risk MDS. Almost 50% of patients experienced a treatment response, ranging from a decreased requirement for red blood cell transfusions to complete remission, after intravenous or subcutaneous injections (108, 109). A subsequent randomized trial of 5-azacytidine at 75 mg/m^2/day subcutaneously for 7 days, every 4 weeks documented the superiority of 5-azacytidine plus supportive care over supportive care alone in terms of responses and delayed progression to AML but not survival advantage (110). The approval summary based on the results of the pivotal randomized trial and two single-arm studies involving 219 patients reports 5.9% complete response (CR), 9.3% partial response (PR), and 19% lesser response rates, with a median response duration of 9 months (111). At least three to four courses were required for optimal response, suggesting the importance of continuing treatment in responding or stable patients.

Fourteen patients with CMML were enrolled in the phase III trial of 5-azacytidine, seven in each arm. Specific results in patients with CMML were not provided, and one is left with the impression of modest improvement of hematological status similar to results in high-risk MDS (110). In the approval report (101), 3 nonspecified responses were reported in 19 CMML patients treated with 5- azacytidine (15.8%). This information, although very limited, suggests a low treatment efficacy in CMML (Table 5.4). Therefore, further studies in larger numbers of patients in various stages and variants of the disease are needed.

The second agent, 5-aza-2-deocytidine (DAC; decitabine, Dacogen^R), demonstrated its ability to induce in vitro differentiation of leukemic cell line (112), AML cells (113) and to elicit trilineage response in poor-prognosis MDS patients (114). Continuous infusion of decitabine (50 mg/m^2 over 24h, daily for 3 days every 6 weeks) was then investigated in 28 patients with progressive MDS and only 1 patient with CMML. After at least two cycles, eight complete and five partial responses were documented. With a progression-free period of 32 weeks, the responses were short and the actuarial median survival from the start of treatment was 12 months (115). Similar activity in MDS was subsequently reported with a less intensive regimen (15 mg/m^2, intravenously, three times daily for 3 days) in a multicenter study that included nine patients with dysplastic CMML (116). In CMML, one CR, one PR, and two hematological improvements suggested an overall response comparable to that of high-risk MDS (116). Using an identical regimen, a randomized, phase III trial in MDS documented the superiority of decitabine over best supportive care, with an overall response rate of 17%, including 9% CRs . The median survival duration was not improved in the decitabine arm (117).

In the study, six and eight CMML patients were assigned to the decitabine and supportive arms, respectively. One of six treated and none of eight supportive care patients achieved a response, which was not specified (117). These results are comparable to those obtained with 5-azacytidine (110, 111) and inferior to a previously reported single-arm study (116). It is possible that further investigations on the effect dose and schedule are necessary for optimal use of decitabine. One study suggested that decitabine might be more active when given at lower daily doses for a longer period of time (118).

The described regimens of 5-azacytidine and decitabine have provided relatively low MDS response rates and no convincing improvement in survival. The results in CMML are essentially nonconclusive. With both drugs, the responses occur gradually (110, 117), and it is now believed that maximal efficacy requires prolonged therapy and perhaps further schedule modification.

Further evidence of the importance of dose schedule and a potential lead was provided by the results of a study that randomized previously untreated high-risk MDS and CMML patients to receive three different regimens of decitabine. Of 95 patients, 34% achieved CR and 72% had an objective response. The CR rate was highest in the 5-day intravenous regimen (39%). The study included 18 patients with CMML, of which 9 (50%) achieved a CR, and three additional patients had objective hematologic responses. The estimated 18-month survival rate was 57% (119). These results in CMML are superior to those in any other study of hypomethylating agents in this disease and compare well with those obtained with single-agent topotecan (105, 120), topotecan–cytarabine combination therapy (121), or more intensive combination regimens used for treatment of AML (122). Patients were first evaluated for response after completion of three courses of therapy, and dose reduction and treatment delays were allowed only for grade 3–4 hematological toxicities. The median number of courses delivered was 6+, with a median number of three courses to response.

A summary of available data and response rates for CMML patients treated with various regimens of 5-azacytidine or decitabine is presented in Table 5.5. Given the limited experience with hypomethylating agents in CMML, the following findings are pertinent. At the present standard dose (110, 111), 5-azacytidine appears less myelosuppressive than decitabine as used in the pivotal study (117). It is also simpler to administer and, with a comparable response rate, it is less toxic (110). For optimal results with either drug, prolonged treatment for six to eight courses might be required. In CMML with organ involvement, a large tumor burden, and proliferative disease, decitabine is a more intensive treatment option, and the recent regimen (119) might offer a higher response rate and better control of disease. Frequent monitoring and extensive supportive care are required.

5.7.5 Drugs Targeting Fusion Tyrosine Kinases

Proliferation of hematopoietic cells expressing TEL/PDGFRβ fusion tyrosine kinase was inhibited in vitro by imatinib mesylate (123), suggesting a potential

Table 5.5 Summary of reported responses of patient with CMML to 5-azacytidine or decitabine

| Drug | No. of patients | Responses (%) | | | | |
		CR	PR	HI	Any	Ref.
5-azacytidine	19				3 (16)	110, 111
	6				1 (17)	117
Decitabine	9	1 (9)	1 (9)	2 (18)	4 (44)	116
	18	9 (50)			12 (67)	119

HI, hematological improvement

therapeutic benefit in patients with this abnormality. Hematological and cytogenetic remissions were achieved by treating patients harboring t(5;12) with a daily oral dose of 400 mg imatinib (57, 124, 125). A rapid normalization of leukocytosis, resolution of eosinophilia and conversion to normal karyotype were achieved after 3–36 weeks. In addition, in a patient with t(5;12)(q33, and unknown partner at q13), skin involvement also subsided in response to imatinib therapy (126). A similar response to imatinib by a patient with CMML expressing RAB5EP/PDGFRβ (126) and an aCML patient with H4/PDGFRβ (127) suggests that most, if not all, fusion protein kinases involving PDGFRβ might be susceptible to imatinib. The duration of the hematological, cytogenetic, and molecular responses is durable (128). In the United States., the use of imatinib at 400 mg/day has been approved for adults with MDS/MPD with PDGFRβ rearrangement and is the initial treatment of choice for these patients. Imatinib should be also considered as the initial treatment for patients with CMML and features associated with the rearrangement of PDGFRβ, such as eosinophilia, with or without monocytosis. In the absence of such abnormalities, empirical treatment of over 30 patients with CMML or aCML with imatinib mesylate yielded no responses (129, 130).

5.7.6   Farnesyl Transferase Inhibitors

With a central position downstream of growth factor receptors and a well-recognized role in malignancy (30), Ras proteins are attractive targets for drugs aimed at disrupting Ras functions. Ras proteins function only when attached to the cell membrane after farnesylation of the precursor proteins by farnesyl transferase. Inhibitors of farnesyl transferase, interfering with this process, such as tipifarnib (R115777; Zarnestra) and lonafarnib (SH66366; Sarasar) have been studied in phase I/II clinical trials. To date, a modest clinical activity of both drugs was observed in CMML and aCML. Of 10 CMML patients treated on a 3 weeks on, 1 week off schedule with daily oral doses of tipifarnib (600–900 mg divided in two doses), hematological improvement was noted in one patient and partial remission in two patients (131). A PR was reported in three of seven patients with aCML and none of two with CMML (132). In a preliminary report of an international study, 82 patients with MDS, including 19 CMML patients, were treated orally, twice daily with near-maximum tolerated doses (MTDs) of tipifarnib. Responses were not given separately for CMML, but the reported medium survival of 15 months for CMML patients is short for a significant clinical benefit (133). In a phase II study, 35 patients with CMML were treated with lonafarnib (200–300 mg orally twice daily; MTD = 200 mg twice daily) until disease progression or unacceptable toxicity. One complete and 7 hematological improvements in 25 evaluable CMML patients were reported (134). With both agents, the response rates in CMML are low and their duration appears short. As in AML (135), with the activity independent of Ras mutational status and of the inhibition of farnesyl transferase (131, 135), the target (s) of these drugs remain elusive. Although these oral agents might hold some promise in CMML, their use as single agents will likely be limited.

5.7.7 Intensive Chemotherapy

Initial experience with intensive chemotherapy originated in occasional inclusion of CMML in the trials of AML, with regimens based on cytosine arabinoside plus other agent(s) and biased toward the treatment of younger patients (136). The experience with intensive chemotherapy has been recently reviewed in detail (137). The largest clinical trial used topotecan and intermediate-dose cytarabine and initially included 27 CMML patients, of which 44% achieved a CR, the majority after one course of therapy (121). The results were later verified in an extended cohort of 39 patients (122). The presence of an abnormal karyotype was not important in achieving a CR. In most such patients, conversion to diploid status was observed (121, 122). The CR rate was higher in patients with <5% bone marrow blasts. The median remission duration was 33 weeks and the median overall survival was 42 weeks (121). Patients who achieved a CR had longer survival than those who did not, but this might be related to the natural history of the disease. To date, there is no convincing evidence that intensive chemotherapy is curative in more than a few patients. A positive impact of intensive chemotherapy on overall survival has yet to be shown in larger trials. A review of various treatment regimens indicates that an intensification of treatment leads to increased morbidity and mortality without a documented survival benefit (122). With the availability of effective single agents such as decitabine, the use of intensive chemotherapy might be limited. Well-tolerated and effective regimens (121) might be considered in younger patients with aggressive disease and extensive organ involvement or in patients with progressive disease that failed to respond to therapy with hypomethylating agents, particularly those awaiting SCT. Induction of complete remission or cytoreduction prior to SCT might reduce the relapse rate after allogeneic SCT in patients with high-risk CMML, and this approach deserves further investigation, preferably in the setting of a clinical trial.

5.7.8 Allogeneic Stem Cell Transplantation

Allogeneic SCT is the only well-documented curative treatment for CMML. The experience remains limited, however, mainly because of the age distribution of CMML patients and lack of a focused approach to CMML as a distinct clinical entity. The reported results must be interpreted cautiously because of the small numbers of patients, variations in patient characteristics, likely selection bias, and use of different conditioning regimens in either matched related or unrelated as well as partially mismatched donors. Overall, the results are still disappointing, with the most significant problem being a high relapse rate (138–140). In the largest reported cohort of 50 adult patients with a median age of 44 years, the 5-year estimated overall and disease-free survival rates were 21% and 16%, respectively. The probability of relapse was 61%, and it was higher in patients without graft versus host disease. No variables were significantly associated with outcome, with the exception of the favorable influence of transplantation soon after diagnosis (138). Slightly better results were reported in a smaller group of 21 patients consisting of both adults and children (139), in which the cumulative relapse rate was 25% at 3 years. In 43 patients with childhood CMML, the 5-year event-free survival rate was 31%, but a 48% relapse rate (141). These results in patients conditioned with myeloablative regimens indicate that although the treatment is feasible in selected patients, it is curative in fewer than one-third, and resistant disease remains a major obstacle. In addition to the improved, risk-based selection of patients, new approaches such as attempting to induce remission or cytoreduction by chemotherapy prior to transplant might improve outcome. Based on the experience with both single-agent and combination chemotherapy, this approach should be safe as well.

Reduced-intensity conditioning regimens that allow full engraftment while significantly reducing toxicity (142–144) offer a new treatment modality in CMML and extend the SCT option to older patients. Cytoreductive chemotherapy prior to stem cell transplantation and posttransplant maintenance with, for example, 5-azacytidine are alternative strategies currently under investigation.

5.8   Future Directions

To optimize and possibly individualize treatment, it is important to improve and validate risk assessments and use a risk score for assignment to clinical trials, paying specific attention to improvement in quality of life in elderly patients with low-risk disease unlikely to affect life expectancy. Continuing efforts to optimize the use of currently available active agents, alone or in combination, should be accompanied by an evaluation of new agents for both clinical and biological activities. An effort should be made to treat patients in the setting of clinical trials. Given the rarity of the disease, cooperative trials would be advantageous. An effective evaluation will require improvement of response criteria, based on, for example, International Working Group (IWG) criteria for MDS, expanded to include response of extramedullary disease and monitoring of cytogenetic and molecular response in CMML with abnormal karyotype and/or molecular markers such as PDGFRβ rearrangement. Most important will be the search for molecular abnormalities present in variants or different stages of the disease, the correlation of new findings with known laboratory and clinical features, and the responses to established and investigational therapies.

Establishment of detailed databases should further facilitate continuous evaluation of the importance of disease features in the response to therapeutic modalities and patient outcomes.

References

1. Bennett JM, Catovsky D, Daniel MT, et al. Proposals for the classification of the myelodysplastic syndromes. Br J Haematol 1982;51:189–199.
2. Bennett JM, Catovsky D, Daniel TM, et al. The chronic myeloid leukaemias: guidelines for distinguishing chronic granulocytic, atypical chronic myeloid, and chronic myelomonocytic leukaemia. Proposals by the French-American-British Cooperative Leukaemia Group. Br J Haematol 1994;87:746–54.
3. Greenberg P, Cox C, Le Beau MM, et al. International scoring system for evaluating prognosis in myelodysplastic syndromes. Blood 1997;89:2079–2088.
4. Onida F, Kantarjian HM, Smith TL, et al. Prognostic factors and scoring systems in chronic myelomonocytic leukemia: a retrospective analysis of 213 patients. Blood 2002;99:840–849.
5. Germing U, Kundgen A, Gattermann N. Risk assessment in chronic myelomonocytic leukemia (CMML). Leuk Lymphoma 2004; 45:1311–1318.
6. Vardiman JW, Harris NL, Banning R. The World Health Organization (WHO) classification of the myeloid neoplasms. Blood 2002;100:2292–2302.
7. Pedersen-Bjergaard J, Pedersen M, Roulston D, et al. Different genetic pathways in leukemogenesis for patients presenting with therapy-related myelodysplasia and therapy-related acute myeloid leukemia. Blood 1995;86:3542–3552.
8. Beran M, Wen S, Shen Y, et al. Prognostic factors and risk assessment in chronic myelomonocytic leukemia: validation study of the M.D. Anderson Prognostic Scoring System. Leuk Lymphoma 2007;48:1150–1160.
9. Fenaux P, Beuscart R, Lai JL, et al. Prognostic factors in adult chronic myelomonocytic leukemia: an analysis of 107 cases. J Clin Oncol 1988;6:1417–1424.
10. Felzmann T, Gisslinger H, Krieger O, et al. Immunophenotypic characterization of myelomonocytic cells in patients with myelodysplastic syndrome.Br J Haematol 1993;84:428–435.
11. Beran M, Shen Y, Onida F, et al. Prognostic significance of monocytosis in patients with myeloproliferative disorders. Leuk Lymphoma 2006;47:417–423
12. Tefferi A, Elliot MA, Pardanani A. Atypical myeloproliferative disorders: diagnosis and management. Mayo Clin Proc 2006;81:553–563.
13. Galton DA. Hematological differences between chronic granulocytic leukemia, atypical chronic myeloid leukemia and chronic myelomonocytic leukemia. Leuk Lymphoma 1992;7:343–350.
14. Nosslinger T, Reisner R, Gruner H, et al. Dysplastic versus proliferative CMML: a retrospective analysis of 91 patients from a single institution. Leuk Res 2001;25:741–747.
15. Germing U, Gattermann N, Minning H, et al. Problems in the classification of CMML: dysplastic versus proliferative type. Leuk Res 1998;22:871–878.
16. Onida F, Beran M. Chronic myelomonocytic leukemia: myeloproliferative variant. Curr Hematol Rep 2004;3:218–226.
17. Voglova J, Chrobak L, Neuwirtova R, et al. Myelodysplastic and myeloproliferative type of chronic myelomonocytic leukemia: distinct subgroups or two stages of the same disease? Leuk Res 2001;25:493–499.
18. Cervera J, Sanz GF, Vallespi T, et al. Does WBC count really define two different subtypes of chronic myelomonocytic leukemia (CMML)? Analysis of a series of 119 patients (Abstract). Leukemia Res 1997;21:7.
19. Rigolin GM, Cuneo A, Roberti MG, et al. Myelodysplastic syndromes with monocytic component: hematologic and cytogenetic characterization. Haematologica 1997;82:25–30.
20. Cuneo A, Tomasi P, Ferrari L, et al. Cytogenetic analysis of different cellular populations in chronic myelomonocytic leukemia. Cancer Genet Cytogenet 1989;37:29–37.
21. Fugazza G, Bruzzone R, Dejana AM, et al. Cytogenetic clonality in chronic myelomonocytic leukemia studied with fluorescence in situ hybridization. Leukemia 1995;9:109–114.

22. Geissler K, Ohler L, Fodinger M, et al. Interleukin 10 inhibits growth and granulocyte/ macrophage colony-stimulating factor production in chronic myelomonocytic leukemia cells. J Exp Med 1996;184:1377–1384.
23. Everson MP, Brown CB, Lilly MB. Interleukin-6 and granulocyte-macrophage colony-stimulating factor are candidate growth factors for chronic myelomonocytic leukemia cells. Blood 1989;74:1472–1476.
24. Ramshaw HS, Bardy PG, Lee MA, et al. Chronic myelomonocytic leukemia requires granulocyte-macrophage colony-stimulating factor for growth *in vitro* and *in vivo*. Exp Hematol 2002;30:1124–1131.
25. Dresh C, Faille A, Poirier O. Bone marrow cell kinetic and culture in chronic and subacute myelomonocytic leukemia. Physiopathological interpretation and prognostic importance. Leuk Res 1979;4:129–133.
26. Yuo A, Miyazono K, Takaku F. Characterization of granulocyte-macrophage colony formation in chronic myelomonocytic leukemia: a comparative study with other myelodysplastic and myeloproliferative disorders. Jpn J Cancer Res 1990;81:820–826.
27. Cambier N, Baruchel A, Schlageter MH, et al. Chronic myelomonocytic leukemia: from biology to therapy. Hematol Cell Ther 1997;39:41–48.
28. Oscier DG, Worsley A, Darlow S, et al. Correlation of bone marrow colony growth in the myelodysplastic syndromes with the FAB classification and the Bournemouth score. Leuk Res 1989;13:833–839.
29. Ugo V, Marzac C, Teyssandier I, et al. Multiple signaling pathways are involved in erythropoietin-independent differentiation of erythroid progenitors in polycythemia vera. Exp Hematol 2004;32:179–187.
30. Emanuel PD, Bates LJ, Castleberry RP, et al. Selective hypersensitivity to granulocyte-macrophage colony-stimulating factor by juvenile chronic myeloid leukemia hematopoietic progenitors. Blood 1991;77:925–929.
31. Shanon KM, LeBeau MM, Largaespada DA, et al. Modelling myeloid leukemia tumor suppressor gene inactivation in the mouse. Am J Med Genet 1999;89:14–22.
32. Le DT, Shannon KM. Ras processing as a therapeutic target in hematological malignancies. Curr Opin Hematol 2002;9:308–315.
33. Akashi K, Shibuya T, Harada M, et al. Interleukine 4 suppresses the spontaneous growth of chronic myelomonocytic leukemia cells. J Clin Invest 1991:88;223–230.
34. Everson MP, Brown CB, Lilly MB. Interleukin-6 and granulocyte-macrophage colony-stimulating factor are candidate growth factors for chronic myelomonocytic leukemia cells. Blood 1989;74:1472–1476.
35. Berkowicz M, Rosner E, Rechavi G, et al. Atypical chronic myelomonocytic leukemia with eosinophilia and translocation (5;12): a new association. Cancer Genet Cytogenet 1991;51:277–278.
36. Wessels JW, Fibbe WE, van der Keur D, et al. t(5;12)(q31;p12). A clinical entity with features of both myeloid leukemia and chronic myelomonocytic leukemia. Cancer Genet Cytogenet 1993;65:7–11.
37. Golub TR, Barker GF, Lovett M, et al. Fusion of PDGF receptor β to a novel ets-like gene, tel, in chronic myelomonocytic leukemia with t(5;12) chromosomal translocation. Cell 1994;77:307–316.
38. Carrol M, Tomasson MH, Barker GF, et al. The TEL/platelet-derived growth factor beta receptor (PDGFbeta R) fusion in chronic myelomonocytic leukemia is a transforming protein that self-associates and activates PDGFbeta R kinase-dependent signaling pathways. Proc Natl Acad Sci USA 1996;93:14,845–14,850.
39. Abe A, Emi N, Tanimoto M, et al. Fusion of the platelet-derived growth factor receptor beta to a novel gene CEV14 in acute myelogenous leukemia after clonal evolution. Blood 1997;90:4271–4277.
40. Ross TS, Bernard OA, Berger R, et al.: Fusion of Huntingtin interacting protein 1 to platelet-derived growth factor beta receptor (PDGFbR) in chronic myelomonocytic leukemia with t(5;7)(q33;q11.2). Blood 1998;91:4419–4426.

41. Kulkermi S, Heath C, Parker S, et al. Fusion of H4/D10S170 to the platelet-derived growth factor receptor beta in BCR-ABL-negative myeloproliferative disorders with a t(5;10)(q33;q21). Cancer Res 2000;60:3592–3598.

42. Schwaller J, Anastasiadou E, Cain D, et al. H4(D10S170), a gene frequently rearranged in papillary thyroid carcinoma, is fused to the platelet-derived growth factor receptor beta gene in atypical chronic myeloid leukemia with t(5;10)(q33;q22). Blood 2001; 97:3910–3918.

43. Magnusson MK, Meade KE, Brown KE, et al. Rabaptin-5 is a novel fusion partner to platelet-derived growth factor beta receptor in chronic myelomonocytic leukemia. Blood 2001;98:2518–2525.

44. Wilkinson K, Velloso ER, Lopes LF, et al. Cloning of the t(1;5)(q23;q33) in a myeloproliferative disorder associated with eosinophilia: Involvement of PDGFRbeta and response to imatinib. Blood 2003;102:4187–4190.

45. Vizmanos JL, Novo FJ, Roman JP, et al. NIN, a gene encoding a CEP110-like centrosomal protein, is fused to PDGFRbeta in a patient with a t(5;14)(q33;q24) and in an imatinib-responsive myeloproliferative disorder. Cancer Res 2004;64:2673–2676.

46. Moreiro C, Acquila M, Rosanda C, et al. HCMOGT-1 is a novel fusion partner to PDGFRbeta in juvenile myelomonocytic leukemia with t(5;17)(q33;p11.2). Cancer Res 2004;64:2649–2651.

47. Levine RL, Wadleigh M, Sternberg DW, et al. KIAA1509 is a novel PDGFRbeta fusion partner in imatinib-responsive myeloproliferative disease associated with a t(5;14)(q33;q32). Leukemia 2005;19:27–30.

48. Grant FH, Burgstaller S, Kuhr T, et al. p53-Binding protein 1 is fused to the platelet-derived growth factor receptor beta in a patient with a t(5;15)(q22;q22) and an imatinib-responsive eosinophilic myeloproliferative disorder. Cancer Res 2004;64:7216–7219.

49. Cross NC, Reiter A. Tyrosine kinase fusion genes in chronic myeloproliferative diseases. Leukemia 2002;16:1207–1212.

50. Baxter EJ, Hochhaus A, Bolufer P, et al. The t(4;22)(q12;q11) in atypical chronic myeloid leukaemia fuses BCR to PDGFRalpha. Hum Mol Genet 2002;11:1391–1397.

51. Peeters, P, Raynaud, SD, Cools, J, et al. Fusion of TEL, the ETS-variant gene 6 (ETV6), to the receptor-associated kinase *JAK2* as a result of t(9;12) in a lymphoid and t(9;15;12) in a myeloid leukemia. Blood 1997;90:2535–2540.

52. Reiter A, Walz C, Watmore A, et al. The t(8;9)(p22;p24) is a recurrent abnormality in chronic and acute leukemia that fuses PCM1 to JAK2. Cancer Res 2005;65:2662–2667.

53. Fenaux P, Jouet JP, Zandecki M, et al. Chronic and subacute myelomonocytic leukemia in the adult: a report of 60 cases with special reference to prognostic factors. Br J Haematol. 1987;65:101–106.

54. Groupe Francais de Cytogenetique Hematologique. Cytogenetics of chronic myelomonocytic leukemia. Cancer Genet Cytogenet 1986;21:11–30.

55. Groupe Francais de Cytogenetique Hematologique. Chronic myelomonocytic leukemia: single entity or heterogenous disorder? A prospective multicenter study of 100 patients. Cancer Genet Cytogenet 1991;55:57–65.

56. Sole F, Espinet B, Sanz GF, et al. Incidence, characterization and prognostic significance of chromosomal abnormalities in 640 patients with primary myelodysplastic syndromes. Grupo Cooperativo Espanol de Citogenetica Hematologica. Br J Haematol 2000;108:346–356.

57. Gunby RH, Camzzaniga G, Tassi E et al. Sensitivity to imatinib but low frequency of TEL/PDGFRbeta fusion protein in chronic myelomonocytic leukemia. Haematologica 2003;88:408–415.

58. Onida F, Glassman A, Estey E et al. Cytogenetics of CMML and Ph-negative CML: a retrospective analysis and comparison with MDS. Blood 1999;84(Suppl 1):273.

59. Onida F, Ball G, Kantarjian HM, et al. Characteristics and outcome of patients with Philadelphia chromosome negative, bcr/abl negative chronic myelogenous leukemia. Cancer 2002;95:1673–1684.

60. Frohling S, Scholl C, Gilliland DG, et al. Genetics of myeloid malignancies: pathogenetic and clinical implications. J Clin Oncol 2005;23:6285–6295.

61. Tsurumi S, Nakamura Y, Maki K, et al. N-ras and p53 gene mutations in Japanese patients with myeloproliferative disorders. Am J Hematol 2002;71:131–133.

62. Janssen JW, Steenvoorden AC, Lyons J, et al. RAS gene mutations in acute and chronic myelocytic leukemias, chronic myeloproliferative disorders, and myelodysplastic syndromes. Proc Natl Acad Sci USA 1987;84:9228–9232.

63. Padua RA, Carter G, Hughes D, et al. RAS mutations in myelodysplasia detected by amplification, oligonucleotide hybridization, and transformation. Leukemia 1988;2:503–510.

64. Collins SJ, Howard M, Andrews DF, et al. Rare occurrence of N-ras point mutations in Philadelphia chromosome positive chronic myeloid leukemia. Blood 1989;73:1028–1032.

65. Hirsch-Ginsberg C, LeMaistre AC, Kantarjian H, et al. RAS mutations are rare events in Philadelphia chromosome-negative/ bcr gene rearrangement-negative chronic myelogenous leukemia, but are prevalent in chronic myelomonocytic leukemia. Blood 1990,76: 1214–1219.

66. Onida F, Kantarjian HM, Ball G, et al. The dysplastic versus proliferative classification dilemma of chronic myelomonocytic leukemia: a retrospective single institution analysis of 273 patients. Blood 2001;98:11(Suppl 1):2607.

67. Onida F, Gatto S, Scappini B, et al. Significance of ras point mutations for prognosis and response to treatment in chronic myelomonocytic leukemia: analysis of 112 patients. Proc Am Soc Clin Oncol 2002;20:abstr 1048.

68. Shih LY, Huang CF, Wang PN, et al. Acquisition of FLT3 or N-ras mutations is frequently associated with progression of myelodysplastic syndrome to acute myeloid leukemia. Leukemia 2004;18:466–475.

69. Ricci C, Onida F, Fermo E, et al. Acquisition of RAS mutations contributes to progression of CMML from the dysplastic to the proliferative variant. Abstract, AACR 2007; in press.

70. Weiss B, Bollag G, Shannon K. Hyperactive Ras as a therapeutic target in neurofibromatosis type 1. Am J Med Genet 1999;89:14–22.

71. Shannon K M, LeBeau M M, Largaespada DA, et al. Modelling myeloid leukemia tumor suppressor gene inactivation in the mouse. Semin Cancer Biol 2001;11:191–200.

72. Lu D, Nounou R, Beran M, et al. The prognostic significance of bone marrow levels of neurofibromatosis-1 protein and RAS oncogene mutations in patients with acute myelogenous leukemia and myelodysplastic syndrome. Cancer 2003;97:441–449.

73. Tartaglia M, Niemeyer CM, Fragale A, et al. Somatic mutations in PTPN11 in juvenile myelomonocytic leukemia, myelodysplastic syndromes and acute myeloid leukemia. Nat Genet 2003;34:148–150.

74. Tartaglia M, Niemeyer CM, Shannon KM, et al. SHP-2 and myeloid malignancies. Curr Opin Hematol 2004;11:44–50.

75. Loh ML, Martinelli S, Cordeddu V, et al. Acquired PTPN11 mutations occur rarely in adult patients with myelodysplastic syndromes and chronic myelomonocytic leukemia. Leuk Res 2005;29:459–462.

76. Johan MF, Bowen DT, Frew ME, et al. Mutations in *PTPN11* are uncommon in adult myelodysplastic syndromes and acute myeloid leukaemia. Br J Haematol 2004;124:843–844.

77. James C, Ugo V, Le Couedic JP, et al. A unique clonal JAK2 mutation leading to constitutive signalling causes polycythaemia vera. Nature 2005;434:1144–1148.

78. Levine RL, Loriaux M, Huntley BJP et al. The JAK2V617F activating mutation occurs in chronic myelomonocytic leukemia and acute myelogenous leukemia, but not in acute lymphoblastic leukemia or chronic lymphocytic leukemia. Blood 2005;106:3377–3379.

79. Steensma DP, Dewald GW, Lasho TL, et al. The JAK2 V617F activating tyrosine kinase mutation is an infrequent event in both atypical myeloproliferative disorders and the myelodysplastic syndrome. Blood 2005;106:1207–1209.

80. Jelinek J, Oki Y, Gharibzan V, et al. JAK2 mutation 1849>T is rare in acute leukemias but can be found in CMML, Philadelphia chromosome-negative CML, and megakaryocytic leukemia. Blood 2005;106:3370–3373.

81. Parganas E, Wang D, Stravopodis D, et al. JAK2 is essential for signaling through a variety of cytokine receptors. Cell 1998;93:385–395.

82. Stirewalt DL, Radich JP. The role of FLT3 in haematopoietic malignancies. Nat Rev Cancer 2003;3:650–665.
83. Kiyoi H, Naoe T, Nakano Y, et al. Prognostic implication of FLT3 and N-RAS gene mutations in acute myeloid leukemia. Blood 1999;93:3074–3080.
84. Frohling S, Schlenk RF, Breitruck J, et al. Prognostic significance of activating FLT3 mutations in younger adults (16 to 60 years) with acute myeloid leukemia and normal cytogenetics: a study of the AML Study Group Ulm. Blood 2002;100:4372–4380.
85. Kottaridis PD, Gale RE, Frew ME, et al. The presence of a FLT3 internal tandem duplication in patients with acute myeloid leukemia (AML) adds important prognostic information to cytogenetic risk group and response to the first cycle of chemotherapy: Analysis of 854 patients from the United Kingdom Medical Research Council AML 10 and 12 trials. Blood 2001;98:1752–1759.
86. Whitman SP, Archer KJ, Feng L, et al. Absence of the wild-type allele predicts poor prognosis in adult de novo acute myeloid leukemia with normal cytogenetics and the internal tandem duplication of FLT3: A cancer and leukemia group B study. Cancer Res 2001;61: 7233–7239.
87. Beran M, Luthra R, Kantarlian H, et al. FLT3 mutation and response to intensive chemotherapy in young adult and elderly patients with normal karyotype. Leuk Res 2004;28: 547–550.
88. Schnittger S, Schoch C, Dugas M, et al. Analysis of FLT3 length mutations in 1003 patients with acute myeloid leukemia: correlation to cytogenetics, FAB subtype, and prognosis in the AMLCG study and usefulness as a marker for the detection of minimal residual disease. Blood 2002;100:59–66.
89. Thiede C, Steudel C, Mohr B, et al. Analysis of FLT3-activating mutations in 979 patients with acute myelogenous leukemia: association with FAB subtypes and identification of subgroups with poor prognosis. Blood 2002;99:4326–4335.
90. Santini V, Kantarjian HM, Issa JP. Changes in DNA methylation in neopasia: pathophysiology and therapeutic implications. Ann Intern Med 2001;134:573–586.
91. Jones PA,Baylin SB. The fundamental role of epigenetic events in cancer. Natl Rev Genet 2002;3:415–428.
92. Leone G, Teofili L,Voso MT, et al. DNA methylation and demethylating drugs in myelodysplastic syndromes and secondary leukemias. Haematologica 2002;87:1324–1341.
93. Aggerholm A, Holm MS, Guldberg P, et al. Promoter hypermethylation of p15^{INK4B}, HIC1, CDH1, and ER is frequent in myelodysplastic syndrome and predicts poor prognosis in earlystage patients. Eur J Haematol 2005;10:1–10.
94. Johan MF, Bowen DT, Frew ME, et al. Aberrant methylation of the negative regulators RASSFIA, SHP-1 and SOCS-1 in myelodysplastic syndromes and acute myeloid leukaemia. Br J Haematol 2005;129:60–65.
95. Shang JW, Ming Y, Wen-Chien C. Clinical implication of SOC1 methylation in myelodysplastic syndrome. Br J Haematol 2006;135:317–323.
96. Tessema M, Langer F, Dingemann J, et al. Aberrant methylation and impaired expression of the p15(INK4b) cell cycle regulatory gene in chronic myelomonocytic leukemia (CMML). Leukemia 2003;17:910–918.
97. Worsley A, Oscier DG, Stevens J, et al. Prognostic features of chronic myelomonocytic leukaemia: a modified Bournemouth score gives the best prediction of survival. Br J Haematol 1988;68:17–21.
98. Aul C, Gattermann N, Heyll A, et al. Primary myelodysplastic syndromes: analysis of prognostic factors in 235 patients and proposals for an improved scoring system. Leukemia 1992;6:52–59.
99. Aul C, Gattersman N, Germing U, et al. Risk assessment in primary myelodysplastic syndromes: validation of the Dusseldorf score. Leukemia 1994;8:1906–1913.
100. Germing U, Strupp C, Aivado M, et al. New prognostic parameters for chronic myelomonocytic leukemia. Blood 2002;100:731–733.
101. Cox DR. Regression models and life tables (with discussion). J Stat Soc 1972;34:187–220.

102. Kerridge I, Spencer A, Azzi A, et al. Response to erythropoietin in chronic myelomonocytic leukaemia. Intern Med J 2001;31:371–2.
103. Wattel E, Guerci A, Hecquet B, et al. A randomized trial of hydroxyurea versus vp16 in adult chronic myelomonocytic leukemia. Blood 1996;88:2480–2487.
104. Beran M, Kantarjian H, O'Brien S, et al. Topotecan, a topoisomerase I inhibitor, is active in the treatment of myelodysplastic syndrome and chronic myelomonocytic leukemia. Blood 1996;88:2473–2479.
105. Beran M, O'Brien S, Thomas DA, et al. Phase I study of prolonged administration of oral topotecan in hematological malignancies. Clin Cancer Res 2003;9:4084–4091.
106. Cortes J, O'Brien S, Beran M, et al. Efficacy of topoisomerase I inhibitor 9-nitro-20-S campthotecin (9-NC, RFS 2000) in chronic myelomonocytic leukemia (CMML) and high-risk myelodysplastic syndromes (MDS) Blood 98;2001,621a.
107. Raza M, Meyer P, Dutt D, et al. Thalidomide produces transfusion independence in ilongstanding refractory anemias of patients with myelodysplastic syndromes. Blood 2001;98: 958–965.
108. Silverman LR, Holland JF, Demakos EP, et al. Azacytidine in myelodysplastic syndromes: CALGB studies 8421 and 8921. Ann Hematol 1994;68:A12.
109. Siverman LR, Demakos EP, Weinberg AS, et al. Effects of treatment with 5-azacytidine on the in vivo and in vitro hematopoiesis in patients with myelodysplastic syndromes. Leukemia 1993;7(Suppl 1):21–29.
110. Silverman LR, Demakos EP, Peterson BL, et al. Randomized controlled trial of azacitidine in patients with the myelodysplastic syndrome: a study of the cancer and leukemia group B. J Clin Oncol 2002;20:2429–2440.
111. Kaminskas E, Farrell A, Abraham S, et al. Approval summary: azacytidine for treatment of myelodysplastic syndrome subtypes. Clin Cancer Res 2005;11:3604–3608.
112. Attadia V, Pinto A, Colombatti A. Stepwise induction of differentiation of the U937 cell line by 5,Aza-2'-deoxycitidine. Exp Hematol 1988;16:474–477.
113. Pinto A, Attadia V, Fusco A, et al. 5-Aza-2,-deoxycytidine induces terminal differentiation of leukemic blasts from patients with acute myeloid leukemias. Blood 1984;64:922–929.
114. Zagonel V, Lo Re G, Marotta G, et al. 5,-Aza-2,-deoxycitidine (Decitabine) induces trilineage response in unfavorable myelodysplastic syndrome. Leukemia 1993;7(Suppl 1); 9–16.
115. Wijermans PW, Krulder JWM, Huijgens PC, et al. Continuous infusion of low dose 5-aza-2 deoxycitidine in elderly patients with high-risk myelodysplastic syndrome. Leukemia 1997;11:1–5.
116. Wijermans P, Lubbet M, Verhoef G, et al. Low-dose 5-ara-2 -deoxycitidine, a DNA hypomethylating agent, for the treatment of high risk myelodysplastic syndrome: a multicenter phase II study in elderly patients. J Clin Oncol 2000;18:956–962.
117. Kantarjian H, Issa JP, Rosenfeld CS, et al. Decitabine improves patient outcomes in myelodysplastic syndromes: results of a phase III randomized study. Cancer 2006;106: 1794–1803.
118. Issa JP, Garcia-Manero G, Giles FJ, et al. Phase I study of low-dose prolonged exposure schedules of the hypomethylating agent 5-aza-2 -deoxycitidine (decitabine) in hematopoeitic malignancies. Blood 2004;103:1635–1640.
119. Kantarjian H, Oki Y, Garcia-Manero G, et al. Results of a randomized study of three schedules of low-dose decitabine in higher risk myelodysplastic syndrome and chronic myelomonocytic leukemia. Blood 2007;109:52–57.
120. Beran M, Estey E, O'Brien S, et al. Results of topotecan single agent therapy in patients with myelodysplastic syndromes and chronic myelomonocytic leukemia. Leuk Lymphoma 1998;31:521–531.
121. Beran M, Estey E, O'Brien S, et al. Topotecan and cytarabine is an active combination regimen in myelodysplastic syndromes and chronic myelomonocytic leukemia. J Clin Oncol 1999;17:2819–2830.
122. Beran M, Onida F, Cortes JE, et al. Chemotherapy of increasing intensity in the treatment of chronic myelomonocytic leukemia. Blood 2001;98:abstr 624a.

123. Carroll M, Ohno-Jones S, Tamura S, et al. CGP 57148, a tyrosine kinase inhibitor, inhibits the growth of cells expressing BCR-ABL, TEL-ABL, and TEL-PDGFR fusion proteins. Blood 1997;90:4947–4952.

124. Apperley JF, Gardembas M, Melo JV, et al. Response to imatinib mesylate in patients with chronic myeloproliferative diseases with rearrangements of the platelet-derived growth factor receptor beta. N Engl J Med 2002;347:481–487.

125. Pitini V, Arrigo C, Teti G, et al. Response to STI571 in chronic myelomonocytic leukemia with platelet derived growth factor beta receptpr involvement: a new case report. Haematologica 2003;88:ECR18.

126. Magnusson MK, Meade KE, Nakamura R, et al. Activity of STI571 in chronic myelomonocytic leukemia with a platelet-derived growth factor beta receptor fusion oncogene. Blood 2002;100:1088–1091.

127. Garcia JL, Font de Mora J, Hernandez JH, et al. Imatinib mesylate elicits positive clinical response in atypical chronic myeloid leukemia involving platelet-derived growth factor receptor beta. Blood 2003;102:2699–2700.

128. David M, Cross NCP, Burgstaller S, et al. Durable responses to imatinib in patients with PDGFRB fusiongene-positive and BCR-ABL-negative chronic myeloproliferative disorders. Blood 2007;109:61–64.

129. Cortes J, Giles F, O'Brien S, et al. Results of imatinib mesylate therapy in patients with refractory or recurrent acute myeloid leukemia, high risk myelodysplastic syndrome, and myeloproliferative disorders. Cancer 2003;97:2760–2766.

130. Raza A, Lisak L, Dutt D, et al. Gleevac (imatinib mesylate) in 16 patients with chronic myelomonocytic leukemia (CMMoL). Blood 2000;96(Suppl 1):abstr 4829.

131. Kurzrock R, Kantarjian H, Cortes JE, et al. Farnesyl transferase inhibitor R115777 in myelodysplastic syndrome: clinical and biological activities in the phase I setting. Blood 2003;102:4527–4534.

132. Gotlib J, Loh M, Vattikuti S, et al. Phase I/II Zarnestra™ (farnesyl transferase inhibitor (FTI) R11577, Tipifarnib) in patients with myeloproliferative disorders (MPDs): preliminary results. Blood 2002;100:abstr 3153.

133. Kurzrock R, Fenaux P, Raza A, et al. High Risk myelodysplastic syndrome (MDS): first result of international Phase 2 study with oral farnesyl transferase inhibitor R22577 (Zarnestra™). Blood 2004;104:abstr 68.

134. Feldman E, Cortes J, Holyoake T, et al. Continuous oral Lonafarnib (Sarasar™) for the treatment of patients with myelodysplastic syndrome. Blood 2003;102:abstr 1531.

135. Karp JE, Lancet JE, Kaufmann SH, et al. Clinical and biologic activity of the farnesyltransferase inhibitor R115777 in adults with refractory and relapsed acute leukemias: a phase 1 clinical-laboratory correlative trial. Blood 2001;97:3361–3369.

136. Seymour J, Cortes J. Chronic myelomonocytic leukemia. In: Talpaz M, Kantarjian H, editors. Medical management of chronic myelogenous leukemia. New York: Marcel Dekker; 1999. p/ 43–48.

137. Beran M. Management of chronic myelomonocytic leukemia and other rare myeloproliferative disorders. In: Sekeres M, editor. Clinical malignant hematology; 2007. p. 487–502.

138. Kroger N, Zabelina T, Guardiola P, et al. Allogeneic stem cell transplantation of adult chronic myelomonocytic leukaemia. A report on behalf of the Chronic Leukaemia Working Party of the European Group for Blood and Marrow Transplantation (EBMT). Br J Haematol 2002;118:67–73.

139. Zang DY, Deeg HJ, Gooley T, et al. Treatment of chronic myelomonocytic leukaemia by allogeneic marrow transplantation. Br J Haematol 2000;110:217–222.

140. Mittal P, Saliba RM, Giralt SA, et al. Allogeneic transplantation: a therapeutic option for myelofibrosis, chronic myelomonocytic leukemia and Philadelphia-negative/BCR-ABL-negative chronic myelogenous leukemia. Bone Marrow Transplant 2004;33:1005–1009.

141. Locatelli F, Niemeyer C, Angelucci E, et al. Allogeneic bone marrow transplantation for chronic myelomonocytic leukemia in childhood: a report from the European Working Group on Myelodysplastic Syndrome in Childhood. J Clin Oncol 1997;15:566–573.

142. Alzea EP, Kim HT, Cutter C, et al. AML and MDS treated with nonmyeloablative stem cell transplantation: overall and progression-free survival comparable to myeloablative transplantation. Blood 2003;102:abstr 266.
143. Giralt S, Anagnastopoulos A, Shahjahauau M, et al. Nonablative stem cell transplantation for older patients with acute leukemias and myelodysplastic syndromes. Semin Hematol 2002;39:57–62.
144. Ho AY, Pagliuca A, Kenyon M, et al. Reduced-intensity allogeneic hematopoietic stem cell transplantation for myelodysplastic syndrome and acute myelogenous leukemia with multi-lineage dysplasia using flufarabin,busulphan, and alemtuzumab (FBC) conditioning. Blood 2004;104:1616–1623.

Chapter 6
The 5q– Syndrome

Aristoteles A.N. Giagounidis and Carlo Aul

6.1 Introduction

In 1956, Tjio and Levan (1) reported in a seminal observation that the correct number of chromosomes in human somatic cells was 46, not 48, as previously thought. Since then, an increasing number of malignant hematological diseases have been directly attributed to abnormalities of the number or the structure of these 46 chromosomes. The first of those disorders, of course, was chronic myeloid leukemia showing a balanced translocation of chromosomal material between chromosomes 9 and 22, reported by Nowell and Hungerford in 1960 (2). In 1973, Rowley identified the translocation t(8;21) in acute myeloid leukemia (AML), a genetic abnormality that today defines this subgroup of AML (3). One year later, in 1974, van den Berghe and colleagues reported three patients with long-standing refractory anemia, macrocytic erythrocyte indices, mild leucopenia, and normal to elevated platelet counts who showed a consistent deletion of the long arm of No. 5 chromosome (4). This disease—now called 5q– syndrome (pronounce 5q "minus" syndrome)—is classified within the myelodysplastic syndromes (MDS) and shares a number of their characteristics. The MDS are a group of bone marrow disorders derived from an abnormal hematopoietic progenitor cell (5). Because of a proliferation advantage, these abnormal stem cells have the ability to clonally expand, leading to the substitution of a variable part of normal bone marrow by malignant hematopoiesis. On the other hand, MDS are characterized by inappropriate activation of growth arrest signals that lead to a high proportion of proliferating cells finally undergoing programmed cell death (6). This impairment in cellular homeostasis explains the paradox of a hypercellular bone marrow and peripheral cytopenias often encountered in MDS. The MDS with a del(5q) chromosomal abnormality are unique because of their defining genetic lesion, their clinical and prognostic features, and their response to immunomodulatory treatments (IMiDs®). Particularly the new treatment options with IMiDs® are exciting, because they seem to target the malignant cell population independent of high-risk morphological or genetic features. This chapter will not only cover the 5q– syndrome itself, but it will also review other forms of MDS with del(5q) chromosomal abnormality that are important to the understanding of this puzzling disease.

6.2   Classification

Myelodysplastic syndromes are classified according to the French-American-British (FAB) or the newer World Health Organization (WHO) classifications (7, 8) (Tables 6.1 and 6.2). Although the WHO classification is becoming increasingly popular with hematologists, many current studies of new compounds in the field are still conceived on the basis of the FAB classification to ensure good comparability with previous investigations. Furthermore, the most widely used prognostic scoring index, the International Prognostic Scoring System (IPSS), is based on the FAB classification (Table 6.3). The FAB classification, of course, is a purely morphological system that categorizes the MDS in five different subtypes: Refractory anemia (RA), refractory anemia with ring sideroblasts (RARS), refractory anemia with excess blasts (RAEB), refractory anemia with excess blasts in transformation (RAEB-T), and chronic myelomonocytic leukemia (CMML). Accordingly, patients with a del(5q) chromosomal abnormality can be classified within the FAB system into any of those subgroups, depending on their bone marrow and peripheral blast count and the number of monocytic cells in the peripheral blood. Del(5q) abnormalities most often present as RA (67%) and rarely as RARS (14%), RAEB (17%), or RAEB-T (1%) (9). Exceptionally, del(5q) MDS might present as CMML (10). The FAB classification does not recognize the notion of 5q– syndrome and considerable confusion has arisen from this fact. Some physicians define the 5q– syndrome as a disease with the characteristics initially reported by van den Berghe (4) [i.e., macrocytic anemia, normal to elevated platelet counts, mild leucopenia, and an isolated deletion del(5q)]. Others use the term in a broader sense, including patients with additional chromosomal abnormalities and elevated blast counts. The WHO classification, instead, taking into account not only morphological but also cytogenetic and immunophenotypic findings of hematological diseases, defined a new entity within the MDS for del(5q) MDS. This classification narrows the notion of "myelodysplastic syndromes with chromosome 5 abnormality" to those patients who have an isolated deletion of del(5q) including bands q31 to q33 and displaying a blast count of <5% both in the bone marrow and the peripheral blood. Although this disease category is certainly helpful in recognizing the existence of a special subtype of MDS with del(5q) abnormality, the inclusion of patients

Table 6.1   The French-American-British classification of myelodysplastic syndromes (7)

Subtype	Blast percentage		Additional features
	Blood	Bone marrow	
Refractory anemia (RA)	<1%	<5%	
RA with ring sideroblasts (RARS)	<1%	<5%	>15% ring sideroblasts
RA with blast excess (RAEB)	<5%	5–20%	
RAEB in transformation (RAEB/T)	≥5%	21–30%	Optional Auer rods
Chronic myelomonocytic leukemia (CMML)	<5%	<20%	Peripheral monocytosis (>1000/µL)

Source. Ref. 7.

Table 6.2 Morphological classification of myelodysplastic syndromes (WHO classification) (8)

Subtype	Blast percentage		Additional features
	Blood	Bone marrow	
Refractory anemia (RA)	<1%	<5%	
RA with ring sideroblasts (RARS)	<1%	<5%	>15% ring sidero-blasts
Refractory cytopenia with multilineage dysplasia (RCMD)	<1%	<5%	Dysplasia >10% of bone marrow cells in ≥2 cell lineages
Refractory cytopenia with multilineage dysplasia and ring sideroblasts (RCMD-RS)	<1%	<5%	Dysplastic features in >10% of bone marrow cells in ≥ 2 cell lineages; >15% ring sideroblasts
Refractory anemia with blast excess (RAEB-I)	<5%	5–9%	
RAEB-II	5–19%	10–19%	Optional Auer rods
5q– Syndrome	<5%	<5%	
MDS, unclassified	<1%	<5%	Dysplasia exclusively in nonerythropoietic lineages

Table 6.3 International Prognostic Scoring System for evaluating prognosis in patients with myelodysplastic syndromes

Prognostic variable	Points				
	0	0.5	1	1.5	2.0
Bone marrow blasts (%)	<5	5–10	—	11–20	21–30
Number of cytopenias[a]	0–1	2–3	—	—	—
Cytogenetic category[b]	Good	Intermediate	Poor	—	—

Risk group	Score	Median survival (years)	25% AML transformation (years)[c]
Low	0	5.7	9.4
Intermediate-1	0.5–1	3.5	3.3
Intermediate-2	1.5–2.0	1.2	1.1
High	≥2.5	0.4	0.2

[a]Cytopenias defined as platelets < 100.000/µL; hemoglobin <10 g/dL; neutrophils <1800/µL.

[b]Good = normal karyotype, 5q–, 20q–, –Y; intermediate = other anomalies; poor = complex (≥3 abnormalities), chromosome 7 anomalies.

[c]Time interval for 25% of the patients to undergo evolution to acute myeloid leukemia.

with a peripheral blood blast count of up to 5% is inconsistent with the rest of the WHO MDS classification. Patients with <5% blasts in the peripheral blast count are considered to have RAEB-I, and it is unclear why patients with low (i.e., < 1%) and higher (i.e., <5%) peripheral blast counts should be grouped together in this special subgroup, as there is ample evidence that patients with del(5q) having a higher blast count (i.e., RAEB) have a worse overall survival than those with a bone marrow blast count <5% and a peripheral blast count <1% (11).

It becomes clear from those considerations that the MDS classification for del(5q) disease needs further improvement. A suggestion for a practical classification is given in Table 6.4. This suggestion is supported by several lines of evidence that are going to be discussed in detail in this chapter:

- Del(5q) is a recurrent chromosomal abnormality in MDS.
- Patients with an isolated del(5q) including bands q31 to q33 in conventional cytogenetic testing and a bone marrow blast count of <5% (and <1% in the peripheral blood) share common clinical, biological, and prognostic characteristics. The notion "5q– syndrome" should be restricted to this subgroup.
- The del(5q) chromosomal aberration occurs early in the development of the hematopoietic stem cell and further abnormalities are later events.
- Patients with additional chromosomal abnormalities have a worse prognosis than those with isolated del(5q).
- Del(5q) MDS patients with an elevated blast count have a worse outcome than those with a limited blast count.
- Del(5q) MDS cases can be effectively treated with IMiDs®, irrespective of additional chromosomal abnormalities or blast percentage.

Taking into account those basic characteristics, it becomes clear that patients sharing a del(5q) including bands q31 to q33 should be categorized as a subgroup of MDS, irrespective of their blast count or additional chromosomal abnormalities. Because of prognostic considerations in the *untreated* del(5q) patient cohort, those with an isolated del(5q) and a normal bone marrow and peripheral blast count should be considered as having the favorable 5q– syndrome. Patients with one additional abnormality but normal blast counts should be grouped into a separate category. Patients with two or more additional chromosomal aberrations (complex karyotype according to IPSS) have an ominous prognosis and should be included in a third group, irrespective of their blast counts, as this does not impact on their prognosis (12). Finally, patients with an increased bone marrow or peripheral blast count and isolated del(5q) or one additional abnormality should accordingly be grouped in another category (Table 6.4).

Table 6.4 A practical classification system for del(5q) MDS

Bone marrow blasts <5% or peripheral blasts <1%	Bone marrow blasts >5% or peripheral blasts >1%	Prognosis
Isolated del(5q) ("The 5q– syndrome")		Good
Del(5q) +1 abnormality		Intermediate
	Isolated del(5q) del(5q) + 1 abnormality	Bad
Del(5q) in association with a complex karyotype		Very bad

Note: A complex karyotype confers a very bad prognosis irrespective of the bone marrow blast count.

6.3   Clinical and Morphological Features

The median age of patients diagnosed with del(5q) MDS is around 70 years, however, patients as young as 30 years might occasionally be encountered (9). The male-to-female ratio has consistently been reported to be shifted to the female sex, with largest series reporting sex ratios between 1:1.6 and 1:5 (9, 13–15). In an analysis of 76 cases, the female preponderance was also found in patients with an increased medullary blast count (9). Both primary and secondary MDS have been identified bearing a del(5q) (9, 16). Usually, the disease is being diagnosed as refractory anemia according to FAB, but all other subtypes have been reported, exceptionally CMML (9, 10). The 5q– syndrome typically presents with macrocytic anemia, mild leukopenia, normal to elevated platelet counts, and erythroid hypoplasia in the bone marrow. Macrocytosis is not necessarily present in all cases; therefore, its presence or absence should not be used to define the "5q– syndrome." Also, a few cases might show erythroid hyperplasia in the bone marrow (9). Patients with a lower than normal platelet count in del(5q) MDS have greater chances to have advanced disease. More than half of those cases were shown to have an elevated blast cell percentage in the bone marrow (9). The morphological hallmark of the disease is the hypolobulation of megakaryocytes in the bone marrow. Those cells show typically one single round to oval nucleus and account for 30–80% of all megakaryocytes. These cells are not micromegakaryocytes because their size exceeds that of a promyelocyte by far. Still, true micromegakaryocytes might be found in del(5q) MDS in about one-third of cases (9). Apart from megakaryocytic dysplasia, morphological irregularities are not very prominent in the other myeloid lineages in the bone marrow. Therefore, if the dysplastic megakaryocytes are missed in cytology, the disease might not be recognized as MDS. For diagnosis with the microscope, low-power magnification reveals to be the most important aspect in diagnosis of del(5q) MDS.

6.4   Laboratory Values

The typical combination of the 5q– syndrome (i.e., female gender, macrocytic anemia, mild leukopenia, and normal to elevated platelet counts) occurs only in about one out of five patients with isolated 5q– deletion (11). Patients with a higher bone marrow blast count or additional abnormalities tend to have lower granulocyte and platelet counts. The reticulocyte count in del(5q) MDS is almost always reduced, even in patients with additional autoimmune hemolysis (17). Erythropoietin (EPO) levels in the syndrome are usually highly elevated, with a median value of 1000 U/L in a series of 60 patients (11). We have seen patients with EPO levels up to 5500 U/L. Interestingly, because all del(5q) patients eventually become transfusion dependent and many are diagnosed a considerable time after their first transfusion, ferritin levels at the time of diagnosis are often elevated. The median value in 41 patients was found to be 540 ng/mL with a range from 37 to 4830 (11).

6.5   Cytogenetics

Del(5q) is a recurrent chromosomal abnormality in MDS. In fact, as many as 15% of MDS cases will display a deletion of variable length at the long arm of No. 5 chromosome, either as the sole abnormality or in combination with other karyotypic anomalies (18). Isolated del(5q) deletions account for half of this figure, and the 5q– syndrome accounts for about 4% of all MDS cases. This deletion consistently involves a region between the bands q31 to q33, but both proximal and distal breakpoints are variable. Three major deletions have been identified. Their frequency is in the same order as the respective length of the lesion: The most common (and the longest) is del(5)(q13q33), the second most common is del(5)(q13q31), and, finally, less common is del(5)(q22q33). A number of other breakpoints have been reported, some as short as del(5)(q31q33) (19, 20). These short deletions in patients with the typical features of del(5q) MDS (and more precisely, the 5q– syndrome) have defined the minimal commonly deleted region (CDR) of the disease (20). The great variability of breakpoints virtually excludes the possibility that formation of a novel oncogene is responsible for the disease by fusion of the proximal and distal breakpoints. Instead, the constant loss of genetic material from 5q in association with a specific syndrome suggests that the mechanism for tumorigenesis is recessive and that loss of a tumor suppressor gene is responsible for the development of del(5q) MDS. However, the exact mechanism by which the chromosomal deletion leads to the disease is unknown. The majority of the genes mapping within the CDR are expressed in CD34+ cells and might, therefore, be at the origin of the disease. However, no inactivating mutation has yet been identified in any candidate gene (11). Another possibility would be that haploinsufficiency contributes to the development of del(5q) MDS (i.e., a gene dosage effect resulting from the loss of one single allele). An alternate possibility is a gene dosage effect caused by the deletion of multiple genes contained in the 5q region, which are functionally related to hematopoiesis (21). Del(5q) seems to occur very early in the differentiation of hematopoietic stem cells. Nilsson et al. (22) purified pluripotent hematopoietic stem cells (CD34+CD38–) from MDS patients with a 5q- deletion between bands 5q13 and 5q33. Virtually all CD34+CD38– cells belonged to the 5q-deleted clone, indicating that a lymphomyeloid hematopoietic stem cell is the primary target of 5q deletions in MDS and that 5q deletions represent an early event in MDS development. Additional cytogenetic abnormalities like trisomy 8 or trisomy 21 are secondary events that are being acquired at later stages (22).

6.6   Molecular Genetics

The molecular basis of del(5q) MDS has been the subject of extensive investigation. The minimal CDR was identified by Boultwood et al. and assigned to a 1.5-Mb interval at 5q32 flanked by *D5S413* and the *GLRA1* gene (20). This CDR contains approximately 48 genes, including putative tumor suppressor genes like

MEGF1 (FAT tumor suppressor homologue 2) and *G3BP* (Ras-GTPase activating protein-binding protein) (20, 21). This region is distinct from and distal to a 1.5-Mb region at 5q31.1 flanked by the genes interleukin (IL)-9 and early growth response 1 (*EGR-1*) that has been found to be commonly deleted in advanced MDS and AML with del(5q) abnormality (23, 24). The identification of more than one CDR of the del(5q) in association with malignant myeloid disorders suggests that different genes might be pathogenetically relevant. Interestingly, however, nearly all of the deletions in del(5q) MDS are large enough to cover both the MDS and AML del(5q) CDR. Molecular profiling with gene expression analysis using a comprehensive array platform (Affymetrix GeneChip U133 Plus 2.0) has yielded additional insight into the pathophysiology of MDS and the del(5q) subgroup (25). In fact, across the MDS spectrum, the two most upregulated genes were found to be the interferon (IFN)-stimulated genes, *IFITM1* and *IFIT1*. IFN-γ is a cytokine that is supposed to exert an inhibitory role on hematopoietic progenitors in the bone marrow of patients with MDS. The expression profile of del(5q) MDS was significantly different from that of patients with MDS and a normal karyotype. This was, of course, partly due to the fact that the deletion of part of chromosome 5 led to underexpression of the genes encoded on 5q. Approximately 40% of the significant probe sets that show lower expression levels in patients with a del(5q) map to chromosome 5, suggesting a gene dosage effect by the loss of one allele. On the other hand, histone genes within the *HIST1* gene cluster on chromosome 6q21 were expressed at significantly higher levels in del(5q) MDS patients. Some of the patients showed a more than 100-fold upregulation of certain *HIST1* genes (25). Other genes with an increased expression level included actin-binding proteins or myosin-related proteins like *ARPC2, CORO1C,* and *CAPZA2*. Disruption of the actin cytoskeleton and, consequently, deregulation of signal transduction pathways has been implicated in tumorigenesis. Other genes overexpressed in del(5q) MDS were *PF4V1, PPBP,* and *CD61*, which are megakaryocyte/platelet associated (25). Interestingly, a recent study on serum protein profiling in MDS revealed PF-4 to be a highly sensitive and stable marker for the recognition of myelodysplastic syndromes (26).

6.7 Prognosis

Patients with del(5q) MDS are usually considered to have a relatively good prognosis. This is true for those patients who have a medullary blast count of <5% and an isolated del(5q) or a del(5q) with not more than one additional chromosomal abnormality (Figure 6.1) (11, 13, 18, 27, 28). In fact, patients with an isolated del(5q) and a normal bone marrow and peripheral blast count (5q– syndrome) have a median overall survival between 70 and 107 months (11, 13, 14, 18). This should, however, be compared to the survival of the general population at the same median age. At the age of 67 years, the general female population in Germany is expected to live for another 244 months, whereas men generally live 188 months (German Federal Office of Statistics, 2004). This shows that even the favorable 5q– syndrome

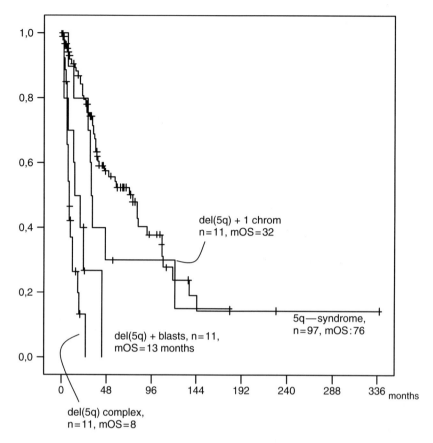

Figure 6.1 Overall survival of patients with del(5q) MDS. Four curves are presented: patients with a bone marrow blast count of <5% (5q– syndrome) and isolated del(5q); patients with a bone marrow blast count <5% and del(5q) plus one additional chromosomal abnormality (del(5q)+1 chrom); patients with isolated del(5q) and a bone marrow blast count >5% (del(5q) + blasts); patients with del(5q) and complex cytogenetic aberrations (del(5q) complex). Median overall survival (mOS) is given in months. No significant difference is found between 5q– syndrome and del(5q)+1 chrom; however, patient numbers are low in the latter group

confers excess mortality compared to the general population. If the patients acquire one additional chromosomal abnormality, the overall survival is reduced to 32–47 months (Figure 6.1) (11, 18). This changes dramatically if the del(5q) comes in association with a complex karyotype. In those cases, the overall survival of the patients is less than 1 year, independent of their medullary blast count (12). Indeed, there is evidence that patients with a complex karyotype involving del(5q) have a worse prognosis than patients with a complex chromosomal abnormality without involvement of chromosome 5. An elevation of the medullary blast count is also an adverse prognostic factor. The median overall survival of 11 patients with an increase in bone marrow blasts and an isolated del(5q) is 13 months (Figure 6.1).

6.8 Therapy

A number of therapeutic approaches have been used in patients with del(5q) disease in the past, generally with little success. Pyridoxine, steroids, and danazol have not shown any effect in a series of patients reported by Mathew et al. (14). More modern approaches are summarized in Table 6.5. A case report has been published in which the use of bortezomib in a patient with del(5q) MDS has resulted in a major hematological response (29).

Erythropoietin or darbepoietin has been given to a small number of del(5q) MDS cases, with some of them showing improvement (30, 31). Its use should be carefully selected, however, because the serum EPO level in this patient subgroup is usually higher than 200–500 U/L, a threshold generally accepted as predictive for EPO responses (32). Indeed, larger series have reported response rates to EPO with or without granulocyte colony-stimulating factor (G-CSF) of only 6–14% (33–36).

The German MDS study group has performed a trial with all-*trans*-retinoic acid (ATRA) in 29 patients with isolated del(5q) with <10% bone marrow blasts. The results were rather disappointing. Overall, 19% of patients showed a reduction in red blood cell transfusions; however, these were not long-lasting and the side effects were serious enough to prompt the authors to conclude that ATRA is not the therapy of choice for this disease entity (37).

Low-dose cytarabine has been used in two small studies for patients with del(5q) MDS, mainly the 5q– syndrome (38, 39). Response rates were 57% and 100%, respectively, with transfusion independence being achieved for up to 30 months. The drug was given at dosages of 20 mg/m^2 twice daily for 14 days as a subcutaneous injection. In most cases, only one course of therapy was given for remission induction. Additional courses were only given in case of relapse, and some of the patients responded again with freedom from transfusion at the time of the second low-dose cytarabine (Ara-C) administration (39). Patients treated with low-dose cytarabine with the above-mentioned schedule will very likely become neutropenic because del(5q) MDS initially often presents with mild to moderate leukopenia. One of our patients experienced life-threatening *Escherichia coli* septicemia after one course of therapy. Therefore, the drug should only be used by experienced hematologists and the patients should be monitored carefully for cytopenias. Supportive therapy with myeloid growth factors might be necessary to prevent serious infection.

Table 6.5 Modern treatment approaches to del(5q) MDS

Erythropoietin and darbepoietin
All-*trans*-retinoic acid
Low-dose cytarabine
Bortezomib
Thalidomide
Lenalidomide
Allogeneic stem cell transplantation

Because of the good overall survival in the 5q– syndrome, hematopoietic stem cell transplantation (HSCT) is considered appropriate only for patients with progressive disease in terms of additional chromosomal abnormalities, peripheral blood cytopenias, or an increase in bone marrow or peripheral blood blast counts (40). Stewart et al. (48) have published a series of 57 patients with del(5q) MDS or secondary AML who underwent HSCT. Seventeen patients had an isolated del(5q) and a blast count of <5%; however, only 5 patients had a low-risk IPSS profile. Hence, 12 of the 17 patients had at least one cytopenia in addition to anemia. Most of the patients with the lower-risk features were referred to the transplantation center because of increasing transfusion dependence. Seven patients with one additional karyotypic abnormality underwent HSCT. Another 30 patients had a poor-risk karyotype, including 12 with chromosome 7 abnormalities and 18 with at least another 2 cytogenetic aberrations. Only 1 of 20 patients with isolated del(5q) relapsed, compared with 15 of 37 patients with additional chromosomal abnormalities. Although patients with additional chromosomal anomalies tended to have more advanced MDS, this result still underlines the unfavorable prognosis of additional karyotypic anomalies in conjunction with del(5q), which is not only true for the natural course of the disease but also in association with HSCT. The nonrelapse mortality, on the other hand, was not statistically significantly different, accounting for 30% in the isolated del(5q) group and 38% in the group of del(5q) with additional chromosomal abnormalities. Although, from a transplantation standpoint, a 30% mortality might not be judged excessive, in patients with an isolated del(5q), 30% of patients would not be expected to die before about 40 months of their natural course (Figure 6.1). Therefore, the decision to proceed with an allogeneic HSCT in patients with isolated del(5q) should be carefully weighed and the patients selected on an individual basis.

Thalidomide is a pleiotropic drug with antiangiogenic, anti-inflammatory, and T-cell costimulatory activity that can effectively treat anemia in MDS, with response rates ranging from 20% to 49% (41). The best results were seen in patients with low-risk or intermediate-1-risk IPSS profiles (42). Strupp et al. (43) reported three cytogenetic responses (19%) out of 16 patients with karyotypic abnormalities, and, interestingly, 2 of those patients had a del(5q) chromosomal abnormality. The first patient had an isolated del(5q)(q22q33) abnormality in 11 out of 20 metaphases and other features of the 5q– syndrome. She was treated with thalidomide doses of 100–400 mg/day and achieved both partial cytogenetic remission (2 out of 20 metaphases remained abnormal) and transfusion independence. Transfusion independence lasted for about 3 years, but the patient eventually had to stop the treatment because of progressive polyneuropathy. The second patient had a complex karyotype including del(5q) and RAEB-T with severe anemia (7.2 g/dL) and thrombocytopenia (22.000/μL). Within 5 months of thalidomide treatment at 200–400 mg/day, this patient achieved transfusion independence (hemoglobin, 12.8 g/dL; platelets, 240.000/μL) and complete cytogenetic remission. However, the patient experienced deep venous thrombosis and pulmonary emboli during treatment with thalidomide. Finally, after 9 months of therapy, he relapsed with RAEB-T and a complex karyotype and died in the further course of the disease.

These observations are of special interest because they show that hematological and cytogenetic remissions might be obtained in del(5q) MDS with an immunomodulatory approach. The consistent activity of thalidomide in MDS provided the rationale for the use of its structural analog lenalidomide in this patient population. Lenalidomide is a 4-amino-substituted thalidomide derivative that has a 20,000–50.000-fold higher activity in suppressing tumor necrosis factor (TNF)-γ, and it is more potent than thalidomide in stimulating T-cell proliferation, natural killer cell activation, and production of IL-2, IL-10 and IFN-α (44). The toxicity profile of lenalidomide is more favorable than that of thalidomide because neither polyneuropathy nor significant constipation or sedation have been reported in MDS patients (45, 46). Most importantly, in the rabbit model most sensitive for thalidomide-associated embryotoxicity, lenalidomide did not show any fetal malformations (44). In the MDS, lenalidomide has been evaluated in a number of clinical studies, the most important being the Lenalidomide-MDS-001, Lenalidomide-MDS-002, and Lenalidomide-MDS-003 studies. In the Lenalidomide-MDS-001 trial, 43 patients with MDS and transfusion-dependent or symptomatic anemia were treated with lenalidomide doses of up to 25 mg. All patients had no response to erythropoietin therapy or were believed to be poor erythropoietin responders because of high endogenous EPO levels. All FAB subtypes could be included, but neutrophil counts were required to be >500/µL and platelet counts >10.000/µL. Responses were defined according to the modified International Working Group criteria (47). Although, according to the natural frequency of del(5q) among all MDS subtypes, one would expect only about 15% of patients with del(5q) in such a trial, 12 out of 43 (28%) of the trial patients displayed a del(5q) chromosomal abnormality. This turned out to be a fortunate event, as 83% of del(5q) patients achieved an erythroid response, defined as a sustained transfusion independence with more than a 2-g/dL hemoglobin increase, compared to 57% of patients with a normal karyotype and 12% of patients with other karyotypic abnormalities (46). Complete cytogenetic remissions occurred in 75% of patients with del(5q). Interestingly, a reduction of bone marrow blast percentages was also observed, as three out of six patients with excess blasts (6–21%) achieved a reduction to ≤5% blasts after treatment. Dose-limiting toxicities were neutropenia and thrombocytopenia of WHO grade 3/4 in 58% and 50%, respectively.

The Lenalidomide-MDS-003 trial (45) was designed to study the effects of lenalidomide in the subgroup of MDS patients with del(5q) cytogenetic abnormalities. The trial included transfusion-dependent del(5q) MDS patients with or without additional chromosomal abnormalities and an IPSS grading of low or intermediate-1. This allowed the authors to study a number of different patient populations with del(5q): the 5q– syndrome, with isolated del(5q), normal blast count, and isolated anemia (e.g., low-risk IPSS), as well as patients with the above features but an increase of medullary blasts of up to 10% and/or two or more peripheral blood cytopenias (e.g., intermediate-1 risk). Also, patients with one additional chromosomal abnormality and a blast count of up to 10% were eligible to participate in the study if the number of cytopenias was <2 (e.g., intermediate-1 IPSS). Finally, patients with a complex karyotype including del(5q) or a chromosome 7 anomaly in addition to del(5q) were eligible if there was only one peripheral cytopenia and the bone marrow blast count was <5%. As a result of the treatment-related neutropenia and thrombocytopenia observed in the Lenalidomide-MDS-001 trial, patients had to have at least 500/μL neutrophils and >50.000/μL platelets to be eligible for the trial. Furthermore, the initial lenalidomide dose was set at 10 mg orally per day ("continuous schedule") or 21 days out of 28 ("syncopated schedule") with possible dose reductions in case of adverse events to 5 mg po daily or 5 mg po every other day. Among 148 patients included, 111 had an isolated del(5q) abnormality and 37 had additional chromosomal abnormalities. Central cytology and cytogenetic review was performed and 120 patients (81%) were confirmed as suffering from low/intermediate-1-risk MDS. The results of this study confirmed the impressive data of the Lenalidomide-MDS-001 trial. Using an intent-to-treat (ITT) analysis, by week 24, 76% of patients achieved at least a 50% reduction of transfusion need compared to pretherapy levels and 67% of patients became entirely transfusion-free for ≥56 days with a rise in hemoglobin of at least 1 g/dL. The median time to response was 4.6 weeks, and the median rise in hemoglobin at maximum response was 5.4 g/dL. After a median follow-up of 2 years, the median duration of transfusion independence was not reached. Fifty-three patients were still on-study and transfusion-free. Cytogenetic responses were very impressive, indeed. Not only did 45% of patients achieve a complete cytogenetic remission and another 28% reduced the number of abnormal metaphases by at least 50%; the trial did not show any significant statistical difference between patients with an isolated del(5q) and those with one or more additional cytogenetic abnormalities. This result is as important as it is astonishing. The natural course of patients with complex cytogenetic abnormalities including del(5q) is very poor indeed, the median overall survival being 8 months (Figure 6.1), independent of the bone marrow blast count (12). The fact that 50% of patients with this adverse feature went into complete cytogenetic remission heralds a new era in the treatment of MDS, as previously no other drug was able to show such impressive remitting activity in such a poor prognosis subgroup. Furthermore, this result suggests that lenalidomide might alter the natural history of disease in patients with a higher-risk del(5q) abnormality. Red blood cell transfusion independence was also unaffected by age, gender, FAB subtype, or IPSS category. The only two variables in multivariate analysis predicting a better response to the drug were a higher peripheral platelet count (because those patients received a higher cumulative lenalidomide dose) and a lower pretreatment transfusion burden.

The most common adverse events were grade 3/4 neutropenia (55%) and thrombocytopenia (44%), necessitating dose adjustment in 91% of patients on the continuous treatment schedule and 67% of patients on the syncopated treatment regimen. The median time to the first dose interruption or reduction was 22 days, and the median duration of this first interruption was also 3 weeks. A third of the patients had to undergo a second dose reduction or interruption. These results emphasize that patients treated with lenalidomide need weekly complete blood count evaluations during the first 8 weeks of therapy and biweekly blood draws thereafter for at least another 4 months. Other adverse effects of lenalidomide included skin rash, pruritus, diarrhea, muscle cramps, and, rarely, hypothyroidism and endocrine hypogonadism. In our experience, pruritus is self-limiting but might require oral antihistamines. In more severe cases, a short course (usually less than 14 days) of 10 mg of prednisone can be given to alleviate symptoms. Diarrhea is difficult to tackle and might require dose reduction. Neither loperamide nor other antidiarrheal drugs are very helpful to treat this complication. Muscle cramps are usually self-limiting. Magnesium supplementation did not show any significant effect, and in some instances, quinine sulfate might be used. Hypothyroidism was always associated with high levels of antithyroid antibodies and needed thyroid supplementation therapy. Deep venous thrombosis, a complication feared with combination lenalidomide and dexamethasone therapy in multiple myeloma, occurred in four patients only (i.e., 2.7% of all patients).

Nine patients progressed to higher MDS subtypes or acute myeloid leukemia, and 11 patients died due to disease complications ($n = 8$) or neutropenic infection ($n = 3$). Interestingly, in contrast to the results of the Lenalidomide-MDS-001 trial, no patient acquired secondary chromosome 7 anomalies.

6.9   Conclusion

Myelodysplastic syndromes with a del(5q) chromosomal abnormality are a heterogeneous group of disorders. The deletion at 5q is acquired early during hematopietic stem cell development (22), and secondary chromosomal abnormalities are later events. Del(5q) is the most common chromosomal abnormality in MDS and might present as an isolated abnormality with or without an increase in bone marrow blasts, and in conjunction with one or several other karyotypic anomalies. The natural course of these patient subgoups can be very different. Only patients with an isolated del(5q) and a normal bone marrow blast count ("the 5q– syndrome") have a truly favorable prognosis, although it is worse than that of the age-matched general population (11). As all patients eventually become red cell transfusion-dependent, therapeutic strategies aimed at reducing the transfusion need should be discussed early in the course of the disease. Erythropoietic agents are not very useful, as most patients display high endogenous EPO levels at the time of transfusion dependence. Lenalidomide has consistently shown high rates of transfusion independence in more than two-thirds of patients treated and has also led to complete cytogenetic remissions in 44% of cases. The induction of cytogenetic remission is independent of the cytogenetic complexity (i.e., additional cytogenetic abnormalities). Lenalidomide has been approved in the Unites States for use in low- and intermediate-1-risk MDS according to the IPSS. For patients with a blast count >10% (i.e., IPSS intermediate-2 or high risk) and a reduced platelet count, a course of low-dose cytarabine could be indicated to reduce the leukemic burden, as the cumulative lenalidomide dose that might be administered might be too low to achieve a response. The treatment should then be followed by maintenance therapy with lenalidomide.

With the advent of powerful molecular techniques, including the microarray technology, proteomics, and single-nucleotide polymorphism scanning, the gene or genes responsible for the disease might soon be identified. This would open the door to a targeted therapy on the molecular level.

Acknowledgment This work was supported by a grant from the German Competence Network "acute and chronic leukemias."

References

1. Tjio JH, Levan A. The chromosome number in man. Hereditas 1956;42:1–6.
2. Nowell PC, Hungerford DA. Chromosome studies on normal and leukemic human leukocytes. J Natl Cancer Inst 1960;25:85–109.
3. Rowley JD. Identificaton of a translocation with quinacrine fluorescence in a patient with acute leukemia. Ann Genet 1973;16(2):109–112.
4. Van den Berghe H, Cassiman JJ, David G, et al. Distinct haematological disorder with deletion of long arm of no. 5 chromosome. Nature 1974;251(5474):437–438.
5. Janssen JW, Buschle M, Layton M, et al. Clonal analysis of myelodysplastic syndromes: evidence of multipotent stem cell origin. Blood 1989;73(1):248–254.
6. Aul C, Bowen DT, Yoshida Y. Pathogenesis, etiology and epidemiology of myelodysplastic syndromes. Haematologica 1998;83(1):71–86.
7. Bennett JM, Catovsky D, Daniel MT, et al. Proposals for the classification of the myelodysplastic syndromes. Br J Haematol 1982;51(2):189–199.
8. Jaffee ES, Harris NL, Stein H, et al.World Health Organization classification of tumours, pathology and genetics of haematopoietic and lymphoid tissues. Lyon: IARC Press; 2001.
9. Giagounidis AA, Germing U, Haase S, et al. Clinical, morphological, cytogenetic, and prognostic features of patients with myelodysplastic syndromes and del(5q) including band q31. Leukemia 2004;18(1):113–119.
10. Washington LT, Doherty D, Glassman A, et al. Myeloid disorders with deletion of 5q as the sole karyotypic abnormality: the clinical and pathologic spectrum. Leuk Lymphoma 2002;43(4):761–765.
11. Giagounidis AA, Germing U, Wainscoat JS, et al. The 5q- syndrome. Hematology 2004;9(4):271–277.
12. Giagounidis AA, Germing U, Strupp C, et al. Prognosis of patients with del(5q) MDS and complex karyotype and the possible role of lenalidomide in this patient subgroup. Ann Hematol 2005;84(9):569–571.
13. Dewald GW, Davis MP, Pierre RV, et al. Clinical characteristics and prognosis of 50 patients with a myeloproliferative syndrome and deletion of part of the long arm of chromosome 5. Blood 1985;66(1):189–197.
14. Mathew P, Tefferi A, Dewald GW, et al. The 5q- syndrome: a single-institution study of 43 consecutive patients. Blood 1993;81(4):1040–1045.
15. Kerkhofs H, Hagemeijer A, Leeksma CH, et al. The 5a-chromosome abnormality in haematological disorders: a collaborative study of 34 cases from the Netherlands. Br J Haematol 1982;52(3):365–381.
16. Van den Berghe H, Vermaelen K, Mecucci C, et al. The 5q-anomaly. Cancer Genet Cytogenet 1985;17(3):189–255.
17. Giagounidis AA, Haase S, Germing U, et al. Autoimmune disorders in two patients with myelodysplastic syndrome and 5q deletion. Acta Haematol 2005;113(2):146–149.
18. Haase D, Germing U, Schanz J, et al. New insights into the prognostic impact of the karyotype in MDS and correlation with subtypes: evidence from a core dataset of 2124 patients. Blood 2007; DOI 10.1182/blood-2007-03-082404.

19. Jaju RJ, Boultwood J, Oliver FJ, et al. Molecular cytogenetic delineation of the critical deleted region in the 5q- syndrome. Genes Chromosomes Cancer 1998;22(3):251–256.
20. Boultwood J, Fidler C, Strickson AJ, et al. Narrowing and genomic annotation of the commonly deleted region of the 5q- syndrome. Blood 2002;99(12):4638–4641.
21. Giagounidis AA, Germing U, Aul C. Biological and prognostic significance of chromosome 5q deletions in myeloid malignancies. Clin Cancer Res 2006;12(1):5–10.
22. Nilsson L, Astrand-Grundström I, Arvidsson I, et al. Isolation and characterization of hematopoietic progenitor/stem cells in 5q-deleted myelodysplastic syndromes: evidence for inolvement at the hematopoietic stem cell level. Blood 2000;96:2012–2021.
23. Horrigan SK, Westbrook CA, Kim AH, et al. Polymerase chain reaction-based diagnosis of del (5q) in acute myeloid leukemia and myelodysplastic syndrome identifies a minimal deletion interval. Blood 1996;88(7):2665–2670.
24. Zhao N, Stoffel A, Wang PW, et al. Molecular delineation of the smallest commonly deleted region of chromosome 5 in malignant myeloid diseases to 1–1.5 Mb and preparation of a PAC-based physical map. Proc Natl Acad Sci USA 1997;94(13):6948–6953.
25. Pellagatti A, Cazzola M, Giagounidis AA, et al. Gene expression profiles of CD34+ cells in myelodysplastic syndromes: involvement of interferon stimulated genes and correlation to FAB subtype and karyotype. Blood 2006;108(1):337–345.
26. Aivado M, Spentzos D, Germing U, et al. From the cover: Serum proteome profiling detects myelodysplastic syndromes and identifies CXC chemokine ligands 4 and 7 as markers for advanced disease. Proc Natl Acad Sci USA 2007;104(4):1307–1312.
27. Germing U, Gattermann N, Strupp C, et al. Validation of the WHO proposals for a new classification of primary myelodysplastic syndromes: a retrospective analysis of 1600 patients. Leuk Res 2000;24(12):983–992.
28. Germing U, Strupp C, Kuendgen A, et al. Prospective validation of the WHO proposals for the classification of myelodysplastic syndromes. Haematologica 2006;91(12):1596–1604.
29. Terpos E, Verrou E, Banti A, et al. Bortezomib is an effective agent for MDS/MPD syndrome with 5q-anomaly and thrombocytosis. Leuk Res 2007;31(4):559–562.
30. Howe RB, Porwit-MacDonald A, Wanat R, et al. The WHO classification of MDS does make a difference. Blood 2004;103(9):3265–3270.
31. Mannone L, Gardin C, Quarre MC, et al. High-dose darbepoetin alpha in the treatment of anaemia of lower risk myelodysplastic syndrome results of a phase II study. Br J Haematol 2006;133(5):513–519.
32. Hellstrom-Lindberg E, Gulbrandsen N, Lindberg G, et al. A validated decision model for treating the anaemia of myelodysplastic syndromes with erythropoietin + granulocyte colony-stimulating factor: significant effects on quality of life. Br J Haematol 2003;120(6):1037–1046.
33. Hellstrom-Lindberg E. Efficacy of erythropoietin in the myelodysplastic syndromes; a meta-analysis of 205 patients from 17 studies. Br J Haematol 1995;89(1):67–71.
34. Group ICS. A randomized double-blind placebo-controlled study with subcutaneous recombinant erythropoietin in patients with low-risk myelodysplastic syndromes. Br J Haematol 1998;103(4):1070–1074.
35. Terpos E, Mougiou A, Kouraklis A, et al. Prolonged administration of erythropoietin increases erythroid response rate in myelodysplastic syndromes; a phase II trial in 281 patients. Br J Haematol 2002;118(1):174–180.
36. Hellstrom-Lindberg E, Ahlgren T, Beguin Y, et al. Treatment of anemia in myelodysplastic syndromes with granulocyte-colony stimulating factor plus erythropoietin; results from a randomized phase II study and long-term follow-up of 71 patients. Blood 1998;92(1):68–75.
37. Giagounidis AA, Haase S, Germing U, et al. Treatment of myelodysplastic syndrome with isolated del(5q) including bands q31–q33 with a combination of all-trans-retinoic acid and tocopherol-alpha: a phase II study. Ann Hematol 2005;84(6):389–394.
38. Giagounidis A, Haase S, Germing U, et al. Low-dose cytarabine in the treatment of patients with the 5q- syndrome. Onkologie 2002;25(Suppl49):XII+304.

39. Juneja HS, Jodhani M, Gardner FH, et al. Low-dose ARA-C consistently induces hematologic responses in the clinical 5q- syndrome. Am J Hematol 1994;46(4):338–342.
40. Cutler CS, Lee SJ, Greenberg P, et al. A decision analysis of allogeneic bone marrow transplantation for the myelodysplastic syndromes: delayed transplantation for low-risk myelodysplasia is associated with improved outcome. Blood 2004;104(2):579–585.
41. Musto P. Thalidomide therapy for myelodysplastic syndromes: current status and future perspectives. Leuk Res 2004;28(4):325–332.
42. Raza A, Meyer P, Dutt D, et al. Thalidomide produces transfusion independence in long-standing refractory anemias of patients with myelodysplastic syndromes. Blood 2001;98(4):958–965.
43. Strupp C, Hildebrandt B, Germing U, et al. Cytogenetic response to thalidomide treatment in three patients with myelodysplastic syndrome. Leukemia 2003;17(6):1200–1202.
44. Mitsiades CS, Mitsiades N. CC-5013 (Celgene). Curr Opin Invest Drugs 2004;5(6): 635–647.
45. List A, Dewald G, Bennett J, et al. Lenalidomide in the myelodysplastic syndrome with chromosome 5q deletion. N Engl J Med 2006;355(14):1456–1465.
46. List A, Kurtin S, Roe DJ, et al. Efficacy of lenalidomide in myelodysplastic syndromes. N Engl J Med 2005;352(6):549–557.
47. Cheson BD, Bennett JM, Kantarjian H, et al. Report of an international working group to standardize response criteria for myelodysplastic syndromes. Blood 2000;96(12):3671–3674.
48. Stewart B, Verdugo M, Guthrie KA, Appelbaum F, Deeg HJ. Outcome following haematopoietic cell transplantation in patients with myelodysplasia and del (5q) karyotypes. Br J Haematol 2003;123(5):879–85.

Chapter 7
Rare Acute Leukemias

Xavier Georges Thomas

7.1 Introduction

Hematopoietic cancers, which arise from various cell types that constitute the blood-forming tissues including the cells of the immune system, belong to the group of nonepithelial tumors. The term leukemia (literally "white blood") refers to malignant derivatives of several of these hematopoietic cell lineages. Acute myeloid leukemia (AML) is a clonal disorder of immature hematopoietic cells and is characterized by aberrant hematopoietic cellular proliferation and maturation. Leukemic blasts might express capabilities for maturation to a variable degree, which leads to morphological heterogeneity. The leukemic transformation might occur at the level of a pluripotent or a less primitive hematopoietic cell. Generally, the transformed leukemic stem cell is committed to the granulocytic lineage, but sometimes a predominance of blast cells from the erythroid or megakaryocytic lineage might be observed.

The decade of the 1990s heralded an era in hematopathology in which traditional morphologic and cytochemical methods would not be sufficient to arrive at accurate diagnoses. The introduction of flow cytometry, cytogenetics, and molecular techniques used in conjunction with traditional methods allowed physicians to recognize rarer disease and clinicopathologic entities. The classification of AML has been recently revised by a group of pathologists and clinicians under the auspices of the World Health Organization (WHO) (Table 7.1) (1). Although elements of the French-American-British (FAB) classification have been retained, the WHO classification incorporates more recent discoveries regarding the genetics and the clinical features of AML in an attempt to define entities that are biologically homogeneous and that have prognostic and therapeutic relevance. The most significant difference between the WHO and FAB classifications is the WHO recommendation that the requisite blast percentage for the diagnosis of AML be at least 20% blasts in the blood or bone marrow, whereas the FAB scheme required a blast percentage of at least 30%. This threshold value eliminated the category "refractory anemia with excess blasts in transformation (RAEB-t)" found in the FAB classification of myelodysplastic syndromes (MDSs). Under the WHO classification, the category "acute myeloid leukemia not otherwise categorized" is

Table 7.1 Classification of AML according to the WHO criteria

- AML with characteristic genetic abnormalities
  AML with t(8;21)(q22;q22); (AML/ETO)
  AML with inv(16)(p13q22) or t(16;16)(p13;q22); (*CBFβ/MYH*11)
  APL (AML with t(15;17)(q22;q12), (*PML/RARα* and variants)
  AML with 11q23 (*MLL*) abnormalities
- AML with FLT3 mutation
- AML with multilineage dysplasia
- AML and MDS, therapy related
  Alkylating agent-related AML and MDS
  Topoisomerase II inhibitor-related AML
- AML not otherwise categorized
  Acute myeloblastic leukemia minimally differentiated (FAB classification M0)
  Acute myeloblastic leukemia without maturation (FAB classification M1)
  Acute myeloblastic leukemia with maturation (FAB classification M2)
  Acute myelomonocytic leukemia (AMML) (FAB classification M4)
  Acute monoblastic leukemia and acute monocytic leukemia (FAB M5a and M5b)
  Acute erythroid leukemias (FAB classification M6a and M6b)
  Acute megakaryoblastic leukemia (FAB classification M7)
  AML/transient myeloproliferative disorder in Down's syndrome
  Acute basophilic leukemia
  Acute panmyelosis with myelofibrosis
  Myeloid sarcoma
- Acute leukemias of ambiguous lineage

AML, acute myeloid leukemia; APL, acute promyelocytic leukemia; MDS, myelodysplastic syndrome.

Source: Data from Brunning et al. (1).

morphology based and reflects the FAB classification with a few significant modifications (2, 3). Among this subgroup, some entities are particularly uncommon, many of which are of unknown clinical significance. Some of these entities are discussed here and the relevant findings are presented.

7.2 Acute Erythroid Leukemia

Erythroleukemia is a myeloproliferative disorder characterized by malignant proliferation of erythroid and myeloid precursors. The disease has a long descriptive history that has gone through different stages of evolution. It was first recognized by Copelli in 1912 as a hematologic disorder named "atypical erythematosis" (4). Copelli's case report described a 60-year-old male with progressive hepatosplenomegaly who died from severe anemia. At autopsy he was found to have both atypical and megaloblastic erythroid cells in the bone marrow, spleen, liver, and lymph nodes. In 1917, Di Guglielmo reported additional observations of a neoplastic disorder with proliferation of the erythroid precursors and involvement of the granulocytic series (5). In the first of several papers he authored on this subject, he described a patient with "erythemia" who showed a marked increase in cells of the erythroid series with immature circulating forms. Additionally, both qualitative and quantitative abnormalities of the white cells and platelets were also observed. In 1923, Di Guglielmo described a "new form of blood disorder involving proliferation purely of the nucleated red blood cell series" and designated this disease "erythemic myelosis" (6). He considered this to be a leukemiclike disease and stressed its purity as "an autonomous pathologic entity of erythropoiesis." In 1940, Moeschlin definitively established the term of "erythroleukemia," (7) and in the late 1950s and 1960s, Dameshek proposed the term "Di Guglielmo's syndrome" to describe a myeloproliferative syndrome striking erythoblastic hyperplasia and a progressive increase of myeloblasts terminating in AML (8, 9). Since 1976, erythroleukemia was no longer considered as a chronic myeloproliferative disorder but, rather, as a form of AML and, as such, was included within the FAB classification system of AML, which designates it as AML-M6 (10). The FAB classification distinguished AML-M6 from MDSs on the basis of the myeloblastic component and erythroblast precursors. Quantitative standards were laid down for its diagnosis. These were revised in 1985: In a differential count of 500 nucleated cells in the marrow, $\geq 50\%$ should be erythroid cells and myeloblasts should constitute at least 30% of the nonerythroid cells (2). However, the FAB did not identify Di Guglielmo syndrome, and only after the publication of Garand et al. (11), the undifferentiated M6 was included within the FAB as M6b (now "pure erythroid" according to WHO). This M6 "variant" is characterized by a unique malignant cell type instead of two distinct clones of blasts (proerythroblasts and myeloblasts).

Other authors described three subtypes of AML-M6 (12,13): (1) Di Guglielmo's syndrome characterized by greater or equal to 30% pronormoblasts, related to the evolution of MDS, and presented few karyotype abnormalities; (2) a second subtype defined by greater than or equal to 30% pronormoblasts and conversely less than 30% of blasts within nonerythrocytic elements, associated with major karyotype abnormalities and highest level of expression of multidrug resistance (MDR)-1 gene product P-glycoprotein; (3) a third subtype characterized by greater or equal to 30% of blasts of nonerythroid cells with greater or equal to 30% pronormoblasts.

Among the various types of AML, acute erythroid leukemia is regarded as a relatively rare disorder and considered as a distinct entity with characteristic features such as complex chromosomal defects and poor prognosis (14–17). According to the recent WHO classification, acute erythroid leukemias are divided into erythroleukemia and pure erythroid leukemia, based on the presence or absence of a significant myeloid component (1).

7.2.1   Epidemiology

AML-M6 constitutes between 2% and 7% of all cases of AML (18–21). Patients of all ages are described with this disease, with a male predominance. However, AML-M6 has been shown to be six times more frequent in patients aged 56 years and above (19). It has therefore been regarded as a disease of the elderly, but a subgroup of younger patients with a significantly improved prognosis is now recognized (17, 22). Erythroleukemia (erythroid/myeloid; M6a) represents the predominant form. Pure erythroid leukemia (M6b) is rare and occurs in all age groups. No racial predilection is known. Several reports of clusterings of erythroleukemia and Di Guglielmo's syndrome in family members have been described (23, 24). No consistent environmental hazards, consanguinity, or cytogenetic abnormalities were identified to explain these cases. AML-M6 can arise *de novo* or from a preexisting myeloproliferative disorder. Occasional cases of chronic myeloid leukemia (CML) might evolve to one of the acute erythoid leukemias. Erythroleukemia might present *de novo* or evolve from an MDS, either refractory anemia with excess blasts (RAEB) or refractory cytopenia with multilineage dysplasia and ringed sideroblasts (RCMD-RS) and refractory cytopenia with multilineage dysplasia (RCMD), respectively (25). AML-M6 might be secondary to previous chemotherapy, immunosuppressive treatment, or radiotherapy given for a wide range of malignant or nonmalignant diseases. It is more commonly associated with exposure to alkylating agents or benzene than other subtypes of AML (26, 27). In addition, several reports described erythroleukemia developing after intense combination chemotherapy with or without radiation in long-term survivors of small cell lung carcinoma (28, 29), Hodgkin's disease (30), and following drug-induced hypoplastic anemia (31). Erythroleukemia has also been reported to complicate immunosuppressive immunotherapy with azathioprine following renal transplant (32). Immunologic aberrations, including increased immunoglobulin levels, or the presence of rheumatoid factor and antinuclear antibodies have also been described in patients with erythroleukemia (33, 34).

Historically, the question has been raised as to whether the erythropoiesis of erythroleukemia is itself malignant or reactive to the presence of a malignant granulocytic precursor (35). Although a few studies support the latter possibility (36, 37), current evidence strongly suggests that the erythropoiesis is malignant and is part of a clonal multilineage myeloid population. The presence of a malignant precursor cell common to erythroid and myeloid lines has been established using glucose 6-phosphate dehydogenase (G6PD) markers (38). Production of fetal hemoglobin, the absence of hemoglobin A2, and the appearance of the I membrane antigen in patients with erythroleukemia also support a neoplastic process (39). Other evidence implicating malignancy include abnormal hemoglobin production such as hemoglobin H (39), defects in globin synthesis (40), and erythrophagocytosis by bizarre erythroid precursors (41).

7.2.2   Criteria for Diagnosis of Acute Erythroid Leukemia

Acute erythroid leukemias are AMLs that are characterized by a predominant erythroid proliferation. They are divided into erythroleukemia and pure erythroid leukemia (1). However, a recent report showed that patients do not always fit the WHO criteria (42).

7.2.2.1   Erythroleukemia

Historically, AML with erythroid features has been designated M6 by the FAB group (10). The FAB criteria for M6 diagnosis include bone marrow erythroblasts ≥50% and blasts ≥30% of nonerythroid cells (2). The WHO has recently recommended that the requisite blast percentage for a diagnosis of AML be 20% or greater, and this includes erythroid leukemia (erythroid/myeloid), which might contain at least 20% of myeloblasts in the nonerythroid cell population and at least 50% of erythroid precursors in the entire nucleated cell population (1). These criteria correspond to the previous M6a AML in the FAB (2), with or without associated multilineage dysplasia. Trilineage dysplasia is then common but is not a requisite for diagnosis. Erythroid dysplasia might manifest as binuclearity, nucleocytoplasmic asynchrony, and vacuolation. The morphological appearance of the myeloblasts is not characteristic (Figures 7.1 and 7.2) and they might contain Auer rods. Myeloperoxidase (MPO) and

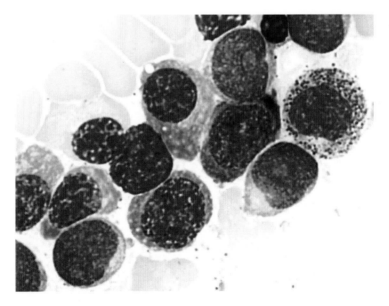

Figure 7.1 Erythroleukemia (bone marrow). Myeloblasts without maturation surrounded by erythroid precursors

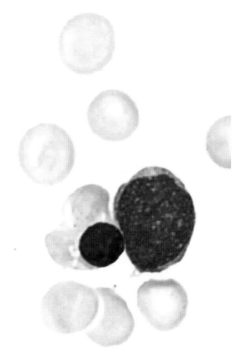

Figure 7.2 Erythroleukemia (peripheral blood). One myeloblast without maturation and one erythroblast

Sudan black B stains might be positive in the myeloblasts. The iron stain might show ringed sideroblasts and periodic acid–Schiff (PAS) might be positive in the erythroid precursors in a block or diffuse pattern (Table 7.2).

The marrow biopsy is usually hypercellular. There might be prominent megakaryocytic dysplasia.

7.2.2.2   Pure Erythroid Leukemia

In addition to the typical erythroleukemia, there is a second subtype of acute erythroid leukemia in which there is a neoplastic proliferation of immature cells entirely committed to the erythroid series (>80% of marrow cells) without evidence of a myeloid component (Figure 7.3). This was termed pure erythroid leukemia by the WHO (1). This pure erythroid leukemia corresponds to the previous M6b of FAB (M6 "variant") and, in part, to the pathology described by Di Guglielmo. Morphology is characterized by medium-sized erythroblasts with fine nuclear chromatin, distinct nucleoli, and deeply basophilic cytoplasm that often have vacuoles (Table 7.2). The erythroid nature of the blasts can be shown by electron

Table 7.2 Morphologic and cytochemical features of acute erythroid leukemias

Morphologic and cytochemical features of erythroleukemia
- ≥ 50% erythoid precursors in the entire nucleated cell population of the bone marrow
- ≥ 20% myeloblasts in the nonerythroid population in the bone marrow
- Dysplastic erythroid precursors with megaloblastoid nuclei
- Multinucleated erythroid cells
- Myeloblasts of medium size, occasionally with Auer rods
- Ringed sideroblasts
- Positive PAS stain in the erythroid precursors
- Hypercellular bone marrow
- Megakaryocytic dysplasia

Morphologic and cytochemical features of pure erythroid leukemia
- Medium- to large-sized erythroblasts with round nuclei, fine chromatin, one or more nucleoli, deeply basophilic cytoplasm, and occasional coalescent vacuoles
- Erythroblasts reactive with alpha-naphthyl acetate esterase
- Acid phosphatase
- PAS

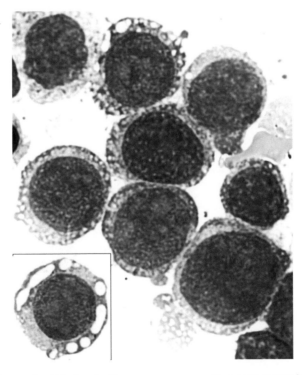

Figure 7.3 Pure erythroid leukemia. Bone marrow smear with numerous very immature erythroid precursors. These cells have cytoplasmic vacuoles that coalesce

microscopy demonstrating free ferritin particles (43). The blasts are negative for Sudan black B And MPO but positive for PAS in a block pattern. Leukemic cells can display a pro-erythroblastlike or an undifferentiated morphology. The morphological features of the latter sometimes lead to an initial diagnosis of an undifferentiated AML (AML-M0), before studying the erythroid markers on leukemic cells. Such cases have been previously reported and have been designated as "cryptic erythroleukemia" (44) or "early erythroblastic leukemia" (45).

In the marrow biopsies, the cells appear undifferentiated. Reactivity with antibody to hemaglobin A varies from a few scattered positive cells to numerous positive cells.

7.2.3   Cytogenetics

There is no unique chromosome abnormality described in acute erythroid leukemia. No specific abnormality has been recognized. A large variety of chromosome abnormalities have been reported. However, complex karyotypes with multiple structural abnormalities are common. Chromosomes 5 and 7 are the most frequently affected (42, 46). These findings are also characteristically found in therapy-related AML and MDS (17). However, loss or deletion of 5q is higher in *de novo* erythroid leukemia, whereas loss or deletion of 7q is higher in therapy-related AML. These abnormalities of chromosome 5 and/or 7 correlate with significantly shorter survival times (17).

The larger study about chromosomal abnormalities of erythroleukemia defined following the WHO classification has been recently performed by the Groupe Francophone de Cytogénétique Hématologique (GFCH) (47). Clonal chromosomal abnormalities were found in 76% of cases at a frequency comparable to other series (16, 17), and distributed in four subgroups according to their ploidy status: pseudodiploid (16%), hypodiploid (47%), hyperdiploid (19%), and 18% mixed cases associating two different clones (hypodiploid + hyperdiploid or pseudodiploid + hyperdiploid). Complex rearrangements and hypodiploid chromosome number were widely dominant (50%). Partial or entire monosomies represented 56% of abnormalities. Chromosome 5 and 7 were confirmed as the most frequently involved, followed by chromosomes 8, 16, and 21 (48). Unbalanced abnormalities were more frequent than balanced, as previously emphasized by others (16, 17, 20) (Table 7.3). All of these kinds of abnormality were observed in *de novo* as well as in secondary erythroleukemia. In an AML-M6 patient with a t(8;9)(p22;p24), the presence of a PCM1-JAK2 fusion was recently demonstrated similar to that observed in myeloproliferative disorders (49).

Pure erythroid leukemia has been frequently associated with complex cytogenetic abnormalities (11, 46, 50–52). If hypodiploidy is one usual cytogenetic characteristic of most erythroleukemia, it is less frequent in pure erythroid erythroleukemia. A high proportion of cases were associated with a BCR-ABL fusion (47, 50, 53) (Table 7.4).

Table 7.3 Cytogenetics of erythroleukemia

Clonal chromosomal abnormalities (76%)
• Pseudodiploid (16%)
• Hypodiploid (47%)
• Hyperdiploid (19%)
• Mixed cases associating two differents clones (hypodiploid + hyperdiploid or pseudodiploid + hyperdiploid) (18%)
Complex rearrangements and hypodiploid chromosome number (50%)
• Partial or entire monosomies (56%)
• Chromosome 5
• Chromosome 7
• Chromosome 8
• Chromosome 16
• Chromosome 21

Source: Data from Lessard et al. (47).

7.2.4 *Immunophenotype*

At present, there are many techniques that enable the recognition of erythroid precursors and progenitors: immunophenotyping with erythroid-specific monoclonal antibodies, ultrastructural detection of ferritin molecules (43), in vitro colony assay and molecular techniques studying mRNA expression of α- or γ-globin, erythroid-specific δ-amino-levulinate synthetase, and GATA1 transcription factor genes (54). Glycophorin A, band 3, and spectrin are specific membrane components of mature erythrocytes. Glycophorin A has been shown on colony-forming unit-erythroid (CFU-E) (55), but also reported first expressed on proerythroblasts (45, 56) or basophilic erythroblasts (57). Band 3 is first expressed on erythroblasts with weak expression (58). Spectrin is first expressed on proerythroblasts (45). In addition to these markers, hemoglobin and carbonic anhydrase 1 are also specific for erythroid hematopoietic cells. Hemoglobin or carbonic anhydrase 1 is first expressed on basophilic-erythroblasts (56) or erythroid progenitors (450, respectively. Two monoclonal antibodies, EP-1 and EP-2, detecting antigenic determinants with restricted expression on erythroid precursors and progenitors have been developed (59). Many other markers, which are not erythroid-specific, are determinants of the differentiation level of erythroid cells: CD36 antigen (thrombospondin receptor or platelet glycoprotein IV), blood group antigens (ABH, M and N, P_1, Lewis, Ii, etc,), CD71 (transferrin receptor), HLA-A, -B, -C and HLA-DR, CD41b, CD33, CD34, and GATA1 transcription factor. Sialyl-Tn antigen and neuron-specific enolase also appear to determine the differentiation level of erythroid cells as well as characteristics of minimally differentiated erythroleukemia blasts (60).

Table 7.4 Cytogenetics of pure "erythroid" leukemia

Reference	Patient	Cytogenetics	Features
Garand et al. (1995) (11)	Child	46,inv(16)(p22q22)	*De novo*
	Child	46,del(5q)	De novo
	Adult	48,XX,del(5)(q31q35),−19,−21,+4 mar [1]/48, idem,−10,+mar5 [4]/49,XX, idem, −10, +mar4,+mar5 [4]/48,XX,idem,−10,+mar6 [3]/46,XX [1]	*De novo*
	Adult	50,XX,+mar4 [4]/46,XX [6]	*De novo*
	Adult	46,XY,del(1)(p22p32)/42,XY,idem,−3,−4,add(7)(q31), der(9)t(3;9) (q24;q31),−10,−13,−15, add(19)(q13.2), add(19)(q12),+mar [23]	Secondary
	Adult	t(9;22)(q34;q11)	Secondary
Cuneo et al. (1996) (53)	Adult	51,XX,+6,t(9;22)(q34;q11),+10,+19,+der(22)t(9;22)(q34;q11)/52,idem,+8	*De novo*
Yamamoto et al. (2000) (50)	Adult	61,XX,−X,−1,−2,−3,−4,−5,−7,t(9;22)(q34;q11)x2, −15,−16,−17,−18,+19, +21,+22/61,idem,−22,+der(22)t(9;22)	Unknown
Hasserjian et al. (2001) (51)	Adult	46,XY	Post-MDS
	Adult	43−44,XY,−5,−7,del(12)(q24),−13,−14,add(16) (p1),−17,−19,add(19)(p1),+4,−5 mar	Unknown
Park et al. (2002) (52)	Adult	46,XY,dup(1)(p?p?) [20]	*De novo*
	Adult	47,del(X)(q22),Y,t(2;7)(q11;p13),del(4)(q21), der(7),der(8),der(9),der(10),der(19) [8]/46,XY [8]	Secondary
Cigudosa et al. (2003) (46)	Child	49,XX,inv(X)(p22.1q13),+5,+8,+18	*De novo*
Lessard et al. (2005) (47)	Adult	48,XX,t(8;9)(p22;p23),del(21)(q21q22),+mar1,+mar2 [14]	*De novo*
	Adult	45,XY,add(4)(q25),del(5)(q13q32)−7,−9,−16,−19,+3 mar [5] 46,XY,−7, ?add(16q),−19,+r,+mar [1]/46,XY [10]	*De novo*
	Adult	47,XX,+8,t(9;22)(q34;q11),der(18)t(18;22) (p11;q11).ish der(6)ins(6;9)(p21;q34)(abl+), t(9;22)(q34;q11)(ABL−;ABL+BCR+),der(18)t(18;22)(p11;q11)(ABL+BCR+)	Secondary
	Adult	36,X,−X,−3,−4,−7,t(9;22)(q34;q11),−12,−16,−17,−18,−22 [3]/36,idem,del(5)(q21q34) [3]/64−68, idem x 2 [cp4]	Post-CML
	Adult	44−46,XY,−7,−8,add(11)(p11),add(12)(p11),−16,−18,−21, −22,+mar,2 dmin [cp5]/46, XY [15] nuc ish7q22 (854E8 × 2),7q32(928C11 × 1) [31%]	*De novo*
	Adult	46,XY,t(9;22)(q34;q11) [4]/63,XY,t(9;22),+1,−5,−7,+8,−9, −12,−14,−16,−17,−18, −20,+21,der22 × 2,+mar1 [6]/62−66,idem,+mar 2 [cp10]	Post-CML
	Adult	46,XX,t(9;22)(q34;q11) [18]/63−83,XXXX,+4,+5,+6,+8,+8,−9, der(9)t(9;22), +10,+12,+13,+16, +16,+21,−22,+mar1,+mar2 [cp6]	Post-CML

7.2.3.1 Erythroleukemia

The myeloid blasts express a variety of myeloid markers, similar to other subtypes of AML: CD13, CD33, CD117 (c-Kit), and MPO. The erythroblasts lack myeloid antigens but are positive to glycophorin A and hemoglobin A.

7.2.3.2 Pure Erythroid Leukemia

Leukemic cells have a HLA DR⁻ CD36⁺⁺ B⁻ T⁻ myeloid⁻ (CD33±) immunopheno-type in addition to a proerythroblastlike or an undifferentiated morphology. Villeval et al. (45) distinguished two main phenotypes that correspond to discrete stages of the normal erythroid differentiation: (1) Erythroid blasts, which have differentiated, will be positive with glycophorin A but negative with MPO and myeloid markers; (2) the more immature blasts are difficult to identify as erythroid because they are usually negative for glycophorin A. Immature erythroid progenitors might be detected using carbonic anhydrase 1 or CD36. Some of them coexpressed CD36 and CD41. This favors the early burst-forming unit-erythroid (BFU-E) type of cells. Although CD36 is not specific for erythroid progenitors, negative markers for megakaryocytes and monocytes will aid the diagnosis.

7.2.4   Clinical and Biological Presentation

7.2.4.1 Clinical Findings

Acute erythroid leukemia presents with symptoms and signs of pancytopenia. Signs and symptoms are usually nonspecific (33, 41, 61, 62). The most common are: fatigue or malaise, weight loss, easy bruising, fever, bone or abdominal pain, dyspnea, and diffuse joint pain. One-third of the patients were reported with symptoms of infection (62). Meningeal signs are very rare and only observed in cases of central nervous system (CNS) involvement. Physical examination can show pallor related to anemia, hemorrhages (ecchymoses, petechiae, gum bleeding, epistaxis, retinal hemorrhage) related to thrombocytopenia, fever and infection related to neutropenia, hepatosplenomegaly (<25% of cases), and lymphadenopathy.

7.2.4.2 Peripheral Blood Findings

Most patients present with pancytopenia. Laboratory evaluation uncovered anemia in virtually all patients (usually normochromic and either normocytic or macro-cytic) (Table 7.5) (33, 41, 61–63). Although the exact cause of the anemia remains unknown, defects in heme synthesis (64), alterations of the transferrin receptor cycle (65), and decreased red blood cell survival (66) have all been implicated.

Table 7.5 Mean initial characteristics and outcome in erythroleukemia

Reference	Pts	Age (years)	Hb (g/L)	WBC (× 10⁹/L)	Platelets (× 10⁹/L)	Secondary AML	Survival (months)
Sheets et al. (1963) (39)	7	56	65	4.8	82	ND	9.2
Scott et al. (1964) (74)	18	37	85	45.5	120	ND	5.9
Bank et al. (1966) (75)	3	57	87	5.7	32	ND	7.8
Karle et al. (1974) (63)	14	51	62	5.8	57	ND	4.4
Bloomfield et al. (1974) (76)	7	39	73	15.7	35	ND	13.6
Sondergaard-Petersen (1975) (41)	17	62	72	ND	ND	ND	3.2
Rosenthal et al. (1977) (77)	7	43	96	56.5	173	ND	2.8
Hetzel and Gee (1978) (33)	32	49	84	12.3	126	ND	11.4
Roggli et al. (1981) (61)	14	58	75	5.4	123	ND	8.7
Olopade et al. (1992) (17)	26	60	66	4.0	92	36%	12.1
Atkinson et al. (1993) (22)	15	57	76	3.1	67	47%	9.4
Goldberg et al. (1998) (82)[a]	26	ND	86	2.6	38	50%	6.0
Wells et al. (2001) (19)[a]	33	39 / 69[b]	84 / 74[b]	6.8 / 5.9[b]	ND	ND	11 / 3[b]
Colita et al. (2001) (73)[a]	54	59	85	3.2	47	26%	9.0
Domingo-Claros et al. (2002) 42[a, c]	62	67	78	2.7	42	11%	6–12

Hb, hemoglobin; ND, not done; Pts, patients; WBC, white blood cell.

[a]Results are expressed not as mean but as median.

[b]Features were given according to age: patients aged less than 56 years (range: 3–53 years)/ patients aged more than 56 years (range: 57–84).

[c]The series comprised two patients classified as having pure erythremia and seven patients who could not be classified according to the WHO criteria.

Few reports have paid particular attention to erythrocytic morphology. Schistocytes and teardrop cells were outstanding features (42, 67, 68). Pincered cells were also found in 60% of cases (42) and might indicate an involvement of the band 3 trans-membrane protein. Nucleated red blood cells were reported with high frequency although reticulocyte counts varied widely between reports (33, 41, 61). Regarding other myeloid lineages, dysplastic features were nonspecific. The peripheral blood differential might vary and include blasts. Thrombocytopenia was generally noted. The megakaryocytic lineage was the second most affected cellular line, with dysplastic features such as micromegakaryocytes, mononuclear elements, and meg-akaryocytes with multiple unconnected nuclei (42). Other peripheral blood findings were Auer rods (41, 63), agranular polymorphonuclear cells, and acquired "pseudo"-Pelger-Huet anomaly in the neutrophils (41, 61).

7.2.4.3 Bone Marrow Findings

Bone marrow findings typically included a hypercellular marrow displaying a decreased M:E ratio and morphologic evidence of trilineage involvement. Morphologic abnormalities of the red cell series included megaloblastoid change with bizarre multilobated nuclei, irregular indented forms, double nuclei and polyploid projections (41, 62, 63, 69). A strongly positive PAS staining reaction of erythroblasts was found to be diagnostically useful (69). Abnormal sideroblasts, including ringed forms, have been described (70). Electron microscopic examination of erythroblasts has shown the presence of cytoplasmic glycogen and numerous mitochondria (71). Multilineage dysplasia is present in most of the reports (72). In a large series, myelodysplastic changes were observed in at least one cell lineage in all cases and in two cell lineages in 86% of cases (25). Increased myeloblasts and promyelocytes displaying large nucleoli and abnormal coarse granules as well as decreased megakaryocytes with atypical forms have been reported (41, 62). The heterogeneity of trilineage dysplasia can be explained by the fact that erythroleukemia includes primary and secondary diseases.

7.2.5   Treatment

Presumably, the published data on AML-M6 include a heterogeneous collection of disorders. Many of the past cases published as erythroleukemia would probably not fulfill the revised FAB or the WHO criteria. Some of these cases would now be classified under another FAB subtype or as RAEB. It has been suggested that AML-M6 patients respond less well to chemotherapy that other AML patients. This remains to be rigorously demonstrated in prospective studies using uniform treatment regimens.

7.2.5.1   Overall Outcomes

The prognosis of acute erythroid leukemia is reported as poor. It is, however, important to differentiate *de novo* from secondary or therapy-related erythroid leukemia, where the latter have a worse prognosis. Remission induction for *de novo* disease is similar to other subtypes of AML. Complete remission (CR) was achieved in about half of the cases (17). This was confirmed in a more recent retrospective larger series showing CR in 54% of cases: 65% and 40% for patients aged less and more than 60 years, respectively (73). In other series, the level of CR did not exceed 10–40%, especially in secondary AML-M6 (52). CR, if obtained, might be brief. The mean survival ranged from 3 months to 13 months (Table 7.5) (17, 22, 33, 39, 41, 42, 61, 63, 73–77). An improved survival has been noted in daunorubicin-treated cases in contrast to those treated with other chemotherapeutic agents (61). The poor outcome has been linked to the short remission duration. Poor prognostic factors for disease-free survival were secondary AML and lower initial platelet counts (73). Poor prognostic factors for overall survival were older age (73), secondary AML (61, 73), splenomegaly (61), morphology of erythroblasts (25), preponderance of proerythroblasts (78), ratio of pronormoblasts to myeloblasts at diagnosis (12), expression of P-glycoprotein (79), and severe initial anemia (73). Patients with complex karyotypes or abnormalities of chromosome 5 and/or 7 have a higher relapse rate than those with normal or simple karyotypes (17, 73, 80). The CR rate in patients with 5q or 7q abnormalities is about 20% and the median survival reaches 16 weeks compared to 77 weeks for patients without these abnormalities (81). Among patients receiving aggressive rather than palliative therapy, higher remission rate (80% vs. 25%) and survival advantage (11.5 vs. 2.5 months) were seen in erythroleukemia compared to Di Guglielmo disease (82). Stem cell transplantation (SCT) in first CR could be considered, particularly in patients with a poor cytogenetics (83).

7.2.5.2 Postremission Therapy

Data indicating the specific outcome of erythroleukemia following allogeneneic or autologous SCT are scarce. The outcome of 19 patients receiving allogeneic or autologous SCT was reported by the Royal Marsden group (83). The overall survival was 66% at 2 years. The only study giving information on hematopoietic SCT in a large series of patients with erythroleukemia is that from the European Group for Blood and Marrow Transplantation (EBMT) registry (84). Erythroleukemia represented 2.9% of patients with *de novo* AML who were registered by the EBMT. In this series, the outcome at 5 years following allogeneic identical sibling SCT showed a leukemia-free survival (LFS) of 57 ± 5% (Table 7.6). Results for the 104 allografted patients matched those of most prospective trials of allogeneic SCT for *de novo* AML in first CR using an HLA-identical family donor (85–89). In contrast, results of autologous SCT in the EBMT study were low. LFS at 5 years was 26%, attributed mainly to a high relapse incidence (RI) of 70% at 5 years (Table 7.6). These results compared unfavorably with the data from the literature for *de novo* AML showing long-term LFS rates between 35% and 67% (85–90). Prognostic factors were not different from those observed in hematopoietic SCT for *de novo* AML. For allogeneic SCT, acute graft-versus-host disease (GVHD) of grade 2 or more was associated with higher treatment-related mortality (TRM),

Table 7.6 Results for autologous and allogeneic transplantation in patients with erythroleukemia from EBMT registry

Outcome	Autologous SCT (103 patients)	Allogeneic SCT[a] (104 patients)
Median follow-up (range)	26 months (1–157)	46 months (2–169)
LFS at 5 years	26% ± 5%	57% ± 5%
RI at 5 years	70% ± 6%	21% ± 5%
TRM at 5 years	13% ± 4%	27% ± 5%
OS at 5 years	34% ± 6%	57% ± 5%

LFS, leukemia-free survival; OS, overall survival; STC, stem cell transplantation; RI, relapse incidence; TRM, treatment-related mortality.

[a]Identical sibling.

Source: Data from Fouillard et al. (84).

and age older than 45 years was associated with lower LFS, higher TRM, and lower overall survival (OS). For autologous SCT, younger age was associated with a better LFS and better OS (84).

7.2.5.3   New Therapeutic Strategies

Alternative therapeutic approaches have been tested in certain cases of AML-M6, including imatinib mesylate in a BCR/ABL-positive AML-M6 (91). CR achievement has been described in certain patients with AML-M6 using highdose recombinant erythropoietin and granulocyte colony-stimulating factor (G-CSF) (92). The use of erythropoietin in AML-M6 patients was however controversial, with studies showing no stimulation of leukemic cells and no interference with the antiproliferative and/or cytotoxic effects of chemotherapy (93) and case reports suggesting a stimulation of leukemic cell population (94).

7.3   Acute Megakaryoblastic Leukemia

Acute megakaryoblastic leukemia is a rare subtype of AML that develops from primitive megakaryoblasts. The term "acute megakaryoblastic leukemia" was introduced in 1931 by von Boros (95). Developments in cytochemistry and immunophenotyping have improved its diagnosis and differentiation from acute myelosclerosis (96). The disease can be identified by antibodies to glycoprotein IIb/IIIa and is often associated with extensive myelofibrosis (96–104). Reports of the natural history of the disease have generally been confined to either sporadic small series (96–103), reports of one or two cases (105–109), or description of the clinical course in infants and children (110–115). In 1985, acute megakaryoblastic leukemia was included in the FAB classification system of hematological neoplasias with the designation of AML-M7 (2). Historically, the lack of specific criteria for the diagnosis has led to reports of patients who likely had AML-M7 but whose disease was labeled acute myelofibrosis or myelosclerosis (116–122). Precise diagnostic criteria were added to the FAB classification only relatively recently. In the WHO classification, AML-M7 is defined by more than 20% (1) of blasts of megakaryocyte lineage in the bone marrow aspirate as determined by morphology and immunoflowcytometry.

7.3.1   Epidemiology

AML-M7 is a rare type of AML and, due to difficulty in diagnosis, its exact incidence is not known. There is no male or female preponderance. AML-M7 occurs in all age groups with two peaks in distribution: One peak is in adults and the other is in children 1–3 years of age (123). It might account for approximately 1–2% of all *de novo* AML in the adult population, but the incidence during childhood is higher (5–15% of AML) (115, 124). Secondary AML-M7, evolving from an antecedent idiopathic myelodysplasia or occurring after exposure to chemotherapeutic agents, such as topoisomerase II inhibitors, is uncommon in children. Several unusual associations with AML-M7 have been identified. First, AML-M7 has been linked to primary mediastinal germ cell tumors (125, 126). Second, a higher than normal proportion of AML-M7 has been reported in children with Down's syndrome (127–129).

7.3.2 Criteria for Diagnosis of Acute Megakaryoblastic Leukemia

The more common types of AML have to be excluded by morphological and cytochemical analyses, whereas immunology is required to exclude acute lymphoblastic leukemia (ALL). By definition, AML-M7 requires confirmation of megakaryocytic lineage in 50% or more of the leukemic blasts (1). The megakaryocytic nature of the leukemia has to be proven by ultrastructural demonstration of platelet peroxidase or by immunological demonstration of CD61, CD42, or CD41 cell surface expression. AML-M7 shows a wide morphologic spectrum (Table 7.7). The blast cell morphology varies from case to case. In some instances, small cells dominate, clearly showing megakaryocytic differentiation with scant amounts of cytoplasm and with nuclei showing dense chromatin. On the other hand, there are cases resembling

Table 7.7 Morphologic and cytochemical features of acute megakaryoblastic leukemia

Acute megakaryoblastic leukemia
- Medium- to large-sized megakaryoblasts with round or indented nucleus and one or more nuclei
- Agranular, basophilic cytoplasm with pseudopod formation
- Lymphoblastlike morphology (high nuclear-cytoplasmic ratio) in some cases
- Circulating micromegakaryocytes, megakaryoblastic fragments, dysplastic large platelets, and hypogranular neutrophils
- Stromal pattern of marrow infiltration mimicking a metastatic tumor in infants
- Negative stains for Sudan black B and MPO
- Blasts reactive with PAS, acid phosphatase, and nonspecific esterase

Variant: AML/transient myeloproliferative disorder in Down syndrome
- Blasts with round to slightly irregular nuclei and a moderate amount of basophilic cytoplasm
- Coarse azurophilic granules in the cytoplasm that resemble basophil granules
- Promegakaryocytes and micromegakaryocytes
- Dyserythropoiesis
- MPO-negative and Sudan black B-negative blasts

ALL-L2 blasts with moderate amounts of rather basophilic cytoplasm, which, in some instances, contain azurophilic granules. In some patients, the blasts are undifferentiated and the diagnosis requires immunophenotyping or electron microscopy studies. Dysmegakaryopoiesis is rather frequent. Other patients might show bleb-forming blasts (Figure 7.4), but this feature is not specific for megakaryoblasts. The nuclei of these cells are round, with more finely reticulated chromatin and with prominent nucleoli. Micromegakaryocytes can be frequently seen. No relationship could be established between morphologic features and cytogenetics. The bone biopsy almost invariably shows fibrosis, which can be extensive in up to 75% of cases (122, 130, 131).

Blast cells exhibit a classical α-naphthyl acetate esterase activity, with a multifocal punctate cytoplasmic staining pattern only partially inhibited by sodium fluoride (124).

The MPO stain is negative by light microscopy, but ultrastructural peroxidase activity with a specific perinuclear staining pattern can be detected at the electron microscopy level (96).

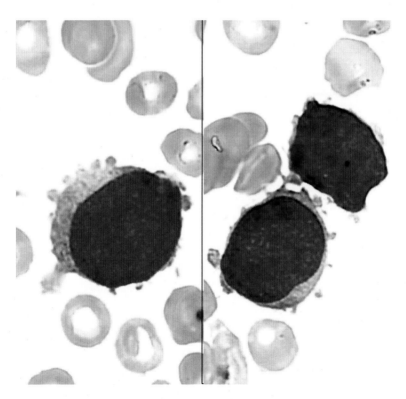

Figure 7.4 Megakaryoblasts of variable size with a round nucleus and a basophilic cytoplasm, which may show distinct blebs or pseudopod formation

7.3.3 Cytogenetics

Compared to other AMLs, AML-M7 is characterized by a higher incidence of abnormalities, a higher complexity of karyotypes, and a different distribution of abnormalities among children and adults (132). Abnormal karyotypes are found in about 94% of cases (132), whereas they represent approximately 80% of cases in *de novo* AMLs in children (133, 134) and 50–60% in adults (135, 136). Poor cytogenetic characteristics are more commonly observed in patients with AML-M7 than in patients with other AML subtypes (137). Complex karyotypes were observed in 39% of children and 53% of adults with AML-M7, whereas they represent 10% of cases in pediatric series (133) and 34% of cases in adults (135) in *de novo* AMLs.

7.3.3.1 Adults

Total or partial deletions of chromosome 5 (-5/5q-) and/or chromosome 7 (-7/7q-) are found in virtually all cases with complex karyotype, which globally account for 70–80% of abnormal cases. Chromosome 3 (q21 or q26) aberrations are found in 20–30% of the cases. The incidence of 3q aberrations in AML-M7 is higher than in *de novo* AMLs (2%) and secondary AMLs (5%) (136). Abnormalities of chromosome 3 [t(3;3) or inv(3)] might be associated with preservation of the peripheral platelet count (138–142). The t(9;22) is another recurrent chromosome aberration in *de novo* AML-M7. Although its genuine incidence is difficult to assess in AML-M7, t(9;22) is probably more frequent in this subgroup than in *de novo* AML, in which probably 1% of patients are Philadelphia-positive (135, 136). Trisomy 19 and 21 might occur in *de novo* as well as in secondary AML-M7 (132). They are the most frequently occurring chromosome gains and they might be associated with any of the cytogenetic anomalies listed above (142). Although pediatric AML-M7 is often associated with t(1;22)(p13;q13), this abnormality has not been reported in adults with AML-M7. No specific association between outcome and chromosome abnormalities has been established in this age group.

7.3.3.2 Children

The t(1;22)(p13;q13) is specifically associated with childhood AML-M7, being found in approximately half of the cases. This translocation occurs primarily during infancy (median age: 4 months). It has seldom been detected in children older than 1 year and occasionally in children with Down's syndrome (143, 144). The t(1;22) has relatively distinct clinicopathologic features. Clinically, it is almost invariably associated with hepatosplenomegaly. Laboratory studies typically demonstrate anemia and thrombocytopenia. Attempts at bone marrow aspiration often result in a "dry tap," and bone marrow biopsy usually shows marked myelofibrosis. The megakaryoblasts often manifest an infiltrative growth pattern suggestive of a metastatic solid tumor (143). The t(1;22) is the sole cytogenetic finding in nearly 60% of cases. The frequency of complex karyotypes increases with age, with approximately 80% of cases in children older than 6 months having complex karyotypes. The exclusive association of the t(1;22) with AML-M7 suggests that this translocation has a critical pathogenetic role in this disorder. The t(1;22)(p13;q13) fuses the One Twenty-Two (*OTT*) or Rna-binding motif protein 15 (*RBM*15) gene on 1p13 to the Megakaryoblastic Acute Leukemia (*MAL*) or Megakaryoblastic Leukemia-1 (*MLK*1) gene on chromosome 22, leading to the *OTT-MAL* fusion gene on the derivative 22 chromosome [der(22)] (145, 146). The OTT-MAL transcript encodes a chimeric protein containing all of the functional domains of both partner proteins and, thus, is believed to encode the oncogenic protein. The t(1;22) likely occurs through a non-homologous, end-joining mechanism (147). The finding of an OTT-MAL transcript in patients with normal karyotype suggests that the frequency of this group is still probably underestimated. The t(1;22) might be cryptic, but it might also be undetected because it is often present in minor clones, as attested by the frequently low numbers of blasts and of abnormal metaphases in these patients (132). Reverse transcriptase–polymerase chain reaction (RT-PCR) could be diagnostically useful in these cases (148). OTT-MAL potentially might deregulate RNA processing and possibly HOX (Homeobox) signaling. However, the exact mechanism by which this chimeric protein affects its oncogenic properties remains unknown.

Other abnormalities account for 40–80% of all primary pediatric AML-M7. Patients are diagnosed at a median age of 2 years and are, therefore, significantly older than those with t(1;22). Cytogenetic studies have identified an array of numeric and structural chromosomal abnormalities, including trisomy 21 (irrespective of the association with Down's syndrome) (149), trisomy 19, and trisomy 8 and abnormalities in chromosome band 3q21q26 (132, 150). Acquired trisomy 21 has a higher incidence in childhood AML-M7 than in other childhood *de novo* AMLs (133, 136) and represents probably one of the characteristics of childhood AML-M7. Partial trisomy 19, involving the q13 band, can be shown to occur at a 20–30% incidence by comparative genomic hybridization (151). Abnormalities of 11q23, targeting the MLL locus, occur in up to 25% of cases (124). The karyotype might be normal in approximately 10% of the cases (132).

7.3.4 *Immunophenotype*

Flow cytometry is the preferred method for immunophenotypic characterization of AML-M7. The blast cells show one or more megakaryocytic markers [i.e., Factor VIII, CD61 (platelet glycoprotein GPIIIa), CD41a (GPIIb), CD41b, or CD42b (GP1bα)] (152–154). They test negative when using the anti-myeloperoxidase monoclonal antibody and never show coordinated expression of lymphoid markers, although isolated CD2 or CD7 positivity can be found. The CD34, CD13, and CD33 markers are positive in a substantial fraction of cases, as is the CD36/thrombospondin receptor (142). AML-M7 blasts typically are dim or negative for CD45 expression and can be negative for all other markers tested when limited antibody panels are used. Indeed, not infrequently, bone marrow aspiration yields an insufficient quantity of cells for complete immunophenotyping due to marrow reticulin fibrosis. Obtaining a bone marrow biopsy and performing appropriate immunohistochemical studies are imperative in these problematic cases to avoid an erroneous diagnosis.

7.3.5 Clinical and Biological Presentation

The presentation is usually acute, although AML-M7 might develop after MDS or CML. In adults, more than half of patients have an antecedent hematologic disorder or MDS or both (137), and one patient in five has previously received chemotherapy for other malignancies. In contrast to adults, there was little evidence to suggest that childhood AML-M7 typically arises as a secondary leukemia, because no dysgranulopoiesis and few of the "hallmark" chromosomal abnormalities were observed. In some cases, acute myelofibrosis is the presentation picture. Extensive bone marrow fibrosis was found in 62% of cases in the study from M. D. Anderson Cancer Center (137). Inaspirable bone marrows have contributed to the difficulty in establishing the diagnosis. AML-M7 is associated more frequently with a lower percentage of bone marrow blasts than other AML subtypes. Main characteristics in adults at presentation are summarized in Table 7.7. In children, AML-M7 is often confused with metastatic solid tumors or MDS. As mentioned earlier, there is an association with Down's syndrome. Splenic enlargement is frequently seen in children (70%) and less frequently in adults (26%), whereas hepatomegaly was observed in 60% and 35%, respectively (132). Lymph node enlargement was rare in children (11%) and never observed in adults. Other sites of disease include periostosis and osteolytic lesions in children (155), mediastinal mass, kidney involvement, chloroma, and the CNS (132).

7.3.6 AML-M7 with Down's Syndrome: A Model for Leukemogenesis

7.3.6.1 AML-M7 with Down's Syndrome

AML-M7 is the most common FAB subtype in cases of leukemia associated with Down's syndrome (156–161). The prevalence rate of AML-M7 with Down's syndrome ranges from 17% to 23% (124, 162, 163). AML-M7 occurs approximately 400–500 times more often in children with Down's syndrome than in the general pediatric population (164) The malignancy is often preceded by a preleukemic phase of few months. If a patient with Down's syndrome has MDS, the condition will ultimately proceed to megakaryoblastic leukemia. Two forms of megakaryoblastic leukemia can be observed in this group of patients. Approximately 10% of newborns with Down's syndrome develop transient leukemia during their first 1–3 months of life, also referred to as transient myeloproliferative disorder and transient abnormal myelopoiesis, a form of megakaryoblastic leukemia specific for Down's syndrome (165–167). Most children with transient myeloproliferative disorder are asymptomatic. Consequently, transient leukemia is detected most frequently in routine blood counts or those ordered for an unrelated clinical indication. The white blood cell count usually is not greatly elevated, although the blast percentage might be quite high. Transient leukemia blasts are morphologically indistinguishable from AML-M7 blasts, contributing to the hypothesis that the second disease is derived from the first (168). Often the karyotype of AML-M7 is more complex than that of the transient leukemia but contains abnormalities observed in the original clone, consistent with clonal evolution (169). In a recent prospective study of 48 infants with Down's syndrome and transient myeloproliferative disorder, 36% had cytogenetic abnormalities in addition to trisomy 21 (170). The frequency of additional karyotypic aberrations was higher in those children with transient leukemia who ultimately progressed to acute leukemia, suggesting that such findings might be of prognostic and pathogenetic significance. A proportion of these blasts also express erythroid-specific mRNAs, such as γ-globin and erythroid δ-aminolevulinate synthetase (171). Although the majority of such infants will show spontaneous and persistent remission within the first 3 months, 20–30% will develop AML-M7 (128, 166, 172). The megakaryoblasts have features of early erythroid precursors, and a higher than normal incidence of erythroleukemia occurs in patients with Down's syndrome. It is likely that in transient leukemia, MDS, and AML-M7 of Down's syndome, the leukemic progenitor cells are able to differentiate into cells of megakaryocytic, mast cell, and erythroid lineage, a phenomenon that is unique to Down's syndrome (173). Megakaryoblasts have an unusual distribution of clonal cytogenetic alterations, suggesting that the molecular and cellular bases for AML-M7 might differ from that occurring in similar patients without Down's syndrome (174). Several cases of transient myeloproliferative disorder have been described in children lacking clinical features of Down's syndrome (175, 176). In these cases, trisomy 21 was documented in only the transient myeloproliferative disorder blasts and was presumably either acquired or arose in a constitutionally mosaic background.

Significant differences were observed in the frequency of expression of the myeloid antigens CD13 and CD11b between Down's syndrome AML-M7 and transient myeloproliferative disorder (177). Nearly all cases of AML-M7 expressed CD13 and CD11b, whereas only few cases of transient leukemia were positive for these markers. More recently, several differentially expressed genes were identified including *MYCN* and *CDKN2C* (cyclin-dependent kinase inhibitor 2C), which can serve as more reliable markers for distinguishing between these disorders (178). One gene, *PRAME* (Preferentially expressed Antigen in Melanoma), was highly expressed in AML-M7 and had virtually undetectable expression in transient leukemia blasts.

Despite its evanescent nature, transient myeloproliferative disorder can be associated with several potentially life-threatening complications. The development *in utero* is a significant cause of morbidity and mortality in Down's syndrome. Hydrops fetalis occurs in 10–15% of cases (179). Hepatic fibrosis also develops in a subset of infants with transient leukemia. Cholestatic liver disease is progressive and fatal in approximately 50% of cases (180). Although its pathogenesis is not well understood, overexpression of platelet-derived growth factor-β (PDGBβ) and transforming growth factor-β1 (TGF-β1) by hepatic parenchymal cells or the _ megakaryocytic cells might have an important pathogenic role in the development of hepatic fibrosis (181). Finally, hemorrhagic or thrombotic complications can occur in occasional cases of transient leukemia secondary to profound cytopenias or hyperleukocytosis.

7.3.6.2 Model for Leukemogenesis

AML-M7 in children with Down's syndrome might be an excellent model for leukemogenesis (182). The genetic background is defined by trisomy 21 and the recently detected mutations in exon 2 of the X-linked *GATA*1 gene in nearly all patients. It encodes a zinc-finger transcription factor that is essential for normal erythroid and megakaryocytic differentiation. Transient leukemia in newborns with trisomy 21 could help to identify leukemogenetic features. Finally, AML-M7 in children without Down's syndrome exhibit similarities in terms of blast phenotype and age at diagnosis but a very high resistance to treatment, providing excellent options for comparison to AML-M7 in children with Down's syndrome.

Trisomy 21 could be assumed to be both a predisposing and first event in leukemogenesis As an increased and prolonged turnover of myelopoiesis and megakaryopoiesis has been demonstrated in these patients. Of note, *RUNX*1 (*AML*1), *ETS*-2, *ERG* (early response genes), and *BACH*1 (all hematopoietic transcription factors involved in early megakaryopoesis) are encoded on chromosome 21 (183). The most interesting candidate leukemia-predisposing gene is *RUNX*1, which is required for the generation of all definitive hematopoietic lineages (184). Mutations in the DNA-binding Runt domain of *RUNX*1 result in a familial platelet disorder with predisposition to AML (185), and are present in about 10% of sporadic cases of *de novo* AML and in myeloid malignancies with acquired trisomy 21 (186).

For the evolution of a leukemic cell, an environment providing a cell survival and proliferation advantage is required. In the trisomy 21 model, an increased megakaryocytic secretion of TGF (187) or platelet-derived growth factor (PDGF) induces an environment with advantages for an increased myelopoiesis and megakaryopoiesis (188). This might be supported by increased levels of thrombopoietin (TPO) (189), which is involved in both early myeloproliferation and megakaryopoiesis. These conditions might cause a positive selection of the preleukemic GATAs clone and favor additional events. The majority of *GATA*1 mutations involved small deletions or insertions. In children with Down's syndrome, the mutation in exon 2 of the *GATA*1 causes the loss of the N-terminal activation domain, leading to a shorter gene product (GATA1s) with decreased activity (190, 191). Similar *GATA*1 mutations were described in patients with transient leukemia and in those with AML-M7 (192). This suggests that *GATA*1 mutations represent an early pathogenic event that occurs prior to the transformation of transient leukemia to AML-M7. Mutations in *GATA*1 were not detected in leukemic cells of Down's syndrome children with other types of acute leukemia or in other patients with AML-M7 who did not have Down's syndrome (191). GATA1s exerts dominant action on early progenitors, leading to hyperproliferation (193). In the absence of *GATA*1, megakaryocytes proliferate excessively and fail to generate platelets (194). A significant increase of GATA1s expression was demonstrated in blasts derived from children with transient leukemia or AML-M7 with Down's syndrome. Because transient leukemia presents in the neonatal period, *GATA*1 mutations almost certainly occur *in utero* (192). Several other members of the GATA family play key roles in specification and maturation of a subset of hematopoietic lineages. *GATA2* participates in the maintenance and proliferation of hematopoietic progenitor cells and was also shown to be increased. By contrast, the chromosome 21-encoded transcription factors RUNX1, ETS-2, and ERG were not differently expressed compared to healthy controls. Due to the loss of the N-terminal site in GATA1s, the binding site of RUNX1 (195), an impaired ability to form a transcription complex with RUNX1 causes an inhibition of megakaryocytic differentiation and maturation but not proliferation. Further, the balance between *GATA*1 and *GATA2* is disturbed (196), and due to the reduced activity of GATA1s, *GATA2* is upregulated. Its increased expression has been shown to stimulate megakaryopoietic and myelopoietic proliferation but to inhibit maturation. Another finding is the reduced expression of *PU.1* in transient leukemia and AML-M7 with Down's syndrome. This loss of expression has been shown to be involved in the development of AML (197). *GATA1* interferes directly with *PU.1* (198). Whereas the stroma cells either in the fetal liver (transient leukemia) or in bone marrow (AML-M7 with Down's syndrome) experience induction of fibrotic changes, the megakaryoblasts seem not to be inhibited by TGF.

All of these observations support the model that Down's syndrome leukemogenesis is a multistep process with acquisition by progenitor cells of multiple genetic lesions during the progression to acute leukemia. Trisomy 21 is the first event but is not sufficient for the expansion of megakaryoblasts seen in transient leukemia. Disruption of wild-type *GATA*1 activity is an essential second step. Mutagenesis of *GATA*1, in conjunction with trisomy 21, is sufficient to promote the transient expansion of immature megakaryoblasts seen in transient leukemia. Additional mutations are involved in the transformation to acute leukemia (Figure 7.5). These additional lesions could be mutations in p*53* (199),

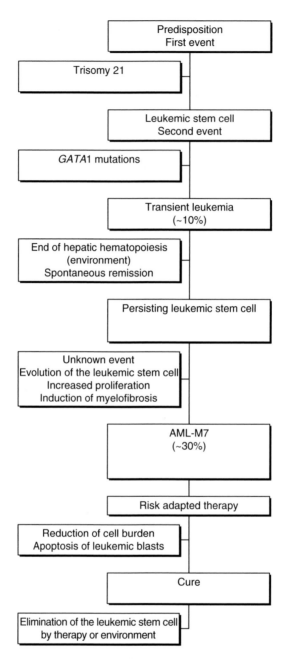

Figure 7.5 Model for the progression of transient leukemia and AML-M7 in Down's syndrome. Trisomy 21 likely represents the initiating event in leukemogenesis of Down's syndrome because it occurs very early in embryogenesis. The subsequent mutagenesis of *GATA*1 and selection of progenitor cells that harbor *GATA*1 mutations might be the second initiating event that leads to the neonatal appearance of transient leukemia in at least 10% of infants with Down's syndrome. In the majority of infants with transient leukemia, the *GATA*1 mutant clone disappears during remission, but 30% of the time, the mutant clones acquire additional mutations that promote the development of acute leukemia by the age of 5 years

altered telomerase activity (200), or additional acquired karyotypic abnormalities (201).

7.3.7 Treatment

7.3.7.1 Overall Outcomes

The prognosis for patients with AML-M7 is poor. Although remission rates are not much lower than those for other myeloid leukemia subtypes, the relapse rate is high. Approximately half of the patient population achieves CR with conventional chemotherapy, but few patients survive beyond 3 years (103, 141, 202, 203). The median overall survival is estimated to be 40 weeks in adults (203), whereas the 2-year event-free survival (EFS) ranges from 0% to 20% in children (124, 156). Because of its rarity and the lack of precise diagnostic criteria in the past, few series of adults treated with contemporary therapy have been reported. A summary of main reports on adult AML-M7 is given in Table 7.8. A histopathologic diagnosis of AML-M7 in adults is an independent adverse prognostic factor for overall survival (137). Thus, the poor prognosis of AML-M7 is not fully dependent on cytogenetic abnormalities. It indicates that distinctive biologic mechanisms play a role in AML-M7. A summary of main reports on children AML-M7 is given in Table 7.9. For patients with secondary AML-M7, the outcome of contemporary treatment appears to be as poor as that for other types of secondary AML. Children with *de novo* AML-M7 in the absence of Down's syndrome have a more than 70% probability of achieving remission with regimens containing dose-intensive cytarabine, but they have a very high rate of relapse if therapy after remission consists only of intensive chemotherapy (124). The prognosis of children with t(1;22) is relatively poor, with only 53% of affected children achieving CR and a median survival of approximately 8 months (143). Children with chromosomal abnormalities other than t(1;22) have a very poor prognosis, with an overall survival of 0–14% (124, 204). Patients treated with chemotherapy alone have a very high rate of relapse. Thus, allogeneic SCT should be considered for patients who enter remission. Children who undergo allogeneic SCT after entering remission have significantly improved survival. However, allogeneic transplantation during active disease is not more advantageous than chemotherapy alone (124).

7.3.7.2 New Therapeutic Strategies

New therapeutic strategies need to be pursued, including biological agents such as interferon (205) and the apoptosis-inducing agent arsenic trioxide, which has been shown to cause an inhibition of growth and survival in megakaryocytic leukemia cell lines (206).

Table 7.8 Summary of main reports on adult AML-M7

Features	MDACC (137) (1987–2003)	ECOG (141) (1984–1997)	GIMEMA (203) (1982–1999)	GFHC (204) (1988–2000)
Characteristics				
Patients	37	20	24	23
Age (years)	54 (21–78)[a]	43 (18–70)	51 (15–76)	58 (19–79)
Male	58%	70%	58%	57%
AHD/MDS	14 (37%)	ND	ND	9 (39%)
Treatment related	5 (13%)	ND	0	2 (9%)
WBC ($\times 10^9$/L)	3.5 (0.5–49.9)	2.0 (0.8–35.2)	7.1 (0.5–162)	4.6 (0.3–72.6)
Hb (g/dL)	7.7 (3.2–10.9)	8.8 (4.0–14)	8.0 (3.6–13)	ND
Platelets ($\times 10^9$/L)	35 (5–2292)	65 (12–1450)	66 (20–572)	48 (4–490)
BM blasts (%)	30 (0–80)	59 (5–59)	75 (30–99)	53 (0–79)
Outcome				
CR rate	43%	50%	50%	50%
DFS (months)	6.5 (3–29)	10.6 (1–160+)	8.2 (2.3–102.9)	ND
OS (months)	5.6 (0.6–37)	10.4 (1–160+)	9.3	4.5 (0.07–53.5)

MDACC, M.D. Anderson Cancer Center; ECOG, Eastern Cooperative Oncology Group; GIMEMA, Gruppo Italiano Malattie Ematologiche dell' Adulto; GFHC, Groupe Français d'Hématologie Cellulaire; AHD, antecedent hematologic disorder; MDS, myelodysplastic syndrome; WBC, white blood cells; Hb, hemoglobin; BM, bone marrow; CR, complete remission; DFS, disease-free survival; OS, overall survival; ND, not done.

[a]Median (range).

Table 7.9 Summary of main reports on children AML-M7 without Down's syndrome

Features	Athale et al. (124)	Athale et al. (124)	Dastugue et al. (132)
Patients	6 children, secondary leukemia	29 children, *de novo* leukemia	23 children, *de novo* leukemia
Clinical features			
Median age (months)	113.3	21.6	10.5
Sex (male/female)	3 / 3	18 / 11	11 / 12
Fever	0%	28%	ND[a]
Lymphadenopathy	0%	38%	11%
Hepatomegaly	0%	55%	60%
Splenomegaly	0%	48%	70%
Biological features			
Hemoglobin (g/dL)	10 (4–13.8)[b]	8.8 (5.9–12.8)	ND
WBC ($\times 10^9$/L)	2.7 (1.1–6.9)	12.1 (3.3–59.2)	14.4
PB blasts (%)	12 (0–43)	16 (0–73)	ND
BM blasts (%)	42 (30–55)	52 (3–100)	ND
Platelets ($\times 10^9$/L)	184 (6–378)	40 (3–528)	ND
Outcome			
CR rate (%)	4 / 6 (X%)	7 / 29 (X%)	(77%)
Overall survival	20% at 2 years	14% at 2 years	36% at 3 years

[a]Not done.

[b]Median (range).

7.3.7.3 Postremission Therapy

Postremission therapy must be improved. Myeloablative treatment followed by allogeneic or autologous SCT represents the best chance of cure, but available clinical data are scant. Published reports are often case reports (100, 107) or small clinical series with inconsistent results (102, 124, 203, 207). In an early study in seven children undergoing bone marrow transplantation, three became long-term survivors (207). In a series of 29 patients with *de novo* AML-M7 but without Down's syndrome, the 2-year EFS rate was significantly higher after allogeneic SCT (26%) than after chemotherapy (0%) and was significantly higher when performed during remission (46%) than during persistent disease (0%) (124). However, in another study, six of seven patients who underwent transplantation during CR died within a few months, three from early toxicity and three from early relapse (203). The EBMT Group has recently evaluated outcomes in 57 children (11 with Down's syndrome) and 69 adults after a first CR following autologous or HLA-identical allogeneic transplantation (162). Results for autologous and allogeneic transplantation are summarized in Table 7.10. After autologous SCT, the relapse rate was high in adults (64% at 3 years, with no plateau). Autologous SCT benefited children more. The relapse rate was also high (45%), but there was a plateau after the first year. However, outcomes seem better than they were with conventional chemotherapy. After allogeneic SCT, TRM was fairly low in children and adults, and relapse rates were lower than after autologous SCT. All relapses in children and more than 90% of relapses in adults occurred within the first year, suggesting a graft-versus-leukemia (GVL) effect. Successful engraftment might be related to the reversal of bone marrow fibrosis by intensive chemotherapy or chemoradiotherapy followed by SCT (100, 107). Time of transplantation was the only significant prognostic factor in the multivariate analysis of adult who underwent allogeneic SCT. Given the dismal outcome of AML-M7 even after achieving CR, allogeneic SCT during the first CR appears to be beneficial in these patients.

Table 7.10 Results for autologous and allogeneic transplantation in children and adults with AML-M7

	Autologous transplantation		Allogeneic transplantation	
	Children (38 patients)	Adults (37 patients)	Children (19 patients)	Adults (32 patients)
Follow-up (months)	56 (5–162)[a]	13 (3–126)	63 (4–166)	47 (1–139)
3-year TRM	3% ± 5%	8% ± 9%	0	26% ± 15%
3-year RI	45% ± 16%	64% ± 18%	34% ± 24%	28% ± 17%
3-year LFS	52% ± 8%	27% ± 8%	66% ± 11%	46% ± 9%
3-year OS	61% ± 8%	30% ± 9%	82% ± 10%	43% ± 10%

TRM, treatment-related mortality; RI, relapse incidence; LFS, leukemia-free survival; OS, overall survival.
[a]Median (range).
Source: Data from Garderet et al. (162).

7.3.8 AML-M7 with Down's Syndrome

In the past, leukemia in patients with Down's syndrome was often treated subop-
timally, and many patients did not receive cytoreductive treatments. Physical
abnormalities, including potentially life-threatening cardiac and intestinal
malformations along with mental retardation and associated psychosocial issues,
high susceptibility to infections, and increased toxicity of chemotherapy might
have prejudiced physicians against the use of standard chemotherapy. The poor
tolerance of cytoreductive regimens in patients with Down's syndrome is well
documented. Their fibroblasts and lymphocytes have increased chromosomal
sensitivity to mutagenic agents and abnormal DNA repair (208). Although
treatment results in the general pediatric population improved greatly in the
1970s, they remained poor in Down's syndrome for a long time. Modern intensive schedules have recently been used to treat patients with Down's syndrome.
Preexisting congenital heart disease did not appear to predispose the patients to
anthracycline cardiac toxicity (157). Major neurotoxicity after high-dose cytarabine was not seen. Patients with Down's syndrome had a significantly higher
2-year EFS estimate (83%) than did other patients with *de novo* AML-M7 (14%)
or with secondary AML-M7 (20%) (124). In one study, EFS at 4 years was nearly
100% (157). A history of prior MDS had no adverse effect on the outcome.
Several patients have even had allogeneic SCT (209). Intensification in these
patients is more toxic, and the conditioning regimen should, therefore, be adjusted
accordingly. In the EBMT study, intensification was well tolerated, and only one
transplant-related death occurred (162). However, 36% of the children with
Down's syndrome had relapses, and there were no differences in outcomes after
autologous and allogeneic SCT.

Differences in prognosis might reflect differences in cellular drug resistance,
pharmacokinetics, or regrowth potential of residual disease. The better prognosis of AML-M7 with Down's syndrome might, at least partially, be explained
by a specific, relatively sensitive drug-resistance profile, reflecting the unique
biology of this disease. AML cells from children with Down's syndrome were
significantly more sensitive to cytarabine, anthracyclines, mitoxantrone, etoposide, and 6-thioguanine than AML cells from children without Down's
syndrome (210–212). Additional studies regarding cytarabine sensitivity
showed higher cytosine arabinoside triphosphate (Ara-CTP) levels and 12-fold
higher cysthationine-β-synthetase (*CBS*, localized to chromosome 21q22.3)
transcript levels (213, 214). In contrast, carbonyl reductase (localized to
21q22.1), which catalyzes the reduction of daunorubicin to daunorubicinol, did
not show higher transcript levels (213).

A specific clinical trial for Down's syndrome AML showed that treatment modification toward less intensive therapy is possible without affecting clinical outcome
(161). Patients with Down's syndrome included in the AML93 protocol of the BFM
(Berlin-Frankfurt-Münster)-AML Study Group were also treated with a less dose-
intensive schedule (dose reduction for anthracyclines and no SCT), resulting in a

5-year EFS rate of 67% ± 8%. The better survival of patients with Down's syndrome coincided with the introduction of the high-dose cytarabine-containing regimens (213). The prevailing opinion is that two or more courses of high-dose cytarabine postremission induction might be necessary for optimal therapy. However, the 100% EFS reported by the Pediatric Oncology Group (POG) investigators, based on the POG 8498 AML regimen 15 (7), has not been duplicated in subsequent studies (164, 215, 216). Subsequent studies eliminated the historic combination course of prednisone, vincristine, methotrexate, and 6-mercaptopurine (POMP), plus the final courses of conventional- dose cytarabine, and sought to intensify the postinduction courses. There was no increase in mortality rate in children with Down's syndrome, but significant pulmonary toxicity during induction was observed, including the need for ventilatory support, and an increased incidence of mucositis and skin toxicity during intensification (158). Undertreated AML children with Down's syndrome had markedly inferior outcomes (164, 215). Moderate-intensity therapy seems to be the most optimal therapy: Results with the intensively timed DCTER (dexamethasone, cytarabine, 6-thioguanine, etoposide, and daunorubicin) chemotherapy arm were worse than with standard-timed DCTER (156); an 80% 8-year EFS was obtained with two to eight courses of conventional-dose daunorubicin or etoposide, and cytarabine in a "3 + 3 + 7"-day combination (161).

7.4. Acute Basophilic Leukemia

Acute basophilic leukemia is an AML that exhibits a primary differentiation to basophils. Acute basophilic leukemia is a rare form of acute leukemia (< 1% of all cases of AML) and has not been included in the FAB classification. In 1991, Dick raised the issue of a place for acute basophilic leukemia in the FAB classification as AML-M8 (217). Many reports have shown increased numbers of basophils in leukemias. Recognition of two types of acute basophilic leukemia has been suggested: (1) a pure monophenotypic acute basophilic leukemia, with or without basophil maturation; (2) an acute leukemia with variable immature basophilic participation (218). Acute basophilic leukemia might be misdiagnosed as acute undifferentiated leukemia or AML-M0. The revised classification of AML under the auspices of the WHO has recently recognized acute basophilic leukemia as a specific entity (1) (Table 7.1).

7.4.1 Epidemiology

Acute basophilic leukemia is a very rare disease with a relatively small number of reported cases, comprising less than 1% of all cases of AML. It occurs in all age groups but might be prominent in patients less than 1 year of age (218).

7.4.2   Criteria for Diagnosis of Acute Basophilic Leukemia

7.4.2.1   Morphologic Criteria

Morphologic features are detailed in Table 7.11. The morphology of leukemic cells varies from undifferentiated large cells, little basophilic cytoplasm, round or slightly indented nuclei with finely dispersed chromatin and frequently one or more prominent nucleoli, to smaller cells resembling lymphoblasts (218). The presence of coarse deep purple granules is highly significant, but it is variable from case to case. The presence of large granules corresponding to basophilic granules observed in 0–70% of the leukemic blasts is very informative. True basophilic maturation is rare (219). The presence of mast cells has sometimes been noted (219, 220). There were generally no dysplastic abnormalities observed in the residual hematopoietic cell lines, although dysplastic erythroid features have been described.

7.4.2.2   Cytochemistry

Basophilic granules are observed on May-Grünwald Giemsa staining and confirmed by using the metachromatic properties of the basophilic granule contents, which can be confirmed by toluidine blue, alcian blue, or astra blue stainings. Basophilic lineage cells are known to be peroxidase negative on light microscopy when studied with the standard method using benzidine as the substrate. However, this issue remains controversial and MPO-positive activity has been shown using diaminobenzidine (221). Acid phosphatase seems to be strongly expressed in most cases(222), and chloracetate esterase is reported to be positive in immature basophils and mast cells as opposed to mature basophils, which are negative (223).

7.4.2.3   Electron Microscopy

The electron microscopic morphology of basophilic cells shows immature cells, frequently with a slightly irregular nucleus. These cells contain two types of

Table 7.11 Morphologic and cytochemical features of acute basophilic leukemia

- Medium-sized blasts with a high nuclear-cytoplasmic ratio and an oval, round, or bilobed nucleus with one or more nuclei
- Moderately basophilic cytoplasm containing a variable number of coarse basophilic granules
- Sparse numbers of mature basophils
- Dysplastic erythroid features
- Blasts with metachromatic positivity, with toluidine blue
- Blasts with acid phosphatase positivity
- Negative by light microscopy for Sudan black B, MPO, and nonspecific esterase
- Hypercellular bone marrow

characteristic granule: immature basophilic granules and theta granules (224). Transmission electron microscopy is the only method that can differentiate basophils from mast cells, with the presence of crystal and scroll formations specific to mast cells (225). Pure mast cell leukemias have been reported, but they are unusual (226, 227). Reports have described leukemic blast cells showing either isolated mast cell granules or mast cell granules associated with immature basophilic granules in the same cell (219). In acute basophilic leukemia, the blast cell identification has been confirmed by the presence of specific granules on electron microscopy. Immature basophil granules have been found to be associated with theta granules, sometimes in a variable number of blast cells. The percentage of granules per blast cell is also highly variable (222). The theta granules are not present in each case and have been associated with basophilic differentiation, whereas all cases also display immature basophilic granules (228).

7.4.2.4 Clonogenic Assays

Clonogenic assays and liquid cultures in the presence of the relevant cytokines might provide help in the diagnosis, especially if electron microscopy is not available. In several cases, these studies have shown the appearance of mature basophils and an important number of cells with metachromatic granules (229, 230).

7.4.2.5 Bone Marrow Biopsy

The bone marrow biopsy shows diffuse replacement by blast cells, sometimes with an increased number of basophil precursors. In cases with mast cell differentiation, differentiated mast cells having a distinct morphology with an oval nucleus and elongated cytoplasm might be identified close to the trabeculi. Reticulin fibrosis is often prominent in the latter cases (1).

7.4.3 Cytogenetics

No consistent chromosome abnormality has been identified for acute basophilic leukemia. Numerous chromosomal abnormalities have been associated with mature basophilic proliferations such as t(9;22), t(6;9)(p23;q34), or the rearrangement of 12p. Several cases with t(X;6)(p11;q23) have been described in infants (229). The candidate genes implicated in this translocation are c-MYB for 6q23, and either ARAF-1 gene or ELK-1 gene (a member of ETS proto-oncogene family) for Xp11. Acute basophilic leukemia with t(3;6) involving the same breakpoint on chromosome 6 at 6q23 has been described (231).

7.4.4   Immunophenotype

Basophils express the panleucocyte antigen CD45, myeloid markers such as CD13, CD33, and CD11b, some activation markers, including CD25 and CD38, the early hematopoietic markers CD34, and class-II HLA-DR (232). Strong expression of CD9 and CD17 is also characteristic. Mast cells are also CD45 positive, but compared to basophils, they only express CD9. CD117 (c-Kit) is also expressed on the mast cell lineage, whereas blood basophils are negative. The Bsp-1 antigen is almost exclusively expressed on basophils (223). However, in published cases of acute basophilic leukemia, a thorough immunological study is rare or incomplete (219, 229). The immunologic study allows for the identification of biphenotypic or multiphenotypic proliferations (218, 233, 234).

7.4.5   Clinical and Biological Presentation

Symptoms and physical findings at the time of presentation are very heterogeneous and the basophil granules that contain acid muccopolysaccharides such as heparin or histamin might be responsible for some of the specific symptoms recorded (235, 236). High blood levels of histamine might give cutaneous signs, including pruritus, edema, urticarial rashes, and areas of hyperpigmentation, and/or digestive signs such as nausea, vomting, diarrhea, dyspeptic symptoms, abdominal swelling, or peptic ulcers. The released heparin might also interfere with coagulation. Actually, despite high histaminemia, which correlates with absolute basophilia, clinical symptoms are very rare (218). However, life-threatening anaphylactoid reactions and coagulopathy have been observed within minutes following the administration of chemotherapy, related to basophilic degranulation, which occurs during blast cell lysis (237). Other clinical features include bone marrow failure, organomegaly, and occasional osseous lytic lesions.

The blood counts vary widely. The leukemic infiltration in the bone marrow is often higher than 80%.

7.4.6   Treatment

Due to its rare incidence, little information regarding survival is available. The therapeutic responses in the cases reported cannot be compared because of the heterogeneity of therapy given. Acute basophilic leukemia with t(X;6)(p11;q23) has been associated with a good response to standard therapy for childhood AML (229). During the treatment of acute basophilic leukemia, potential complications related to basophilic degranulation should be anticipated, and antihistamine prophylaxis might be of value.

References

1. Brunning RD, Matutes E, Harris NL, et al. Acute myeloid leukaemia: introduction. In: Jaffe ES, Harris NL, Stein H, et al., editors. Pathology and genetics of tumours of haematopoietic and lymphoid tissues. Lyon: IARC Press; 2001. vol. 3, p. 77–80.
2. Bennett JM, Catovsky D, Daniel MT, et al. Proposed revised criteria for the classification of acute myeloid leukaemia: a report of the French-American-British Cooperative group. Ann Intern Med 1985,103:620–25.
3. Cheson BD, Cassileth PA, Head DR, et al. Report of the National Cancer Institut-sponsored workshop on definitions of diagnosis and response in acute myeloid leukemia. J Clin Oncol 1990;8:813–819.
4. Copelli M. Di una emopatia sistemizzata rapresentata da una iperplasia eritroblastica (eritromatosi). Pathologica 1912;4:460–465.
5. Di Guglielmo G. Richerche di ematologica. Folia Med 1917;3:386–396.
6. Di Guglielmo G. Eritremie acute. Bollettino-Societa medico chirurgica, 1926;1:665–73.
7. Moeschlin S. Erythroblastosen, erythroleukamien und erythroblastemien. Folia Haematol (Leipz) 1940 64:262.
8. Dameshek W. The Di Guglielmo syndrome. Blood 1958;13:192.
9. Dameshek W. The Di Guglielmo syndrome revisited. J Hematol 1969;34:567–572.
10. Bennett JM, Catovsky D, Daniel MT, et al. Proposals for the classification of the acute leukemias. Br J Haematol 1976;33:451–458.
11. Garand R, Duchayne E, Blanchard D, et al. Minimally differentiated erythroleukaemia (AML M6 'variant'): a rare subset of AML distinct from AML M6. Groupe Français d'Hématologie Cellulaire. Br J Haematol 1995;90:868–875.
12. Mazzella FM, Kowal-Vern A, Shrit MA, et al. Acute erythroleukemia: evaluation of 48 cases with reference to classification, cell proliferation, cytogenetics, and prognosis. Am J Clin Pathol 1998;110:590–598.
13. Kowal-Vern A, Mazzella FM, Cotelingam JD, et al. Diagnosis and characterization of acute erythroleukemia subsets by determining the percentages of myeloblasts and proerythroblasts in 69 cases. Am J Hematol 2000;65:5–13.
14. Sakurai M, Sandberg AA. Chromosomes and causation of human cancer and leukemia. XIII. An evaluation of karyotypic findings in erythroleukemia. Cancer 1976;37:790–804.
15. Trent JM, Durie BGM, Davis JR, et al. Cytogenetic and clinical assessment of six patients with erythroleukemia. Anti-cancer Res 1983;3:111–116.
16. Cuneo A, Van Orshoven A, Michaux JL, et al. Morphologic, immunologic and cytogenetic studies in erythroleukemia: evidence for multilineage involvement and identification of two distinct cytogenetic-clinicopathological types. Br J Haematol 1990;75:346–354.
17. Olopade OI, Thangavelu M, Larson RA, et al. Clinical, morphologic, and cytogenetic characteristics of 26 patients with erythroblastic leukemia. Blood 1992;80:2873–2882.
18. Mitelman F, editor. ISCN 1995: an international system for human cytogenetic nomenclature. Basel: S Karger; 1995.
19. Wells AW, Bown N, Reid MM, et al. Erythroleukaemia in the north of England: a population based study. J Clin Pathol 2001;54:608–612.
20. Preiss BS, Kerndrup GB, Schmidt KG, et al. AML Study Group Region of Southern Denmark. Cytogenetic findings in adult de novo acute myeloid leukaemia. A population based study of 303/337 patients. Br J Haematol 2003;123:219–234.
21. Kuriyama K, Tomonaga M, Kobayashi T, et al. Japan Adult Leukemia Study Group. Morphological diagnoses of the Japan adult leukemia study group acute myeloid leukemia protocols: central review. Int J Hematol 2001;73:93–99.
22. Atkinson JA, Hrisinko MA, Weil SC. Erythroblastoma: a review of 15 cases meeting 1985 FAB criteria and survey of the literature. Blood Rev 1993;6:204–214.
23. Peterson HR, Bowlds CF, Yam LT. Familial Di Gugliemo syndrome. Cancer 1984;54: 932–938.

24. Novik Y, Marino P, Makower DF, et al. Familial erythroleukemia: a distinct clinical and genetic type of familial leukemias. Leuk Lymphoma 1998;30:395–401.
25. Davey FR, Abraham N Jr, Brunetto VL, et al. Morphological characteristics of erythroleukaemia/acute myeloid leukemia: FAB-M6: a CALGB Study. Am J Hematol 1995;45:29–38.
26. Forni A, Moreo L. Chromosome studies in a case of benzene-induced erythroleukaemia. Eur J Cancer 1969;5:459–463.
27. Rozman C, Woessner S, Saez-Serrania J. Acute erythromyelosis after benzene poisoning. Acta Haematol 1968;40:234–237.
28. Bradley EL, Schechter GP, Matthews MJ, et al. Erythroleukemia and other hematologic complications of intensive therapy in long-term survivors of small cell lung cancer. Cancer 1982;49:221–223.
29. Whang-Peng J, Lee EC, Minna JD, et al. Deletion of 3(p14p23) in secondary erythroleukamie arising in long-term survivors of small cell lung cancer. J Natl Cancer Instit 1988;80: 1253–1255.
30. Mantovani G, Del Giacco GS, Marongiu F, et al. Acute erythroblastic leukemia as a terminating event in a very long survivor (27 years) with Hodgkin's disease. Haematologica 1982;67:411–417.
31. Ellims P, van der Weyden MB, Brodie GN, et al. Erythroleukemia following drug induced hypoplastic anemia. Cancer 1979;44:2140–2146.
32. Ellerton JA, DeVeber GA, Baker MA. Erythroleukemia in a renal transplant recipient. Cancer 1979;43:1924–1926.
33. Hetzel P, Gee TS. A new observation in the clinical spectrums of erythroleukemia. Am J Med 1978;64:765–772.
34. Finkel HE, Brauer MJ, Taub RN, et al. Immunologic aberrations in Di Guglielmo syndrome. Blood 1966;28:634–649.
35. Bernheim A, Berger R, Daniel MT, et al. Malignant and reactive erythroblasts in erythroleukemia (M6). Cancer Genet Cytogenet 1983;10:1–10.
36. Inoue S, Ravindranath Y, Zuelzer WW. Cytogenetic analysis of erythroleukemia in two children: evidence of nonmalignant nature of erythron. Scand J Haematol 1975;14:129–139.
37. Roloff JN, Lukens JN. Dissociation of erythroblastic and myeloblastic proliferation in erythroleukemia. Am J Dis Child 1972;123:11.
38. Ferraris AM, Canepa L, Mareni C, et al. Reexpansion of normal stem cells in erythroleukemia during remission. Blood 1983;62:177–179.
39. Sheets RF, Drevets CC, Hamilton HE. Erythroleukemia (Di Guglielmo syndrome): a report of clinical observations and experimental studies in seven patients. Arch Intern Med 1963;111:296–306.
40. Necheles TF, Dameshek W. The Di Guglielmo syndrome: studies in hemoglobin synthesis. Blood 1967;29:550.
41. Sondergaard-Petersen H. The Di Guglielmo syndrome: a study of 17 cases. Acta Med Scand 1975;198:165–174.
42. Domingo-Claros A, Larriba I, Rozman M, et al. Acute erythroid neoplastic proliferations. A biological study based on 62 patients. Haematologica 2002;87:148–153.
43. Breton-Gorius J, Villeval JL, Mitjavila MT, et al. Ultrastructural and cytochemical characterization of blasts from early erythroblastic leukaemias. Leukemia 1987;1:173–181.
44. Greaves MF, Sieff C, Edwards PAW. Monoclonal antiglycophorin as a probe for erythroleukemias. Blood 1983;61:645–651.
45. Villeval JL, Cramer P, Lemoine F, et al. Phenotype of early erythroblastic leukemias. Blood 1986;68:1167–1174.
46. Cigudosa JC, Odero MD, Calasanz MJ, et al. De novo erythroleukemia chromosome features include multiple rearrangements, with special involvement of chromosomes 11 and 19. Genes Chromosomes Cancer 2003;36:406–412.

47. Lessard M, Struski S, Leymarie V, et al. Cytogenetic study of 75 erythroleukemias. Cancer Genet Cytogenet 2005;163:113–122.
48. Rowley JD, Alimena G, Garson OM, et al. A collaborative study of the relationship of the morphological type of acute non-lymphocytic leukemia with patient age and karyotype. Blood 1982;59:1013–1022.
49. Murati A, Gelsi-Boyer V, Adélaïde J, et al. PCM1-JAK2 fusion in myeloproliferative disorders and acute erythroid leukemia with t(8;9) translocation. Leukemia 2005;19:1692–1696.
50. Yamamoto K, Nakamura Y, Arai H, et al. Triple Philadelphia chromosomes with major-bcr rearrangement in hypotriploid erythroleukaemia. Eur J Haematol 2000;65:182–187.
51. Hasserjian RP, Howard J, Wood A, et al. Acute erythremic myelosis (true erythroleukaemia): a variant of AML FAB-M6. J Clin Pathol 2001;54:205–209.
52. Park S, Picard F, Azgui Z, et al. Erythroleukemia: a comparison between the previous FAB approach and the WHO classification. Leuk Res 2002;26:423–429.
53. Cuneo A, Ferrant A, Michaux JL, et al. Philadelphia chromosome-positive acute myeloid leukemia: cytoimmunologic and cytogenetic features. Haematologica 1996;81:423–427.
54. Eckert H, Sievers EL, Tan A, et al. GATA-1 is expressed in acute erythroblastic leukaemia. Br J Haematol 1994;86:410–412.
55. Loken MR, Shah VO, Dattilio KL, et al. Flow cytometric analysis of human bone marrow: I. Normal erythroid development. Blood 1987;69:255–263.
56. Okumura N, Tsuji K, Nakahata T. Changes in cell surface antigen expressions during proliferation and differentiation of human erythroid progenitors. Blood 1992;80:642–650.
57. Gahmberg CG, Jokinen M, Andersson LC. Expression of the major sialoglycoprotein (glycophorin) on erythroid cells in human bone marrow. Blood 1978;52:379–387.
58. Fukuda M, Fukuda MN, Papayannopoulou T, et al. Membrane differentiation in human erythroid cells: unique profiles of cell surface glycoproteins expressed in erythroblasts in vitro from three ontogenic stages. Proc Natl Acad Sci USA 1980;77:3474–3478.
59. Yokochi T, Brice M, Rabinovitch PS, et al. Monoclonal antibodies detecting antigenic determinants with restricted expression on erythroid cells: from the erythroid committed progenitor level to the mature erythroblast. Blood 1984;63:1376–1384.
60. Muroi K, Suda T, Nakamura M, et al. Expression of sialosyl-Tn in colony-forming unit-erythroid, erythroblasts, B cells, and a subset of CD4+ cells. Blood 1994;83:84–91.
61. Roggli VL, Subach J, Saleem A. Prognostic factors and treatment effects on survival in erythroleukemia: a retrospective study of 134 cases. Cancer 1981;48:1101–1105.
62. Schwartz AD, Zelson JH, Pearson HA. AML with compensatory but ineffective erythropoiesis: Di Guglielmo's syndrome. J Pediatr 1970;77:653–657.
63. Karle H, Killmann SA, Jensen MK, et al. The vagaries of erythroleukaemia. Acta Med Scand 1974;196:245–253.
64. Steiner M, Baldini M, Dameshek W. Heme synthesis in refractory anemias with ineffective erythropoiesis. Blood 1963;22:810a.
65. Muta K, Nishimura J, Yamamoto M. Possible mechanisms of ineffective erythropoiesis by an altered transferrin receptor cycle in erythroleukemia. Eur J Haematol 1988;40:309–314.
66. Baldini M, Fudenberg HH, Fukutake K, et al. The anemia of the Di Guglielmo syndrome. Blood 1959;14:334–363.
67. Atkins JN, Muss HB. Schistocytes in erythroleukemia. Am J Med Sci 1985;289:110–113.
68. Acin P, Woessner S, Florensa L, et al. Spiculated red cells in erythroleukemia. Eur J Haematol 1997;59:190–193.
69. Roggli VL, Saleem A. Erythroleukemia: a study of 15 cases and literature review. Cancer 1982;49:101–108.
70. Adamson JW, Finch CA. Erythropoietin and the regulation of erythropoiesis in Di Guglielmo's syndrome. Blood 1970;36:590–597.
71. Zucker-Franklin D, Greaves MF, Grossi CE, et al. Atlas of blood cells function and pathology. 2nd ed. Philadelphia: Lea & Febiger; 1988. p. 124.

72. Park S, Picard F, Dreyfus F. Erythroleukemia: a need for a new definition. Leukemia 2002;16:1399–1401.
73. Colita A, Belhabri A, Chelghoum Y, et al. Prognostic factors and treatment effects on survival in acute myeloid leukemia of M6 subtype: a retrospective study of 54 cases. Ann Oncol 2001;12:451–455.
74. Scott RB, Ellison RR, Ley AB. A clinical study of twenty cases of erythroleukemia (Di Guglielmo's syndrome). Am J Med 1964;37:162–171.
75. Bank A, Larsen PR, Anderson HM. Di Guglielmo's syndrome after polycythemia. N Engl J Med 1966;275:489–490.
76. Bloomfield CD, Brunning RD, Kennedy BJ. Daunorubicin-prednisone treatment of erythroleukemia. Ann Intern Med 1974;81:746–750.
77. Rosenthal S, Cancellos GP, Gralnick HP. Erythroblastic transformation of chronic granulocytic leukemia. Am J Med 1977;63:116–124.
78. Kowal-Vern A, Cotelingam J, Schumacher HR. The prognostic significance of proerythroblasts in acute erythroleukemia. Am J Clin Pathol 1992;98:34–40.
79. Mazzella FM, Kowal-Vern A, Shrit MA, et al. Effects of multidrug resistance gene expression in acute erythroleukemia. Mod Pathol 2000;13:407–413.
80. Nakamura H. Cytogenetic heterogeneity in erythroleukemia defined as M6 by the French-American-British Cooperative Group criteria. Leukemia 1989;3:305–309.
81. Olufunmilayo O, Thangavelu M, Larson RA, et al. Clinical, morphologic and cytogenetic characteristics of 26 patients with acute erythroblastic leukemia. Blood 1992;80: 2873–2882.
82. Goldberg SL, Noel P, Klumpp TR, et al. The erythroid leukemias: a comparative study of erythroleukemia (FAB M6) and Di Guglielmo disease. Am J Clin Oncol 1998;21:42–47.
83. Killick S, Matutes E, Powles RL, et al. Acute erythroid leukemia (M6): outcome of bone marrow transplantation. Leuk Lymphoma 1999;35:99–107.
84. Fouillard L, Labopin M, Gorin NC, et al. Hematopoietic stem cell transplantation for de novo erythroleukemia: a study of the European Group for Blood and Marrow Transplantation (EBMT). Blood 2002;100:3135–3140.
85. Reiffers J, Stoppa AM, Attal M, et al. Allogeneic vs autologous stem cell transplantation in patients with acute myeloid leukemia in first remission: the BGMT 87 study. Leukemia 1996;10:1874–1882.
86. Zittoun RA, Mandelli F, Willemze R, et al. Autologous or allogeneic bone marrow transplantation compared with intensive chemotherapy in acute myelogenous leukemia. N Engl J Med 1995;332:217–223.
87. Harousseau JL, Cahn JY, Pignon B, et al. Comparison of autologous bone marrow transplantation and intensive chemotherapy as postremission therapy in adult acute myeloid leukemia. Blood 1997;90:2978–2986.
88. Cassileth PA, Harrington DP, Appelbaum FR, et al. Chemotherapy compared with autologous or allogeneic bone marrow transplantationin the management of acute myeloid leukemia in first remission. N Engl J Med 1998;339:1649–1656.
89. Löwenberg B, Verdonck LJ, Dekker AW, et al. Autologous bone marrow transplantation in acute myeloid leukemia in first remission: results of a Dutch prospective study. J Clin Oncol 1990;8:287–294.
90. Sierra J, Brunet S, Granena A, et al. Feasibility and results of bone marrow transplantation after remission induction and intensification chemotherapy in de novo acute myeloid leukemia. J Clin Oncol 1996;14:1353–1363.
91. Pompetti F, Spadano A, Sau A, et al. Long-term remission in BCR/ABL-positive AML-M6 patient treated by imatinib mesylate. Leuk Res 2007;31:563–7.
92. Camera A, Volpicelli M, Villa MR, et al. Complete remission induced by high dose erythropoietin and granulocyte colony-stimulating factor in acute erythroleukemia (AML-M6) with maturation. Haematologica 2002;87:1225–1227.
93. Gewirtz DA, Di X, Walter TD, et al. Erythropoietin fails to interfere with the antiproliferative and cytotoxic effects of antitumor drugs. Clin Cancer Res 2006;12:2232–2238.

94. Coleman TA, Hamill RL, Ford SM. Erythroleukemia following erythropoietin therapy, extramedullary hematopoiesis, and splenectomy in a patient with myelofibrosis and myeloid metaplasia. Am J Hematol 2001;67:214–215.

95. Von Boros J, Korenyi A. Uber einen fall von akuter megakaryoblasten leukämie: zugleich einige bemerkungen zum problem der akuten leukämie. Z Klein Med 1931;118:697–718.

96. Breton-Gorius J, Reyes F, Duhamel G, et al. Megakaryoblastic acute leukemia: identification by the ultrastructural demonstration of platelet peroxidase. Blood 1978;51:45–60.

97. Bain BJ, Catovsky D, O'Brien M, et al. Megakaryoblastic leukemia presenting as acute myelofibrosis: a study of four cases with the platelet-peroxidase reaction. Blood 1981;58:206–213.

98. Bevan D, Rose M, Greaves M. Leukaemia of platelet precursors: diverse features in four cases. Br J Haematol 1982;51:147–164.

99. Innes DJ, Mills SE, Walker GK, et al. Megakaryocytic leukemia: Identification utilizing antifactor VIII immunoperoxidase. Am J Clin Pathol 1982;77:107–110.

100. Mehta AB, Baughan AS, Catovsky D, et al. Reversal of marrow fibrosis in acute megakaryoblastic leukaemia after remission-induction and consolidation chemotherapy followed by bone marrow transplantation. Br J Haematol 1983;53:445–449.

101. Mirchandani I, Palutke M. Acute megakaryoblastic leukemia. Cancer 1983;50:2866–2872.

102. Huang MJ, Li CY, Nichols WL, et al. Acute leukemia with megakaryocytic differentiation: a study of 12 cases identified immunocytochemically. Blood 1984;64:427–439.

103. Ruiz-Arguelles GJ, Marin-Lopez A, Lobato-Mendizabal E, et al. Acute megakaryoblastic leukemia: a prospective study of its identification and treatment. Br J Haematol 1986;62:55–63.

104. Bloomfield CD, Brunning RD. FAB M7: acute megakaryoblastic leukaemia: beyond morphology. Ann Intern Med 1985;103:450–452.

105. Reilly JT, Barnett D, Dolan G, et al. Characterization of an acute micromegakaryocytic leukemia: evidence for the pathologenesis of myelofibrosis. Br J haematol 1993;83:58–62.

106. Slarc I, Urban C, Haas OA, et al. Acute megakaryocytic leukemia in children: clinical, immunologic and cytogenetic findings in two patients. Cancer 1991;68:2266–2272.

107. Bullorsky EO, Shanley CM, Stemmelin G, et al. Acute megakaryoblastic leukemia with massive myelofibrosis: complete remission and reversal of marrow fibrosis with allogeneic bone marrow transplantation as the only treatment. Bone Marrow Transplant 1990;6:449–452.

108. Johansson B, Mertens F, Heim S, et al. Cytogenetic findings in acute megakaryoblastic leukemia (ANLL-M7). Cancer Genet Cytogenet 1990;218:119–123.

109. Akahoshi M, Oshimi K, Mizoguchi H, et al. Myeloproliferative disorders terminating in acute megakaryoblastic leukemia with chromosome 3 or 26 abnormality. Cancer 1987;60:2654–2661.

110. Brissette MD, Duval-Arnold BJ, Gordon BG, et al. Acute megakaryoblastic leukemia following transient myeloproliferative disorder in a patient without Down syndrome. Am J Hematol 1994;47:316–319.

111. Chan WC, Carrol A, Alvarado CS, et al. Acute megakaryoblastic leukemia in infants with t(1;22)(p13;q13) abnormality. Am J Clin Pathol 1992;98:2114–2121.

112. Lion T, Haas OA, Harbott J, et al. The translocation t(1;22)(p13;q13) is a nonrandom marker specifically associated with acute megakaryocytic leukemia in young children. Blood 1992;79:3325–3330.

113. Carroll A, Civin C, Schneider N, et al. The t(1;22)(p13;q13) is nonrandom and restricted to infants with acute megakaryocytic leukemia: a Pediatric Oncology Group study. Blood 1991; 78:748–752.

114. Gavel D, Mielot F, Gauland P, et al. Acute megakaryocytic leukemia (AMKL) with major myelofibrosis in an infant: diagnosis by liver biopsy and response to treatment. Nouv Rev Fr Hematol 1991;33:5–8.

115. Windebank KP, Tefferi A, Smithson WA, et al. Acute megakaryoblastic leukaemia (M7) in children. Mayo Clin Proc 1989;64:1339–1351.

116. Den Ottolander GJ, Te Veide J, Brederoo P, et al. Megakaryoblastic leukemia (acute myelofibrosis): a report of three cases. Br J Haematol 1979;42:9–20.

117. Ali NO, Janes WO. Malignant myelofibrosis (acute myelofibrosis): report of 2 cases following cytotoxic chemotherapy. Cancer 1979;43:1211–1215.

118. Sultan C, Sigaux F, Imber TM, et al. Acute myelodysplasia with myelofibrosis: a report of eight cases. Br J Haematol 1981;49:11–16.
119. Weisenburger DD. Acute myelofibrosis terminating as acute myeloblastic leukemia. Am J Clin Pathol 1980;73:128–132.
120. Bearman RM, Pangalis GA, Rappaport H. Acute ("malignant") myelosclerosis. Cancer 1979;43:279–293.
121. Bird T, Proctor SJ. Malignant myelosclerosis: myeloproliferative disorder or leukemia? Am J Clin Pathol 1977;67:512–520.
122. Cuneo A, Mecuci C, Kerim S, et al. Multipotent stem cell involvement in megakaryoblastic leukemia: cytologic and cytogenetic evidence in 15 patients. Blood 1989;74:1781–1790.
123. Gassman W, Löffler H. Acute megakaryoblastic leukaemia. Leuk Lymphoma 1995; 18(Suppl 1):69–73.
124. Athale UH, Razzouk BI, Raimondi SC, et al. Biology and outcome of childhood acute megakaryoblastic leukemia: a single institution's experience. Blood 2001;97:3727–3732.
125. Nichols CR, Hoffman R, Glant MD, et al. Malignant disorders of megakaryocytes associated with primary germ cell tumors. Prog Clin Biol Res 1986;215:347–353.
126. Domingo A, Romagosa V, Callis M, et al. Mediastinal germ cell tumor and acute megakaryo-blastic leukemia (Letter). Ann Intern Med 1989;111:539.
127. Zipursky A, Peeters M, Poon A. Megakaryoblastic leukemia and Down's syndrome: a review. Pediatr Hematol Oncol 1987;4:211–230.
128. Zipursky A, Poon A, Doyle J. Leukemia in Down syndrome: a review. Pediatr Hematol Oncol 1992;9:139–149.
129. Kojima S, Matsuyama T, Sato T, et al. Down's syndrome and acute leukemia in children: an analysis of phenotype by use of monoclonal antibodies and electron microscopic platelet peroxidase reaction. Blood 1990;76:2348–2353.
130. San Miguel JF, Gonzales M, Canizo MC, et al. Leukemia with megakaryoblastic involvement: clinical, hematological and immunological characteristics. Blood 1988;72:402–407.
131. Kolke T, Urushiyama M, Narita M, et al. Target cell of leukemic transformation in acute megakaryoblastic leukemia. Am J Hematol 1990;34:252–258.
132. Dastugue N, Lafage-Pochitaloff M, Pages MP, et al. Cytogenetic profile of childhood and adult megakaryoblastic leukemia (M7): a study of the Groupe Français de Cytogénétique Hématologique (GFCH). Blood 2002;100:618–626.
133. Raimondi SC, Chang MN, Ravindranah Y, et al. Chromosomal abnormalities in 478 children with acute myeloid leukemia: clinical characteristics and treatment outcome in a cooperative Pediatric Oncology Group study–POG 8821. Blood 1999;94:3707–3716.
134. Berger M, Ferrero I, Vassallo E, et al. Stem cell Transplantation as consolidation therapy for children in First-remission AML: a single-center report. Pediatr Hematol Oncol 2005; 22:597–608.
135. Dastugue N, Payen C, Lafage-Pochitaloff M, et al. Prognostic significance of karyotype in de novo adult acute myeloid leukemia. Leukemia 1995;9:1491–1498.
136. Grimwade D, Walker H, Oliver F, et al. The importance of diagnostic cytogenetics on outcome in AML: analysis of 1,612 patients entered into the MRC AML 10 trial. Blood 1998;2: 2322–2333.
137. Oki Y, Kantarjian HM, Zhou X, et al. Adult acute megakaryocytic leukemia: an analysis of 37 patients treated at M.D. Anderson Cancer Center. Blood 2006;107:880–884.
138. Fonatsch C, Gudat H, Lengfelder E, et al. Correlation of cytogenetic findings with clinical features in 18 patients with inv(3)(q21;q26) or t(3;3)(q21;q26). Leukemia 1994;8:1318–1326.
139. Lu G, Alton AJ, Benn PA. A review of the cytogenetic changes in acute megakaryoblastic leukemia: one disease or several? Cancer Genet Cytogenet 1993;67:81–89.
140. Jotterand Bellomo M, Parlier V, Muhlematter D, et al. Three new cases of chromosome 3 rearrangement in bands q21 and q26 with abnormal thrombopoiesis bring further evidence to the existence of a 3q21q26 syndrome. Cancer Genet Cytogenet 1992;59:138–160.
141. Tallman MS, Neuberg D, Bennett JM, et al. Acute megakaryocytic leukemia: the Eastern Cooperative Oncology Group experience. Blood 2000;96:2405–2411.

142. Cuneo A, Cavazzini F, Castoldi GL. Acute megakaryoblastic leukemia (AMegL), M7 acute non lymphocytic leukemia (M7-ANLL). Atlas Genet Cytogenet Oncol Haematol. November 2003. URL: http://www.infobiogen.fr/services/chromcancer/Anomalies/M7ANLLID1100.html.

143. Bernstein J, Dastugue N, Haas OA, et al. Nineteen cases of the t(1;22)(p13;q13) acute megakaryoblastic leukaemia of infants/children and a review of 39 cases: report from a t(1;22) study group. Leukemia 2000;14:216–218.

144. Arana Trejo RM, Paredes Aguilera R, Nieto S, et al. t(1;22)(p13;q13) in four children with acute megakaryo-blastic leukemia (M7), two with Down syndrome. Cancer Genet Cytogenet 2000;120:160–162.

145. Ma Z, Morris SW, Valentine V, et al. Fusion of two novel genes, RBM15 and MKL1, in the t(1;22)(p13;q13) of acute megakaryoblastic leukemia. Nat Genet 2001;28:220–221.

146. Mercher T, Coniat MB, Monni R, et al. Involvement of a human gene related to the *Drosophila spen* gene in the recurrent t(1;22) translocation of acute megakaryoblastic leukemia. Proc Natl Acad Sci USA 2001;98:5776–5779.

147. Mercher T, Busson-Le Coniat M, Khac FN, et al. Recurrence of OTT-MAL fusion in t(1;22) of infant AML-M7. Genes Chromosomes Cancer 2002;33:22–28.

148. Ballerini P, Blaise A, Mercher T, et al. A novel real-time RT-PCR assay for quantification of OTT-MAL fusion transcript reliable for diagnosis of t(1;22) and minimal residual disease (MRD) detection. Leukemia 2003;17:1193–1196.

149. Cosson A, Despres P, Gazengal C, et al. Nouveau-né trisomique 21, prolifération trisomique 21, prolifération mégacaryocyto-plaquettaire: syndrome de coagulation intravasculaire diffuse. Nouv Rev Fr Hematol 1974;14:181–198.

150. Nimer SD, MacGrogan D, Jhanwar S, et al. Chromosome 19 abnormalities are commonly seen in AML, M7. Blood 2002;100:3838.

151. Alvarez S, MacGrogan D, Calasanz MJ, et al. Frequent gain of chromosome 19 in megakaryoblastic leukemias detected by comparative genomic hybridization. Genes Chromosomes Cancer 2001;32:285–293.

152. Debili N, Issaad C, Masse JM, et al. Expression of CD34 and platelet glycoproteins during human megakaryocytic differentiation. Blood 1992;80:3022–3035.

153. Zucker-Franklin D, Yang JS, Grusky G. Characterization of glycoprotein IIb/IIIa–positive cells in human umbilical cord blood: their potential usefulness as megakaryocyte progenitors. Blood 1992;79:347–355.

154. Helleberg C, Knudgen H, Hansen PB, et al. CD34+ megakaryoblastic leukemic cells are CD38–, but CD61+ and glycoprotein A+: improved criteria for diagnosis of AML-M7? Leukemia 1997;11:830–834.

155. Athale UH, Kaste SC, Razzouk BI, et al. Skeletal manifestations of pediatric acute megakaryoblastic leukemia. J Pediatr Hematol Oncol 2002;24:561-565.

156. Lange BJ, Kobrinsky N, Barnard DR, et al. Distinctive demography, biology, and outcome of acute myeloid leukemia and myelodysplastic syndrome in children with Down syndrome: Children's Cancer Group Studies 2861 and 2891. Blood 1998;91:608–615.

157. Ravindranath Y, Abella E, Krischer JP, et al. Acute myeloid leukemia (AML) in Down's syndrome is highly responsive to chemotherapy: experience of Pediatric Oncology Group AML Study 8498. Blood 1992;80:2210–2214.

158. Gamis AS, Alonzo TA, Buxton A, et al. Increased age at diagnosis has a significantly negative effect on outcome in children with Down's syndrome and acute myeloid leukemia: a report from the Children's Cancer Group Study, CCG-2891. J Clin Oncol 2003;21:3415–3422.

159. Creutzig U, Reinhardt D, Diekamp S, et al. AML patients with Down syndrome have a high cure rate with AML-BFM therapy with reduced dose intensity. Leukemia 2005;19:1355–1360.

160. Zeller B, Gustafsson G, Forestier E, et al. Acute leukaemia in children with Down syndrome: a population-based Nordic study. Br J Haematol 2005;128:797–804.

161. Kojima S, Sako M, Kato K, et al. An effective chemotherapeutic regimen for acute myeloid leukemia and myelodysplastic syndrome in children with Down's syndrome. Leukemia 2000;14:786–791.

162. Garderet L, Labopin M, Gorin CN, et al. Hematopoietic stem cell transplantation for de novo acute megkaryocytic leukemia in first complete remission: a retrospective study of the European Group for Blood and Marrow Transplantation (EBMT). Blood 2005;105:405–409.
163. Ribeiro RC, Oliveira MS, Fairclough D, et al. Acute megakaryocytic leukemia in children and adolescents: a retrospective analysis of 24 cases. Leuk Lymphoma 1993;10:299–306.
164. Creutzig U, Ritter J, Vormoor J, et al. Myelodysplasia and acute myelogenous leukemia in Down's syndrome: a report of 40 children of the AML-BFM study group. Leukemia 1996;10:1677–1686.
165. Zipursky A. Transient leukemia: a benign form of leukemia in newborn infants with trisomy 21. Br J Haematol 2003;120:930–938.
166. Gamis AS, Hilden JM. Transient myeloproliferative disorder, a disorder with too few data and many unanswered questions: does it contain an important piece of the puzzle to understanding hematopoiesis and acute myelogenous leukemia? J Pediatr Hematol Oncol 2002;24:2–5.
167. Taub JW, Ravindranath Y. Down syndrome and the transient myeloproliferative disorder: Why is it transient? J Pediatr Hematol Oncol 2002;24:6–8.
168. Taub JW. Relationship of chromosome 21 and acute leukemia in children with Down syndrome. J Pediatr Hematol Oncol 2001;23:175–178.
169. Wong KY, Jones MM, Srivastava AK, et al. Transient myeloproliferative disorder and acute nonlymphoblastic leukemia in Down syndrome. J Pediatr 1988;112:18–22.
170. Massey G, Zipursky A, Doyle JJ, et al. A prospective study of the natural history of transient leukemia (TL) in neonates with Down syndrome (DS): a Pediatric Oncology Group (POG) study. Blood 2004;100:87a.
171. Ito E, Kasai M, Hayashi Y, et al. Expression of erythroid-specific genes in acute megakaryoblastic leukaemia and transient myeloproliferative disorder in Down's syndrome. Br J Haematol 1995;90:607–614.
172. Homans AC, Verissimo AM, Viacha V. Transient abnormal myelopoiesis of infancy associated with trisomy 21. Am J Pediatr Hematol Oncol 1993;15:392–399.
173. Zipursky A, Christensen H, De Harven E. Ultrastructural studies of the megakaryoblastic leukemia of Down's syndrome. Leuk Lymphoma 1995;18:341–347.
174. Iselius L, Jacobs P, Morton N. Leukemia and transient leukemia in Down syndrome. Hum Genet 1990;85:477–485.
175. Ridgway D, Benda GI, Magenis E, et al. Transient myeloproliferative disorder of the Down type in the normal newborn. Am J Dis Child 1990;144:1117–1119.
176. Kalousek DK, Chan KW. Transient myeloproliferative disorder in chromosomally normal newborn infant. Med Pediatr Oncol 1987;15:38–41.
177. Karandikar NJ, Aquino DB, McKenna RW, et al. Transient myeloproliferative disorder and acute myeloid leukemia in Down syndrome: an immunophenotypic analysis. Am J Clin Pathol 2001;116:204–210.
178. McElwaine S, Mulligan C, Groet J, et al. Microarray transcript profiling distinguishes the transient from the acute type of megakaryoblastic leukaemia (M7) in Down's syndrome, revealing PRAME as a specific discriminating marker. Br J Haematol 2004;125:729–742.
179. Smrcek JM, Baschat AA, Germer U, et al. Fetal hydrops and hepatosplenomegaly in the second half of pregnancy: a sign of myeloproliferative disorder in fetuses with trisomy 21. Ultrasound Obstet Gynecol 2001;17:403–409.
180. Al Kasim F, Doyle JJ, Massey GV, et al. Incidence and treatment of potentially lethal diseases in transient leukemia of Down syndrome: Pediatric Oncology Group Study. J Pediatr Hematol Oncol 2002;24:9–13.
181. Hattori H, Matsuzaki A, Suminoe A, et al. High expression of platelet-derived growth factor and transforming growth factor-beta 1 in blast cells from patients with Down syndrome suffering from transient myeloproliferative disorder and organ fibrosis. Br J Haematol 2001;115:472–475.
182. Gurbuxani S, Vyas P, Crispino JD. Recent insights into the mechanisms of myeloid leukemogenesis in Down syndrome. Blood 2004;103:399–406.
183. Bourquin JP, Subramanian A, Langebrake C, et al. Identification of distinct molecular phenotypes in acute megakaryoblastic leukemia by gene expression profiling. Proc Natl Acad Sci USA 2006;103:3339–3344.

184. Okuda T, van Deursen J, Hiebert SW, et al. AML1, the target of multiple chromosomal trans-locations in human leukemia, is essential for normal fetal liver hematopoiesis. Cell 1996;84:321–330.

185. Michaud J, Wu F, Osato M, et al. In vitro analyses of known and novel RUNX1/AML1 mutations in dominant familial platelet disorder with predisposition to acute myelogenous leukemia: implications for mechanisms of pathogenesis. Blood 2002;99:1364–1372.

186. Preudhomme C, Warot-Loze D, Roumier C, et al. High incidence of biallelic point mutations in the Runt domain of the AML1/PEBP2 alpha B gene in M0 acute myeloid leukemia and in myeloid malignancies with acquired trisomy 21. Blood 2000;96:2862–2869.

187. Bromage SJ, Lang AK, Atkinson I, et al. Abnormal TGFbeta levels in the amniotic fluid of Down syndrome pregnancies. Am J Reprod Immunol 2000;44:205–210.

188. Pierelli L, Marone M, Bonanno G, et al. Transforming growth factor-beta1 causes transcriptional activation of CD34 and preserves haematopoietic stem/progenitor cell activity. Br J Haematol 2002;118:627–637.

189. Tamiolakis D, Papadopoulos N, Karamanidis D, et al. The immunophenotypic profile of hemopoiesis in fetuses with Down's syndrome during the second trimester of development. Clin Exp Obstet Gynecol 2001;28:153–156.

190. Hitzler JK. GATA1-a player in normal and leukemic megakaryopoiesis. Pediatr Res 2002;52:831.

191. Wechsler J, Greene M, McDewitt MA, et al. Acquired mutations in GATA1 in the megakaryoblastic leukemia of Down syndrome. Nat Genet 2002;32:148–152.

192. Hitzler JK, Cheung J, Li Y, et al. GATA1 mutations in transient leukemia and acute megakaryoblastic leukemia of Down syndrome. Blood 2003;101:4301–4304.

193. Li Z, Godinho FJ, Klusmann JH, et al. Developmental stage-selective effect of somatically mutated leukemogenic transcription factor GATA1. Nat Genet 2005;37:613–619.

194. Shivdasani RA, Fujiwara Y, McDevitt MA, et al. A lineage-selective knockout establishes the critical role of transcription factor GATA-1 in megakaryocyte growth and platelet development. EMBO J 1997;16:3965–3973.

195. Elagib KE, Racke FK, Mogass M, et al. RUNX1 and GATA-1 coexpression and cooperation in megakaryocytic differentiation. Blood 2003;101:4333–4341.

196. Persons DA, Allay JA, Allay ER, et al. Enforced expression of the GATA-2 transcription factor blocks normal hematopoiesis. Blood 1999;93:488–499.

197. Rosenbauer F, Wagner K, Kutok JL, et al. Acute myeloid leukemia induced by graded reduction of a lineage-specific transcription factor, PU.1. Nat Genet 2004;36:624–630.

198. Cantor AB, Orkin SH. Transcriptional regulation of erythropoiesis: an affair involving multiple partners. Oncogene 2002;21:3368–3376.

199. Malkin D, Brown EJ, Zipursky A. A role of p53 in megakaryocyte differentiation and the megakaryocyte leukemias of Down syndrome. Cancer Genet Cytogenet 2000;116:1–5.

200. Holt SE, Brown EJ, Zipursky A. Telomerase and the benign and malignant megakaryoblastic leukemias of Down syndrome. J Pediatr Hematol Oncol 2002;24:14–17.

201. Ma SK, Lee AC, Wan TS, et al. Trisomy 8 as a secondary genetic change in acute megakaryoblastic leukemia associated with Down's syndrome. Leukemia 1999;13:491–492.

202. Ruiz-Arguelles GJ, Lobato-Mendizabal E, San Miguel JF, et al. Long-term treatment results for acute megakaryoblastic leukaemia patients: a multicentre study. Br J Haematol 1992;82:671–675.

203. Pagano L, Pulsoni A, Vignetti M, et al. Acute megakaryoblastic leukemia: experience of GIMEMA trials. Leukemia 2002;16:1622–1626.

204. Duchayne E, Fenneteau O, Pages MP, et al. Acute megakaryoblastic leukaemia: a national clinical and biological study of 53 adult and childhood cases by the Groupe Français d'Hématologie Cellulaire (GFHC). Leuk Lymphoma 2003;44:49–58.

205. Hassan HT, Grell S, Bormann-Danso U, et al. Effect of recombinant human interferons in inducing differentiation of acute megkaryoblastic leukemia blast cells. Leuk Lymphoma 1995;16:329–333.

206. Lu M, Levin J, Sulpice E, et al. Effect of arsenic trioxide on viability, proliferation and apoptosis in human megakaryoblastic leukemia cell lines. Exp Hematol 1999;27:845–852.

207. De Oliveira JS, Sale GE, Bryant EM, et al. Acute megakaryoblastic leukemia in children: treatment with bone marrow transplantation. Bone Marrow Transplant 1992;10:399–403.
208. Schwaiger H, Weirich HG, Brunner P, et al. Radiation sensitivity of Down's syndrome fibroblasts might be due to overexpressed Cu/Zn-superoxidase dismutase (EC 1.15.1.1). Eur J Cell Biol 1989;48:79–87.
209. Arenson EB, Forbe MD. Bone marrow transplantation for acute leukemia and Down syndrome: report of a successful case and results of a national survey. J Pediatr 1989;114: 69–72.
210. Zwaan CM, Kaspers GJL, Pieters R, et al. Different drug sensitivity profiles of acute myeloid and lymphoblastic leukemia and normal peripheral blood mononuclear cells in children with or without Down syndrome. Blood 2002;99:245–251.
211. Taub JW, Stout ML, Buck SA, et al. Myeloblasts from Down syndrome children with acute myeloid leukemia have increased in vitro sensitivity to cytosine arabinoside and daunorubicin (Letter). Leukemia 1997;11:1594–1595.
212. Frost BM, Gustafsson G, Larsson R, et al. Cellular cytotoxic drug sensitivity in children with acute leukemia and Down's syndrome: an explanation to differences in clinical outcome (Letter). Leukemia 2000;14:943–944.
213. Taub JW, Huang X, Matherly LH, et al. Expression of chromosome 21-localized genes in acute myeloid leukemia: differences between Down syndrome and non-Down syndrome blast cells and relationship to in vitro sensitivity to cytarabine arabinoside and daunorubicin. Blood 1999;94:1393–1400.
214. Taub JW, Matherly LH, Stout ML, et al. Enhanced metabolism of 1-β-D-arabinofuranosyl-cytosine in Down syndrome cells: a contributing factor to the superior event free survival of Down syndrome children with acute myeloid leukemia. Blood 1996;87:3395–3403.
215. Lie SO, Jonmundsson G, Mellander L, et al. A population-based study of 272 children with acute myeloid leukaemia treated on two consecutive protocols with different intensity: best outcome in girls, infants, and children with Down's syndrome: Nordic Society of Paediatric Haematology and Oncology (NOPHO). Br J Haematol 1996;94:82–88.
216. Craze JL, Harrison G, Wheatley K, et al. Improved outcome of acute myeloid leukaemia in Down's syndrome. Arch Dis Child 1999;81:32–37.
217. Dick FR. Evolution of the French-American-British (FAB) proposals. Am J Clin Pathol 1991;96:153–155.
218. Duchayne E, Demur C, Rubie H, et al. Diagnosis of acute basophilic leukemia. Leuk Lymphoma 1999;32:269–278.
219. Peterson LC, Parkin JL, Arthur DC, et al. Acute basophilic leukemia: a clinical, morphological and cytogenetic study of eight cases. Am J Clin Pathol 1991;96:160–170.
220. Wick MR, Li CY, Pierre RV. Acute non lymphocytic leukemia with basophilic differentiation. Blood 1982;60:38–45.
221. Ackerman GA, Clark MA. Ultrastructural localization of peroxydase in human basophil leucocytes. Acta Haematol 1971;45:280–284.
222. Kurosawa H, Eguchi M, Sakakibara H, et al. Ultrastructural cytochemistry of congenital basophilic leukemia. Am J Pediatr Hematol/Oncol 1987;9:27–32.
223. Bodger MP, Newton LA. The purification of human basophils: their immunophenotype and cytochemistry. Br J Haematol 1987;67:281–284.
224. Zucker-Franklin D. Electron microscopic studies of human basophils. Blood 1967;29:878–900.
225. Parkin LJ, McKenna RW, Brunning RD. Philadelphia chromosome-positive leukaemia: ultrastructural and ultracytochemical evidence of basophil and mast cell differentiation. Br J Haematol 1982;52:663–677.
226. Daniel MT, Flandrin G, Bernard J. Leucémie aiguë à mastocytes. Nouv Rev Fr Hematol 1975;15:319–332.
227. Coser P, Quaglino D, DePasquale A, et al. Cytobiological and clinical aspects of tissue mast cells leukaemia. Br J Haematol 1980;45:5–12.
228. Soler J, O'Brien M, Tavares de Castro J, et al. Blast crisis of chronic granulocytic leukemia with mast cell and basophilic precursors. Am J Clin Pathol 1984;10:254–259.

229. Dastugue N, Duchayne E, Kuhlein E, et al. Acute basophilic leukaemia and translocation t(X;6)(p11;q23). Br J Haematol 1997;98:170–176.
230. Teshima T, Kondo S, Harada M, et al. Characterization of leukaemic basophil progenitors from chronic myelogenous leukeamia. Br J Haematol 1991;78:55–59.
231. Alvarez Y, Ortega M, Escudero T, et al. Translocation t(3;6)(p21;q23) y trisomia 8 en un caso de leucemia aguda de precursores mieloides de basofilos. Reunion Nacional de la AEHH. Malaga, 7–9 Noviembre 1996; poster 38.
232. Valent P, Bettelheim P. Cell surface structures on human basophils and mast cells: biochemical and functional characterization. Adv Immunol 1992;52:333–423.
233. San Miguel JF, Tavares de Castro J, Matutes E, et al. Characterization of blast cells in chronic granulocytic leukaemia in transformation, acute myelofibrosis and undifferentiated leukaemia II: studies with monoclonal antibodies and terminal transferase. Br J Haematol 1985;59:297–309.
234. Lawlor E, McCann SR, Willoughby R, et al. Basophilic differentiation in Ph-positive blast cell leukaemia. Br J Haematol 1983;54:157–160.
235. Youman JD, Taddeini ML, Cooper T. Histamine excess symptoms in basophilic chronic granulocytic leukemia. Arch Intern Med 1973;131:560–562.
236. Rosenthal S, Schwartz JH, Canellos GP. Basophilic chronic granulocytic leukemia with hyperhistaminemia. Br J Haematol 1977;36:367–372.
237. Bernini JC, Timmons CF, Sandler ES. Acute basophilic leukemia in a child. Cancer 1995;75:110–114.

Chapter 8
Hairy Cell Leukemia

Paul Timothy Fanta and Alan Saven

8.1 Introduction

Hairy cell leukemia (HCL) is a rare, chronic, B-cell lymphoproliferative disorder with well-defined diagnostic criteria and successful treatment outcomes. HCL, classified as an indolent non-Hodgkin's lymphoma in the World Health Organization (WHO) classification, typically presents with the diagnostic triad of pancytopenia, splenomegaly, and circulating cells with characteristic cytoplasmic villous projections. In this chapter, we will review insights pertaining to the historical aspects, epidemiology, pathogenesis, biology, clinical presentation, diagnosis, and treatments of this uncommon but fascinating hematologic entity.

8.2 Historical Perspectives

Leukemic reticuloendotheliosis was first recognized by Eswald in 1923 and later detailed by Bouroncle in 1958. Bouroncle described the clinicopathologic entity, now known as HCL, in her review of 26 such patients. Thorough review of peripheral and bone marrow samples noted the characteristic "hyperplasia of the reticulum tissue in the blood-forming organs with the appearance of reticuloendothelial cells in the bloodstream" (1).

Typical presentations were characterized by splenomegaly, malaise, spontaneous hemorrhagic manifestations, abdominal pain, and infectious complications. Thrombocytopenia, normocytic anemia, and leukopenia with an absolute and relative neutropenia were seen in the majority of patients. A variable clinical course was described, which proved resistant to then known treatments of the time, including nitrogen mustard, radiation, and steroids. In 1966, Schrek and Donnelly (2) named this lymphoproliferative disorder hairy cell leukemia based on the characteristic cytoplasmic projections seen on light microscopy. These early observations formed the basis for the systematic characterization of the pathology, biology, and treatment of HCL.

8.3   Epidemiology

Morton et al. (3) reported on lymphoma incidence patterns during the period 1992–2001. The diagnosis of 114,548 lymphoid neoplasms were reported to the 12 Surveillance, Epidemiology, and End Results (SEER) registries using the WHO 2001 criteria for lymphoma classification. Among 1,116 HCL patients, there was a predominance of males, with the majority of cases in the Caucasian population. Incidence rates were age-adjusted to the 2000 US population and were reported as 0.33 cases per 100,000 person-years, with an annual change in the incidence rate of −1.84% during the period of evaluation. HCL is a rare disease accounting for 2–3% of all adult leukemias, and with about 600 new cases in the United States annually (4). Mean age at presentation was 52 years.

8.4   Pathogenesis and Biology

The cause of HCL is unknown. Exposure to ionizing radiation, Epstein-Barr virus, organic solvents, woodworking, and farming (in the setting of petrol/diesel use) has been proposed as potential antecedents (5). Two siblings with similar haplotypes have been reported, suggesting a HLA- linked etiology (6).

In a review of the cytogenetics of lymphoma, Campbell (7) summarized the known cytogenetic data in HCL. Abnormalities in chromosomes 5 (trisomy, 5q13 deletions), 7, and 14 were the most commonly cited structural and numerical abnormalities (8). Another study by Sambini et al. (9) identified rearrangements of 14q, the most common abnormality in patients with HCL. No specific cytogenetic marker has been discovered that might aid in the diagnosis and prognosis of HCL.

Hairy cell leukemia represents the clonal expansion of mature B-cells; however, it lacks reciprocal chromosomal translocations (10, 11). The cellular origin of HCL has been debated. HCL cells lack morphologic similarity to any known peripheral B-cell population. They are indeed of mature, monoclonal, B-cell derivation without terminal differentiation (12, 13) and express surface light chain-restricted surface immunoglobulin. HCL cells express the B-lineage-specific antigens CD19, CD20, and CD22. They also demonstrate bright expression of CD40 and CD79a in almost all patients, along with HCL-specific CD103 and CD11c (14–19). HCL cells express switched immunoglobulin isotypes and harbor somatic mutations in their rearranged immunoglobulin variable genes in 85% of cases (20–24), which indicates that the cell of origin transits through the germinal center. Exposure to somatic hypermutation (IgVH) and isotype switch recombination, characteristic of the HCL cell, are the hallmarks of cells derived from the germinal center (25). Based on studies of comparative expressed sequence hybridization (CESH), HCL cells displayed a genomewide expression signature. This, combined with its mutated immunoglobulin genes, seems to suggest that the derivation of HCL cells is from memory B-cells, perhaps from the splenic marginal zone (26–29). Other data suggest a pregerminal cell B-cell origin lacking mutations or a postgerminal cell that escaped mutation (24).

Inhibition of apoptosis by bcl-2 has been suggested in HCL clonal expansion. HCL cells have a low proliferation rate and express bcl-2 (30). However, frequent upregulation of cyclin D1, involved in the cell cycle advance from G1 to S phase, is seen in HCL cells (31, 32). Speculation for HCL survival prolongation through the phosphatidylinositol 3 kinase (PI3K)-AKT stimulated pathways, related to both cyclin D1 and G1-S cell cycling (33, 34), via HCL-specific overexpression of interleukin (IL)-3 receptor alpha (IL-3Rα) (31) and overexpression of receptor tyrosine kinase FLT3 (31), have been proposed as antiapoptotic signals (35).

Unique to HCL is the pattern of dissemination into bone marrow, peripheral blood, splenic red pulp, and hepatic sinusoids, with relative sparing of the peripheral lymph nodes (29). $\alpha_4\beta_1$ integrin (VLA4) and its ligand, vascular cell adhesion molecule 1(VCAM 1), might play a role in the preferential homing patterns of hairy cells (36). The splenic red pulp is highly enriched with vitronectin. HCL cells express the corresponding ligand, vitronectin receptor $\alpha_v\beta_3$, again allowing for preferential localization of HCL cells (37). Overexpression of matrix metalloproteinases inhibitors, including TIMP1, TIMP4, RECK, and thrombospondin-1, have been seen in HCL cells and are thought to represent a mechanism for degradation of tissue matrix (31).

The hairy cell has a characteristic morphologic appearance with numerous membrane projections. These are composed of F-actin and lamellipodia-like structures (38). It is thought that cytoskeletal rearrangements are controlled by the Rho family of GTPases, a subfamily of the Ras superfamily, through overexpression of cell division cycle 42 (CDC42), and RAC1, both through their GTPase functions with regulation via p53 (39).

Characteristic of HCL is the development of bone marrow reticulin-induced fibrosis. Although the composition of these fibers has not been defined, the process of induction of fibrosis has been proposed (40). Levels of transforming growth factor (TGF) β_1 levels, a fibrogenic cytokine, were found to be present at higher concentration in patients with HCL measured both by both mRNA and protein levels. It is thought that the overexpression of TGFβ_1 significantly enhanced the production and deposition of reticulin and collagen by bone marrow fibroblasts. Autocrine secretion of basic fibroblast growth factor (bFGF) also has a role in fibronectin synthesis in HCL cells, and with TGFB$_1$ are the main determinants of fibrosis in HCL (29).

8.5   Pathology and Immunophenotypic Analysis

Accurate diagnosis of HCL is essential and relies on the characteristic morphology of the peripheral cells, the immunophenotypic pattern, examination of bone marrow morphology, including reticulin deposition, and cytochemical staining. The typical hairy cell is 1.5–2 times the size of a mature lymphocyte, with a smooth, contoured, round nucleus with a rim of textured cytoplasm with circumferential hairlike projections (41) (see Figure 8.1A). The chromatin pattern is uniformly granular, without evidence of nucleoli. The characteristic ultrastructural finding of the

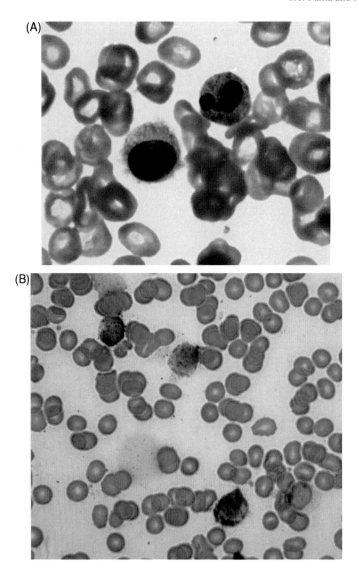

Figure 8.1 (A) Classic hairy cell (left) with rounded, smooth, nuclear contours, conspicuous textured cytoplasm, and circumferential villous projections (peripheral blood, Wright's stain, original magnification × 100). (B) HCL cells stained with a TRAP preparation displaying granular appearance in positive cells (bone marrow aspirate, tartrate-treated acid phosphatase stain, original magnification × 100)

ribosome–lamella complex has been well described (42–45). HCL cells are resistant to treatment with tartaric acid through the expression of isoenzyme 5 of acid phosphatase. Tartrate-resistant acid phosphatase (TRAP) activity is seen in almost all cases. Although TRAP activity is not unique to HCL, bright expression of TRAP activity is almost pathognomonic of HCL (41) (see Figure 8.1B).

Immunophenotypic analysis by flow cytometry of HCL provides a distinctive profile to complement morphology and cytochemical stains. Typical expression patterns demonstrate bright CD20 and CD22, both B-cell markers, CD5 negativity, with approximately 10% of cases being CD10 positive (46). Expression of CD11c, CD103, and CD25 is the diagnostic pattern seen in typical HCL (18) (see Figure 8.2). ANXZ1 overexpression (annexin A1) is preferentially seen in HCL, but not in HCL-variant or splenic marginal zone lymphoma (47). Immunohistochemical stains suggestive of HCL include TRAP and DBA.44. A DBA.44 and TRAP positive profile is 97% specific for HCL (41).

Neutropenia, lymphopenia, and monocytopenia are common. Often, hairy cells are categorized as monocytes in the automated differential (48). Circulating hairy cells are usually present in small, variable numbers and typically seen in the thin portion of the preparation. Buffy coat preparations may be useful in concentrating the hairy cells in suspected cases. Reticulin fibrosis, as a result of fibronectin deposition, and an inaspirable marrow are typical (1) (see Figure 8.3A). Histologic preparations display a distinctive patchy or diffuse mononuclear infiltrate (49). Bone marrow review of HCL samples display patchy infiltrates, often paratrabecular and intramedullary in location (41). Their characteristic pattern of pale-staining cytoplasm and round nuclei has been described as a "fried-egg" appearance (see Figure 8.3B). Splenic involvement is typically isolated to the red pulp, with the same pattern of infiltration seen in the bone marrow, with characteristic blood-filled spaces called "blood lakes." Liver infiltration is characterized by the "angiomatoid focus" and hepatic sinus and portal tract involvement (41). Up to one-third of patients might have lymphadenopathy on computed tomography (CT) scan, which may be associated with a more aggressive clinical course (50).

8.6   Differential Diagnosis

The histopathological and clinical differential diagnosis of HCL includes hairy cell leukemia variant (HCL-v), splenic marginal zone lymphoma (SMZL), acute monocytic leukemia, systemic mast cell disease, multiple myeloma, melanoma, aplastic anemia, large granulocytic leukemia, B-cell prolymphocytic leukemia,

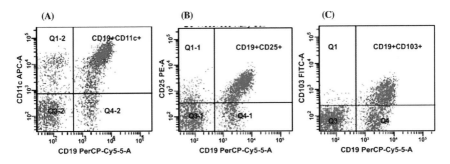

Figure 8.2 The diagnosis of HCL is established by immunophenotypic characterization using flow cytometry. Hairy cells show concordant expression of CD11c (**A**), CD25 (**B**), and CD103 (**C**)

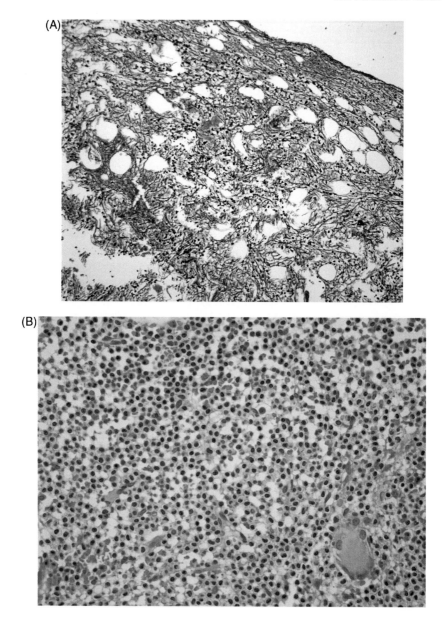

Figure 8.3 (**A**) Marrow reticulin fibrosis from fibronectin secreted by hairy cells (bone marrow, silver stain, original magnification × 40). (**B**) Classic infiltrative pattern of the bone marrow seen in HCL cells with conspicuous cytoplasm and central nuclei, termed the "fried egg" appearance (bone marrow, hematoxylin-eosin, original magnification × 40)

hypoplastic myelodysplastic syndrome, paroxysmal nocturnal hemoglobinuria, atypical chronic lymphocytic leukemia, and idiopathic myelofibrosis (51). The major pathologic differential diagnosis is among HCL-v, SMZL, and prolymphocytic leukemia (52).

Hairy cell leukemia variant generally presents at an older age, typically the eighth decade, less than 2:1 male predominance, with splenomegaly, lymphocytosis, as well as anemia, and thrombocytopenia (44). Morphologically, HCL-v possesses a higher nuclear-to-cytoplasmic ratio, more condensed chromatin, and more prominent nuclei than classic HCL (52). HCL-v is CD25-negative and CD103-negative, with weak to absent TRAP staining. HCL-v tends to follow a more aggressive course, is more chemorefractory, has median survivals of 10 years, and might ultimately undergo transformation to a large-cell process in 5–10% of cases with pronounced splenomegaly, leukocytosis, and B-symptoms and decreased survival (53, 54).

Splenic marginal zone lymphoma likewise might mimic the presentation of HCL with massive splenomegaly without lymphadenopathy. It is distinguished from HCL by its profound lymphocytosis, basophilic cytoplasm, subtle polar cytoplasmic projections, weak to absent TRAP staining, CD11c positivity, and CD103 negativity (52).

8.7   Clinical Manifestations

Approximately 80% of patients present with anemia, thrombocytopenia, and neutropenia at time of diagnosis (55) usually in the evaluation for fatigue, bruising, opportunistic infection, early satiety, or an incidentally discovered enlarged spleen. Skeletal complications, including lytic lesions and osteosclerosis, have been reported and are more typical of a high tumor burden (56). Opportunistic infections include *Mycobacterium kansasii*, *Pneumoncystis carinii*, *aspergillus*, *histoplasma*, and *Toxoplasma gondii* (57).

8.8   Indications for Treatment

Indications for treatment include cytopenias [absolute neutrophil count less than $(0.5–1.0) \times 10^9/L$, hemoglobin less than $9\,g/dL$ or platelet counts less than $(50–100 \times 10^9/L)$], symptomatic splenomegaly, rarely leukocytosis greater than $20.0 \times 10^9/L$, bulky or painful lymphadenopathy, constitutional symptoms (fevers, night sweats, weight loss, fatigue), significant autoimmune disease (vasculitis), recurrent infections, and/or bony involvement (52). Asymptomatic patients or those who lack significant cytopenias should be observed, as no survival or response benefit is to be gained from early intervention. Results of treatment in symptomatic patients are summarized in Table 8.1.

Table 8.1 Systemic treatments in HCL

Agent/investigator	Total	CR	PR	Minor/NR
Pentostatin				
Else et al. (63)	185	150	28	7
Dearden et al. (83)	165	135	25	5
Grever et al. (84)	154	117	4	33
Grem et al. (85)	66	37	15	14
Cassileth et al. (68)	50	32	10	8
Ho et al. (86)	33	11	15	7
Kraut et al. (87)	23	20	1	2
Total	676	502 (74%)	98 (14%)	76 (12%)
Cladribine				
Saven et al. (71)	349	319	22	8
Tallman et al. (88)	50	40	9	1
Hoffman et al. (89)	49	37	12	0
Estey et al. (90)	46	36	5	5
Dearden et al. (83)	45	38	7	0
Else et al. (63)	34	28	6	0
Juliusson and Liliemark (91)	16	12	0	4
Total	589	510 (87%)	62 (10%)	18 (3%)
Interferon				
Golomb et al. (92)	195	7	152	36
Grever et al. (84)	159	17	43	99
Quesada et al. (93)	30	9	17	4
Rai et al. (94)	25	7	6	12
Foon et al. (95)	14	1	12	1
Total	423	41 (10%)	230 (54%)	152 (36%)
Rituximab				
Nieva et al. 73	24	3	3	18
Thomas et al. 74	15	10	2	3
Hagberg and Lundholm (96)	11	6	1	4
Total	50	19 (38%)	6 (12%)	25 (50%)

CR = Complete response; PR = partial response; NR = no response.

8.9 Cladribine

Cladribine (2-CdA, 2-chlorodeoxyadenosine, Leustatin; Ortho Biotech, Raritan, NJ) is an adenosine deaminase-resistant deoxyadenosine analog directly toxic to both resting and proliferating human lymphocytes and monocytes (58). Since the initial demonstration of its significant activity by Carrera et al. in 1987 (59), cladribine has emerged as the treatment of choice for HCL, with overall response rates of 97% and complete responses of 87% (52). Oral, subcutaneous, and intravenous dosing have been evaluated, with the optimal route and method of administration not clarified in randomized trials; however, intravenous administration is the preferred route.

An update on 209 patients with HCL treated with cladribine by continuous infusion for 7 days at a dose of 0.1 mg/kg/day, reported 95% complete responses and 5% partial responses, for a 100% overall response rate. With over 7 years of follow-up, the median first-response duration was 98 months, with 37% experiencing relapse after their first course of cladribine. The median time to relapse for all responders was recorded as 42 months, and the overall survival rate was 97% at 108 months (60). Twenty-two percent of patients developed secondary malignancies, with the observed-to-expected ratio of second malignancies, compared to NCI SEER data, reported as 2.03 [95% confidence interval (CI): 1.19–2.71]. Other studies displayed an incidence of second malignancy not significantly higher than the expected standardized incidence ratio of 1.01 (95% CI: 0.74–1.33); however, the standardized incidence ratio of non-Hodgkin's lymphomas was higher at 5.3% (95% CI: 1.9–11.5) in a single study (61).

A smaller study of 86 HCL patients reported a 79% complete and a 21% partial response rate, for an overall response rate of 100%. Progression-free survival after 12 years was 54%. At a median of 9.7 years, 36% of patients had relapsed. Of these patients, 23 were retreated with cladribine with 52% complete responses and 30% partial responses, for an overall response rate of 82% (62). Else et al. (63) documented an overall response to cladribine in the first-line setting of 100%, with a complete response rate of 82% and a disease-free survival greater than 11 years. The observed relapsed rates in the study were 24% and 42% at 5 and 10 years, respectively (63). Alternative treatment regimens of cladribine using 5 consecutive days at 0.14 mg/kg/ day, or once weekly at 0.14 mg/kg for five cycles, were reported to have a projected 13-year overall survival and relapse-free survival of 96% and 52%, respectively. Relapse rates were not significantly different between treatment groups (24% vs. 30%, respectively), and weekly administration reported a decreased incidence of grade 3 to 4 neutropenia (64).

Fever is the principal toxicity of cladribine, occurring in approximately 42% of patients treated (52) and is related to tumor cell burden in its severity. Immunosuppression, profound and prolonged CD4 lymphopenia, and subsequent infectious complications have been reported, primarily dermatomal herpes zoster reactivation. Filgrastim (Neupogen; Amgen, Thousand Oaks, CA) increases the absolute neutrophil count and shortens the duration of severe neutropenia in cladribine-treated patients; however, it failed to demonstrate a clinical advantage with respect to percentage of febrile patients, number of febrile days, and admissions for antibiotics when compared to historical controls. Accordingly, the use of filgrastim as an adjunct to cladribine-induced neutropenia in HCL is not routinely recommended (65).

8.10 Pentostatin

Pentostatin (2′-deoxycoformycin, Nipent; Supergen, Dublin, CA), a purine nucleoside analogue, is a potent inhibitor of adenosine deaminase, which causes the accumulation of deoxyadenosine triphosphates, is thought responsible for its activity in HCL (66, 67). Pentostatin, a potently toxic agent to lymphocytes, particularly T-cells, displayed significant activity, with reported overall response rates of 84% and complete responses of 64%, with maximum responses at 6 months (68). The dosing of pentostatin in HCL is $4\,mg/m^2$ IV every other week, for 3–6 months, or until maximum response (52).

Fever, nausea, vomiting, photosensitivity, prolonged immunosuppression, and keratoconjunctivitis are pentostatin's major toxicities. Pentostatin should be avoided in patients with poor performance status, active infections, or chronic kidney disease. Pentostatin has activity in prior interferon-treated patients as well as in splenectomized patients, with overall response rates of 96%, complete responses of 81%, and a disease-free survival of 15 years (63). In a separate review, an overall response rate of 86%, with 72% complete responses, was reported in 491 HCL patients (52).

8.11   Interferon

In 1984, interferon was reported as an effective therapy in splenectomy-failed patients. It has been widely used in the treatment of HCL; however, it does not induce the same magnitude of complete response seen with purine analogue therapy (52). Interferon-α-2B (Intron A; Schering Corporation, Kenilworth, NY, USA) is given at a dose of 2 million units/m² subcutaneously 3 times a week for 12 months. Recombinant interferon-α-2A (Roferon; Hoffman-La Roche, Nutley, NJ, USA) is given at a dose of 3 million units/m² subcutaneously daily for 6 months and then decreased to 3 times per week for an additional 6 months. Flulike symptoms, anorexia, nausea, vomiting, peripheral neuropathies, clinical depression, elevated transaminases, and myelosuppression may complicate therapy. A recent summary of 423 cases of HCL treated with interferon reported a 64% overall response rate, with only 10% of patients achieving complete responses. Treatment with interferon should be reserved for patients with active infections or who are not candidates for purine analogue therapy, because of concerns regarding T-cell immunosuppression, or in purine analogue refractory disease (52).

8.12   Splenectomy

Historically, splenectomy was the first standard treatment for HCL and has a role in the rapid normalization of blood counts when clinically warranted. Indications now include active infections, symptomatic splenomegaly, bleeding in the setting of severe thrombocytopenia, purine analogue refractory disease, and rarely in symptomatic pregnant patients (52, 69). Median response is approximately 20 months, and overall survival at 5 years was reported as 65% (70).

8.13   Relapsed or Refractory Disease

An optimal treatment approach for relapsed/refractory HCL has been hindered by the lack of prospective, randomized clinical trials, as well as the inability to directly compare studies due to differences in trial design. Several studies support the use of the same nucleoside analogue in the second or third relapse setting provided that the preceding response had been durable (52, 65) (see Table 81). Patients initially treated with cladribine have achieved response rates of 88% with repeat courses of cladribine (71). When resistance to one purine analogue has been established, treatment with a different purine analogue (62) is recommended because there was lack of cross-resistance between cladribine and pentostatin, despite mechanistic similarities (71, 72) (see Figure 8.4). Care must be taken to limit the reinstitution of purine analogue therapy within a 12-month interval due to concerns for cumulative marrow damage.

Anti-CD20 immunotherapy, rituximab (Rituxan; Biogen-IDEC Pharmaceuticals, San Diego, CA) is a reasonable therapeutic option in patients with relapsed or refractory HCL. In a study of 24 HCL patients with purine-analogue refractory or relapsed disease, rituximab at $375\,mg/m^2$ weekly for 4 doses displayed a 26% overall response rate and a complete response of 13% (73). Thomas et al. treated 15 patients with relapsed or refractory HCL with rituximab at $375\,mg/m^2$ weekly for 8 doses, with 4 additional doses administered to responders who had not achieved a complete response (74). In that study, an overall response rate of 80% was achieved, with 67% of those responses being complete. Rituximab is generally well tolerated.

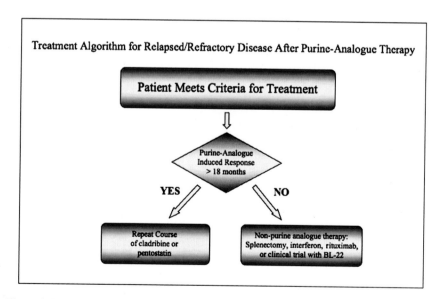

Figure 8.4 Treatment algorithm for relapsed/refractory disease after purine-analogue therapy

Splenectomy and alpha-interferon are also reasonable treatment options for selected patients with purine analogue- and rituximab-resistant patients. A single patient report on the use of thalidomide (Thalomed; Celgene, Summit, NJ) in a purine analogue-naïve patient demonstrated a partial response of 11 months (75).

BL22, an anti-CD22 variable domain (Fv) monoclonal antibody fused to a truncated immunotoxin *Pseudomonas* exotoxin (PE38), showed promise in cladribine-resistant HCL (76). Kreitman et al. (77) treated 16 cladribine-resistant patients with a dose escalation of BL22. Eleven of 16 patients had a complete remission and two achieved a partial response. Common toxicities included transient hypoalbuminemia and elevated transaminases. Two patients experienced reversible hemolytic-uremic syndromes (77). An anti-CD25 antibody linked to a truncated form of pseudomonas exotoxin (LMB-2) demonstrated clinical activity in a phase I study of four patients with cladribine- and interferon-resistant disease; all achieved major responses (78, 79).

8.14   Minimal Residual Disease

Despite the spectacular advances in the treatment of HCL, most patients treated will eventually relapse. In an early study, patients with evidence of minimal residual disease (MRD) by immunohistochemistry had a shorter relapse-free survival (80). Strategies to further improve initial response rates, to achieve maximum disease eradication, and to formulate a curative strategy have been investigated. In this regard, Ravandi et al. (81) evaluated the addition of rituximab at a dose of 375 mg/m² for 8 weeks to cladribine (5.6 mg/m² given intravenously over 2 h daily for 5 days); in a study of 13 previously treated and untreated HCL patients, all patients (2 cladribine-failures, 11 newly diagnosed) achieved complete responses. MRD by consensus primer polymerase chain reaction (PCR) or flow cytometry was undetectable in 11 of 12 patients and in 12 of 13 patients, respectively (81). Compared to flow cytometry, assessment of MRD using the clone-specific PCR (RQ-PCR) was more sensitive (100%), and in another study, it correlated with disease status and remission duration (82). Elimination of MRD appears to be attainable, which might translate into an improved disease-free survival or perhaps even cure.

8.15   Summary

Hairy cell leukemia is an indolent B-cell non-Hodgkin's lymphoma with a characteristic presentation of pancytopenia, splenomegaly, and circulating hairy cells. An immunophenotypic pattern of CD11c, CD25, and CD103 expression, TRAP staining, reticulin deposition, and morphology of bone marrow and circulating cells help establish the diagnosis. Although up to 10% of patients might not require systemic treatment, for the vast majority effective treatments are available with the purine-nucleoside analogues cladribine and pentostatin. Cladribine is considered the drug of choice in the first-line setting due to the very high complete remission rate and prolonged duration of response following a single 7-day infusion. Cladribine and pentostatin both have unique but different mechanisms of action, with a lack of cross-resistance between them, which might be exploited in the relapsed or refractory disease setting. Therapy for relapsed and refractory patients also includes novel biologic agents as well as splenectomy. Despite the effective treatment options, the prospect of cure remains elusive due to the frequent presence of MRD even in complete responders. Future studies employing combination therapies targeting the eradication of MRD will hopefully improve relapse-free survivals as well as overall survival, and might even offer the prospect of cure.

Acknowledgment The authors thank Robert W. Sharpe, M.D., Division of Hematopathology, Department of Pathology, Scripps Clinic, La Jolla, California, for providing pathologic and flow cytometry materials for Figures 1–3.

References

1. Bouroncle BA, Wiseman BK, Doan CA. Leukemic reticuloendotheliosis. Blood 1958;13: 609–630.
2. Schrek R, Donnelly WJ. "Hairy" cells in blood in lymphoreticular neoplastic disease and "flagellated" cells of normal lymph nodes. Blood 1966;27:199–211.
3. Morton LM, Wang SS, Devesa SS, et al. Lymphoma incidence patterns by WHO subtype in the United States, 1992–2001. Blood 2006; 107:265–276.
4. O'Brien S, Keating MJ. Chronic lymphoid leukemias. In: DeVita VT, Hellman S, Rosenberg SA, editors. Cancer: Principles and practice of oncology. 7th ed. Philadelphia: Lippincott Williams & Wilkins, 2005. p. 2133–2143.
5. Oleske D, Golomb HM, Farber MD, et al. A case-control inquiry into the etiology of hairy cell leukemia. Am J Epidemiol 1985;121:675–683.
6. Ward FT, Baker J, Krishnan J, et al. Hairy cell leukemia in two siblings. A human leukocyte antigen-linked disease? Cancer 1990;65:319–321.
7. Campbell LJ. Cytogenetics of lymphomas. Pathology 2005;37:493–507.
8. Kluin-Nelemans HC, Beverstock GC, Mollevanger P, et al. Proliferation and cytogenetic analysis of hairy cell leukemia upon stimulation via the CD40 antigen. Blood 1994;84:3134–3141.
9. Sambani C, Trafalis DT, Mitsoulis-Mentzikoff C, et al. Clonal chromosome rearrangements in hairy cell leukemia: personal experience and review of literature. Cancer Genet Cytogenet 2001;129:138–144.
10. Korsmeyer SJ, Greene WC, Cossman J, et al. Rearrangement and expression of immunoglobulin genes and expression of Tac antigen in hairy cell leukemia. Proc Natl Acad Sci USA 1983;80:4522–526.
11. Foucar K, Catovsky D. Hairy cell leukaemia. In: Jaffe ES, Harris NL, Stein H, et al., editors. Pathology and genetics of tumours of haematopoietic and lymphoid tissues: World Health Organization classification of tumours. Lyon: IARC Press; 2001. p. 138–141.
12. Anderson KC, Boyd AW, Fisher DC, et al. Hairy cell leukemia: A tumor of pre-plasma cells. Blood 1985;65:620–629.
13. Polliack A. Hairy cell leukemia: Biology, clinical diagnosis, unusual manifestations and associated disorders. Rev Clin Exp Hematol 2002;6:366–388; discussion 449–450.

14. Golde DW, Stevens RH, Quan SG, et al. Immunoglobulin synthesis in hairy cell leukaemia. Br J Haematol 1977;35:359–365.
15. Jansen J, Schuit HR, Meijer CJ, et al. Cell markers in hairy cell leukemia studied in cells from 51 patients. Blood 1982;59:52–60.
16. Falini B, Schwarting R, Erber W, et al. The differential diagnosis of hairy cell leukemia with a panel of monoclonal antibodies. Am J Clin Pathol 1985;83:289–300.
17. Matutes E, Morilla R, Owusu-Ankomah K, et al. The immunophenotype of hairy cell leukemia (HCL). Proposal for a scoring system to distinguish HCL from B-cell disorders with hairy or villous lymphocytes. Leuk Lymphoma 1994;14(Suppl 1):57–61.
18. Robbins BA, Ellison DJ, Spinosa JC, et al. Diagnostic application of two-color flow cytometry in 161 cases of hairy cell leukemia. Blood 1993;82:1277–1287.
19. Matutes E, Owusu-Ankomah K, Morilla R, et al. The immunological profile of B-cell disorders and proposal of a scoring system for the diagnosis of CLL. Leukemia 1994;8: 1640–1645.
20. Golomb HM, Davis S, Wilson C, et al. Surface immunoglobulins on hairy cells of 55 patients with hairy cell leukemia. Am J Hematol 1982;12:397–401.
21. Maloum K, Magnac C, Azgui Z, et al. VH gene expression in hairy cell leukaemia. Br J Haematol 1998;101:171–178.
22. Forconi F, Sahota SS, Raspadori D, et al. Hairy cell leukemia: At the crossroad of somatic mutation and isotype switch. Blood 2004;104:3312–3317.
23. Vanhentenrijk V, Tierens A, Wlodarska I, et al. V(H) gene analysis of hairy cell leukemia reveals a homogeneous mutation status and suggests its marginal zone B-cell origin. Leukemia 2004;18:1729–1732.
24. Thorselius M, Walsh SH, Thunberg U, et al. Heterogeneous somatic hypermutation status confounds the cell of origin in hairy cell leukemia. Leuk Res 2005;29:153–158.
25. MacLennan IC. Germinal centers. Annu Rev Immunol 1994;12:117–139.
26. Tangye SG, Liu YJ, Aversa G, et al. Identification of functional human splenic memory B cells by expression of CD148 and CD27. J Exp Med 1998;188:1691–1703.
27. Dunn-Walters DK, Isaacson PG, Spencer J. Analysis of mutations in immunoglobulin heavy chain variable region genes of microdissected marginal zone (MGZ) B cells suggests that the MGZ of human spleen is a reservoir of memory B cells. J Exp Med 1995;182:559–566.
28. Vanhentenrijk V, De Wolf-Peeters C, Wlodarska I, et al. Comparative expressed sequence hybridization studies of hairy cell leukemia show uniform expression profile and imprint of spleen signature. Blood 2004;104:250–255.
29. Tiacci E, Liso A, Piris M, et al. Evolving concepts in the pathogenesis of hairy-cell leukaemia. Nat Rev Cancer 2006;6:437–448.
30. Zaja F, Di Loreto C, Amoroso V, et al. BCL-2 immunohistochemical evaluation in B-cell chronic lymphocytic leukemia and hairy cell leukemia before treatment with fludarabine and 2-chloro-deoxy-adenosine. Leuk Lymphoma 1998;28:567–572.
31. Basso K, Liso A, Tiacci E, et al. Gene expression profiling of hairy cell leukemia reveals a phenotype related to memory B cells with altered expression of chemokine and adhesion receptors. J Exp Med 2004;199:59–68.
32. Bosch F, Campo E, Jares P, et al. Increased expression of the PRAD-1/CCND1 gene in hairy cell leukaemia. Br J Haematol 1995;91:1025–1030.
33. Brennan P, Babbage, JW, Burgering BM, et al. Phosphatidylinositol 3-kinase couples the interleukin-2 receptor to the cell cycle regulator E2F. Immunity 1997;7:679–689.
34. Liang J, Slingerland JM. Multiple roles of the PI3K/PKB (Akt) pathway in cell cycle progression. Cell Cycle 2003;2:339–345.
35. Jonsson M, Engstrom M, Jonsson JI. FLT3 ligand regulates apoptosis through AKT-dependent inactivation of transcription factor FoxO3. Biochem Biophys Res Commun 2004;318:899–903.
36. Vincent AM, Burthem J, Brew R, et al. Endothelial interactions of hairy cells: The importance of alpha 4 beta 1 in the unusual tissue distribution of the disorder. Blood 1996;88:3945–3952.
37. Nanba K, Soban EJ, Bowling MC, et al. Splenic pseudosinuses and hepatic angiomatous lesions. Distinctive features of hairy cell leukemia. Am J Clin Pathol 1977;67:415–426.

38. Caligaris-Cappio F, Bergui L, Tesio L, et al. Cytoskeleton organization is aberrantly rearranged in the cells of B chronic lymphocytic leukemia and hairy cell leukemia. Blood 1986;67:233–239.

39. Chaigne-Delalande B, Deuve L, Reuzeau E, et al. RhoGTPases and p53 are involved in the morphological appearance and interferon-alpha response of hairy cells. Am J Pathol 2006;168:562–573.

40. Shehata M, Schwarzmeier JD, Hilgarth M, et al. TGF-beta1 induces bone marrow reticulin fibrosis in hairy cell leukemia. J Clin Invest 2004;113:676–685.

41. Sharpe RW, Bethel KJ. Hairy cell leukemia: Diagnostic pathology. Hematol Oncol Clin North Am 2006; 20:1023–1049.

42. Katayama I, Li CY, Yam LT. Ultrastructural characteristics of "hairy cells" of leukemic reticuloendotheliosis. Am J Pathol 1972;67:361–370.

43. Schnitzer B, Kass L. Hairy-cell leukemia. A clinicopathologic and ultrastructural study. Am J Clin Pathol 1974;61:176–187.

44. Katayama I, Schneider GB. Further ultrastructural characterization of hairy cells of leukemic reticuloendotheliosis. Am J Pathol 1977;86:163–182.

45. Burke JS, Mackay B, Rappaport H. Hairy cell leukemia (leukemic reticuloendotheliosis) II. Ultrastructure of the spleen. Cancer 1976;37:2267–2274.

46. Jasionowski TM, Hartung L, Greenwood JH, et al. Analysis of CD10+ hairy cell leukemia. Am J Clin Pathol 2003;120:228–235.

47. Falini B, Tiacci E, Liso A, et al. Simple diagnostic assay for hairy cell leukaemia by immunocytochemical detection of annexin A1 (ANXA1). Lancet 2004;363:1869–1870.

48. Seshadri RS, Brown EJ, Zipursky A. Leukemic reticuloendotheliosis: a failure of monocyte production. N Engl J Med 1976;295:181–184.

49. Catovsky D, Pettit JE, Galton DA, et al. Leukaemic reticuloendotheliosis ('Hairy cell leukaemia'): a distinct clinico-pathologic entity. Br J Haematol 1974;26:9–27.

50. Mercieca J, Matutes E, Moskovic E, et al. Massive abdominal lymphadenopathy in hairy cell leukemia: a report of 12 cases. Br J Haematol 1992;82:547–554.

51. Wanko S, de Castro C. Hairy cell leukemia: an elusive but treatable disease. Oncologist 2006;11:780–789.

52. Saven A. Chapter 99: Hairy cell leukemia. In: Lichtman MA, Beutler E, Kaushansky K, et al., editors. Williams' hematology. 7th ed. New York: McGraw-Hill; 2006. p. -:1385–1392.

53. Matutes E, Wotherspoon A, Brito-Babapulle V, et al. The natural history and clinicopathological features of the variant form of hairy cell leukemia. Leukemia 2001;15:184–186.

54. Matutes E, Wotherspoon A, Catovsky D. The variant form of hairy cell leukemia. Best Pract Res Clin Haematol 2003;16:41–56.

55. Turner A, Kjeldsberg CR. Hairy cell leukemia: a review. Medicine (Balt) 1978;57:477–499.

56. Quesada JR, Keating MJ, Libshitz HI, et al. Bone involvement in hairy cell leukemia. Am J Med 1983;74:228–231.

57. Kraut EH, Neff JC, Bouroncle BA, et al. Immunosuppressive effects of pentostatin. J Clin Oncol 1990;8:848–855.

58. Greyz N, Saven A. Cladribine: from the bench to the bedside—focus on hairy cell leukemia. Expert Rev Anticancer Ther 2004;4:745–757.

59. Carrera CJ, Piro LD, Miller WE, et al. Remission induction in hairy cell leukemia by treatment with 2-chlorodeoxyadenosine: role of DNA strand breaks and NAD depletion ([Abstract). Clin Res 1987;35:597A.

60. Goodman G, Burian C, Koziol JA, et al. Extended follow-up of patients with hairy cell leukemia after treatment with cladribine. J Clin Oncol 2003;21:891–896.

61. Kampmeier P, Spielberger R, Dickstein J, et al. Increased incidence of second neoplasms in patients treated with interferon alpha 2b for hairy cell leukemia: a clinicopathologic assessment. Blood 1994;83:2931–2938.

62. Chadha P, Rademaker AW, Mendiratta P, et al. Treatment of hairy cell leukemia with 2-chlorodeoxyadenosine (2-CdA): long-term follow-up of the Northwestern University experience. Blood 2005;106:241–246.

63. Else M, Ruchlemer R, Osuji N, et al. Long remissions in hairy cell leukemia with purine analogs: a report of 219 patients with a median follow-up of 12.5 years. Cancer 2005;104:2442–2448.
64. Zinzani PL Tani M, Marchi E, et al. Long-term follow-up of front-line treatment of hairy cell leukemia with 2-chlorodeoxyadenosine. Haematologica 2004;89:309–313.
65. Saven A, Burian C, Adusumalli J, et al. Filgrastim for cladribine-induced neutropenic fever in patients with hairy cell leukemia. Blood 1999;93:2471–2477.
66. Carson DA, Wasson DB, Kaye J, et al. Deoxycytidine kinase-mediated toxicity of deoxyadenosine analogs toward malignant lymphoblasts in vitro and toward murine L1210 leukemia in vivo. Proc Natl Acad Sci USA 1980;77:6865–6869.
67. Seto S, Carrera CJ, Kubota M, et al. Mechanism of deoxyadenosine and 2-chlorodeoxyadenosine toxicity to dividing and non-dividing human lymphocytes. J Clin Invest 1985;75:377–383.
68. Cassileth PA, Cheuvart B, Spiers AS, et al. Pentostatin induces durable remissions in hairy cell leukemia. J Clin Oncol 1991;9:243–246.
69. Stiles GM, Stanco LM, Saven A, et al. Splenectomy for hairy cell leukemia in pregnancy. J Perinatol 1998;18:200–201.
70. Golomb HM, Vardiman JW. Response to splenectomy in 65 patients with hairy cell leukemia: an evaluation of spleen weight and bone marrow involvement. Blood 1983;61:349–352.
71. Saven A, Burian C, Koziol JA, et al. Long-term follow-up of patients with hairy cell leukemia after cladribine treatment. Blood 1998;92:1918–1926.
72. Saven A, Piro LD. Complete remissions in hairy cell leukemia with 2-chlorodeoxyadenosine after failure with 2'-deoxycoformycin. Ann Intern Med 1993;119:278–283.
73. Nieva J, Bethel K, Saven A. Phase 2 study of rituximab in the treatment of cladribine-failed patients with hairy cell leukemia. Blood 2003;102:810–3.
74. Thomas D, O'Brien S, Bueso-Ramos C, et al. Rituximab in relapsed or refractory hairy cell leukemia. Blood 2003;102:3906–3911.
75. Strupp C, Fenk R, Kundgen A, et al. Hairy cell leukemia (HCL) with extensive myelofibrosis responds to thalidomide. Leuk Res 2005;29:967–969.
76. Tallman MS. Monoclonal antibody therapies in leukemias. Semin Hematol 2002;39:12–19.
77. Kreitman RJ, Wilson WH, Bergeron K. Efficacy of the anti-CD22 recombinant immunotoxin BL22 in chemotherapy-resistant hairy-cell leukemia. N Engl J Med 2001;345:241–247.
78. Kreitman RJ, Wilson WH, White JD, et al. Phase I trial of recombinant immunotoxin anti-Tac(Fv)-PE38 (LMB-2) in patients with hematologic malignancies. J Clin Oncol 2000;18:1622–1636.
79. Robbins DH, Margulies I, Stetler-Stevenson M, et al. Hairy cell leukemia, a B-cell neoplasm that is particularly sensitive to the cytotoxic effect of anti-Tac(Fv)-PE38 (LMB-2). Clin Cancer Res 2000;6:693–700.
80. Wheaton S, Tallman MS, Hakimian D, et al. Minimal residual disease may predict bone marrow relapse in patients with hairy cell leukemia treated with 2-chlorodeoxyadenosine. Blood 1996;87:1556–1560.
81. Ravandi F, Jorgensen JL, O'Brien SM, et al. Eradication of minimal residual disease in hairy cell leukemia. Blood 2006;107:4658–4662.
82. Arons E. Margulies I, Sorbara L, et al. Minimal residual disease in hairy cell leukemia patients assessed by clone-specific polymerase chain reaction. Clin Cancer Res 2006;12:2804–2811.
83. Dearden CE, Matutes E, Hilditch BL, et al. Long-term follow-up of patients with hairy cell leukaemia after treatment with pentostatin or cladribine. Br J Haematol 1999;106:515–559.
84. Grever M, Kopecky K, Foucar MK, et al. Randomized comparison of pentostatin versus interferon alfa-2a in previously untreated patients with hairy cell leukemia: An intergroup study. J Clin Oncol 1995;13:974–982.
85. Grem J, King S, Cheson B, et al. Pentostatin in hairy cell leukemia: treatment by the special exception mechanism. J Natl Cancer Inst 1989;81:448–453.
86. Ho AD, Thaler J, Stryckmans P, et al. Pentostatin in refractory chronic lymphocytic leukemia: a phase II trial of the European Organization for Research and Treatment of Cancer. J Natl Cancer Inst 1990;82:1416–420.

87. Kraut EH, Bouroncle BA, Grever MR. Pentostatin in the treatment of advanced hairy cell leukemia. J Clin Oncol 1989;7:168–172.
88. Tallman MS, Hakimian D, Rademaker AW, et al. Relapse of hairy cell leukemia after 2-chlorodeoxyadenosine: long-term follow-up of the Northwestern University experience. Blood 1996;88:1954–1959.
89. Hoffman MA, Janson D, Rose E, et al. Treatment of hairy cell leukemia with cladribine: response, toxicity, and long-term follow-up. J Clin Oncol 1997;15:1138–1142.
90. Estey EH, Kurzrock R, Kantarjian HM, et al. Treatment of hairy cell leukemia with 2-chlorodeoxyadenosine (2-CdA). Blood 1992;79:882–887.
91. Juliusson G, Liliemark J. Rapid recovery from cytopenia in hairy cell leukemia after treatment with 2-chloro-2'-deoxyadenosine(CdA): relation to opportunistic infections. Blood 1992;79:888–894.
92. Golomb H, Fefer A, Golde D, et al. Update of a multi-institutional study of 195 patients with hairy cell leukemia (HCL) treated with interferon alfa-2b (IFN) (Abstract). Proc Am Soc Clin Oncol 1990;6:215.
93. Quesada JR, Reuben J, Manning JT, et al. Alpha interferon for induction of remission in hairy-cell leukemia. N Eng J Med 1984;310:15–18.
94. Rai K, Mick R, Ozer H, et al. Alpha-interferon therapy in untreated active hairy cell leukemia: a Cancer and Leukemia Group B (CALGB) study (Abstract). Proc Am Soc Clin Oncol 1987;6:159.
95. Foon KA, Maluish AE, Abrams PG, et al. Recombinant leukocyte A interferon therapy for advanced hairy cell leukemia. Therapeutic and immunologic results. Am J Med 1986;80:351–356.
96. Hagberg H, Lundholm L. Rituximab, a chimaeric anti-CD20 monoclonal antibody, in the treatment of hairy cell leukaemia. Br J Haematol 2001;115:609–611.

Chapter 9
Waldenstrom's Macrogloblinemia/ Lymphoplasmacytic Lymphoma

Steven P. Treon, Evdoxia Hatjiharissi, and Giampaolo Merlini

9.1 Introduction

Waldenström's macroglobulinemia (WM) is a distinct clinicopathological entity resulting from the accumulation, predominantly in the bone marrow, of clonally related lymphocytes, lymphoplasmacytic cells, and plasma cells that secrete a monoclonal IgM protein (Figure 9.1) (1). This condition is considered to correspond to the lymphoplasmacytic lymphoma (LPL) as defined by the Revised European American Lymphoma (REAL) and World Health Organization (WHO) classification systems (2, 3). Most cases of LPL are WM, with less than 5% of cases made up of IgA, IgG, and nonsecreting LPL.

9.2 Epidemiology and Etiology

Waldenström's macroglobulinemia is an uncommon disease, with a reported age-adjusted incidence rate of 3.4 per million among males and 1.7 per million among females in the United States and a geometrical increase with age (4, 5). The incidence rate for WM is higher among Caucasians, with African descendants representing only 5% of all patients. Genetic factors appear to be important in the pathogenesis of WM. Approximately 20% of WM patients have an Ashkenazi (Eastern European) Jewish ethnic background, and there have been numerous reports of familiar disease, including multigenerational clustering of WM and other B-cell lymphoproliferative diseases (6–10). In a recent study, approximately 20% of 257 serial WM patients presenting to a tertiary referral had a first- degree relative with either WM or another B-cell disorder (7). Frequent familiar association with other immunological disorders in healthy relatives, including hypogammaglobulinemia and hypergammaglobulinemia (particularly polyclonal IgM), autoantibody (particularly to thyroid) production, and manifestation of hyperactive B-cells have also been reported (9, 10). Increased expression of the *bcl-2* gene with enhanced B-cell survival might underlie the increased immunoglobulin synthesis in familial WM (9). The role of environmental factors in WM remains to be clarified,

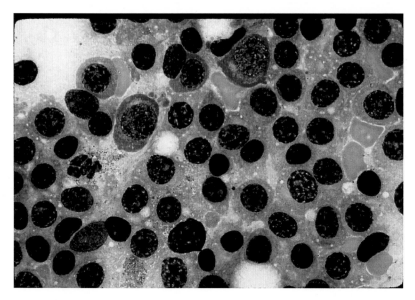

Figure 9.1 Aspirate from a patient with Waldenstrom's macroglobulinemia demonstrating excess mature lymphocytes, lymphoplasmacytic cells, and plasma cells. (Courtesy of Marvin Stone M.D.)

but chronic antigenic stimulation from infections, certain drug, and Agent Orange exposures remain suspect. An etiological role for hepatitis C virus (HCV) infection has been suggested though in a recent study examining 100 consecutive WM patients; no association could be established using both serological and molecular diagnostic studies for HCV infection (11–13).

9.3 Biology

9.3.1 Cytogenetic Findings

Several studies, usually performed on limited series of patients, have been published on cytogenetic findings in WM demonstrating a great variety of numerical and structural chromosome abnormalities. Numerical losses involving chromosomes 17, 18, 19, 20, 21, 22, X, and Y have been commonly observed, although gains in chromosomes 3, 4, and 12 have also been reported (7, 14–19). Chromosome 6q deletions encompassing 6q21–22 have been observed in up to half of WM patients and at a comparable frequency among patients with and without a familial history (7, 19). Several candidate tumor suppressor genes in this region are under study, including BLIMP-1, a master regulatory gene implicated in lymphoplasmacytic differentiation. Notable, however, is the absence of IgH switch region rearrangements in WM, a finding that might be used to discern cases of IgM myeloma where IgH switch region rearrangements are a predominant feature (20).

9.3.2 Nature of the Clonal Cell

The WM bone marrow B-cell clone shows intraclonal differentiation from small lymphocytes with large focal deposits of surface immunoglobulins, to lymphoplasmacytic cells, to mature plasma cells that contain intracytoplasmic immunoglobulins (21). Clonal B-cells are detectable among blood B-lymphocytes, and their number increases in patients who fail to respond to therapy or who progress (22). These clonal blood cells present the peculiar capacity to differentiate spontaneously, in in vitro culture, to plasma cells. This is through an interleukin-6 (IL-6)-dependent process in IgM monoclonal gammopathy of undetermined significance (MGUS) and mostly an IL-6-independent process in WM patients (23). All of these cells express the monoclonal IgM present in the blood and a variable percentage of them also express surface IgD. The characteristic immunophenotypic profile of the lymphoplasmacytic cells in WM includes the expression of the pan B-cell markers CD19, CD20, CD22, CD79, and FMC7.2 (24–26). Expression of CD5, CD10, and CD23 might be found in 10–20% of cases and does not exclude the diagnosis of WM (27).

The phenotype of lymphoplasmacytic cells in WM cell suggests that the clone is a postgerminal center B-cell. This indication is further strengthened by the results of the analysis of the nature (silent or amino acid replacing) and distribution (in framework or Complement Determinant Regions (CDR)) of somatic mutations in Ig heavy- and light-chain variable regions performed in patients with WM (28, 29). This analysis showed a high rate of replacement mutations, compared with the closest germline genes, clustering in the CDR regions and without intraclonal variation. Subsequent studies showed a strong preferential usage of VH3/JH4 gene families, no intraclonal variation, and no evidence for any isotype-switched transcripts (30, 31). These data indicate that WM might originate from a IgM+ and/or IgM+ IgD+ memory B-cell. Normal IgM+ memory B-cells localize in bone marrow, where they mature to IgM-secreting cells (32).

9.3.3 Bone Marrow Microenvironment

Increased numbers of mast cells are found in the bone marrow of WM patients, wherein they are usually admixed with tumor aggregates (26, 33). Recent studies have helped clarify the role of mast cells in WM. Coculture of primary autologous or mast cell lines with WM LPC resulted in dose-dependent WM cell proliferation and/or tumor colony, primarily through CD40 ligand (CD40L) signaling. Furthermore, WM cells through elaboration of soluble CD27 (sCD27) induced the upregulation of CD40L on mast cells derived from WM patients and mast cell lines (34).

9.4 Clinical Features

The clinical and laboratory findings at time of diagnosis of WM in one large institutional study (7) are presented in Table 9.1. Unlike most indolent lymphomas, splenomegaly and lymphadenopathy are prominent in only a minority of patients

Table 9.1 Clinical and laboratory findings for 149 consecutive newly diagnosed patients with the consensus panel diagnosis of WM presenting to the Dana Farber Cancer Institute

	Median	Range	Institutional normal reference range
Age (years)	59	34–84	NA
Gender (male/female)	85/64		NA
Bone marrow involvement	30%	5–95%	NA
Adenopathy	16%		NA
Splenomegaly	10%		NA
IgM (mg/dL)	2,870	267–12,400	40–230
IgG (mg/dL)	587	47–2770	700–1600
IgA (mg/dL)	47	8–509	70–400
Serum viscosity (cp)	2.0	1.4–6.6	1.4–1.9
Hct (%)	35.0%	17.2–45.4%	34.8–43.6
Plt (× 10^9/L)	253	24–649	155–410
WBC (×10^9/L)	6.0	0.3–13	3.8–9.2
B_2M (mg/dL)	3.0	1.3–13.7	0–2.7
LDH	395	122–1,131	313–618

NA = not applicable.

($\leq$15%). Purpura is frequently associated with cryoglobulinemia and more rarely with AL amyloidosis, whereas hemorrhagic manifestations and neuropathies are multifactorial (see later). The morbidity associated with WM is caused by the concurrence of two main components: tissue infiltration by neoplastic cells and, more importantly, the physicochemical and immunological properties of the monoclonal IgM. As shown in Table 9.2, the monoclonal IgM can produce clinical manifestations through several different mechanisms related to its physicochemical properties, nonspecific interactions with other proteins, antibody activity, and tendency to deposit in tissues (35–37).

9.5 Morbidity Mediated by the Effects of IgM

9.5.1 Hyperviscosity Syndrome

Blood hyperviscosity is effected by increased serum IgM levels leading to hyperviscosity-related complications (38). The mechanisms behind the marked increase in the resistance to blood flow and the resulting impaired transit through the microcirculatory system are rather complex (38–40). The main determinants are (1) a high concentration of monoclonal IgMs, which might form aggregates and might bind water through their carbohydrate component, and (2) their interaction with blood cells. Monoclonal IgMs increase red cell aggregation (*rouleaux* formation) and red cell internal viscosity while reducing deformability. The possible presence of cryoglobulins can contribute to increasing blood viscosity as well as to the tendency to induce erythrocyte aggregation. Serum viscosity is proportional

Table 9.2 Physicochemical and immunological properties of the monoclonal IgM protein in Waldenstrom's macroglobulinemia

Properties of IgM monoclonal protein	Diagnostic condition	Clinical manifestations
Pentameric structure	Hyperviscosity	Headaches, blurred vision, epistaxis, retinal hemorrhages, leg cramps, impaired mentation, intracranial hemorrhage
Precipitation on cooling	Cryoglobulinemia (Type I)	Raynaud's phenomenom, acrocyanosis, ulcers, purpura, cold urticaria
Autoantibody activity to myelin associated glycoprotein (MAG), ganglioside M1 (GM1), sulfatide moieties on peripheral nerve sheaths	Peripheral neuropathies	Sensorimotor neuropathies, painful neuropathies, ataxic gait, bilateral foot drop
Autoantibody activity to IgG	Cryoglobulinemia (Type II)	Purpura, arthralgias, renal failure, sensorimotor neuropathies
Autoantibody activity to red blood cell antigens	Cold agglutinins	Hemolytic anemia, Raynaud's phenomenom, acrocyanosis, livedo reticularis
Tissue deposition as amorphous aggregates	Organ dysfunction	Skin: bullous skin disease, papules, Schnitzler's syndrome
		GI: diarrhea, malabsorption, bleeding
		Kidney: proteinuria, renal failure (light-chain component)
Tissue deposition as amyloid fibrils (light-chain component most commonly)	Organ dysfunction	Fatigue, weight loss, edema, hepatomegaly, macroglossia, organ dysfunction of involved organs: heart, kidney, liver, peripheral sensory and autonomic nerves

to an IgM concentration up to 30 g/L, then increases sharply at higher levels. Plasma viscosity and hematocrit are directly regulated by the body. Increased plasma viscosity might also contribute to inappropriately low erythropoietin production, which is the major reason for anemia in these patients (41). Clinical manifestations are related to circulatory disturbances that can be best appreciated by ophthalmoscopy, which shows distended and tortuous retinal veins, hemorrhages, and papilledema (42) (Figure 9.2). Symptoms usually occur when the monoclonal IgM concentration exceeds 50 g/L or when serum viscosity is > 4.0 centipoises (cp), but there is a great individual variability, with some patients

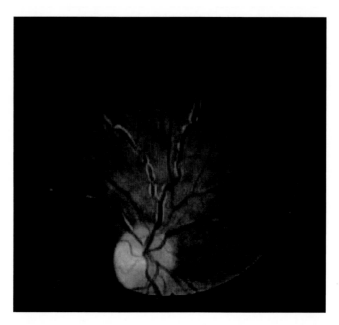

Figure 9.2 Funduscopic examination of a patient with Waldenstrom's macroglobulinemia demonstrating hyperviscosity related changes including dilated retinal vessels, peripheral hemorrhages, and "venous sausaging." (Courtesy of Marvin Stone M.D.)

showing no evidence of hyperviscosity even at 10 cp (38). The most common symptoms are oronasal bleeding, visual disturbances due to retinal bleeding, and dizziness that might rarely lead to coma. Heart failure can be aggravated, particularly in the elderly, owing to increased blood viscosity, expanded plasma volume, and anemia. Inappropriate transfusion can exacerbate hyperviscosity and might precipitate cardiac failure.

9.5.2 Cryoglobulinemia

In up to 20% of WM patients, the monoclonal IgM can behave as a cryoglobulin (type I), but it is symptomatic in 5% or less of the cases (43). Cryoprecipitation is mainly dependent on the concentration of monoclonal IgM; for this reason, plasmapheresis or plasma exchange are commonly effective in this condition. Symptoms result from impaired blood flow in small vessels and include Raynaud's phenomenon, acrocyanosis, and necrosis of the regions most exposed to cold (tip of the nose, ears, fingers, and toes), malleolar ulcers, purpura, and cold urticaria. Renal manifestations might occur but are infrequent.

9.5.3 Autoantibody Activity

Monoclonal IgM might exert its pathogenic effects through specific recognition of autologous antigens, the most notable being nerve constituents, immunoglobulin determinants, and red blood cell antigens.

9.5.4 IgM-Related Neuropathy

In a series of 215 patients with WM, Merlini et al. (43) reported the clinical presence of peripheral neuropathy in 24% of WM patients, although prevalence rates ranging from 5% to 38% have been reported in other series (44, 45). An estimated 6.5–10% of idiopathic neuropathies are associated with a monoclonal gammopathy, with a preponderance of IgM (60%) followed by IgG (30%) and IgA (10%) (reviewed in Refs. 46 and 47). In WM patients, the nerve damage is mediated by diverse pathogenetic mechanisms: IgM antibody activity toward nerve constituents causing demyelinating polyneuropathies; endoneurial granulofibrillar deposits of IgM without antibody activity, associated with axonal polyneuropathy; occasionally by tubular deposits in the endoneurium associated with IgM cryoglobulin and, rarely, by amyloid deposits or by neoplastic cell infiltration of nerve structures (48). Half of the patients with IgM neuropathy have a distinctive clinical syndrome that is associated with antibodies against a minor 100-kDa glycoprotein component of nerve, myelin-associated glycoprotein (MAG). Anti-MAG antibodies are generally monoclonal IgMκ and usually also exhibit reactivity with other glycoproteins or glycolipids that share antigenic determinants with MAG (49–51). The anti-MAG-related neuropathy is typically distal and symmetrical, affecting both motor and sensory functions; it is slowly progressive, with a long period of stability (45, 52). Most patients present with sensory complaints (paresthesias, aching discomfort, dysesthesias, or lancinating pains), imbalance and gait ataxia, owing to lack proprioception, and leg muscles atrophy in the advanced stage. Patients with predominantly demyelinating sensory neuropathy in association with monoclonal IgM to gangliosides with disialosyl moieties, such as GD1b, GD3, GD2, GT1b, and GQ1b, have also been reported (53, 54). Anti-GD1b and anti-GQ1b antibodies were significantly associated with predominantly sensory ataxic neuropathy (58). These antiganglioside monoclonal IgMs present core clinical features of chronic ataxic neuropathy with variably present ophthalmoplegia and/or red blood cell cold agglutinating activity. The disialosyl epitope is also present on red blood cell glycophorins, thereby accounting for the red cell cold agglutinin activity of anti-Pr2 specificity (55, 56). Monoclonal IgM proteins that bind to gangliosides with a terminal trisaccharide moiety, including GM2 and GalNac-GD1A, are associated with chronic demyelinating neuropathy and severe sensory ataxia, unresponsive to corticosteroids (57). Antiganglioside IgM proteins might also cross-react with lipopolysaccharides of *Campylobacter jejuni*, whose infection is known to precipitate the Miller Fisher syndrome, a variant of the Guillain–Barré syndrome (58). This finding indicates that molecular mimicry might play a role in this condition. Antisulfatide monoclonal IgM proteins, associated with sensory/sensorimotor neuropathy, have been detected in 5% of patients with IgM monoclonal gammopathy and neuropathy (59). Motor neuron disease has been reported in patients with WM, and monoclonal IgM disease has been reported in patients with anti-GM1 and sulfoglucuronyl paragloboside activity (60). POEMS (polyneuropathy, organomegaly, endocrinopathy, M protein, and skin changes) syndrome is rarely associated with WM (61).

9.5.5 Cold Agglutinin Hemolytic Anemia

Monoclonal IgM might present with cold agglutinin activity; that is, it can recognize specific red cell antigens at temperatures below physiological, producing chronic hemolytic anemia. This disorder occurs in < 10% of WM patients (62) and is associated with cold agglutinin titers > 1:1000 in most cases. The monoclonal component is usually an IgMκ and reacts most commonly with I/i antigens, with complement fixation and activation (63, 64). Mild chronic hemolytic anemia can be exacerbated after cold exposure but rarely does hemoglobin drop below 70 g/L. The hemolysis is usually extravascular (removal of C3b opsonized cells by the reticuloendotelial system, primarily in the liver) and rarely intravascular from complement destruction of red blood cell (RBC) membrane. The agglutination of RBCs in the cooler peripheral circulation also causes Raynaud's syndrome, acrocyanosis, and livedo reticularis. Macroglobulins with the properties of both cryoglobulins and cold agglutinins with anti-Pr specificity have been reported. These properties might have as a common basis the immune binding of the sialic acid-containing carbohydrate present on RBC glycophorins and on Ig molecules. Several other macroglobulins with various antibody activities toward autologous antigens (i.e., phospholipids, tissue and plasma proteins, etc.) and foreign ligands have also been reported.

9.5.6 Tissue Deposition

The monoclonal protein can deposit in several tissues as amorphous aggregates. Linear deposition of monoclonal IgM along the skin basement membrane is associated with bullous skin disease (65). Amorphous IgM deposits in the dermis determine the so-called IgM storage papules on the extensor surface of the extremities—macroglobulinemia cutis (66). Deposition of monoclonal IgM in the lamina propria and/or submucosa of the intestine might be associated with diarrhea, malabsorption, and gastrointestinal bleeding (67, 68). It is well known that kidney involvement is less common and less severe in WM than in multiple myeloma, probably because the amount of light chain excreted in the urine is generally lower in WM than in myeloma and because of the absence of contributing factors, such as hypercalcemia, although cast nephropathy has also been described in WM (69).

On the other hand, the IgM macromolecule is more susceptible to being trapped in the glomerular loops, where ultrafiltration presumably contributes to its precipitation, forming subendothelial deposits of aggregated IgM proteins that occlude the glomerular capillaries (70). Mild and reversible proteinuria might result and most patients are asymptomatic. The deposition of monoclonal light chain as fibrillar amyloid deposits (AL amyloidosis) is uncommon in patients with WM (71). Clinical expression and prognosis are similar to those of other AL patients with involvement of the heart (44%), kidneys (32%), liver (14%), lungs (10%), peripheral/autonomic nerves (38%), and soft tissues (18%). However, the incidence of cardiac and pulmonary involvement is higher in patients with monoclonal IgM than with other immunoglobulin isotypes. The association of WM with reactive amyloidosis (AA) has been documented rarely (72, 73) Simultaneous occurrence of fibrillary glomerulopathy, characterized by glomerular deposits of wide noncongophilic fibrils and amyloid deposits, has been reported in WM (74).

9.5.7 Manifestations Related to Tissue Infiltration by Neoplastic Cells

Tissue infiltration by neoplastic cells is rare and can involve various organs and tissues, from the bone marrow (described later) to the liver, spleen, lymph nodes, and possibly the lungs, gastrointestinal tract, kidneys, skin, eyes, and central nervous system. Pulmonary involvement in the form of masses, nodules, diffuse infiltrate, or pleural effusions is relatively rare, as the overall incidence of pulmonary and pleural findings reported for WM is only 3–5% (75–77). Cough is the most common presenting symptom, followed by dyspnea and chest pain. Chest radiographic findings include parenchymal infiltrates, confluent masses, and effusions. Malabsorption, diarrhea, bleeding, or obstruction might indicate involvement of the gastrointestinal tract at the level of the stomach, duodenum, or small intestine (78–81). In contrast to multiple myeloma, infiltration of the kidney interstitium with lymphoplasmacytoid cells has been reported in WM (82), whereas renal or perirenal masses are not uncommon (83). The skin can be the site of dense lymphoplasmacytic infiltrates, similar to that seen in the liver, spleen, and lymph nodes, forming cutaneous plaques and, rarely, nodules (84). Chronic urticaria and IgM gammopathy are the two cardinal features of the Schnitzler syndrome, which is not usually associated initially with clinical features of WM (85), although evolution to WM is not uncommon. Thus, close follow-up of these patients is warranted. Invasion of articular and periarticular structures by WM malignant cells is rarely reported (86). The neoplastic cells can infiltrate the periorbital structures, lacrimal gland, and retro-orbital lymphoid tissues, resulting in ocular nerve palsies (87, 88). Direct infiltration of the central nervous system by monoclonal lymphoplasmacytic cells as infiltrates or as tumors constitutes the rarely observed Bing–Neel syndrome, characterized clinically by confusion, memory loss, disorientation, and motor dysfunction (reviewed in Ref. 89).

9.6   Laboratory Investigations and Findings

9.6.1   Hematological Abnormalities

Anemia is the most common finding in patients with symptomatic WM and is caused by a combination of factors: mild decrease in red cell survival, impaired erythropoiesis, hemolysis, moderate plasma volume expansion, and blood loss from the gastrointestinal tract. Blood smears are usually normocytic and normochromic, and rouleaux formation is often pronounced. Electronically measured mean corpuscular volume might be elevated spuriously because of erythrocyte aggregation. In addition, the hemoglobin estimate can be inaccurate (i.e., falsely high) because of interaction between the monoclonal protein and the diluent used in some automated analyzers (90). Leukocyte and platelet counts are usually within the reference range at presentation, although patients might occasionally present with severe thrombocytopenia. As reported earlier, monoclonal B-lymphocytes expressing surface IgM and late-differentiation B-cell markers are uncommonly detected in blood by flow cytometry. A raised erythrocyte sedimentation rate is almost constantly observed in WM and might be the first clue to the presence of the macroglobulin. The clotting abnormality detected most frequently is prolongation of thrombin time. AL amyloidosis should be suspected in all patients with nephrotic syndrome, cardiomyopathy, hepatomegaly, or peripheral neuropathy. Diagnosis requires the demonstration of green birefringence under polarized light of amyloid deposits stained with Congo red.

9.6.2   Biochemical Investigations

High-resolution electrophoresis combined with immunofixation of serum and urine are recommended for identification and characterization of the IgM monoclonal protein. The light chain of the monoclonal IgM is κ in 75–80% of patients. A few WM patients have more than one M-component. The concentration of the serum monoclonal protein is very variable but, in most cases, lies within the range of 15–45 g/L. Densitometry should be adopted to determine IgM levels for serial evaluations because nephelometry is unreliable and shows large intralaboratory as well as interlaboratory variation. The presence of cold agglutinins or cryoglobulins might affect the determination of IgM levels; therefore, testing for cold agglutinins and cryoglobulins should be performed at diagnosis. If present, subsequent serum samples should be analyzed under warm conditions for the determination of the serum monoclonal IgM level. Although Bence Jones proteinuria is frequently present, it exceeds 1 g/24 h in only 3% of cases. IgA and IgG levels are most often depressed in patients with WM and do not demonstrate recovery even after successful treatment (91). In recent studies by Hunter et al., mutations in the receptor TACI were demonstrated in WM patients akin to those demonstrated in patients with common variable deficiency disorder (CVID), suggesting a possible CVID background for WM patients (92).

9.6.3   Serum Viscosity

Because of its large size (almost 1×10^6 Daltons), most IgM molecules are retained within the intravascular compartment and can exert an undue effect on serum viscosity. Therefore, serum viscosity should be measured if the patient has signs or symptoms of hyperviscosity syndrome. Fundoscopy remains an excellent indicator of clinically relevant hyperviscosity (see Figure 9.2). Among the first clinical signs of hyperviscosity is the appearance of peripheral and mid-peripheral dot and blotlike hemorrhages in the retina, which are best appreciated with indirect ophthalmoscopy and scleral depression (42). In more severe cases of hyperviscosity, dot, blot, and flame-shaped hemorrhages can appear in the macular area along with markedly dilated and tortuous veins with focal constrictions resulting in "venous sausaging," as well as papilledema.

9.6.4   Bone Marrow Findings

Bone marrow is always involved in WM. Central to the diagnosis of WM is the demonstration, by trephine biopsy, of bone marrow infiltration by a lymphoplasmacytic cell population constituted by small lymphocytes with evidence of plasmacytoid/plasma cell differentiation (Figure 9.1). The pattern of bone marrow infiltration might be diffuse, interstitial, or nodular, showing usually an intertrabecular pattern of infiltration. A solely paratrabecular pattern of infiltration is unusual and should raise the possibility of follicular lymphoma (1). The bone marrow infiltration should routinely be confirmed by immunophenotypic studies (flow cytometry and/or immunohistochemistry) showing the following profile: sIgM⁺CD19⁺CD20⁺CD22⁺CD79⁺ (24–26). Up to 20% of cases might express either CD5, CD10, or CD23 (27). In these cases, care should be taken to satisfactorily exclude chronic lymphocytic leukemia, and mantle cell lymphoma (1). "Intranuclear" periodic acid-Schiff (PAS)-positive inclusions (Dutcher-Fahey bodies) consisting of IgM deposits in the perinuclear space and sometimes in intranuclear vacuoles might be seen occasionally in lymphoid cells in WM. An increase number of mast cells, usually in association with the lymphoid aggregates, is commonly found in WM, and their presence might help in differentiating WM from other B-cell lymphomas (2, 3).

9.6.5   Other Investigations

Magnetic resonance imaging (MRI) of the spine in conjunction with computed tomography (CT) of the abdomen and pelvis are useful in evaluating the disease status in WM (94). Bone marrow involvement can be documented by MRI studies of the spine in over 90% of patients, whereas CT of the abdomen and pelvis demonstrated enlarged nodes in 43% of WM patients (94). Lymph node biopsy might show preserved architecture or replacement by infiltration of neoplastic cells with lymphoplasmacytoid, lymphoplasmacytic, or polymorphous cytological patterns.

The residual disease after high-dose chemotherapy with allogeneic or autologous stem cell rescue can be monitored by polymerase chain reaction (PCR)-based methods using primers specific for the monoclonal Ig variable regions.

9.7 Prognosis

Waldenström's macroglobulinemia typically presents as an indolent disease, although considerable variability in prognosis can be seen. The median survival reported in several large series has ranged from 5 to 10 years (95–101). Age is consistently an important prognostic factor (>60–70 years) (95, 96, 98, 101), but this factor is often impacted by unrelated morbidities. Anemia, which reflects both marrow involvement and the serum level of the IgM monoclonal protein (due to the impact of IgM on intravascular fluid retention), has emerged as a strong adverse prognostic factor with hemoglobin levels of <9–12 g/dL associated with decreased survival in several series (95–98, 101). Cytopenias have also been regularly identified as a significant predictor of survival (96). However, the precise level of cytopenias with prognostic significance remains to be determined (98). Some series have identified a platelet count of < 100–150 × 10⁹/L and a granulocyte count of < 1.5 × 10⁹/L as independent prognostic factors (95, 96, 98, 101). The number of cytopenias in a given patient has been proposed as a strong prognostic factor (96). Serum albumin levels have also correlated with survival in WM patients in certain but not all studies using multivariate analyses (96, 98, 99). High beta-2 microglobulin levels (>3–3.5 mg/L) were shown in several studies (97–101), a high serum IgM M-protein (>7 g/dL) (101), as well as a low serum IgM M-protein (<4 g/dL) (99), and the presence of cryoglobulins (95) as adverse factors. A few scoring systems have been proposed based on these analyses (Table 9.3).

9.8 Treatment of Waldenström's Macroglobulinemia

As part of the 2nd International Workshops on WM, a consensus panel was organized to recommend criteria for the initiation of therapy in patients with WM (98). The panel recommended that initiation of therapy should not be based on the IgM level *per se*, as this might not correlate with the clinical manifestations of WM. The consensus panel, however, agreed that initiation of therapy was appropriate for patients with constitutional symptoms, such as recurrent fever, night sweats, fatigue due to anemia, or weight loss. The presence of progressive symptomatic lymphadenopathy or splenomegaly provides additional reasons to begin therapy. The presence of anemia with a hemoglobin value of ≤ 10 g/dL or a platelet count ≤ 100 × 10⁹/L resulting from marrow infiltration also justifies treatment. Certain complications, such as

Table 9.3 Prognostic scoring systems in Waldenstrom's macroglobulinemia

Study	Adverse prognostic factors	No. of groups	Survival
Gobbi et al. (95)	Hb <9 g/dL	0–1 prognostic factors	Median: 48 months
	Age >70 years	2–4 prognostic factors	Median: 80 months
	Weight loss		
	Cryoglobulinemia		
Morel et al. (96)	Age ≥ 65 yearrs	0–1 prognostic factors	5 years: 87%
	Albumin < 4 g/dL	2 prognostic factors	5 yearsr: 62%
	Number of cytopenias:	3–4 prognostic factors	5 yearsr: 25%
	Hb < 12 g/dL		
	Platelets <150 × 10⁹/L		
	WBC < 4 × 10⁹/L		
Dhodapkar et al, (97)	$\beta_2M \geq 3$ mg/L	$\beta_2M < 3$ mg/L + Hb ≥ 12 g/dL	5 years: 87%
	Hb < 12 g/dL	$\beta_2M < 3$ mg/L + Hb < 12 g/dL	5 years: 63%
	IgM < 4 g/dL	$\beta_2M \geq 3$ mg/L + IgM ≥ 4 g/dL	5 years: 53%
		$\beta_2M \geq 3$ mg/L + IgM < 4 g/dL	5 years: 21%
Application of International Staging System Criteria for Myeloma to WM Dimopoulos et al. (99)	Albumin ≤3.5 g/dL	Albumin ≥ 3.5 g/dL + $\beta_2M \geq 3.5$ mg/L	Median: NR
	$\beta_2M < 3.5$ mg/L	Albumin ≤ 3.5 g/dL + $\beta_2M < 3.5$ or β_2M 3.5–5.5 mg/L	Median: 116 months
		$\beta_2M > 5.5$ mg/L	Median: 54 months
International Prognostic Scoring System for WM Morel et al. (101)	Age > 65 yr	0–1 prognostic factors[a]	5 years: 87%
	Hb <11.5 g/dL	2 prognostic factors[b]	5 years: 68%
	Platelets <100 × 10⁹/L	3–5 prognostic factors	5 years: 36%
	$\beta_2M > 3$ mg/L		
	IgM > 7 g/dL		

[a]Excluding age.

[b]or age >65 years.

hyperviscosity syndrome, symptomatic sensorimotor peripheral neuropathy, systemic amyloidosis, renal insufficiency, or symptomatic cryoglobulinemia, might also be indications for therapy (98).

9.9   Front-Line Therapy

Although a precise therapeutic algorithm for therapy of WM remains to be defined given the paucity of randomized clinical trials, consensus panels composed of experts who treat WM were organized as part of the 2nd and 3rd

International Workshop on Waldenström's macroglobulinemia and have formulated recommendations for both frontline and salvage therapy of WM based on the best available clinical trials evidence. Among front-line options, the panels considered alkylator agents (e.g., chlorambucil), nucleoside analogues (cladribine or fludarabine), the monoclonal antibody rituximab. as well as combinations thereof as reasonable choices for the upfront therapy of WM (102, 103). Importantly, the panel felt that individual patient considerations, including the presence of cytopenias, need for more rapid disease control, age, and candidacy for autologous transplant therapy, should be taken into account in making the choice of a first-line agent. For patients who are candidates for autologous transplant therapy and in whom such therapy is seriously considered, the panel recommended that exposure to alkylator or nucleoside analogue therapy should be limited.

9.9.1   Alkylator-Based Therapy

Oral alkylating drugs, alone and in combination therapy with steroids, have been extensively evaluated in the upfront treatment of WM. The greatest experience with oral alkylator therapy has been with chlorambucil, which has been administered on both a continuous (i.e., daily dose) schedule as well as an intermittent schedule. Patients receiving chlorambucil on a continuous schedule typically receive 0.1 mg/kg/day, whereas on the intermittent schedule, patients will typically receive 0.3 mg/kg for 7 days, every 6 weeks. In a prospective randomized study, Kyle et al. (104) reported no significant difference in the overall response rate between these schedules, although, interestingly, the median response duration was greater for patients receiving intermittent versus continuously dosed chlorambucil (46 vs. 26 months). Despite the favorable median response duration in this study for use of the intermittent schedule, no difference in the median overall survival was observed. Moreover, an increased incidence for development of myelodysplasia and acute myelogenous leukemia with the intermittent (3 of 22 patients) versus the continuous (0 of 24 patients) chlorambucil schedule prompted the authors of this study to express preference for use of continuous chlorambucil dosing. The use of steroids in combination with alkylator therapy has also been explored. Dimopoulos and Alexanian (105) evaluated chlorambucil (8 mg/m^2) along with prednisone (40 mg/m^2) given orally for 10 days, every 6 weeks, and reported a major response (i.e., reduction of IgM by greater than 50%) in 72% of patients. Non-chlorambucil-based alkylator regimens employing melphalan and cyclophosphamide in combination with steroids have also been examined by Petrucci et al. (106) and Case et al. (107), producing slightly higher overall response rates and response durations, although the benefit of these more complex regimens over chlorambucil remains to be demonstrated. Facon et al.

(108) have evaluated parameters predicting for response to alkylator therapy. Their studies in patients receiving single-agent chlorambucil demonstrated that age 60, male sex, symptomatic status, and cytopenias (but, interestingly, not high tumor burden and serum IgM levels) were associated with poor response to alkylator therapy. Additional factors to be taken into account in considering alkylator therapy for patients with WM include necessity for more rapid disease control given the slow nature of response to alkylator therapy, as well as consideration for preserving stem cells in patients who are candidates for autologous transplant therapy.

9.9.2 Nucleoside Analogue Therapy

Both cladribine and fludarabine have been extensively evaluated in untreated as well as previously treated WM patients. Cladribine administered as a single agent by continuous intravenous infusion, by 2-h daily infusion, or by subcutaneous bolus injections for 5–7 days has resulted in major responses in 40–90% of patients who received primary therapy, whereas in the salvage setting, responses have ranged from 38% to 54%. (108–115) The median time to achievement of response in responding patients following cladribine ranged from 1.2 to 5 months. The overall response rate with daily infusional fludarabine therapy administered mainly on 5-day schedules in previously untreated and treated WM patients has ranged from 38% to 100% and from 30% to 40%, respectively (116–121), which are on par with the response data for cladribine. The median time to achievement of response for fludarabine was also on par with cladribine at 3–6 months. In general, response rates and durations of responses have been greater for patients receiving nucleoside analogues as first-line agents, although in several of the above studies wherein both untreated and previously treated patients were enrolled, no substantial difference in the overall response rate was reported. Myelosuppression commonly occurred following prolonged exposure to either of the nucleoside analogues, as did lymphopenia with sustained depletion of both $CD4^+$ and CD8+ T-lymphocytes observed in WM patients 1 year following initiation of therapy (108, 110). Treatment-related mortality due to myelosuppression and/or opportunistic infections attributable to immunosuppression occurred in up to 5% of all treated patients in some series with either nucleoside analogue. Factors predicting for response to nucleoside analogues in WM included age at start of treatment (<70 years), pretreatment hemoglobin >95 g/L, platelets >75,000/mm³, disease relapsing off therapy, patients with resistant disease within the first year of diagnosis, and a long interval between first-line therapy and initiation of a nucleoside analogue in relapsing patients (108, 114, 120). There are limited data on the use of an alternate nucleoside analogue to salvage patients whose disease relapsed or demonstrated resistance off cladribine or fludarabine therapy (122, 123). Three of four (75%) patients responded to cladribine to salvage patients who progressed following an unmaintained remission to fludarabine, whereas only 1 of 10 (10%) with disease resistant to fludarabine responded to cladribine (122). However, Lewandowski et al. (123) reported a response in two of six patients (33%) and disease stabilization in the remaining patients to fludarabine, in spite of an inadequate response or progressive disease following cladribine therapy. The long-term safety of nucleoside analogues in WM was recently examined by Leleu et al. (124) in a large series of WM patients. A sevenfold increase in transformation to an aggressive lymphoma, and a three-fold increase in the development of acute myelogenous leukemia/myelodysplasia was observed among patients who received a nucleoside analogue versus other therapies for their WM.

9.9.3 CD20-Directed Antibody Therapy

Rituximab is a chimeric monoclonal antibody that targets CD20, a widely expressed antigen on lymphoplasmacytic cells in WM (125). Several retrospective and prospective studies have indicated that rituximab, when used at standard dosimetry (i.e., 4 weekly infusions at $375 \, mg/m^2$) induced major responses in approximately 27–35% of previously treated and untreated patients (126–132). Furthermore, it was shown in some of these studies that patients who achieved minor responses or even sTable disease benefited from rituximab as evidenced by improved hemoglobin and platelet counts and reduction of lymphadenopathy and/or splenomegaly. The median time to treatment failure in these studies was found to range from 8 to 27+ months. Studies evaluating an extended rituximab schedule consisting of 4 weekly courses at $375 mg/m^2$/week, repeated 3 months later by another 4-week course have demonstrated major response rates of 44–48%, with time to progression estimates of 16+ to 29+ months (132, 133).

In many WM patients, a transient increase of serum IgM may be noted immediately following initiation of treatment. Such an increase does not herald treatment failure, and while most patients will return to their baseline serum IgM level by 12 weeks some continue to show prolonged spiking despite demonstrating a reduction in their bone marrow tumor load (134–136). However, patients with baseline serum IgM levels of $>50 g/L$ or serum viscosity of $>3.5 cp$ may be particularly at risk for a hyperviscosity related event and in such patients plasmapheresis should be considered in advance of rituximab therapy (135). Because of the decreased likelihood of response in patients with higher IgM levels, as well as the possibility that serum IgM and viscosity levels may abruptly rise, rituximab monotherapy should not be used as sole therapy for the treatment of patients at risk for hyperviscosity symptoms.

Time to response after rituximab is slow and exceeds 3 months on average. The time to best response in one study was 18 months (133). Patients with baseline serum IgM levels of $<60 g/dL$ are more likely to respond, irrespective of the underlying bone marrow involvement by tumor cells (132, 133). A recent analysis of 52 patients who were treated with single-agent rituximab has indicated that the objective response rate was significantly lower in patients who had either low serum albumin ($<35\,g/L$) or elevated serum monoclonal protein ($>40\,g/L$ M-spike). Furthermore, the presence of both adverse prognostic factors was related to a short time to progression (3.6 months). Moreover, patients who had normal serum albumin and relatively low serum monoclonal protein levels derived a substantial benefit from rituximab, with a time to progression exceeding 40 months (137).

The genetic background of patients might also be important for determining the response to rituximab. In particular, a correlation between polymorphisms at position 158 in the FcγRIIIa receptor (CD16), an activating Fc receptor on important effector cells that mediate antibody-dependent cell-mediated cytotoxicity (ADCC), and rituximab response was observed in WM patients. Individuals might encode either the amino acid valine or phenylalanine at position 158 in the FcγRIIIa receptor. WM patients who carried the valine amino acid (either in a homozygous or heterozygous pattern) had a fourfold higher major response rate (i.e., 50% decline in serum IgM levels) to rituximab versus those patients who expressed phenylalanine in a homozygous pattern (138).

9.9.4   Combination Therapies

Because rituximab is an active and a nonmyelosuppressive agent, its combination with chemotherapy has been explored in WM patients. Weber et al. (139) administered rituximab along with cladribine and cyclophosphamide to 17 previously untreated patients with WM. At least a partial response was documented in 94% of WM patients, including a complete response in 18%. With a median follow-up of 21 months, no patient has relapsed. In a study by the Waldenstrom's Macroglobulinemia Clinical Trials Group (WMCTG), the combination of rituximab and fludarabine was evaluated in 43 WM patients, 32 (75%) of whom were previously untreated (140). Ninety-one percent of patients demonstrated at least a 25% decrease in serum IgM levels, and response rates were as follows: complete response (CR), 7%; partial response (PR), 74.4%; major response (MR), 9.3%. Hematological toxicity was common with grade 3/4 neutropenia observed in 58% of patients. Two deaths occurred in this study, which might have been related to therapy-induced immunosuppression. With a median follow-up of 17 months, 34/39 (87%) remain in remission. The addition of rituximab to fludarabine and cyclophosphamide has also been explored in the salvage setting by Tam et al. (141), wherein four of five patients demonstrated a response141. In another combination study with rituximab, Hensel et al. (142) administered rituximab along with pentostatin and cyclophosphamide to 13 patients with untreated and previously treated WM or lymphoplasmacytic lymphoma. A major response was observed in 77% or patients. In a study by Dimopoulos et al., the combination of rituximab, dexamethasone, and cyclophosphamide was used as primary therapy to treat 70 patients with WM (143). On an intent-to-treat basis, at least a major response was observed in 70% of patients. With a median follow-up of 24 months, 60% of patients are progression-free. Therapy was well tolerated, although one patient died of interstitial pneumonia.

In addition to nucleoside analogue-based trials with rituximab, two studies have examined CHOP (cyclophosphamide, doxorubicin, vincristine, prednisone) in combination with rituximab (CHOP-R). In a randomized front-line study by the German Low Grade Lymphoma Study Group (GLSG) involving 72 patients (71% of whom had lymphoplasmacytic lymphoma), a significantly higher response rate (94% vs. 69%) was observed among patients receiving CHOP-R versus CHOP, respectively (144). Treon et al. (145) have also evaluated CHOP-R in 13 WM patients, 8 and 5 of whom were relapsed or refractory to nucleoside analogues and single-agent rituximab, respectively. Among 13 evaluable patients, 10 patients achieved a major response (77%) including 3 CR and 7 PR, and two patients achieved a minor response.

The addition of alkylating agents to nucleoside analogues has also been explored in WM. Weber et al. administered two cycles of oral cyclophosphamide along with subcutaneous cladribine to 37 patients with previously untreated WM (139). At least a partial response was observed in 84% of patients and the median duration of response was 36 months. Dimopoulos et al. (146) examined fludarabine in combination with intravenous cyclophosphamide and observed partial responses in 6 of 11 (55%) WM patients with either primary refractory disease or who had relapsed on treatment. The combination of fludarabine plus cyclosphosphamide was also evaluated in a recent study by Tamburini et al. (147) involving 49 patients, 35 of whom were previously treated. Seventy-eight percent of the patients in this study achieved a response, and median time to treatment failure was 27 months. Hematological toxicity was commonly observed and three patients died of treatment-related toxicities. Two interesting findings in this study was the development of acute leukemia in two patients, histologic transformation to diffuse large-cell lymphoma in one patient, and two cases of solid malignancies (prostate and melanoma), as well as failure to mobilize stem cells in four of six patients.

In view of the above data, the consensus panel on therapeutics amended its original recommendations for the therapy of WM to include the use of combination therapy with either nucleoside analogues and alkylator agents, or rituximab in combination with nucleoside analogues, nucleoside analogues plus alkylator agents, or combination chemotherapy such as CHOP as reasonable therapeutics options for the treatment of WM (103).

9.10   Salvage Therapy Including Novel Agents

For patients in relapse or who have refractory disease, the consensus panels recommended the use of an alternative first-line agent as defined earlier, with the caveat that for those patients for whom autologous transplantation was being seriously considered, further exposure to stem-cell-damaging agents (i.e., many alkylator agents and nucleoside analogue drugs) should be avoided, and a non-stem-cell toxic agent such as should be considered if stem cells had not previously been harvested (102, 103). Recent studies have also demonstrated activity for several novel agents, including bortezomib, thalidomide alone or in combination, and alemtuzumab, and can be considered in the treatment of relapsed/refractory WM. Finally, autologous stem cell transplant remains an option for the salvage therapy of WM, particularly among younger patients who have had multiple relapses or have primary refractory disease.

9.10.1 Proteosome Inhibitor

Bortezomib, a stem-cell-sparing agent (148, 149), is a proteosome inhibitor that induces apoptosis of primary WM lymphoplasmacytic cells, as well as the WM-WSU WM cell line at pharmacologically achievable levels (150). Moreover, bortezomib might also impact on bone marrow microenvironmental support for lymphoplasmacytic cells (151). In a multi-enter study of the Waldenstrom's Macroglobulinemia Clinical Trials Group (WMCTG) (152), 27 patients received up to 8 cycles of bortezomib at $1.3 \, mg/m^2$ on days 1, 4, 8, and 11. All but one patient had relapsed/or refractory disease. Following therapy, median serum IgM levels declined from 4660 to 2092 mg/dL ($p < 0.0001$). The overall response rate was 85%, with 10 and 13 patients achieving a minor response (<25% decrease in IgM) and major (<50% decrease in IgM) response, respectively. Responses were prompt and occurred at a median of 1.4 months. The median time to progression for all responding patients in this study was 7.9 (range: 3–21.4+) months, and the most common grade 3/4 toxicities occurring in ≥5% of patients were sensory neuropathies (22.2%), leukopenia (18.5%), neutropenia (14.8%), dizziness (11.1%), and thrombocytopenia (7.4%). Importantly, sensory neuropathies resolved or improved in nearly all patients following cessation of therapy. As part of an NCI-Canada study, Chen et al. (153) treated 27 patients with both untreated (44%) and previously treated (56%) disease. Patients in this study received bortezomib utilizing the standard schedule until they either demonstrated progressive disease or two cycles beyond a complete response or sTable disease. The overall response rate in this study was 78%, with major responses observed in 44% of patients. Sensory neuropathy occurred in 20 patients, 5 with grade >3, and occurred following two to four cycles of therapy. Among the 20 patients developing a neuropathy, 14 patients resolved and 1 patient demonstrated a one-grade improvement at 2–13 months. In addition to the above experiences with bortezomib monotherapy in WM, Dimopoulos et al. (154) observed major responses in 6 of 10 (60%) previously treated WM patients, whereas Goy et al. (155) observed a major response in 1 of 2 WM patients included in a series of relapsed or refractory patients with non-Hodgkin's lymphoma.

9.10.2 CD52-Directed Antibody Therapy

Alemtuzumab is a humanized monoclonal antibody that targets CD52, an antigen widely expressed on bone marrow lymphoplasmacytic cells (LPC) in WM patients as well as on mast cells that are increased in the BM of patients with WM and provide growth and survival signals to WM LPC through several tumor necrosis factor (TNF) family ligands (CD40L, APRIL, BLYS). As part of a WMCTG effort (156), 28 subjects with the REAL/WHO clinicopathological diagnosis of LPL, including 27 patients with IgM (WM) and 1 with IgA monoclonal gammopathy, were enrolled in this prospective, multicenter study. Five patients were untreated and 23 were previously treated, all of whom had previously received rituximab. Patients received 3 daily test doses of alemtuzumab (3, 10, and 30 mg IV) followed by 30 mg alemtuzumab IV three times a week for up to 12 weeks. All patients received acyclovir and bactrim or equivalent prophylaxis for the duration of therapy plus 8 weeks following the last infusion of alemtuzumab. Among 25 patients evaluable for response, the overall response rate was 76%, which included 8 (32%) major responders and 11 (44%) minor responders. Hematological toxicities were common among previously treated (but not untreated) patients and included grade 3/4 neutropenia (39%), thrombocytopenia (18%), and anemia (7%.) Grade 3/4 nonhematological toxicity for all patients included dermatitis (11%), fatigue (7%), and infection (7%). Cytomegalovirus (CMV) reactivation and infection was commonly seen among previously treated patients and might have been etiological for one death on study. With a median follow-up of 8.5+ months, 11/19 responding patients remain free of progression. High rates of response with the use of alemtuzumab as salvage therapy have also been reported by Owen et al. (157) in a small series of heavily pretreated WM patients (with a median prior therapies of four) who received up to 12 weeks of therapy (at 30 mg IV three times a week) following initial dose escalation. Among the seven patients receiving alemtuzumab, five patients achieved a partial response and one patient achieved a complete response. Infectious complications were common, with CMV reactivation occurring in three patients requiring ganciclovir therapy, and hospitalization for three patients for bacterial infections. Opportunistic infections occurred in two patients and were responsible for their deaths. An upfront study by the WMCTG examining the role of alemtuzumab in combination with rituximab is anticipated, given the efficacy results of the above studies.

9.10.3   Thalidomide and Lenalidomide

Thalidomide as a single agent, and in combination with dexamethasone and clarithromycin, has also been examined in patients with WM, in view of the success of these regimens in patients with advanced multiple myeloma. Dimopoulos et al. (158) demonstrated a major response in 5 of 20 (25%) previously untreated and treated patients who received single-agent thalidomide. Dose escalation from the thalidomide start dose of 200 mg daily was hindered by the development of side effects, including the development of peripheral neuropathy in five patients obligating discontinuation or dose reduction. Low doses of thalidomide (50 mg orally daily) in combination with dexamethasone (40 mg orally once a week) and clarithromycin (250 mg orally twice a day) have also been examined, with 10 of 12 (83%) previously treated patients demonstrating at least a major response (159). However, in a follow-up study by Dimopoulos et al. (160) using a higher thalidomide dose (200 mg orally daily) along with dexamathasone (40 g orally once a week) and clarithromycin (500 mg orally twice a day), only 2 of 10 (20%) previously treated patients responded. In a previous study, the immunomodulators thalidomide and its analogue lenalidomide significantly augmented rituximab-mediated antibody-dependent cell-mediated cytotoxicity (ADCC) against lymphoplasmacytic cells (161). Moreover, an expansion of natural killer cells has been observed with thalidomide, which, in previous studies, have been shown to be associated with rituximab response (162, 163). In view of these data, the WMCTG conducted two phase II clinical trials in symptomatic patients with WM combining thalidomide or lenalidomide with rituximab (164). Intended therapy for patients on the phase II study of thalidomide plus rituximab consisted of thalidomide administered at 200 mg daily for 2 weeks, followed by 400 mg daily thereafter for 1 year. Patients received four weekly infusions of rituximab at 375 mg/m^2 beginning 1 week after initiation of thalidomide, followed by four additional weekly infusions of rituximab at 375 mg/m^2 beginning at week 13. Twenty-three of 25 patients were evaluable in this study and responses included the following: CR, $n = 1$; PR $n = 15$; MR, $n = 2$; Stable Disease (SD), $n = 1$, for an overall (ORR) and a major response rate of 78% and 70%, respectively. Median serum IgM levels decreased from 3670 (924–8610 mg/dL) to 1590 (36–5230 mg/dL) ($p < 0.001$), whereas the median hematocrit rose from 33.0 (23.6–42.6%) to 37.6 (29.3–44.3%) ($p = 0.004$) at best response. With a median follow-up of 42+ months, the median Time to Progression (TTP) for evaluable patients on this study was 35 months, and it was 38+ months for responders. Responses were associated with a median cumulative thalidomide dose: CR/PR/MR (29,275 mg) vs. SD/NR (7400 mg); $p = 0.004$. Responses were unaffected by FcγRIIIA-158 polymorphism status (81% vs. 71% for Valine/Valine (VV)/Phenylalanine/Valine (FV) vs. Phenylalanine/Phenylalanine (FF); IgM (78% vs. 80% for <6000 vs. ≥6000 mg/dL); and B$_2$M (71% vs. 89% for <3 vs. ≥3 g/dL). Dose reduction of thalidomide occurred in all patients and led to discontinuation in 11 patients. Among 11 patients experiencing grade ≥2 neuroparesthesias, 10 demonstrated resolution to grade 1 ($n = 3$) or complete resolution ($n = 7$) at a median of 6.7 (range: 0.4–22.5 months).

In a phase II study of lenalidomide and rituximab in WM (165), patients were initiated on lenalidomide at 25 mg daily on a syncopated schedule wherein therapy was administered for 3 weeks, followed by a 1-week pause for an intended duration of 48 weeks. Patients received 1 week of therapy with lenalidomide, after which rituximab (375 mg/m^2) was administered weekly on weeks 2–5, then weeks 13–16. Twelve of 16 patients were evaluable and responses included the following: PR, $n = 4$; MR, $n = 4$; SD, $n = 3$; and NR, $n = 1$ for an overall and a major response rate of 67% and 33%, respectively, and a median TTP of 15.6 months. In two patients with bulky disease, significant reduction in node/spleen size was observed. Acute decreases in hematocrit were observed during first 2 weeks of lenalidomide therapy in 13/16 (81%) patients with a median hematocrit decrease of 4.4% (1.7–7.2%), resulting in hospitalization in 4 patients. Despite reduction of initiation doses to 5 mg daily, anemia continued to be problematic without evidence of hemolysis or more general myelosuppression. Therefore, the mechanism for pronounced anemia in WM patients receiving lenalidomide remains to be determined and the use of this agent among WM patients remains investigational.

9.11   High-Dose Therapy and Stem Cell Transplantation

The use of transplant therapy has also been explored in patients WM. Desikan et al. (166) reported their initial experience of high-dose chemotherapy and autologous stem cell transplant, which has more recently been updated by Munshi et al. (167) Their studies involved eight previously treated WM patients between the ages of 45 and 69 years, who received either melphalan at 200 mg/m^2 ($n = 7$) or melphalan at 140 mg/m^2 along with total-body irradiation. Stem cells were successfully collected in all eight patients, although a second collection procedure was required for two patients who had extensive previous nucleoside analogue exposure. There were no transplant-related mortalities and toxicities were manageable. All eight patients responded, with seven of eight patients achieving a major response and one patient achieving a complete response, with durations of response raging from 5+ to 77+ months. Dreger et al. (168) investigated the use of the DEXA-BEAM (dexamethasone, BCNU, etoposide, cytarabine, melphalan) regimen followed by myeloablative therapy with cyclophosphamide, and total-body irradiation and autologous stem cell transplantation in seven WM patients, which included four untreated patients. Serum IgM levels declined by >50% following DEXA-BEAM and myeloablative therapy for six of seven patients, with progression-free survival ranging from 4+ to 30+ months. All three evaluable patients, who were previously treated, also attained a major response in a study by Anagnostopoulos et al. (169) in which WM patients received various preparative regimens and showed event-free survivals of 26+, 31, and 108+ months. Tournilhac et al. (170) recently reported the outcome of 18 WM patients in France who received high-dose chemotherapy followed by autologous stem cell transplantation. All patients were previously treated with a median of three (range: 1–5) prior regimens. Therapy was well tolerated with an improvement in response status observed for seven patients (six PR to CR; one SD to PR), whereas only one patient demonstrated progressive disease. The median event-free survival for all nonprogressing patients was 12 months. Tournilhac et al. (170) have also reported the outcome of allogeneic transplantation in 10 previously treated WM patients (ages: 35–46 years) who received a median of 3 prior therapies, including 3 patients with progressive disease despite therapy. Two of three patients with progressive disease responded, and an improvement in response status was observed in five patients. The median event-free survival for nonprogressing, evaluable patients was 31 months. Involved in this series was the death of three patients as a result of transplantation-related toxicity. Anagnostopoulos et al. (171) have also reported on a retrospective review of WM patients who underwent either autologous or allogeneic transplantation and whose outcomes were reported to the Center for International Blood and Marrow Transplant Research. Seventy-eight percent of patients in this cohort had two or more previous therapies and 58% of them were resistant to their previous therapy. The relapse rate at 3 years was 29% in the allogeneic group and 24% in the autologous group. Nonrelapse mortality, however, was 40% in the allogeneic group and 11% in the autologous group in this series. In view of the high rate of nonrelapse mortality associated with high-dose chemotherapy and allogeneic transplantation, Maloney et al. (172) have evaluated the use of nonmyeloablative allogeneic transplantation in five patients with refractory WM. In this series, three of three evaluable patients (all of whom had matched sibling donors) responded with two in CR and one in PR at 1–3 years posttransplant. In view of the above data, the consensus panel on therapeutics for WM has recommended that autologous transplantation in WM be considered in the relapsed setting, particularly among younger patients who have had multiple relapses or primary refractory disease, whereas allogeneic and mini-allogeneic transplantation should be undertaken ideally in the context of a clinical trial (102, 103).

9.12 Response Criteria in Waldenstrom's Macroglobulinemia

Assessment of response to treatment for WM has been widely heterogeneous. As a consequence, studies using the same regimen have reported significantly different response rates. As part of the 2nd and 3rd International Workshops on WM, consensus panels developed guidelines for uniform response criteria in WM (173, 174). The category of minor response was adopted at the 3rd International Workshop of WM, given that clinically meaningful responses were observed with newer biological agents and is based on ≥25% to <50% decrease in serum IgM level, which is used as a surrogate marked of disease in WM. In distinction, the term *major response* is used to denote a response of ≥50% in serum IgM levels and includes partial and complete responses (174). Response categories and criteria for progressive disease in WM based on consensus recommendations are summarized in Table 9.4. An important concern with the use of IgM as a surrogate marker of disease is that it can fluctuate, independent of tumor cell killing, particularly with newer biologically targeted agents such as rituximab and bortezomib (134–136, 152, 175). Rituximab induces a spike or flare in serum IgM levels that can last for months, whereas bortezomib can suppress IgM levels independent of tumor cell killing in certain patients. In circumstances where the serum IgM levels appear out of context with the clinical progress of the patient, a bone marrow biopsy should be considered in order to clarify the patient's underlying disease burden. Soluble CD27 is currently being investigated by Ho et al. (34) as an alternative surrogate marker in WM.

Table 9.4 Summary of updated response criteria from the 3rd International Workshop on Waldenstrom's Macroglobulinemia (174)

Complete response	CR	Disappearance of monoclonal protein by immunofixation; no histological evidence of bone marrow involvement, and resolution of any adenopathy/organomegaly (confirmed by CT scan), along with no signs or symptoms attribuTable to WM. Reconfirmation of the CR status is required at least 6 weeks apart with a second immunofixation.
Partial response	PR	A ≥50% reduction of serum monoclonal IgM concentration on protein electrophoresis and ≥50% decrease in adenopathy/organomegaly on physical examination or on CT scan. No new symptoms or signs of active disease.
Minor response	MR	A ≥25% but <50% reduction of serum monoclonal IgM by protein electrophoresis. No new symptoms or signs of active disease.
Stable disease	SD	A <25% reduction and <25% increase of serum monoclonal IgM by electrophoresis without progression of adenopathy/organomegaly, cytopenias or clinically significant symptoms due to disease and/or signs of WM.
Progressive disease	PD	A ≥25% increase in serum monoclonal IgM by protein electrophoresis confirmed by a second measurement or progression of clinically significant findings due to disease (i.e., anemia, thrombocytopenia, leukopenia, bulky adenopathy/organomegaly) or symptoms (unexplained recurrent fever ≥38.4°C, drenching night sweats, ≥10% body weight loss, or hyperviscosity, neuropathy, symptomatic cryoglobulinemia or amyloidosis) attributable to WM.

References

1. Owen RG, Treon SP, Al-Katib A, et al. Clinicopathological definition of Waldenström's macroglobulinemia: Consensus Panel Recommendations from the Second International Workshop on Waldenström's macroglobulinemia. Semin Oncol 2003;30:110–115.
2. Harris NL, Jaffe ES, Stein H, et al. A revised European-American classification of lymphoid neoplasms: a proposal from the International Lymphoma Study Group. Blood 1994;84:1361–1392.
3. Harris NL, Jaffe ES, Diebold J, et al. The World Health Organization classification of neoplastic diseases of the hematopoietic and lymphoid tissues. Report of the Clinical Advisory Committee meeting, Airlie House, Virginia, November, 1997. Ann Oncol 1999;10:1419–1432.
4. Groves FD, Travis LB, Devesa SS, et al. Waldenström's macroglobulinemia: incidence patterns in the United States, 1988–1994. Cancer 1998;82:1078–1081.
5. Herrinton LJ, Weiss NS. Incidence of Waldenström's macroglobulinemia. Blood 1993;82:3148–3150.
6. Bjornsson OG, Arnason A, Gudmunosson S, et al. Macroglobulinaemia in an Icelandic family. Acta Med Scand 1978;203:283–288.
7. Treon SP, Hunter ZR, Aggarwal A, et al. Characterization of familial Waldenstrom's macroglobulinemia. Ann Oncol 2006;17:488–494.
8. Renier G, Ifrah N, Chevailler A, et al. Four brothers with Waldenström's macroglobulinemia. Cancer 1989;64:1554–1559.

9. Ogmundsdottir HM, Sveinsdottir S, Sigfusson A, et al. Enhanced B cell survival in familial macroglobulinaemia is associated with increased expression of Bcl-2. Clin Exp Immunol 1999;117:252–260.
10. Linet MS, Humphrey RL, Mehl ES, et al. A case-control and family study of Waldenström's macroglobulinemia. Leukemia 1993;7:1363–1369.
11. Santini GF, Crovatto M, Modolo ML, et al. Waldenström macroglobulinemia: a role of HCV infection? Blood 1993;82:2932.
12. Silvestri F, Barillari G, Fanin R, Zaja F, Infanti L, Patriarca F, et al. Risk of hepatitis C virus infection, Waldenström's macroglobulinemia, and monoclonal gammopathies. Blood 1996; 88:1125–1126.
13. Leleu X, O'Connor K, Ho A, et al. Hepatitis C viral infection is not associated with Waldenstrom's macroglobulinemia. Am J Hematol 2007;82:83–84.
14. Carbone P, Caradonna F, Granata G, et al. Chromosomal abnormalities in Waldenström's macroglobulinemia. Cancer Genet Cytogenet 1992;61:147–151.
15. Mansoor A, Medeiros LJ, Weber DM, et al. Cytogenetic findings in lymphoplasmacytic lymphoma/Waldenström macroglobulinemia. Chromosomal abnormalities are associated with the polymorphous subtype and an aggressive clinical course. Am J Clin Pathol 2001;116:543–549.
16. Han T, Sadamori N, Takeuchi J, et al. Clonal chromosome abnormalities in patients with Waldenstrom's and CLL-associated macroglobulinemia: significance of trisomy 12. Blood 1983;62(3):525–531.
17. Rivera AI, Li MM, Beltran G, et al. Trisomy 4 as the sole cytogenetic abnormality in a Waldenstrom macroglobulinemia. Cancer Genet Cytogenet 2002;133:172–173.
18. Wong KF, So CC, Chan JC, et al. Gain of chromosome 3/3q in B-cell chronic lymphoproliferative disorder is associated with plasmacytoid differentiation with or without IgM overproduction. Cancer Genet Cytogenet 2002;136:82–85.
19. Schop RF, Kuehl WM, Van Wier SA, et al. Waldenström macroglobulinemia neoplastic cells lack immunoglobulin heavy chain locus translocations but have frequent 6q deletions. Blood 2002;100:2996–3001.
20. Avet-Loiseau H, Garand R, Lode L, et al. 14q32 translocations discriminate IgM multiple myeloma from Waldenstrom's macroglobulinemia. Semin Oncol 2003;30:153–155.
21. Preud'homme JL, Seligmann M. Immunoglobulins on the surface of lymphoid cells in Waldenström's macroglobulinemia. J Clin Invest 1972;51:701–705.
22. Smith BR, Robert NJ, Ault KA. In Waldenstrom's macroglobulinemia the quantity of detecTable circulating monoclonal B lymphocytes correlates with clinical course. Blood 1983;61:911–914.
23. Levy Y, Fermand JP, Navarro S, et al. Interleukin 6 dependence of spontaneous in vitro differentiation of B cells from patients with IgM gammopathy. Proc Natl Acad Sci USA 1990;87:3309–3313.
24. Owen RG, Barrans SL, Richards SJ, Waldenström macroglobulinemia. Development of diagnostic criteria and identification of prognostic factors. Am J Clin Pathol 2001;116:420–428.
25. Feiner HD, Rizk CC, Finfer MD, et al. IgM monoclonal gammopathy/Waldenström's macroglobulinemia: a morphological and immunophenotypic study of the bone marrow. Mod Pathol 1990;3:348–356.
26. San Miguel JF, Vidriales MB, Ocio E, et al. Immunophenotypic analysis of Waldenstrom's macroglobulinemia. Semin Oncol 2003;30:187–195.
27. Hunter ZR, Branagan AR, Manning R, et al. CD5, CD10, CD23 expression in Waldenstrom's macroglobulinemia. Clin Lymph 2005; 5:246–249.
28. Wagner SD, Martinelli V, Luzzatto L. Similar patterns of V kappa gene usage but different degrees of somatic mutation in hairy cell leukemia, prolymphocytic leukemia, Waldenström's macroglobulinemia, and myeloma. Blood 1994;83:3647–3653.
29. Aoki H, Takishita M, Kosaka M, et al. Frequent somatic mutations in D and/or JH segments of Ig gene in Waldenström's macroglobulinemia and chronic lymphocytic leukemia (CLL) with Richter's syndrome but not in common CLL. Blood 1995;85:1913–1919.

30. Shiokawa S, Suehiro Y, Uike N, Muta K, Nishimura J. Sequence and expression analyses of mu and delta transcripts in patients with Waldenström's macroglobulinemia. Am J Hematol 2001; 68:139–143.
31. Sahota SS, Forconi F, Ottensmeier CH, et al. Typical Waldenström macroglobulinemia is derived from a B-cell arrested after cessation of somatic mutation but prior to isotype switch events. Blood 2002;100:1505–1507.
32. Paramithiotis E, Cooper MD. Memory B lymphocytes migrate to bone marrow in humans. Proc Natl Acad Sci USA 1997;94:208–212.
33. Tournilhac O, Santos DD, Xu L, et al. Mast cells in Waldenstrom's macroglobulinemia support lymphoplasmacytic cell growth through CD154/CD40 signaling. Ann Oncol 2006;17: 1275–1282.
34. Ho A, Leleu X, Hatjiharissi E, et al. A novel functional role for soluble CD27 in the pathogenesis of Waldenstrom's macroglobulinemia. Blood 2005;106:4701.
35. Merlini G, Farhangi M, Osserman EF. Monoclonal immunoglobulins with antibody activity in myeloma, macroglobulinemia and related plasma cell dyscrasias. Semin Oncol 1986;13:350–365.
36. Farhangi M, Merlini G. The clinical implications of monoclonal immunoglobulins. Semin Oncol 1986;13:366–379.
37. Marmont AM, Merlini G. Monoclonal autoimmunity in hematology. Haematologica 1991;76:449–459.
38. Mackenzie MR, Babcock J. Studies of the hyperviscosity syndrome. II. Macroglobulinemia. J Lab Clin Med 1975;85:227–234.
39. Gertz MA, Kyle RA. Hyperviscosity syndrome. J Intens Care Med 1995;10:128–141.
40. Kwaan HC, Bongu A. The hyperviscosity syndromes. Semin Thromb Hemost 1999;25:199–208.
41. Singh A, Eckardt KU, Zimmermann A, et al. Increased plasma viscosity as a reason for inappropriate erythropoietin formation. J Clin Invest 1993;91:251–256.
42. Menke MN, Feke GT, McMeel JW, et al. Hyperviscosity-related retinopathy in Waldenstrom's macroglobulinemia. Arch Opthalmol 2006;124:1601–1606.
43. Merlini G, Baldini L, Broglia C, et al. Prognostic factors in symptomatic Waldenström's macroglobulinemia. Semin Oncol 2003;30:211–215.
44. Dellagi K, Dupouey P, Brouet JC, et al. Waldenström's macroglobulinemia and peripheral neuropathy: a clinical and immunologic study of 25 patients. Blood 1983; 62:280–285.
45. Nobile-Orazio E, Marmiroli P, Baldini L, et al. Peripheral neuropathy in macroglobulinemia: incidence and antigen-specificity of M proteins. Neurology 1987;37:1506–1514.
46. Nemni R, Gerosa E, Piccolo G, et al. Neuropathies associated with monoclonal gammapathies. Haematologica 1994;79:557–566.
47. Ropper AH, Gorson KC. Neuropathies associated with paraproteinemia. N Engl J Med 1998;338:1601–1607.
48. Vital A. Paraproteinemic neuropathies. Brain Pathol 2001;11:399–407.
49. Latov N, Braun PE, Gross RB, et al. Plasma cell dyscrasia and peripheral neuropathy: identification of the myelin antigens that react with human paraproteins. Proc Natl Acad Sci USA 1981;78:7139–42.
50. Chassande B, Leger JM, Younes-Chennoufi AB, et al. Peripheral neuropathy associated with IgM monoclonal gammopathy: correlations between M-protein antibody activity and clinical/electrophysiological features in 40 cases. Muscle Nerve 1998;21:55–62.
51. Weiss MD, Dalakas MC, Lauter CJ, et al. Variability in the binding of anti-MAG and anti-SGPG antibodies to target antigens in demyelinating neuropathy and IgM paraproteinemia. J Neuroimmunol 1999;95:174–184.
52. Latov N, Hays AP, Sherman WH. Peripheral neuropathy and anti-MAG antibodies. Crit Rev Neurobiol 1988;3:301–332.
53. Dalakas MC, Quarles RH. Autoimmune ataxic neuropathies (sensory ganglionopathies): are glycolipids the responsible autoantigens? Ann Neurol 1996; 39:419–422.
54. Eurelings M, Ang CW, Notermans NC, et al. Antiganglioside antibodies in polyneuropathy associated with monoclonal gammopathy. Neurology 2001;57:1909–1912.

55. Ilyas AA, Quarles RH, Dalakas MC, et al. Monoclonal IgM in a patient with paraproteine-mic polyneuropathy binds to gangliosides containing disialosyl groups. Ann Neurol 1985;18:655–659.
56. Willison HJ, O'Leary CP, Veitch J, et al. The clinical and laboratory features of chronic sensory ataxic neuropathy with anti-disialosyl IgM antibodies. Brain 2001; 124:1968–1977.
57. Lopate G, Choksi R, Pestronk A. Severe sensory ataxia and demyelinating polyneuropathy with IgM anti-GM2 and GalNAc-GD1A antibodies. Muscle Nerve 2002;25:828–836.
58. Jacobs BC, O'Hanlon GM, Breedland EG, et al. Human IgM paraproteins demonstrate shared reactivity between Campylobacter jejuni lipopolysaccharides and human peripheral nerve disialylated gangliosides. J Neuroimmunol 1997;80:23–30.
59. Nobile-Orazio E, Manfredini E, Carpo M, et al. Frequency and clinical correlates of antineural IgM antibodies in neuropathy associated with IgM monoclonal gammopathy. Ann Neurol 1994;36:416–424.
60. Gordon PH, Rowland LP, Younger DS, et al. Lymphoproliferative disorders and motor neuron disease: an update. Neurology 1997;48:1671–1678.
61. Pavord SR, Murphy PT, Mitchell VE. POEMS syndrome and Waldenström's macroglobulinaemia. J Clin Pathol 1996;49:181–182.
62. Crisp D, Pruzanski W. B-cell neoplasms with homogeneous cold-reacting antibodies (cold agglutinins). Am J Med 1982;72:915–922.
63. Pruzanski W, Shumak KH. Biologic activity of cold-reacting autoantibodies (first of two parts). N Engl J Med 1977;297:538–542.
64. Pruzanski W, Shumak KH. Biologic activity of cold-reacting autoantibodies (second of two parts). N Engl J Med 1977;297:583–589.
65. Whittaker SJ, Bhogal BS, Black MM. Acquired immunobullous disease: a cutaneous manifestation of IgM macroglobulinaemia. Br J Dermatol 1996;135:283–286.
66. Daoud MS, Lust JA, Kyle RA, et al. Monoclonal gammopathies and associated skin disorders. J Am Acad Dermatol 1999;40:507–535.
67. Gad A, Willen R, Carlen B, Gyland F, et al. Duodenal involvement in Waldenström's macroglobulinemia. J Clin Gastroenterol 1995;20:174–176.
68. Mural MR, Kratz A, Fiberg KE. Case records of the Massachusetts General Hospital. Weekly clinicopathological exercises. Case 3–1990. A 66-year-old woman with Waldenström's macroglobulinemia, diarrhea, anemia, and persistent gastrointestinal bleeding. N Engl J Med 1990;322:183–192.
69. Isaac J, Herrera GA. Cast nephropathy in a case of Waldenström's macroglobulinemia. Nephron 2002;91:512–515.
70. Morel-Maroger L, Basch A, Danon F, et al. Pathology of the kidney in Waldenström's macroglobulinemia. Study of sixteen cases. N Engl J Med 1970;283:123–129.
71. Gertz MA, Kyle RA, Noel P. Primary systemic amyloidosis: a rare complication of immunoglobulin M monoclonal gammopathies and Waldenström's macroglobulinemia. J Clin Oncol 1993;11:914–920.
72. Moyner K, Sletten K, Husby G, et al. An unusually large (83 amino acid residues) amyloid fibril protein AA from a patient with Waldenström's macroglobulinaemia and amyloidosis. Scand J Immunol 1980;11:549–554.
73. Gardyn J, Schwartz A, Gal R, et al. Waldenström's macroglobulinemia associated with AA amyloidosis. Int J Hematol 2001;74:76–78.
74. Dussol B, Kaplanski G, Daniel L, et al. Simultaneous occurrence of fibrillary glomerulopathy and AL amyloid. Nephrol Dial Transplant 1998;13:2630–2632.
75. Rausch PG, Herion JC. Pulmonary manifestations of Waldenström macroglobulinemia. Am J Hematol 1980;9:201–209.
76. Fadil A, Taylor DE. The lung and Waldenström's macroglobulinemia. South Med J 1998;91:681–685.
77. Kyrtsonis MC, Angelopoulou MK, Kontopidou FN, et al. Primary lung involvement in Waldenström's macroglobulinaemia: report of two cases and review of the literature. Acta Haematol 2001;105:92–96.

78. Kaila VL, el Newihi HM, Dreiling BJ, et al. Waldenström's macroglobulinemia of the stomach presenting with upper gastrointestinal hemorrhage. Gastrointest Endosc 1996;44:73–75.
79. Yasui O, Tukamoto F, Sasaki N, et al. Malignant lymphoma of the transverse colon associated with macroglobulinemia. Am J Gastroenterol 1997;92:2299–2301.
80. Rosenthal JA, Curran WJ Jr, Schuster SJ. Waldenström's macroglobulinemia resulting from localized gastric lymphoplasmacytoid lymphoma. Am J Hematol 1998;58:244–245.
81. Recine MA, Perez MT, Cabello-Inchausti B, et al. Extranodal lymphoplasmacytoid lymphoma (immunocytoma) presenting as small intestinal obstruction. Arch Pathol Lab Med 2001;125:677–679.
82. Veltman GA, van Veen S, Kluin-Nelemans JC, et al. Renal disease in Waldenström's macroglobulinaemia. Nephrol Dial Transplant 1997;12:1256–1259.
83. Moore DF Jr, Moulopoulos LA, Dimopoulos MA. Waldenström macroglobulinemia presenting as a renal or perirenal mass: clinical and radiographic features. Leuk Lymphoma 1995;17:331–334.
84. Mascaro JM, Montserrat E, Estrach T, et al. Specific cutaneous manifestations of Waldenström's macroglobulinaemia. A report of two cases. Br J Dermatol 1982;106:17–22.
85. Schnitzler L, Schubert B, Boasson M, et al. Urticaire chronique, lésions osseuses, macroglobulinémie IgM: Maladie de Waldenström? Bull Soc Fr Dermatol Syphiligr 1974;81:363–368.
86. Roux S, Fermand JP, Brechignac S, et al. Tumoral joint involvement in multiple myeloma and Waldenström's macroglobulinemia: report of 4 cases. J Rheumatol 1996;23:2175–2178.
87. Orellana J, Friedman AH. Ocular manifestations of multiple myeloma, Waldenström's macroglobulinemia and benign monoclonal gammopathy. Surv Ophthalmol 1981;26:157–69.
88. Ettl AR, Birbamer GG, Philipp W. Orbital involvement in Waldenström's macroglobulinemia: ultrasound, computed tomography and magnetic resonance findings. Ophthalmologica 1992;205:40–45.
89. Civit T, Coulbois S, Baylac F, et al. [Waldenström's macroglobulinemia and cerebral lymphoplasmocytic proliferation: Bing and Neel syndrome. Apropos of a new case.] Neurochirurgie 1997;43:245–249.
90. McMullin MF, Wilkin HJ, Elder E. Inaccurate haemoglobin estimation in Waldenström's macroglobulinaemia. J Clin Pathol 1995;48:787.
91. Treon SP, Branagan AR, Hunter Z, et al. IgA and IgG hypogammaglobulinemia persists in most patients with Waldenstrom's macroglobulinemia despite therapeutic responses, including complete remissions. Blood 2004;104:306b.
92. Hunter Z, Leleu X, Hatjiharissi E, et al. IgA and IgG hypogammaglobulinemia are associated with mutations in the APRIL/BLYS receptor TACI in Waldenstroms macroglobulinemia (WM). Blood 2006;108:228.
93. Dutcher TF, Fahey JL. The histopathology of macroglobulinemia of Waldenström. J Natl Cancer Inst 1959;22:887–917.
94. Moulopoulos LA, Dimopoulos MA, Varma DG, et al. Waldenström macroglobulinemia: MR imaging of the spine and CT of the abdomen and pelvis. Radiology 1993;188:669–673.
95. Gobbi PG, Bettini R, Montecucco C, et al. Study of prognosis in Waldenström's macroglobulinemia: a proposal for a simple binary classification with clinical and investigational utility. Blood 1994;83:2939–2945.
96. Morel P, Monconduit M, Jacomy D, et al. Prognostic factors in Waldenström macroglobulinemia: a report on 232 patients with the description of a new scoring system and its validation on 253 other patients. Blood 2000;96:852–858.
97. Dhodapkar MV, Jacobson JL, Gertz MA, et al. Prognostic factors and response to fludarabine therapy in patients with Waldenström macroglobulinemia: results of United States intergroup trial (Southwest Oncology Group S9003). Blood 2001;98:41–48.
98. Kyle RA, Treon SP, Alexanian R, et al. Prognostic markers and criteria to initiate therapy in Waldenström's macroglobulinemia: Consensus Panel Recommendations from the Second International Workshop on Waldenström's macroglobulinemia. Semin Oncol 2003;30:116–120.
99. Dimopoulos M, Gika D, Zervas K, et al. The international staging system for multiple myeloma is applicable in symptomatic Waldenstrom's macroglobulinemia. Leuk Lymph 2004; 45:1809–1813.

100. Anagnostopoulos A, Zervas K, Kyrtsonis M, et al. Prognostic value of serum beta 2-microglobulin in patients with Waldenstrom's macroglobulinemia requiring therapy. Clin Lymph Myeloma 2006;7:205–209.

101. Morel P, Duhamel A, Gobbi P, et al. International prognostic scoring system (IPSS) for Waldenstrom's macroglobulinemia. Blood 2006;108:42a.

102. Gertz M, Anagnostopoulos A, Anderson KC, et al. Treatment recommendations in Waldenström's macroglobulinemia: Consensus Panel Recommendations from the Second International Workshop on Waldenström's macroglobulinemia. Semin Oncol 2003;30:121–126.

103. Treon SP, Gertz MA, Dimopoulos M, et al. Update on treatment recommendations from the Third International Workshop on Waldenstrom's Macroglobulinemia. Blood 2006;107:3442–3446.

104. Kyle RA, Greipp PR, Gertz MA, et al. Waldenström's macroglobulinaemia: a prospective study comparing daily with intermittent oral chlorambucil. Br J Haematol 2000;108:737–742.

105. Dimopoulos MA, Alexanian R. Waldenstrom's macroglobulinemia. Blood 1994;83:1452–1459.

106. Petrucci MT, Avvisati G, Tribalto M, et al. Waldenström's macroglobulinaemia: results of a combined oral treatment in 34 newly diagnosed patients. J Intern Med 1989;226:443–447.

107. Case DC Jr, Ervin TJ, Boyd MA, et al. Waldenström's macroglobulinemia: long-term results with the M-2 protocol. Cancer Invest 1991;9:1–7.

108. Facon T, Brouillard M, Duhamel A, et al. Prognostic factors in Waldenström's macroglobulinemia: a report of 167 cases. J Clin Oncol 1993;11:1553–1558.

109. Dimopoulos MA, Kantarjian H, Weber D, et al. Primary therapy of Waldenström's macroglobulinemia with 2-chlorodeoxyadenosine. J Clin Oncol 1994;12:2694–2698.

110. Delannoy A, Ferrant A, Martiat P, et al. 2-Chlorodeoxyadenosine therapy in Waldenström's macroglobulinaemia. Nouv Rev Fr Hematol 1994;36:317–320.

111. Fridrik MA, Jager G, Baldinger C, et al. First-line treatment of Waldenström's disease with cladribine. Arbeitsgemeinschaft Medikamentose Tumortherapie. Ann Hematol 1997;74:7–10.

112. Liu ES, Burian C, Miller WE, et al. Bolus administration of cladribine in the treatment of Waldenström macroglobulinaemia. Br J Haematol 1998;103:690–695.

113. Hellmann A, Lewandowski K, Zaucha JM, et al. Effect of a 2-hour infusion of 2-chlorodeoxyadenosine in the treatment of refractory or previously untreated Waldenström's macroglobulinemia. Eur J Haematol 1999;63:35–41.

114. Betticher DC, Hsu Schmitz SF, Ratschiller D, et al. Cladribine (2-CDA) given as subcutaneous bolus injections is active in pretreated Waldenström's macroglobulinaemia. Swiss Group for Clinical Cancer Research (SAKK). Br J Haematol 1997;99:358–363.

115. Dimopoulos MA, Weber D, Delasalle KB, et al. Treatment of Waldenström's macroglobulinemia resistant to standard therapy with 2-chlorodeoxyadenosine: identification of prognostic factors. Ann Oncol 1995;6:49–52.

116. Dimopoulos MA, O'Brien S, Kantarjian H, et al. Fludarabine therapy in Waldenström's macroglobulinemia. Am J Med 1993;95:49–52.

117. Foran JM, Rohatiner AZ, Coiffier B, et al. Multicenter phase II study of fludarabine phosphate for patients with newly diagnosed lymphoplasmacytoid lymphoma, Waldenström's macroglobulinemia, and mantle-cell lymphoma. J Clin Oncol 1999;17:546–553.

118. Thalhammer-Scherrer R, Geissler K, Schwarzinger I, et al. Fludarabine therapy in Waldenström's macroglobulinemia. Ann Hematol 2000;79:556–559.

119. Dhodapkar MV, Jacobson JL, Gertz MA, et al. Prognostic factors and response to fludarabine therapy in patients with Waldenström macroglobulinemia: results of United States intergroup trial (Southwest Oncology Group S9003). Blood 2001;98:41–48.

120. Zinzani PL, Gherlinzoni F, Bendandi M, et al. Fludarabine treatment in resistant Waldenström's macroglobulinemia. Eur J Haematol 1995;54:120–123.

121. Leblond V, Ben Othman T, Deconinck E, et al. Activity of fludarabine in previously treated Waldenström's macroglobulinemia: a report of 71 cases. Groupe Cooperatif Macroglobulinemie. J Clin Oncol 1998;16:2060–2064.

122. Dimopoulos MA, Weber DM, Kantarjian H, et al. 2-Chlorodeoxyadenosine therapy of patients with Waldenström macroglobulinemia previously treated with fludarabine. Ann Oncol 1994;5:288–289.

123. Lewandowski K, Halaburda K, Hellmann A. Fludarabine therapy in Waldenström's macroglobulinemia patients treated previously with 2-chlorodeoxyadenosine. Leuk Lymphoma 2002;43:361–363.
124. Leleu XP, Manning R, Soumerai JD, et al. Increased incidence of disease transformation and development of MDS/AML in Waldenstrom's Macroglobulinemia patients treated with nucleoside analogues. Proc Am Soc Clin Oncol 2007;25: 445s.
125. Treon SP, Kelliher A, Keele B, et al. Expression of serotherapy target antigens in Waldenstrom's macroglobulinemia: therapeutic applications and considerations. Semin Oncol 2003;30:248–252.
126. Treon SP, Shima Y, Preffer FI, et al. Treatment of plasma cell dyscrasias with antibody-mediated immunotherapy. Semin Oncol 1999;26(Suppl 14):97–106.
127. Byrd JC, White CA, Link B, et al. Rituximab therapy in Waldenstrom's macroglobulinemia: preliminary evidence of clinical activity. Ann Oncol 1999;10:1525–527.
128. Weber DM, Gavino M, Huh Y, et al. Phenotypic and clinical evidence supports rituximab for Waldenstrom's macroglobulinemia. Blood 1999;94:125a.
129. Foran JM, Rohatiner AZ, Cunningham D, et al. European phase II study of rituximab (chimeric anti-CD20 monoclonal antibody) for patients with newly diagnosed mantle-cell lymphoma and previously treated mantle-cell lymphoma, immunocytoma, and small B-cell lymphocytic lymphoma. J Clin Oncol 2000;18:317–324.
130. Treon SP, Agus DB, Link B, et al. CD20-Directed antibody-mediated immunotherapy induces responses and facilitates hematologic recovery in patients with Waldenstrom's macroglobulinemia. J Immunother 2001;24:272–279.
131. Gertz MA, Rue M, Blood E, et al. Multicenter phase 2 trial of rituximab for Waldenstrom macroglobulinemia (WM): an Eastern Cooperative Oncology Group Study (E3A98) Leuk Lymphoma 2004;45:2047–2055.
132. Dimopoulos MA, Zervas C, Zomas A, et al. Treatment of Waldenstrom's macroglobulinemia with rituximab. J Clin Oncol 2002;20:2327–2333.
133. Treon SP, Emmanouilides C, Kimby E, et al. Extended rituximab therapy in Waldenström's Macroglobulinemia. Ann Oncol 2005;16:132–138.
134. Donnelly GB, Bober-Sorcinelli K, Jacobson R, et al. Abrupt IgM rise following treatment with rituximab in patients with Waldenstrom's macroglobulinemia. Blood 2001;98:240b.
135. Treon SP, Branagan AR, Anderson KC. Paradoxical increases in serum IgM levels and serum viscosity following rituximab therapy in patients with Waldenstrom's macroglobulinemia. Blood 2003;102:690a.
136. Ghobrial IM, Fonseca R, Greipp PR, et al. The initial "flare" of IgM level after rituximab therapy in patients diagnosed with Waldenstrom macroglobulinemia: an Eastern Cooperative Oncology Group Study. Blood 2003;102:448α.
137. Dimopoulos MA, Anagnostopoulos A, Zervas C, et al. Predictive factors for response to rituximab in Waldenstrom's macroglobulinemia. Clin Lymphoma 2005;5:270–272.
138. Treon SP, Hansen M, Branagan AR, et al. Polymorphisms in FcγRIIIA (CD16) receptor expression are associated with clinical responses to Rituximab in Waldenstrom's macroglobulinemia. J Clin Oncol 2005;23:474–481.
139. Weber DM, Dimopoulos MA, Delasalle K, et al. 2-chlorodeoxyadenosine alone and in combination for previously untreated Waldenstrom's macroglobulinemia. Semin Oncol 2003;30:243–247.
140. Treon SP, Branagan A, Wasi P, et al. Combination therapy with Rituximab and Fludarabine in Waldenstrom's macroglobulinemia. Blood 2004;104:215a.
141. Tam CS, Wolf MM, Westerman D, et al. Fludarabine combination therapy is highly effective in first-line and salvage treatment of patients with Waldenstrom's macroglobulinemia. Clin Lymphoma Myeloma 2005;6:136–139.
142. Hensel M, Villalobos M, Kornacker M, et al. Pentostatin/cyclophosphamide with or without rituximab: an effective regimen for patients with Waldenstrom's macroglobulinemia/lymphoplasmacytic lymphoma. Clin Lymphoma Myeloma 2005;6:131–135.

143. Dimopoulos MA, Anagnostopoulos A, Kyrtsonis MC, et al. Primary treatment of Waldenstrom's macroglobulinemia with Dexamethasone, Rituximab and Cyclophosphamide. Blood 2006;108:42a.
144. Buske C, Dreyling MH, Eimermacher H, et al. Combined immuno-chemotherapy (R-CHOP) results in significantly superior response rates and time to treatment failure in first line treatment of patients with lymphoplasmacytoid/ic immunocytoma. Results of a prospective randomized trial of the German Low Grade Lymphoma Study Group. Blood 2004;104:162a.
145. Treon SP, Hunter Z, Branagan A. CHOP plus rituximab therapy in Waldenström's Macroglobulinemia. Clin Lymphoma Myeloma 2005; 5:273–277.
146. Dimopoulos MA, Hamilos G, Efstathiou E, et al: Treatment of Waldenstrom's macroglobulinemia with the combination of fludarabine and cyclophosphamide. Leuk Lymphoma 2003;44:993–996.
147. Tamburini J, Levy V, Chateilex C, et al. Fludarabine plus cyclophosphamide in Waldenstrom's macroglobulinemia: results in 49 patients. Leukemia 2005;19:1831–1834.
148. Jagannath S, Durie BG, Wolf J, et al. Bortezomib therapy alone and in combination with dexamethasone for previously untreated symptomatic multiple myeloma. Br J Haematol 2005;129:776–783.
149. Oakervee HE, Popat R, Curry N, et al. PAD combination therapy (PS-341/bortezomib, doxorubicin and dexamethasone) for previously untreated patients with multiple myeloma. Br J Haematol 2005;129:755–762.
150. Harousseau JL, Attal M, Leleu X, et al. Bortezomib plus dexamethasone as induction treatment prior to autologous stem cell transplantation in patients with newly diagnosed multiple myeloma. Preliminary results of an IFM Phase II Study. Blood 2004;104:416a.
151. Mitsiades CS, Mitsiades N, McMullan CJ, et al. The proteasome inhibitor bortezomib (PS-341) is active against Waldenstrom's macroglobulinemia. Blood 2003;102:181a.
152. Treon SP, Hunter ZR, Matous J, et al. Multicenter Clinical Trial of Bortezomib in Relapsed/Refractory Waldenstrom's macroglobulinemia: Results of WMCTG Trial 03–248. Clin Cancer Res 2007;13:3320–3325.
153. Chen CI, Kouroukis CT, White D, et al. Bortezomib is active in patients with untreated or relapsed Waldenstrom's macroglobulinemia: A phase II study of the National Cancer Institute of Canada Clinical Trials Group. J Clin Oncol 2007;25:1570–1575.
154. Dimopoulos MA, Anagnostopoulos A, Kyrtsonis MC, et al. Treatment of relapsed or refractory Waldenstrom's macroglobulinemia with bortezomib. Haematologica 2005;90:1655–1657.
155. Goy A, Younes A, McLaughlin P, et al. Phase II study of proteasome inhibitor bortezomib in relapsed or refractory B-cell non-Hodgkin's lymphoma. J Clin Oncol 2005;23:667–675.
156. Hunter ZR, Boxer M, Kahl B, et al. Phase II study of alemtuzumab in lymphoplasmacytic lymphoma: Results of WMCTG trial 02-079.Proc Am Soc Clin Oncol 2006 24:427s.
157. Owen RG, Rawstron AC, Osterborg A, et al. Activity of alemtuzumab in relapsed/refractory Waldenstrom's macroglobulinemia. Blood 2003;102:644a.
158. Dimopoulos MA, Zomas A, Viniou NA, et al. Treatment of Waldenström's macroglobulinemia with thalidomide. J Clin Oncol 2001;19:3596–3601.
159. Coleman C, Leonard J, Lyons L, et al. Treatment of Waldenström's macroglobulinemia with clarithromycin, low-dose thalidomide and dexamethasone. Semin Oncol 2003;30:270–274.
160. Dimopoulos MA, Zomas K, Tsatalas K, et al. Treatment of Waldenström's macroglobulinemia with single agent thalidomide or with combination of clarithromycin, thalidomide and dexamethasone. Semin Oncol 2003;30:265–269.
161. Hayashi T, Hideshima T, Akiyama M, et al. Molecular mechanisms whereby immunomodulatory drugs activate natural killer cells: clinical application. Br J Haematol 2005;128:192–203.
162. Davies FE, Raje N, Hideshima T, et al. Thalidomide and immunomodulatory derivatives augment natural killer cell cytotoxicity in multiple myeloma. Blood 2001;98:210–216.
163. Janakiraman N, McLaughlin P, White CA, et al. Rituximab: correlation between effector cells and clinical activity in NHL. Blood 1998;92:337a.

164. Soumerai JD, Branagan AR, Patterson CJ, et al. Long term responses to thalidomide and rituximab in Waldenstrom's macroglobulinemia. Proc Am Soc Clin Oncol 2007;25: 445s.
165. Treon S, Patterson C, Hunter Z, et al. Phase II Study of CC-5013 (Revlimid) and rituximab in Waldenström's macroglobulinemia: preliminary safety and efficacy results. Blood 2005;106:2443.
166. Desikan R, Dhodapkar M, Siegel D, et al. High-dose therapy with autologous haemopoietic stem cell support for Waldenström's macroglobulinaemia. Br J Haematol 1999;105:993–996.
167. Munshi NC, Barlogie B. Role for high dose therapy with autologous hematopoietic stem cell support in Waldenström's macroglobulinemia. Semin Oncol 2003;30:282–285.
168. Dreger P, Glass B, Kuse R, et al. Myeloablative radiochemotherapy followed by reinfusion of purged autologous stem cells for Waldenström's macroglobulinaemia. Br J Haematol 1999;106:115–118.
169. Anagnostopoulos A, Dimopoulos MA, Aleman A, et al. High-dose chemotherapy followed by stem cell transplantation in patients with resistant Waldenström's macroglobulinemia. Bone Marrow Transplant 2001;27:1027–1029.
170. Tournilhac O, Leblond V, Tabrizi R, et al. Transplantation in Waldenström's macroglobulinemia: the French experience. Semin Oncol 2003;30:291–296.
171. Anagnostopoulos A, Hari PN, Perez WS, et al. Autologous or allogeneic stem cell transplantation in patients with Waldenstrom's macroglobulinemia. Biol Blood Marrow Transplant 2006;12: 845–854.
172. Maloney DG, Sandmaier B, Maris M, et al. The use of non-myeloablative allogeneic hematopoietic cell transplantation for patients with refractory Waldenström's macroglobulinemia: replacing high-dose cytotoxic therapy with graft versus tumor effects. Proceedings of the Second International Workshop on Waldenström's Macroglobulinemia, Athens, 2002.
173. Weber D, Treon SP, Emmanouilides C, et al. Uniform response criteria in Waldenstrom's macroglobulinemia: Consensus panel recommendations from the Second International Workshop on Waldenstrom's Macroglobulinemia. Semin Oncol 2003;30:127–131.
174. Kimby E, Treon SP, Anagnostopoulos A, et al. Update on recommendations for assessing response from the Third International Workshop on Waldenstrom's Macroglobulinemia. Clin Lymphoma Myeloma 2006;6:380–383.
175. Strauss SJ, Maharaj L, Hoare S, et al. Bortezomib therapy in patients with relapsed or refractory lymphoma: Potential correlation of in vitro sensitivity and tumor necrosis factor alpha response with clinical activity. J Clin Oncol 2006;24:2105–2112.

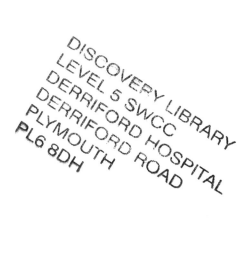

Chapter 10
Rare B-cell Lymphomas

Primary Mediastinal, Intravascular, and Primary Effusion Lymphoma

Kerry J. Savage

10.1   Introduction

Diffuse large B-cell lymphoma (DLBCL) is the most common type of non-Hodgkin lymphoma. This group of diseases is defined pathologically by a diffuse infiltrate of large neoplastic B-cells and clinically by aggressive presentations. Variants and subtypes of DLBCL are recognized in the REAL (Real European-American Lymphoma Classification) and WHO (World Health Classifications) based on unique pathologic features and clinical presentations. Herein are described the three clinical subtypes of DLBCL.

10.2   Primary Mediastinal Large B-Cell Lymphoma

Primary mediastinal large B-cell lymphoma (PMBCL) is recognized as a unique clinical subtype of DLBCL based on distinct clinical and pathologic features and it is believed to arise from thymic medullary B-cells, suggesting a unique histogenesis (1). It accounts for approximately 2% of patients with non-Hodgkin's lymphoma with a propensity to affect young adults. Although morphologically it resembles DLBCL, it has distinct morphologic, immunophenotypic, and genetic features. Further, it has long been appreciated that there is considerable clinical and pathologic overlap with nodular sclerosis Hodgkin's lymphoma and recent microarray studies confirm that PMBCL nasa gene signature with striking similarities to that of classical Hodgkin's lymphoma (CHL)(2).

10.2.1   Pathology

The tumor is composed of diffuse large cells with pale or 'clear' cytoplasm and variable degrees of sclerosis (Figure 10.1). PMBCL is derived from B-cells and the malignant cells express pan-B-cell antigens (CD19, CD20, CD22). However,

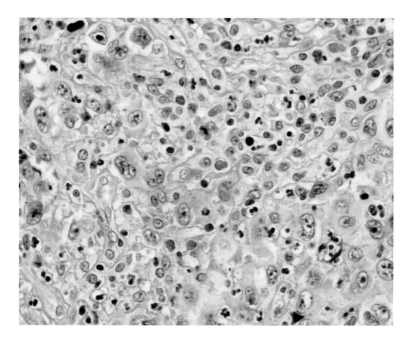

Figure 10.1 PMBCL large malignant cells with clear cytoplasm compartmentalized by fine delicate bands of fibrosis.

unlike other B-cell lymphomas, the malignant cells often lack surface immunoglobulin (sIg) (1), despite expression of the Ig coreceptor CD79a. CD30 expression is often weak and inhomogeneous in contrast to uniform and strong expression seen in classical Hodgkin's lymphoma or anaplastic large-cell lymphoma.

The mediastinal location of PMBCL in addition to the finding of Hassall's corpuscles and thymic lobules in some cases suggest a thymic origin. Although it is primarily a site of T-cell maturation, the thymus does contain a small number of B-cells that are positive for CD19, CD20, CD22, IgM, and lack CD21 (3). Hypermutated VH and BCL6 genes of a similar pattern have been observed in both PMBCL tumor cells and thymic B-cells, supporting derivation from the thymus and suggesting exposure to the germinal center at some point in histogenesis (4).

10.2.2   Molecular Genetics

Primary mediastinal large B-cell lymphoma is characterized by distinctive chromosomal aberrations, including consistent gains in chromosome 9p and 2p corresponding to JAK2 and c-REL, respectively (5, 6). Gains in chromosome 9 are highly specific for PMBCL and occur only sporadically in other B-cell lymphomas.

Aberrations in chromosome X are also observed at a high frequency, but the significance is unknown. Conversely, BCL2 and BCL6 rearrangements found in a subset of DLBCL are notably absent in PMBCL. More recently, a more sensitive technique than standard CGH (comparative genomic hybridization) using a tiling resolution array CGH has also demonstrated a significant number of chromosomal losses, including 1p13.2 and 17p12 (7), but the corresponding genes involved are unknown.

Biallelic mutations of SOCS1 (suppressor in cytokine signaling) in the MedB1, a PMBCL cell line, were recently discovered that result in sustained activity of phospho-JAK2 through delayed protein turnover (8). Mutations in the SOCS1 gene are seen at a relatively high frequency in PMBCL tumors correlating with gains at 9p24, the JAK2 locus (8). Similarly, Karpas 1106, another PMBCL cell line, harbors a homozygous deletion at 16p13.13 and absent expression of SOCS1, providing further evidence that SOCS1 qualifies as a novel tumor suppressor in PMBCL (9).

10.2.3 Relationship of Primary Mediastinal Large B-Cell lymphoma with Nodular Sclerosis Classical Hodgkin's Lymphoma

Although PMBCL is considered a subtype of DLBCL, it has several notable overlapping clinical and pathologic features that are shared with the nodular sclerosis subtype of classical Hodgkin's lymphoma (NScHL) (2). Both occur most often in young adults who present with a prominent mediastinal mass but lack extrathoracic disease. Pathologically, sclerosis is prominent in both tumors and Reed-Sternberg-like cells can be seen in PMBCL. Further, the Hodgkin Reed-Sternberg cells (HRS) are typified by the absence of surface immunoglobulin (sIg) and, similarly, the malignant B-cells of PMBCL lack sIg in up to 70% of cases. Classical Hodgkin's lymphoma also harbors gains in chromosome 2p and 9p and, in addition, SOCS1 mutations have also recently been found in cHL, resulting in accumulation of phospho-STAT5, supporting the hypothesis that this pathway might be critical in both tumors (2). MAL, a lipid raft component, is differentially expressed in PMBCL compared to DLBCL and is found in some cases of NScHL (10–12) and might be associated with a worse prognosis (13). In addition to these striking clinical, immunologic, and molecular similarities, there are rare reported cases of composite or sequential NScHL and PMBCL in addition to "mediastinal gray zone lymphomas" with features between NScHL and PMBCL. (14). In cases of sequential lymphoma, IgH rearrangements of a similar size have been found, confirming a common origin (14).

Despite these similarities, there are still important differences between PMBCL and NScHL. Unlike HRS cells, PMBCL tumor cells retain several B-cell differentiation markers and histologically appear more similar to other DLBCLs. The brisk inflammatory background seen in cHL is not usually seen in PMBCL.

These observations support the notion that PMBCL may be pathogenetically related to NScHL. This hypothesis of an overlapping relationship is further supported by two recent gene expression profiling studies that demonstrated that the molecular signature of PMBCL had a striking resemblance to the expression profile of HRS cell lines (12, 15) (Figures 10.2A and 10.2B). A prominent cytokine pathway with over-expression of IL13Rα1, JAK2, and STAT1 were present (15) (Figures 10.2A and 10.2B), in addition to chemokines TARC and RANTES, both of which have been identified in HRS cells (16). Further, a prominent tumor necrosis factor (TNF) signature was identified in both cHL and PMBCL, including the adaptor protein TRAF1 (12, 15). Nuclear factor (NF) κB promotes HRS cell survival and, similarly, nuclear localization of c-REL, consistent with activation, was seen in the majority of cases of

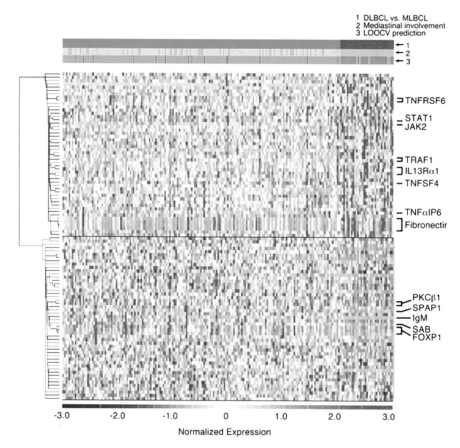

Figure 10.2 (**A**) Comparative gene expression profiles of DLBCL and PMBCL. At the top, the actual clinical/pathologic diagnosis of DLBCL versus PMBCL (green vs. red), presence or absence of mediastinal disease (pink vs. light green), and molecular prediction of DLBCL versus PMBCL (green vs. red) are compared. Genes are clustered using hierarchical clustering. Expression profiles of 176 DLBCLs are on the left; profiles of the 34 PMBCL are on the right. Note: Red = high relative expression, blue = low expression. Column = sample, row = gene. (Copyright American Society of Hematology, adapted and used with permission) (15)

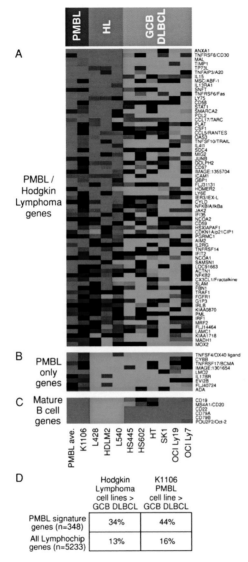

Figure 10.2 (B) Relationship of PMBCL to Hodgkin lymphoma. Relative gene expression is shown in primary PMBCLs (average of all biopsy samples), the PMBCL cell line K1106, three Hodgkin's lymphoma (HL) cell lines, and six GCB DLBCL cell lines, according to the color scale shown in (A) PMBCL signature genes that are also expressed at high levels in Hodgkin's lymphoma cell lines compared with GCB DLBCL cell lines. (B) PMBCL signature genes not expressed in Hodgkin lymphoma cell lines. (C) Mature B-cell markers expressed in PMBCL and GCB DLBCL but not in Hodgkin's lymphoma. (D) Enrichment within the set of PMBCL signature genes of genes highly expressed in Hodgkin's lymphoma cell lines or in the K1106 PMBCL cell line relative to GCB DLBCL cell lines. (Adapted from the *Journal of Experimental Medicine*, by copyright permission of The Rockefeller University Press)

PMBCL (15). Further, increased expression of downstream targets of NFKB is also seen in PMBCL, supporting that this pathway might also be critical in disease pathogenesis (15, 17).

The expression of TRAF1 and nuclear c-REL together may also aid in differentiating PMBCL from the morphologically similar DLBCL (18). These and other markers that can reliably and reproducibly differentiate PMBCL will also facilitate future study comparisons.

10.2.4   Clinical Features

Patients with PMBCL are typically females in their third to fourth decade who present with large, often bulky, anterior mediastinal masses with associated respiratory symptoms (Figures 10.3A and 10.3B). Superior vena caval syndrome can occur with facial swelling, dyspnea, headache, neck vein distention, and, occasionally, thrombosis. Most patients have bulky, stage I or II disease at diagnosis, often

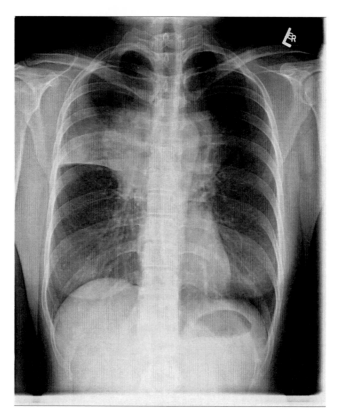

Figure. 10.3 **(A)** Chest X-ray of a patient with a bulky anterior mediastinal mass; **(B)** CT scan of a patient with a bulky anterior mediastinal mass.

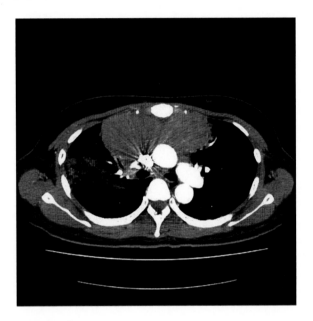

Figure. 10.3 (B) (continued)

accompanied by intrathoracic extension into the lung, chest wall, and pericardial and pleural effusions can occur. Extrathoracic disease, including bone marrow involvement, at presentation is rare. However, at relapse, disease in unusual extranodal sites such as the liver, kidneys and central nervous system (CNS) can occur (2).

10.2.5 Prognostic Features

There have been varied reports regarding survival in PMBCL that might, in part, be due to diagnostic imprecision and the difficulty in separating PMBCL from DLBCL with secondary mediastinal involvement because there are no definitive biological markers of PMBCL. This diagnostic uncertainty can influence reports on biological characteristics and survival analyses, complicating comparisons between studies. This problem is highlighted in earlier studies in which a more aggressive course was observed (19–21), with cure rates in some cases worse than DLBCL despite the younger age of presentation. In contrast, more recent analyses have demonstrated outcome patterns at least equivalent to or superior than DLBCL (22–26) (Table 10.1 and Figure 10,4A and 10.4B). Further, using a refined molecular signature to diagnose PMBCL, a more favorable survival is observed, supporting the notion that PMBCL might have a different natural history than DLBCL (12). This is further highlighted by the clear plateau seen in the progression-free survival (PFS) curve of PMBCL with rare relapses seen beyond 2 years (26) in distinct comparison to DLBCL (Figure 10.4A).

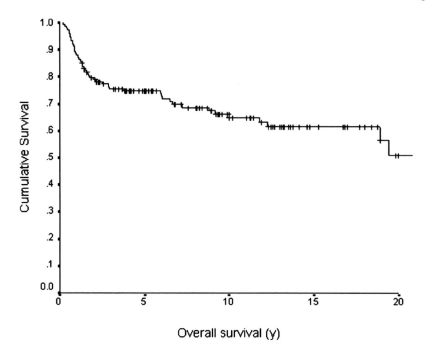

Overall survival (y)

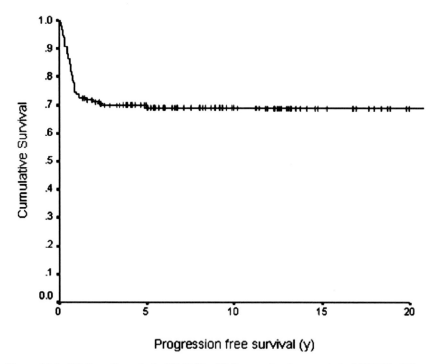

Progression free survival (y)

Figure 10.4 **(A)** Overall survival of PMBCL; **(B)** Progression-free survival of PMBCL (26)

The International Prognostic Index (IPI) was originally developed in diffuse large-cell lymphoma prior to the recognition of PMBCL. Subsequent studies evaluating the IPI or the aaIPI (age-adjusted) have been discrepant in PMBCL (23, 25–27). This may reflect differences between studies assigning patient as stage IV or stage IIE if multiple but contiguous extranodal sites are involved. In the few studies that have found the index useful, it has been the IPI that was applied, suggesting that it is primarily age that drives the poor prognosis. Even if the aaIPI is used, which eliminates the number of extranodal sites as a risk factor, most patients will have an elevated lactate dehydrogenase (LDH), again reducing the usefulness of its discrimatory power (27). Other factors that in individual studies have been found to prognosticate also include pleural or pericardial involvement and poor performance status (26, 28).

10.2.6 Primary Treatment of PMBCL

The optimal type of chemotherapy and role of consolidative radiotherapy in the management of PMBCL is unknown. Treatments at various study centers have been extremely heterogeneous with respect to the choice of chemotherapy regimen and whether radiotherapy was utilized in the primary therapy (Table 10.1). In several retrospective analyses, there is emerging evidence that dose-intensified therapy using Methotrexate, doxorubicin, cyclophosphamide, vincristine, prednisone, bleomycin (MACOPB) or Etoposide, doxorubicin, cyclophosphamide, vincristine, prednisone, bleomycin (VACOPB) may be superior to cyclophosphamide doxorubicin, vincristine, prednisone (CHOP) chemotherapy (23, 25) (Table 10.1). Survival using CHOP ranges from 40% to 71%, and for MACOPB/VACOPB, it ranges from 71% to 93% (Table 10.1). The large retrospective SWOG study comparing CHOP to second- and third-generation regimens, including MACOPB, in the treatment of diffuse large-cell lymphoma was performed prior to the recognition of PMBCL as a distinct entity; thus, information regarding the superiority of these intensified regimens over CHOP from a randomized trial are not available (29). The group at Memorial Sloan-Kettering recently reported a retrospective series comparing "CHOP-like" chemotherapy, which included second and third-generation regimens, to an intensified regimen, NHL-15 (dose dense sequential induction with doxorubicin followed by cyclophosphamide with GCSF support) (Table 10.1). NHL-15 was associated with a more favorable outcome in multivariate analysis (Table 10.1). However, the number of patients receiving specific regimens was too small for individual comparisons. Further, in general there is an inherent selection bias of patients chosen to be treated with more intensive regimens.

Some researchers support using autologous stem cell transplant in the primary treatment of PMBCL with one small report of 15 patients with high–intermediate- or high-risk disease achieving a disease-free survival (DFS) of 93% after a median follow-up of 35 months with transplant (30). However, all but two patients were in a complete remission (CR) or partial remission (PR) prior to transplant with induction

Table 10.1 Recent studies in the last 10 years of the treatment and survival in PMBCL

Reference	No. of patients	Mediastinal radiation planned	Chemotherapy (n)	PFS/EFS (%)	OS (%)	Comment
Zinzani et al. (1996) (40)	22	Yes (100 %)	MACOPB F-MACHOP	86 (2 years)	66	Similar oucome vs. "nonmediastinal"
Cazals-Hatem et al. (1996)(24)	141	No	Intensive regimens[a]	61 (2 years)	100	Only 1 patient received RT
			Group 1 (14)	—		Treatment regimens were not formally compared
			Group 2 (104)	59	60	
			Group 3 (23)	58	69	
Lazzarino et al. (1997) (19)	106	Yes (77%)	CHOP (36)[b] MACOPB/VACOPB (29) CHOP-like Intensive(41)	N/A	52 (3 years)	
Martelli et al. (1998) (54)	37	Yes (89%) No	MACOPB F-MACHOP	91 (2 years) 60 (2 years) $p < 0.02$	93 70 $p = ns$	
Abou-Ellela et al. (1998) (55)	43	Not reported	CHOP-like regimens[c]	38 (5 years)	46 (5 years)	Similar outcome vs. "nonmediastinal" Heterogeneous tx; some with non-anthracycline regimens
Zinzani et al. (1999) (22)	50	Yes (94%)	MACOPB	82 (8 years)	93 (8y)	Type of chemotherapy ("Intensive") improved PFS in MVA
Bieri et al. (1999) (39)	27	No (41%)	CHOP (11)[d] CHOP-like (intensified) (12) CVP (4 elderly)	44 (5 years)	55 (5 years)	RT improved PFS in MVA but no XRT group also includes induction failures
Nguyen et al. (2000) (56)	40	Yes (85%)	CHOP (12)[e] CHOP-like (intensified) (13) Doxorubicin/salvage-type (14)	67 (5 years)	72 (5 years)	

Study	N	RT	Chemotherapy (n)			Comments
Zinzani et al. (2002) (25)	426	Yes (80%)	All	62 (10 years)	65 (10 years)	Type of chemotherapy (CHOP vs. intensive) improved OS but not PFS in MVA
			CHOP (105)	35	44	
			MACOPB (204) / VACOPB (34) or ProMACE CytaBOM (39)	67	71	
			High-dose sequential (27) or ASCT (17)	78 $p = .0003$	77 $p = .0001$	
Todeschini et al. (2004) (23)	138	Yes Yes If CR or Cru 75%	CHOP (43)	39.5		Type of chemo (MACOPB/VACOPB) improved OS in MVA
			MACOPB/VACOPB (95)	76 $p<.001$		RT improved EFS in pts in CR
Hamlin et al. (2005) (27)	141	Variable (23%)	All	50	66	Type of chemo NHL-15/ASCT improved EFS/OS in MVA
			CHOP/CHOP-like (intensive)[f]	34	51	
			NHL-15	60		
			ASCT	60 $p < .001$	84 $p < .001$	
Savage et al. (2006) (26)	153	Before 1998 variable After 1998 routine	All	69	78	Type of treatment not significant in MVA
			MACOPB/VACOPB (47)[g]		75	Addition of radiation did not improve PFS or OS
			CHOP/CHOP-like (intensive) (63)		87	
			CHOPR (18)		71	
					82 $p = 0.048$	Improved PFS and OS compared to DLBCL

RT = radiation therapy; MVA = multivariate analysis; OS = overall survival; PFS progression-free survival; EFS = event-free survival

[a] Three treatment groups (24)
No poor prognostic factors and < 70
1. ACVBP v mBACOD
Adverse prognostic factors and <55
2. ACVBP vs, NCVBP (N = mitoxatrone)—pts achieving CR randomized condolidation chemotherapy

(continued)

Table 10.1 (continued)

LNH-84 vs. intensive consolidation with CBV + autologous stem cell transplant

Adverse prognostic factors and >55

Adverse prognostic factor = bulky disease ≥ 10 cm, bone marrow or CNS involvement, 2 extranodal sites, PS ≥ 2

3. LNH-84 vs. VIM3

[b]Three treatment groups (19)

1. CHOP

2. MACOPB or VACOPB

3. CHOP-like Intensive (CH2OP (11) (doxorubicin repeated day 2); CHOEP (10); hCHOP (high-dose cyclophosphamide)/IVEP (ifosfamide, vindesine, etoposide, prednisone) or CHOP/VIM (etoposide, ifosfamide, methotrexate, prednisone) (13)

[c]Four treatment groups (55)

1. Cyclophosphamide, doxorubicin, vincristine, procarbazine, prednisone, bleomycin

2. Cyclophosphamide, doxorubicin, vincristine, procarbazine, dexamethasone, bleomycin

3. Cyclophosphamide, mitoxantrone, vincristine, procarbazine, prednisone

4. M mitoxantrone, vincristine, prednisone

[d]Three treatment groups (39)

1. CHOP

2. "Third-generation" CHOP-like intensive (doxorubicin D1/8, cyclophosphamide D1/D8, vincristine D1/D8, methotrexate alternating Q 22 days with etoposide, AraC, bleomycin, procarbazine

3. CVP (elderly)

[e]Three treatment groups (56)

1. CHOP

2. CHOP-like Intensive (CHOP-Bleo; CHOP-Bleo/OPEN (vincristine, prednisone, etoposide, mitroxantrone)

3. ASHAP (doxorubicin, methylprednisone, AraC, cisplatin)/MBACOS (methotrexate, bleomycin, doxorubicin, cyclophosphamide, vincristine, methylprednisolone) and MINE (Mesna, ifosfamide, mitroxantrone, etoposide)

[f]Three treatment groups (27)

a. Includes CHOP and CHOP-like (CHOP-bleomycin, ProMACE-CytaBom, MACOPB)

b. Dose –dense sequential chemotherapy with GCSF support

c. TBI and upfront transplant— this patient group were from a trial comparing ASCT to MACOPB for patients with bulky disease or LDH > 2.5 times ULN

[g]Three treatment groups (26)

1. CHOP or CHOP-like [ACOP12, ECV (CHOP ×4 then high dose etoposide, cyclophosphamide, vincristine)]

2. MACOPB/VACOPB

3. CHOPR

therapy consisting of VACOPB, and due to the high frequency of residual masses in this disease, many of the PR patients by imaging might be in a pathological CR; thus, the true impact of consolidative autologous stem cell transplant (ASCT) is unknown.

Further complicating the evaluation of the effectiveness of dose-dense and dose-intensive regimens is that these studies were undertaken in the "pre-rituximab" era. The addition of rituximab to CHOP chemotherapy has been shown in multiple studies to improve cure rates in DLBCL over CHOP alone (31–33). The value of adding rituximab to CHOP (R-CHOP) in PMBCL is unknown; however, it is likely that the same magnitude of benefit will be observed. Dose-adjusted Etoposide, vincristine, doxorubicin, bolus cyclophosphamide, prednisone (EPOCH) (DA-EPOCH) was recently evaluated in 36 patients with PMBCL, 22 of whom received DA-EPOCH in combination with rituximab (DA-EPOCH-R). This regimen administers the natural product chemotherapy agents by continuous infusion (etoposide, doxorubicin, vincristine) in addition to bolus cyclophosphamide and oral prednisone with dose adjustments based on the neutrophil nadir (34). With a median follow-up of 8.6 years, patients treated with DA-EPOCH-R had a 2-year event-free survival (EFS) that was superior to DA-EPOCH alone (94% vs. 64%, respectively, $p = 0.036$) (35). However, the utility of more intensive chemotherapy regimens in the treatment of PMBCL can only be evaluated in a well-designed randomized clinical trial that includes the addition of rituximab to each regimen. Until such studies are available, it is reasonable to consider R-CHOP chemotherapy as the standard treatment in PMBCL.

10.2.7 Consolidative Radiotherapy in the Treatment of PMBCL

A major challenge in the management of PMBCL is the evaluation of a residual mass postchemotherapy. There is poor correlation between the size of a residual mass on computerized tomography (CT) and risk of relapse (36, 37). In many instances, the residual density represents fibrotic tissue rather than active lymphoma, similar to the problem encountered in bulky mediastinal NScHL (36). Many patients are given mediastinal radiotherapy as consolidative treatment for this reason; however, it is unclear whether this impacts relapse or cure rates. There is also an inherent concern regarding the long-term toxicities of mediastinal radiotherapy, including an increased risk of cardiovascular disease and secondary malignancies, particularly given the young population at risk (38), akin to treatment considerations in NScHL. Although some studies have suggested that radiotherapy improves EFS (23, 25, 39) (Table 10.1), other analyses have demonstrated that chemotherapy alone is effective in many cases (24, 26, 27, 35), suggesting that radiotherapy is not mandatory in all patients. An improvement in EFS was reported in one study when radiotherapy is given to patients achieving a CR (23). However, a recent analysis evaluating the impact on PFS with a policy recommending routine radiotherapy following primary chemotherapy failed to demonstrate a benefit (26). The retrospective nature of such analyses, including definitions of response rates, is problematic and randomized studies addressing this question are lacking. Improved identification of patients who might benefit from the addition of radiotherapy is needed.

^{67}Ga scintigraphy has been used to detect persistent viable tumor in patients with a residual mass after therapy (40). However, Fluorine-18 fluorodeoxyglucose (^{18}F-FDG) positron emission tomography (PET) is superior to ^{67}Ga for the detection of residual disease (41). Therefore, future studies are needed to that evaluate the utility of ^{18}F-FDG PET to select patients with PMBCL who might benefit from radiotherapy and, alternatively, identify those cases where it can be safely withheld without compromising cure rates, with the goal of reducing secondary long-term complications.

10.2.8 Salvage Therapy

Treatment failures in PMBCL tend to occur within the first 6–12 months after treatment completion, with recurrences rare beyond 2 years (25, 26). Like DLBCL, chemosensitivity to the salvage regimen is predictive of a more favorable outcome to ASCT (42). Limited data suggest that PMBCL patients might be less likely to respond to salvage chemotherapy and proceed to ASCT than DLBCL; however, in those patients who could be transplanted, outcomes appear to be similar (43). It is unclear what the outcome of patients with refractory disease is. Some studies have suggested that survival is comparable to relapsed patients (42); however, other studies have found that they might be less likely to respond to salvage chemotherapy (19, 26), with a lower likelihood of survival compared to those with relapsed disease (27).

10.3 Intravascular Lymphoma

Intravascular or "angiotropic" lymphoma (IVL) is a rare clinical subtype of diffuse large B-cell lymphoma characterized by the presence of neoplastic B-cell lymphocytes within the microvasculature (44). It has only recently been included as a clinical subtype of DLBCL in the WHO classification. It typically is widely disseminated at presentation involving multiple, often subclinical, extranodal sites including the **CNS**, skin, lung, kidney, and adrenals.

10.3.1 Pathology

A tissue biopsy is essential for the diagnosis to highlight the intravascular growth pattern. Clinically uninvolved organs such as the spleen and bone marrow can demonstrate IVL, and in some instances, a random skin biopsy might yield a diagnosis (44, 45). The "classic variant" of IVL is typified by large neoplastic cells with prominent nucleoli and frequent mitotic figures that are found in the

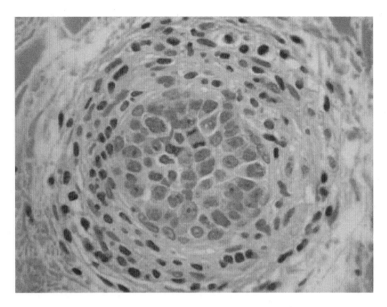

Figure 10.5 H&E stain of intravascular lymphoma with large neoplastic cells detected in a blood vessel lumen.

lumina of small vessels (Figure 10.5). In the bone marrow, sinusoidal involvement occurs. A so-called "Asian variant" has also been described that often has, in addition, a rich infiltrate of non-neoplastic cells, predominantly hemophagocytic histiocytes.

The most distinctive property of IVL malignant cells is their propensity to grow within the lumina of blood vessels. It is hypothesized that the intraluminal growth pattern is secondary to a defect in homing receptors of the neoplastic cells. In support of this, the malignant cells appear to lack CD29 (beta 1 integrin) and CD54 (ICAM-1) adhesion molecules (44).

The majority of IVL display a B-cell phenotype expressing CD20 and/or CD79a. In the Western series, approximately 20% of cases display a germinal center (GC) phenotype (CD10+ or BCL6+), and CD5+ cells can also be seen (46). A recent Japanese series also described CD5 expression in 38% of cases, however, there was no immunophenotypic or clinical differences between the CD5- and CD5+ subgroups. Similar to the classic variant, almost all Asian cases display a non-GCB phenotype (CD10-,BCL6-/+, MUM1) (47).

Rare cases with a T-cell immunophenotype have been reported, occasionally in the setting of HIV infection (48). Anecdotal cases of Natural killer (NK) IVL have also been seen (44).

10.3.2 Molecular Genetics

Due to disease rarity, there have been no large-scale studies evaluating cytogenetic abnormalities in IVL. Aberrations in chromosomes 1, 6, and 18, including 1p and trisomy 6, were frequently observed in one small series. Somatic hypermutation of the Ig heavy chain is apparent in most cases, supporting that exposure to the GC occurred at some point in pathogenesis, but BCL-2 rearrangements are typically absent.

10.3.3 Clinical Features

The median age at diagnosis is approximately 70 years with equal prevalence in both sexes. The clinical presentation can be heterogeneous because virtually any organ might be involved; however, nodal involvement is rare. Fever is common and IVL should always be considered in cases of fever of unknown origin. Patients might also have other B symptoms in addition to a rapid decline in performance status Patients usually present with high or high–intermediate IPI scores (Table 10.2). Even those cases with apparent limited stage disease can often be found at autopsy to have disseminated disease, highlighting some of the limitations of standard staging techniques for the diagnosis of IVL. In more recent series, more patients were diagnosed "in vivo" (versus at autopsy) compared to older reports, consistent with a growing recognition of IVL in recent times.

Interestingly, IVL cases in Western populations display distinct differences compared to those reported in Japanese series (Table 10.2). In Japanese patients, IVL is more often associated with bone marrow involvement with evidence of hematophagocytosis as well as hepato-splenomegaly with thrombocytopenia and anemia, whereas CNS and cutaneous involvement is uncommon, supporting the notion that the "Asian variant" might be a distinct clinical entity (47). Whether other non-Japanese Asian patients have a similar clinical presentation is unknown.

The "cutaneous variant" refers to cases that are exclusively found in the skin after extensive staging procedures and appears to be confined to Western populations. Patients are predominantly female have a good performance status (PS), lack B symptoms, and present at a younger age. In addition, they are less likely to have cytopenias than patients with more widespread disease.

Patients with neurologic involvement can have very heterogeneous symptoms at presentation from sensory and motor neuropathies to seizures and altered consciousness. There are no pathognomonic neuroradiologic findings. Ischemic foci are the most common and it can often be confused with vasculitis.

Additional laboratory findings in both the classic and the Asian variant include an elevated LDH and B2 microglobulin in over 80%. A monoclonal protein is seen in 15% and altered hepatic and renal function can be observed in some cases.

Table 10.2 Comparison of presenting clinical features in the Western or "classic variant" and the "Asian variant"

Clinical or laboratory feature	Western "classic variant" n (%) Total n = 38 (49)	Japanese "Asian variant" n (%) Total n = 96 (47)
Median age	70	67
Sex (M:F)	.9	~1.1
PS > 1	95% (> 1)	79 (82)
High LDH	25 (86) Total n= 29	89 (93)
EN > 1	N/A	65 (68)
IPI		
Low 0, 1	6 (16)	2 (2)
Low-int 2	16 (2 and 3) (42)	6 (6)
High-int 3		17 (17)
High 4, 5	16 (42)	75 (75)
B symptoms	21 (55)	73 (76)
Liver involved	10 (26)	53 (55)
Spleen involved	10 (26)	64 (67)
Neurologic signs/symptoms	13 (34)	26 (27)
CNS	15 (39)	26 (27)
Cutaneous lesions	15 (39)	14 (15)
"Cutaneous variant"	10	0
Advanced stage	5	14 (15)
Bone marrow	12 (32)	67 (75) n = 89
Hemophagocytosis		54 (61)
Peripheral Blood	2 (5)	23 (24)
Anemia < 12 g/dL	24 (63)	63 (66)
Thrombocytopenia <150	11 (29)	56 (58)
Leukopenia	9 (24)	26 (27)
Hypoalbuminemia <36 g/L	81(96)	7 (18)
Event-free survival 3 years	27% (n = 30)[a]	27%[a] (n = 81)
Overall survival	32%[a]	—

[a]Outcome of patients with in vivo diagnosis. For whole series, 3 years overall survival as 25% for all patients.

Approximately 15% of patients with IVL have a prior history or concomitant malignancy, most often a prior non-Hodgkin's lymphoma. Among solid tumors, renal cell carcinoma has been observed and, occasionally, IVL cells can be seen within the tumor associated vasculature (44).

10.3.4 Primary Treatment of IVL

Typically, IVL has an aggressive course and the median survival is approximately 6 months, with no significant differences observed between Western and Japanese reports. Regimens without anthracyclines appear to be associated with an inferior prognosis (44). It is unknown whether rituximab improves survival rates, given the rarity of this condition however, CNS penetration is poor. Over half of the patients will ultimately relapse, usually within the first year of diagnosis. Relapses typically involve extranodal sites, and CNS disease can occur in approximately one-third of patients.

Several small series report improved outcome using high dose chemotherapy (HDC) and ASCT as consolidation therapy, however, it remains experimental in this setting. Anecdotal reports using methotrexate-containing chemotherapy (MACOP-B) followed by HDC and ASCT in a patient with initial CNS involvement has resulted in long-term remission (44).

10.3.5 Prognostic Factors

Regardless of the country of origin, the survival of patients with intravascular lymphoma is uniformly poor with a 3-year EFS of 30%, with similar approximations for overall survival (OS), suggesting that salvage therapy is usually ineffective in this population (47, 49). In the Western series, patients with the cutaneous variant, low IPI, and limited stage disease and who are able to receive multiagent anthracyline-based chemotherapy have a more favorable prognosis in multivariate analysis (49). In the Japanese series, older age, thrombocytopenia, and lack of anthracycline-based chemotherapy was associated with a worse outcome (47). In this analysis, there was no difference in outcome regardless of their immunophenotype (i.e., CD5+ vs. CD5– or GC vs. non-GCB) (47).

10.4 Primary Effusion Lymphoma

Primary effusion lymphoma (PEL) is also a recently recognized clinical subtype of DLBCL presenting as a serous effusion composed of large B-cells. It is universally associated with HHV-8/KSHV (human herpes virus 8/Kaposi sarcoma herpes virus) and usually occurs in the setting of HIV (50), but rare cases have been reported in the absence of HIV infection.

10.4.1 Pathology

Malignant B-cells are isolated from the serous effusion and show a range of appearances from large immunoblastic or plasmablastic cells to those with a more anaplastic morphology. The neoplastic cells are positive for HHV8/KSHV in all cases and many are coinfected with Epstein-Barr virus (EBV). The cells usually express leukocyte common antigen (CD45) but are negative for B-cell markers CD19, CD20, and CD79a; however, immunoglobulin rearrangements present, confirming a clonal B-cell origin. Activation (CD30, CD38, EMA) and plasma cell markers (CD138, MUM-1/IRF4) are typically present (50).

Recently, gene expression profiling has been performed on PEL cells and expression patterns have similarities to both plasma cells and EBV-transformed immunoblasts, suggesting that PEL might represent a variant of plasmablastic lymphoma (51). Supervised analysis revealed that PEL has a unique gene expression compared to other B-cell NHL and AIDS-related lymphomas with underexpression of many genes that are B-cell or lymphoid specific.

10.4.2 Clinical Features

Primary effusion lymphoma accounts for approximately 3% of all HIV-related NHL. The majority of patients are homosexual white men with a median age of approximately 40 years. Cases in HIV-negative individuals typically occur in elderly patients from endemic areas of high prevalence of HHV8 or in allograft recipients. Effusions are seen most commonly in the pleural, pericardial, or peritoneal cavities, usually without nodal disease. A recent series of 28 patients reported simultaneous involvement of all serous cavities in 25%, and 43% had extracavitary disease localization, including occasional involvement of lymph nodes, bone marrow, CNS, pancreas, and sinus (52). Some cases might occur in association with Castleman's disease.

10.4.3 Primary Treatment of PEL

Since the widespread use of HAART (highly active antiretroviral therapy), the overall outcome of HIV-associated NHLs has improved; however, it remains poor in PEL. Some exceptional cases have been shown to respond to antiretroviral therapy alone. Most patients are treated with CHOP-like regimens and HAART in the setting of HIV. In most published series, the clinical course is usually aggressive, with a median survival of 6 months. Given that CD20 is negative in these tumors, rituximab will not impact the prognosis and should not be utilized in this disease.

10.4.4 Prognostic Factors

A recent study of clinical factors associated with prognosis PEL demonstrated that poor performance status (> 2) and the absence of HAART before the PEL diagnosis were associated with a poor outcome (52) in multivariate analysis. Other researchers have found that a high HHV-8 viral load correlates inversely with CD4 count and is associated with a shorter survival time; however, this requires validation in a larger analysis (53).

References

1. Banks PM, Warnke RA. Mediastinal (thymic) large B-cell lymphoma. In: Jaffe ES, Harris NL, Stein H, et al., editors. World Health Organization classification of tumours: pathology and genetics of tumours of hematopoetic and lymphoid tissues, Lyon: IARC Press; 2001. p. 175–178.
2. Savage KJ. Primary mediastinal large B-cell lymphoma. Oncologist 2006;11(5): 488–48895.
3. Isaacson P, Norton A, Addis B. The human thymus contains a novel population of B-lymphocytes. Lancet 1987;ii:1488–1490.
4. Csernus B, Timar B, Fulop Z, et al. Mutational analysis of IgVH and BCL-6 genes suggests thymic B-cells origin of mediastinal (thymic) B-cell lymphoma. Leuk Lymphoma 2004;45(10):2105–2110.
5. Bentz M, Barth TF, Bruderlein S, et al. Gain of chromosome arm 9p is characteristic of primary mediastinal B-cell lymphoma (MBL): comprehensive molecular cytogenetic analysis and presentation of a novel MBL cell line. Genes Chromosomes Cancer 2001r;30(4):393–401.
6. Joos S, Otano-Joos MI, Ziegler S, et al. Primary mediastinal (thymic) B-cell lymphoma is characterized by gains of chromosomal material including 9p and amplification of the REL gene. Blood 1996;87(4):1571–1578.
7. deLeeuw RJ, Savage KJ, Gascoyne RD, et al. Identification of copy number alterations in primary mediastinal B-cell lymphoma by tiling resolution array comparative genomic hybridization. Proc AACR 2005;46:4476a.
8. Melzner I, Bucur AJ, Bruderlein S, et al. Biallelic mutation of SOCS-1 impairs JAK2 degradation and sustains phospho-JAK2 action in the MedB-1 mediastinal lymphoma line. Blood 2005;105(6):2535–2542.
9. Mestre C, Rubio-Moscardo F, Rosenwald A, et al. Homozygous deletion of SOCS1 in primary mediastinal B-cell lymphoma detected by CGH to BAC microarrays. Leukemia 2005;19(6):1082–1084.
10. Copie-Bergman C, Gaulard P, Maouche-Chretien L, et al. The MAL gene is expressed in primary mediastinal large B-cell lymphoma. Blood 1999;94(10):3567–3575.
11. Copie-Bergman C, Plonquet A, Alonso MA, et al. MAL expression in lymphoid cells: Further evidence for MAL as a distinct molecular marker of primary mediastinal large B-cell lymphomas. Mod Pathol. 2002;15(11):1172–1180.
12. Rosenwald A, Wright G, Leroy K, et al. Molecular diagnosis of primary mediastinal B cell lymphoma identifies a clinically favorable subgroup of diffuse large B cell lymphoma related to Hodgkin lymphoma. J Exp Med 2003;198(6):851–862.
13. Hsi ED, Sup SJ, Alemany C, MAL is expressed in a subset of Hodgkin lymphoma and identifies a population of patients with poor prognosis. Am J Clin Pathol 2006;125(5): 776–782.
14. Traverse-Glehen A, Pittaluga S, et al. Mediastinal gray zone lymphoma: the missing link between classic Hodgkin's lymphoma and mediastinal large B-cell lymphoma. Am J Surg Pathol 2005;29(11):1411–1421.
15. Savage KJ, Monti S, Kutok JL, et al. The molecular signature of mediastinal large B-cell lymphoma differs from that of other diffuse large B-cell lymphomas and shares features with classical Hodgkin lymphoma. Blood 2003;102(12):3871–389.
16. Maggio E, van den Berg A, Diepstra A, et al. Chemokines, cytokines and their receptors in Hodgkin's lymphoma cell lines and tissues. Ann Oncol 2002;13(Suppl 1):52–56.
17. Feuerhake F, Kutok JL, Monti S, et al. NFkappaB activity, function, and target-gene signatures in primary mediastinal large B-cell lymphoma and diffuse large B-cell lymphoma subtypes. Blood 2005;106(4):1392–1399.
18. Rodig SJ, Savage KJ, Harris NL, et al. Expression of TRAF1 and nuclear C-Rel distinguishes primary mediastinal large B-cell lymphoma from nodal diffuse large B-cell lymphoma. Mod Pathol 2006;19(1):244a.

19. Lazzarino M, Orlandi E, Paulli M, Strater J, Klersy C, Gianelli U, et al. Treatment outcome and prognostic factors for primary mediastinal (thymic) B-cell lymphoma: a multicenter study of 106 patients. J Clin Oncol. 1997 Apr;15(4):1646–1653.
20. Todeschini G, Ambrosetti A, Meneghini V, et al. Mediastinal large-B-cell lymphoma with sclerosis: a clinical study of 21 patients. J Clin Oncol 1990;8(5):804–808.
21. Lavabre-Bertrand T, Donadio D, Fegueux N, et al. A study of 15 cases of primary mediastinal lymphoma of B-cell type. Cancer 1992;69(10):2561–2566.
22. Zinzani PL, Martelli M, Magagnoli M, et al. Treatment and clinical management of primary mediastinal large B-cell lymphoma with sclerosis: MACOP-B regimen and mediastinal radiotherapy monitored by (67)gallium scan in 50 patients. Blood.1999; 94(10):3289–3293.
23. Todeschini G, Secchi S, Morra E, et al. Primary mediastinal large B-cell lymphoma (PMLBCL): long-term results from a retrospective multicentre Italian experience in 138 patients treated with CHOP or MACOP-B/VACOP-B. Br J Cancer 2004;90(2):372–376.
24. Cazals-Hatem D, Lepage E, Brice P, et al. Primary mediastinal large B-cell lymphoma. A clinicopathologic study of 141 cases compared with 916 nonmediastinal large B-cell lymphomas, a GELA ("Groupe d'Etude des Lymphomes de l'Adulte") study. Am J Surg Pathol 1996;20(7):877–888.
25. Zinzani PL, Martelli M, Bertini M, et al. Induction chemotherapy strategies for primary mediastinal large B-cell lymphoma with sclerosis: a retrospective multinational study on 426 previously untreated patients. Haematologica 2002;87(12):1258–1264.
26. Savage KJ, Al-Rajhi N, Voss N, et al. Favorable outcome of primary mediastinal large B-cell lymphoma in a single institution: the British Columbia experience. Ann Oncol 2006;17(1):123–130.
27. Hamlin PA, Portlock CS, Straus DJ, et al. Primary mediastinal large B-cell lymphoma: optimal therapy and prognostic factor analysis in 141 consecutive patients treated at Memorial Sloan Kettering from 1980 to 1999. Br J Haematol 2005130(5):691–699.
28. van Besien K, Kelta M, Bahaguna P. Primary mediastinal B-cell lymphoma: a review of pathology and management. J Clin Oncol 2001;19(6):1855–1864.
29. Fisher RI, Gaynor ER, Dahlberg S, et al. Comparison of a standard regimen (CHOP) with three intensive chemotherapy regimens for advanced non-Hodgkin's lymphoma. N Engl J Med. 1993;328(14):1002–1006.
30. Cairoli R, Grillo G, Tedeschi A, et al. Efficacy of an early intensification treatment integrating chemotherapy, autologous stem cell transplantation and radiotherapy for poor risk primary mediastinal large B cell lymphoma with sclerosis. Bone Marrow Transplant 2002;29(6): 473–477.
31. Sehn LH, Donaldson J, Chhanabhai M, et al. Introduction of combined CHOP-rituximab therapy dramatically improved outcome of diffuse large B-cell lymphoma in British Columbia. J Clin Oncol 2005; 23(22):5027–33.
32. Coiffier B, Lepage E, Briere J, Herbrecht R, Tilly H, Bouabdallah R, et al. CHOP chemotherapy plus rituximab compared with CHOP alone in elderly patients with diffuse large-B-cell lymphoma. N Engl J Med 2002;346(4):235–242.
33. Pfreundschuh M, Trumper L, Ma D. Randomized intergroup trial of first line treatment for patients < = 60 years with diffuse large B-cell non-Hodgkin's lymphoma with a CHOP-like regimen with or without the anti-CD20 antibody rituximab: early stopping after the first interim analysis. Proc Annu Meet Am Soc Clin Oncol 2004;23:556a.
34. Wilson WH, Grossbard ML, Pittaluga S, et al. Dose-adjusted EPOCH chemotherapy for untreated large B-cell lymphomas: a pharmacodynamic approach with high efficacy. Blood 2002;99(8):2685–2693.
35. Dunleavy K, Pittaluga S, Janik J, et al. Primary mediastinal large B-cell lymphoma (PMBL) outcome is signficantly improved by the addition of rituximab to dose adjusted (DA)-EPOCH and overcomes the need for radiation. Blood. 2005;106(11):929a.
36. Canellos GP. Residual mass in lymphoma may not be residual disease. J Clin Oncol 1988;6(6):931–933.

37. Jerusalem G, Beguin Y, Fassotte MF, et al. Whole-body positron emission tomography using 18F-fluorodeoxyglucose for posttreatment evaluation in Hodgkin's disease and non-Hodgkin's lymphoma has higher diagnostic and prognostic value than classical computed tomography scan imaging. Blood 1999;94(2):429–433.
38. Aleman BM, van den Belt-Dusebout AW, et al. Long-term cause-specific mortality of patients treated for Hodgkin's disease. J Clin Oncol 2003;21(18):3431–3439.
39. Bieri S, Roggero E, Zucca E, et al. Primary mediastinal large B-cell lymphoma (PMLCL): the need for prospective controlled clinical trials. Leuk Lymphoma 1999;35(1–2):139–146.
40. Zinzani PL, Bendandi M, Frezza G, et al. Primary mediastinal B-cell lymphoma with sclerosis: clinical and therapeutic evaluation of 22 patients. Leuk Lymphoma 1996;21(3–4):311–316.
41. Kostakoglu L, Goldsmith SJ. Fluorine-18 fluorodeoxyglucose positron emission tomography in the staging and follow-up of lymphoma: is it time to shift gears? Eur J Nucl Med 2000; 27(10):1564–1578.
42. Sehn LH, Antin JH, Shulman LN, et al. Primary diffuse large B-cell lymphoma of the mediastinum: outcome following high-dose chemotherapy and autologous hematopoietic cell transplantation. Blood 1998;91(2):717–723.
43. Kuruvilla J, Nagy T, Pintilie M, et al. Outcomes of salvage chemotherapy and autologous stem cell transplanatation for relapsed or refractory primary medistianal large B-cell lymphoma (PMLCL) are inferior to diffuse large B-cell lymphoma. . Blood 2005;106(11):2085a.
44. Ponzoni M, Ferreri AJ. Intravascular lymphoma: a neoplasm of 'homeless' lymphocytes? Hematol Oncol 2006;24(3):105–112.
45. Gill S, Melosky B, Haley L, et al. Use of random skin biopsy to diagnose intravascular lymphoma presenting as fever of unknown origin. Am J Med 2003;114(1):56–58.
46. Yegappan S, Coupland R, Arber DA, et al. Angiotropic lymphoma: an immunophenotypically and clinically heterogeneous lymphoma. Mod Pathol 2001;14(11):1147–1156.
47. Murase T, Yamaguchi M, Suzuki R, et al. Intravascular large B-cell lymphoma (IVLBCL): a clinicopathologic study of 96 cases with special reference to the immunophenotypic heterogeneity of CD5. Blood 2007;109(2):478–85.
48. Malicki DM, Suh YK, Fuller GN, et al. Angiotropic (intravascular) large cell lymphoma of T-cell phenotype presenting as acute appendicitis in a patient with acquired immunodeficiency syndrome. Arch Pathol Lab Med 1999;123(4):335–357.
49. Ferreri AJ, Campo E, Seymour JF, et al. Intravascular lymphoma: clinical presentation, natural history, management and prognostic factors in a series of 38 cases, with special emphasis on the 'cutaneous variant'. Br J Haematol. 2004;127(2):173–183.
50. Carbone A, Gloghini A. AIDS-related lymphomas: from pathogenesis to pathology. Br J Haematol 2005;130(5):662–670.
51. Klein U, Gloghini A, Gaidano G, et al. Gene expression profile analysis of AIDS-related primary effusion lymphoma (PEL) suggests a plasmablastic derivation and identifies PEL-specific transcripts. Blood 2003;101(10):4115–4221.
52. Boulanger E, Gerard L, Gabarre J, et al. Prognostic factors and outcome of human herpesvirus 8-associated primary effusion lymphoma in patients with AIDS. J Clin Oncol 2005;23(19):4372–4380.
53. Simonelli C, Tedeschi R, Gloghini A, et al. Characterization of immunologic and virological parameters in HIV-infected patients with primary effusion lymphoma during antiblastic therapy and highly active antiretroviral therapy. Clin Infect Dis 2005;40(7):1022–1027.
54. Martelli MP, Martelli M, Pescarmona E, et al. MACOP-B and involved field radiation therapy is an effective therapy for primary mediastinal large B-cell lymphoma with sclerosis. Ann Oncol 1998;9(9):1027–1029.
55. Abou-Elella AA, Weisenburger DD, Vose JM, et al. Primary mediastinal large B-cell lymphoma: a clinicopathologic study of 43 patients from the Nebraska Lymphoma Study Group. J Clin Oncol 1999;17(3):784–790.
56. Nguyen LN, Ha CS, Hess M, et al. The outcome of combined-modality treatments for stage I and II primary large B-cell lymphoma of the mediastinum. Int J Radiat Oncol Biol Phys 2000;47(5):1281–1285.

Chapter 11
Lymphomatoid Granulomatosis

Ryan B. Lundell, Roger H. Weenig, and Lawrence E. Gibson

11.1   Introduction

Lymphomatoid granulomatosis (LG) is a rare, Epstein-Barr virus (EBV)-positive, B-cell lymphoproliferative disorder often accompanied by an exuberant reactive but cytotoxic T-cell infiltrate. The density of the T-cell infiltrate led to the initial impression that LG was a T-cell malignancy. Also, LG used to be included under the rubric of angiocentric lymphomas and shares many features with nasal-type, extranodal, natural killer (NK)/T-cell lymphoma (NKL). Both LG and NKL can present in the airways/nasal cavity, both are associated with an angiocentric, angiodestructive, and cytotoxic lymphoid infiltrate, and both are associated with EBV infection. However, the neoplastic, EBV-infected lymphoid cells of LG are of B-cell lineage and NK cell lineage in NKL. A broad clinical and pathologic spectrum is observed for LG, ranging from indolent and regressive disease to an aggressive large B-cell lymphoma. Consequently, controversy still surrounds the precise nosologic designation of LG as a reactive, inflammatory versus a neoplastic lymphoid process. Some cases of LG would be well characterized as immunosupression-related or posttransplant lymphoproliferative disorders and reduction of immunosuppression in many of these cases has been associated with resolution of disease. Other cases require aggressive chemotherapeutic agents to halt disease progression.

11.2   Pathogenesis

Lymphomatoid granulomatosis represents an EBV-driven B-cell lymphoma resulting in recruitment and activation of cytotoxic, CD8-positive T-lymphocytes. A remarkably low number of neoplastic B-cells might be observed in a given LG infiltrate and it is the non-neoplastic, cytotoxic T-lymphocytes that mediate vascular destruction and tissue necrosis.

S.M. Ansell (ed.), *Rare Hematological Malignancies.*
© Springer 2008

11.3   Clinical Features

Nodular mass lesions predominate and are characteristically angiocentric and angiodestructive, which frequently results in necrosis of affected tissue. The most common sites of involvement are the lungs (great majority of patients affected during the course of the disease). Other commonly involved sites include the skin (25–50%), kidney (30–40%), liver (29%), central nervous system (CNS) (26%), upper respiratory system, and peripheral nervous system (PNS) (1–4). Spleen, lymph node, and gastrointestinal involvement are less common (<20% of cases) (1).

Disease onset is in the fifth to sixth decade of life for the majority of patients; however, it rarely presents in childhood immunodeficiency states (5, 6). Males are more commonly affected than females (ratio 2:1). The clinical course of LG varies widely from a "benign" or regressing indolent process to an aggressive, rapidly progressive disease. Approximately 15–25% of patients might have the disease resolve spontaneously; however, mortality rates approach 65% in previously published series. Common causes of death include extensive destruction of pulmonary parenchyma, infection, development of an aggressive large B-cell lymphoma, and CNS disease (1, 2).

Patients might present with lung involvement (cough, dyspnea, and chest pain), and constitutional symptoms occur in 35–58% of patients (fever, weight loss, myalgias, and neurological symptoms) (1, 7). Varying sized pulmonary nodules are typical and most often involve the mid and lower lung fields. Larger nodules might demonstrate central necrosis. Signs and symptoms of mass lesions might also occur elsewhere depending on the extent of involvement. Ataxia, hemiparesis, and

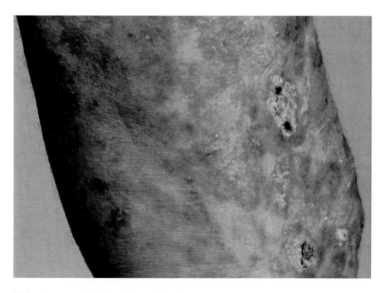

Figure 11.1 Cutaneous LG involving skin of lateral thigh and knee. Note indurated violaceous to focally necrotic plaques and nodules

seizures might accompany CNS involvement. Although hepatic and renal lesions are fairly frequent, the lesions themselves are usually asymptomatic and are only identified on radiographic imaging (4). Skin involvement by LG usually manifests as indurated, red nodules or plaques (Figure 11.1). Necrotic skin ulceration might also be observed and results from the attendant vascular destruction.

Patients with underlying immunodeficiency are at increased risk of developing LG. Predisposing immunodeficient states include history of organ transplant, HIV, Wiskott-Aldrich syndrome, other preceding lymphoproliferative disorders, and immunosuppressive medications. Upon close examination, most patients without an underlying specific immunodeficiency will manifest decreased immune function. Defects in cytotoxic T-cell function or reduced numbers of CD8+ T-cells have been implied. Decreased cellular immunity is important in propagating the disease by incomplete eradication of EBV and the EBV-infected B-cell clone (4).

The differential diagnosis of LG includes Wegener's granulomatosis (WG), angiocentric NK/T-cell lymphoma, posttransplant lymphoproliferative disease (LPD), as well as other Hodgkin's and non-Hodgkin's lymphomas. Table 11.1 lists the distinctive clinical and histologic differences among these entities (4, 11).

Table 11.1 Differential Diagnosis and Distinguishing features of lymphomatic granulomatosis

	Lymphomatoid granulomatosis	Wegener's granulomatosis	NK/T-cell lymphoma	Posttransplant LPD	Hodgkin's lymphoma
Primary involvement	Lungs	Upper respiratory tract; lungs	Nasal cavity	Variable	Cervical Lymph Nodes, Mediastinum
Renal findings	Nodular mass lesions	Segmental glomerulonephritis	Rare	Might involve allograft	Rare
EBV association	Yes	No	Yes	Yes	Variable
Typical histology	Variable number of EBV-positive atypical B-cells	Necrotizing granuloma formation	Sheets of atypical cells	Variable (early, pleomorphic, monomorphic)	Occasional multinucleate; Hodgkin and Reed-Sternberg cells
Angiocentric, angiodestructive	Yes	Yes	Yes	No	No
Background inflammatory infiltrate	Predominantly T-cells; eosinophils and neutrophils rare	Prominent multinucleate giant cells and neutrophils	Usually mixed	Predominantly plasmacytoid B-cells	Usually mixed with numerous eosinophils
Neoplastic cell phenotype	CD20+	N/A	CD2+ CD56+	Usually CD20+	CD15+ CD30+

11.4   Diagnosis

Definitive diagnosis of LG requires careful clinical workup and tissue biopsy. Open lung biopsies are recommended, as only approximately 30% of transbronchial biopsies are diagnostic [8]. Histologically, LG is characterized by varying numbers of large atypical CD20-positive B-cells set within a nodular polymorphous inflammatory cell background (Figure 11.2). The inflammatory milieu includes small lymphocytes, plasma cells, histiocytes (some might contain karyorrhectic debris), and larger reactive lymphocytes. Numerous CD3-positive T-cells are usual, and consist of an admixture of CD4 and CD8-positive cells (Figure 11.3). The inflammatory infiltrate is generally centered around bronchovascular structures in the lung and perivascularly in other sites. EBV is demonstrated within the large atypical B-cells by *in situ* hybridization studies, and these cells might resemble immunoblasts or Hodgkin cells. Occasional multinulcleate cells might also be seen. Vascular damage by neoplastic and non-neoplastic lymphoid cells is remarkable and includes transmural lymphocytic infiltration and necrosis of vessel walls. Associated coagulative tissue necrosis is common and was observed in 93% of cases in one study (7). Well-formed granulomas are not present (1, 4, 7–9). Biopsies of involved skin usually demonstrate a dense perivascular, often angiodestructive lymphohistiocytic infiltrate within the mid to deep dermis (Figure 11.4). Neoplastic EBV-positive B-lymphocytes might be rare or absent in LG skin lesions. Therefore,

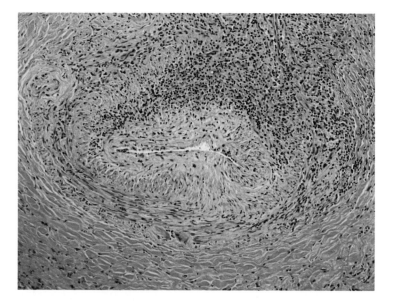

Figure 11.2   Pulmonary LG. An angioinvasive lymphocytic infiltrate composed of predominantly small cells (T-cells by immunophenotyping) is present (H&E, 20×)

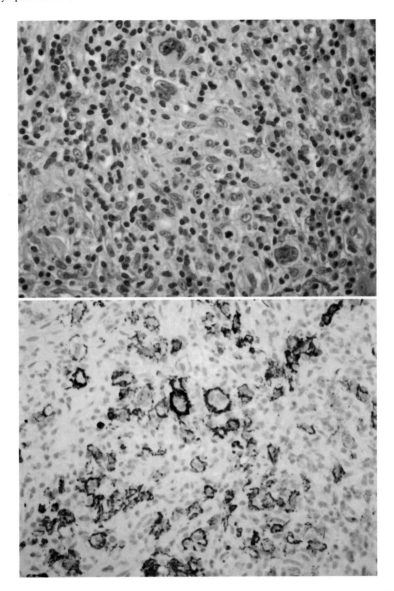

Figure 11.3 Pulmonary LG. **(A)** Grade III lesion with several large severely atypical cells (Reed-Sternberg-like appearance) admixed with background small round lymphocytes (H&E, 60×). **(B)** The large cells were B-lymphocytes that showed positive immunoreactivity with CD20 (60×).

a diagnosis of LG is precarious for patients with skin lesions that histiologically resemble LG but do not have evidence of internal organ (usually lung) involvement. These patients require close longitudinal follow-up and repeat biopsy is often needed.

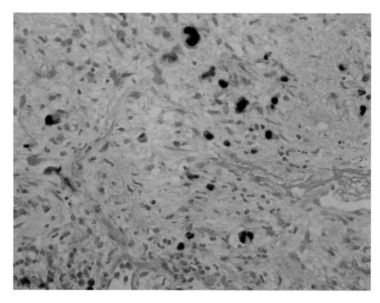

Figure 11.3 (continued) **(C)** Many of the large cells demonstrate EBV-positivity by *in-situ* hybridization (40×)

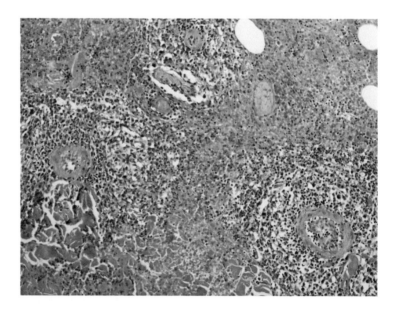

Figure 11.4 Cutaneous LG. Skin biopsy highlighting prominent angiocentric and angiodestructive nature of LG with surrounding tissue necrosis (H&E, 20×)

11.5 Prognosis

The clinical prognosis is variable in LG and poor prognostic findings include neurologic involvement and higher pathologic grade (1). Histologic grading of LG depends on the number of large atypical B-cells present in the infiltrate and on the degree of tissue necrosis. Grade I lesions contain a polymorphous angiocentric and angiodestructive lymphoid infiltrate with rare transformed EBV-positive lymphocytes (< 5 per high-power field). Tissue necrosis is minimal. Grade II lesions also demonstrate a polymorphous infiltrate, including occasional transformed lymphoid cells, and EBV-positive cells are easily identified (5–20 per high-power field) by EBV *in situ* hybridization studies. Grade III disease is considered a subtype of diffuse large B-cell lymphoma with sheets of large EBV-infected pleomorphic B-cells present (> 20 per high–power field). Extensive necrosis might be observed in grade III lesions (4, 8–11). Recurrent disease often demonstrates a higher histologic grade. Most cases of grade II and III lesions demonstrate monoclonal immunoglobulin gene rearrangement studies. Grade I lesions might be polyclonal, which might reflect low numbers of neoplastic B-cells or, in some cases, a truly polyclonal infiltrate.

11.6 Therapy

Due to the rarity of LG, standard treatments have not been established. Current treatment depends on histologic grade and clinical aggressiveness. Observation or corticosteroids might be reasonable in clinically indolent cases of grade I or II lesions. Reduction or discontinuation of immunosuppressive agents is prudent if clinically feasible. Interestingly, interferon = -α-2b has been used successfully in a small number of patients with grade I and II disease (12). More aggressive grade I or II cases might require single-agent or combination chemotherapy. Grade III disease should be treated as an aggressive lymphoma with combination chemotherapy such as R-CHOP (rituximab, cyclophosphamide, doxorubicin, vincristine, and prednisone). Rituximab has shown mixed results as a monotherapy (13–15). Bone marrow transplantation is a therapeutic option in patients failing chemotherapy and was associated with a prolonged remission in a recently published case (16).

11.7 Conclusions

In summary, LG is should be considered along a clinicopathologic continuum of disease ranging from a spontaneously regressing, immunosuppression-related lymphoproliferative disorder with rare neoplastic B-cells to an overtly malignant and clinically aggressive large B-cell lymphoma. Careful clinical workup and follow-up is often required to establish a diagnosis of LG as well as to distinguish between the extremes of this disease.

References

1. Katzenstein, AL, Carrington CB, Liebow AA. Lymphomatoid granulomatosis: a clinicopathologic study of 152 cases. Cancer, 1979;43(1):360–373.
2. Fauci AS, Haynes BF, Costa J, et al. Lymphomatoid Granulomatosis. Prospective clinical and therapeutic experience over 10 years. New England Journal of Medicine, 1982;306(2):68–74.
3. Cuadra-Garcia I, Proulx GM, Wu CL, et al., Sinonasal lymphoma: a clinicopathologic analysis of 58 cases from the Massachusetts General Hospital. American Journal of Surgical Pathology, 1999;23(11):1356–1369.
4. Jaffe ES, Wilson WH. Lymphomatoid granulomatosis: pathogenesis, pathology and clinical implications. Cancer Surveys, 1997;30:233–248.
5. Mazzie JP, Price AP, Khullar P, et al., Lymphomatoid granulomatosis in a pediatric patient. Clinical Imaging, 2004;28(3):209–213.
6. Sebire NJ, Haselden S, Malone M, et al. Isolated EBV lymphoproliferative disease in a child with Wiskott-Aldrich syndrome manifesting as cutaneous lymphomatoid granulomatosis and responsive to anti-CD20 immunotherapy. Journal of Clinical Pathology, 2003;56(7):555–557.
7. Koss, MN, Hochholzer L, Langloss JM, et al. Lymphomatoid granulomatosis: a clinicopathologic study of 42 patients. Pathology, 1986;18(3):283–288.
8. Koss, MN, Malignant and benign lymphoid lesions of the lung. Annals of Diagnostic Pathology, 2004;8(3):167–187.
9. Guinee DG, Perkins SL, Travis WD, et al. Proliferation and cellular phenotype in lymphomatoid granulomatosis: implications of a higher proliferation index in B cells. [see comment]. American Journal of Surgical Pathology, 1998;22(9):1093–1100.
10. Lipford EH, Margolick JB, Longo DL, et al. Angiocentric immunoproliferative lesions: a clinicopathologic spectrum of post-thymic T-cell proliferations. Blood, 1988;72(5): p. 1674–1681.
11. Jaffe ES, W. W. Lymphomatoid granulomatosis, in Pathology and Genetics. Tumours of Haematopoietic and Lymphoid Tissues, H.N. Jaffe ES, Stein H, Vardiman J, Editor. 2001, IARC Press, 2001: Lyon, France, p. 185–187.
12. Wilson WH, Kingma DW, Raffeld M, et al. Association of lymphomatoid granulomatosis with Epstein-Barr viral infection of B lymphocytes and response to interferon-alpha 2b. Blood, 1996;87(11):4531–4537.
13. Jordan K, Grothey A, Grothe W, et al. Successful treatment of mediastinal lymphomatoid granulomatosis with rituximab monotherapy. [see comment]. European Journal of Haematology, 2005;74(3):263–266.
14. Polizzotto MN, Dawson MA, Opat SS. Failure of rituximab monotherapy in lymphomatoid granulomatosis. [comment]. European Journal of Haematology, 2005;75(2):172–173.
15. Zaidi A, Kampalath B, Peltier WL, et al. Successful treatment of systemic and central nervous system lymphomatoid granulomatosis with rituximab. Leukemia & Lymphoma, 2004;45(4):777–780.
16. Johnston AL, Coyle L, Nevell D. Prolonged remission of refractory lymphomatoid granulomatosis after autologous hemopoietic stem cell transplantation with post-transplantation maintenance interferon. Leukemia & Lymphoma, 2006;47(2):323–328.

Chapter 12
Posttransplant Lymphoproliferative Disorders

Thomas M. Habermann

12.1 Introduction

In 1968, Starzl reported the clinical observation that transplant patients are prone to develop lymphomatous growths (1). The term *posttransplant lymphoproliferative disorder* (PTLD) is applied to a group of lymphoproliferative disorders arising in a pharmacologically immunocompromised host after solid-organ or allogeneic stem cell transplantation. Among iatrogenic immune deficiency states, PTLD is quite common (2). PTLDs are the most serious complications of chronic immunosuppression and represent one of the most commonly observed fatal consequences of immunosuppression in patients undergoing solid-organ transplantation. PTLDs are the most common malignancy complicating organ transplantation after nonmelanomatous skin cancer and *in situ* cervical cancer (3). PTLDs represent 21% of all malignancies versus 5% of malignancies in immunocompetent patients (not sure what this means?). Clinically, this group of disorders might be slow growing or aggressive, localized or mulitcentric, associated with symptoms or no symptoms, more characteristically involve extranodal sites, and disease in the allograft organ is more common (4–6). The biology, diagnosis, and management of this heterogeneous group of disorders have nuances that are different than other non-Hodgkin's lymphomas.

The issues in evaluating published PTLD data involve multiple variables, including Epstein-Barr virus (EBV) serostatus prior to the organ transplant in the donor and the recipient, stages of disease, types and doses of immunosuppressive agents utilized in the course of the transplant, initial PTLD management strategies (surgery, immunosuppression reduction strategies), types of treatment (rituximab as monotherapy, etc.), the timing and incorporation of treatment regimens, the timing of treatment after the PTLD diagnosis, presentation from the time of transplant, pathology reporting, locations of extranodal involvement, and comorbid conditions [other vital organ involvement, performance status, active infections (Cytomegalovirus (CMV), fungal), etc.. Two International Consensus Development meetings were held in 1997 and 1998 that addressed different issues in PTLD in working groups, recommended management guidelines, and set the stage for future directions (7). This review will focus on adult solid-organ PTLD.

12.2   Incidence

The incidence of PTLD is related to the organ transplanted and is dependent on the duration of follow-up. In various publications, the incidence in renal transplantation is 0.8–1.2%, lung 4.5–7.9%, pancreas 0.6%, hepatic 1.0–5.4%, cardiac 1.8–13%, heart/lung 1.8–9.4%, and T-cell-depleted allogeneic bone marrow transplantation 24% (8). Reported durations of follow-up vary in different series. Previous reports in orthotic liver transplantation reported frequencies in the 2–3.5% range (8). The type of survival analysis influences this interpretation. Competing risk survival analysis, which simultaneously estimates the two competing outcomes of PTLD and death without (before) PTLD, yields an accurate estimate of the probability of PTLD as a function of time since transplant. This is in contrast to Kaplan-Meier estimates, which estimates the probability of a patient developing PTLD conditional upon the patient not dying until they have developed PTLD. Utilizing competing risk analysis, Kremers et al. observed that the cumulative incidence of PTLD varies by year of follow-up (9). At 5 years, the incidence is 2.1%; 10 years, 4.2%; 15 years, 4.7%; and 19 3/4 years, 5.4%. Data on other types of organ transplant with accounting for the length of follow-up and the competing risk of death in estimating PTLD has not been published.

12.3   Clinical Presentation of PTLD

The signs and symptoms are quite variable in patients with PTLD. PTLD lymphomas might be slow growing versus aggressive. They might be localized versus multicentric. Patients might be asymptomatic or symptomatic. Some present with the classical symptoms of lymphoma, including fevers, night sweats, and weight loss. Patients might also present with the classical sign of lymphoproliferative disorders, which is lymphadenopathy (10). However, the presentation of PTLD is often different to that of *de novo* NHL (non-Hodgkin's lymphoma). These disorders are characteristically extranodal, involving organs such as the central nervous system, gastrointestinal tract, lung, liver, kidney, skin, and other organs versus primarily being nodal in immunocompetent patients with NHL. This accounts for a high incidence of stage IV disease in PTLD. Extranodal disease has been reported to correlate with poor prognosis (11). The high incidence of extranodal lymphoma in patients with PTLDs compared with patients who develop lymphoma in the immunocompetent state is not well understood. Tumor burden is a poor prognostic factor in PTLD (12, 13). Involvement of one or more extranodal sites was predictive of poor survival (11). In addition, the allograft itself is involved in a significant number of patients and has been reported to influence survival. Ghobrial et al. reported that 80% of patients had extranodal disease including the grafted organ (14). Ghobrial and colleagues reported that extranodal disease with or without the presence of nodal disease was a strong predictor of poor prognosis ($p < 0.01$); however, graft organ involvement, which was present in 28% of patients, was a stronger adverse predictor of survival than other extranodal disease (14).

12.4   Etiology of PTLD

Posttransplant lymphoproliferative disorder is highly associated with immunosuppressive treatments and EBV infection. EBV has been implicated in 78–93% of all cases of PTLD. EBV infection is associated with rare consequences in the normal population, but in organ transplant recipients, EBV is associated with a range of disorders from reactive polyclonal hyperplasia to monoclonal malignant lymphomas (15). Early reports of PTLD were frequently reported to be EBV positive. Ho first reported that the presence of pretransplantation EBV seronegativity was a significant risk factor for the development of PTLD (16). More recent reports suggest an increasing frequency of EBV-negative PTLD (16–18). These are viewed as distinct from the EBV-positive PTLD because they tend to occur later after transplantation and have a worse prognosis (6, 16–19). Primary EBV infection typically occurs in childhood or early adolescence and can be asymptomatic or associated with a benign mononucleosis syndrome, implying that most patients are not aware of a past infection (20). *In situ* hybridization studies on paraffin section tissues are now routinely utilized to determine EBV status (21). Although transmission of EBV to naïve seronegative EBV transplant recipients might occur by infection through community-acquired contacts, patients are at highest risk after transplantation of an organ from an EBV-positive donor into an EBV-negative recipient (22). The EBV undergoes lytic replication due to lack of an EBV-specific immune surveillance. This increase in EBV burden in the naïve recipient is postulated to infect the recipient's blood cells, allowing their transformation. These EBV-infected B-cells would normally be eliminated by cytotoxic T-cells (4, 24, 25). However, immunosuppression creates a state of impaired T-cell immunity allowing for an uncontrolled expansion of an EBV-transformed B-cell clone (23, 24). Because not all cases demonstrate EBV by *in situ* hybridization studies, further studies are necessary to further elucidate the etiology of PTLD.

12.5   Origin of PTLD

The origin of PTLD in solid-organ transplantation is usually the recipient rather than the donor. The majority of PTLD cases in solid-organ transplant recipients arise from the recipient's B-lymphocytes based on HLA typing, sex chromosome analysis, minisatellite DNA analysis, restriction fragment polymorphism DNA analysis, DNA fingerprinting, *in situ* hybridization, and polymerase chain reaction (PCR) amplification (13, 25–28)]. However, the involvement of the grafted organ with PTLD might be related to development of donor origin PTLD that usually presents early after transplantation and is more characteristically confined to the transplanted organ (27). In contrast, in allogeneic transplantation, the origin of PTLD is the donor in over 80% of cases (28). Detection of donor- or recipient-origin PTLD by short tandem repeat analysis for DNA polymorphism might be performed in early PTLD patients to detect the origin of the tumor (29).

12.6   Classification

The classification of PTLD has evolved over time, including the early descriptions of "reticulum cell sarcoma" in 1968, "pseudolymphomas" recognizing the ability to undergo regression, and the Frizzera classification recognizing the histologic variability (1, 30, 31). The World Health Organization has classified PTLD (Table 12.1) (32). The spectrum of PTLDs include early lesions, which are reactive plasmacytic hyperplasia, that are infectious mononucleosislike lesions, polymorphic PTLD, monomorphic PTLD, and Hodgkin's lymphoma or Hodgkin-like PTLD. Monomorphic PTLD includes B-cell lymphomas, which are most commonly diffuse large B-cell lymphoma and Burkitt lymphoma. The T-cell disorders include peripheral T-cell lymphoma, nonspecified, CD30 large-cell anaplastic lymphoma, hepatosplenic T-cell lymphoma, and other types of lymphoma.

As PTLDs are highly associated with the EBV, the diagnosis is established by *in situ* hybridization analysis of the pathology tissue. PTLD tumors are characteristically EBV-positive by *in situ* hybridization but might be EBV-negative (16, 33). The patterns of EBV gene expression demonstrate that PTLD mirrors acquired immune deficiency syndrome (AIDS) in EBV genes expressed with a type 3 latency (EBNA1, 2, 3a, 3b, 3c, LP; LMP1, 2a, 2b, and EVR) (34). However, not all occurrences of PTLDs are associated with EBV infection. EBV-negative occurrences have been reported to occur in 20 – 30% of adult patients (16). In adults, EBV is characteristically a result of reactivation of latent EBV infection. In contrast, in the pediatric population, PTLD usually arises as a result of primary EBV infection in children who have not yet had a primary EBV infection.

Table 12.1   WHO classification of PTLD; categories of PTLD

1. Early lesions
   Reactive plasmacytic hyperplasia
   Infectious mononucleosis-like
2. Polymorphic PTLD
3. Monomorphic PTLD (classify according to lymphoma classification)
   B-cell neoplasms
   Diffuse large B-cell lymphomas (immunoblastic, centroblastic, anaplastic)
   Burkitt/Burkitt-like lymphoma
   Plasma cell myeloma
   Plasmacytoma-like lesion
   T-cell neoplasms
   Peripheral T-cell lymphoma, not otherwise specified
   Other types
4. Hodgkin lymphoma (HL) and Hodgkin lymphoma-like PTLD

12.7   Surveillance for Early Detection and Prevention Strategies

At this time, there are no standard monitoring strategies. Different strategies have been reported, including measuring monoclonal proteins in the serum. In one series, a monoclonal protein was detected in 28% of patients of 201 patients following a solid-organ transplant (35). Seventy-one percent of patients went on to develop PTLD, and 27% did not. In these patients, the serum protein electrophoresis was abnormal ($p = 0.04$) and urine protein electrophoresis was abnormal ($p = 0.01$). Although protein electrophoresis studies might be helpful in disease surveillance, they are not routinely recommended for this purpose.

Epstein-Barr virus viral load studies have been analyzed (36, 37) as a way to detect evolving PTLD. Gera et al. evaluated 957 patients who had a kidney transplant (37). One hundred thirty-three of 957 (14%) were EBV mismatches as defined by positive IgG to EBNA in the donor and negative in the recipient in this renal transplant series (37). Seventy percent of these mismatch patients had sequential EBV DNA performed by LightCycler PCR as well as EBV serostatus by serum Elisa Assays (EIA) monthly for 1 year, quarterly for the second year, and semiannually thereafter. In the absence of PTLD, no reduction in immunosuppression or other interventions were carried out in viremic patients. Sixteen of 74 (22%) converted to EBV-positive serostatus. Viremia was detected in 38/93 (41%) of the patients beginning at a mean of 7.5 months posttransplant. Viremia occurred in 10/16 (63%) of seroconverters versus 28/58 (48%) nonconverters ($p = 0.01$). The maximum viral load was higher among those who developed PTLD than those who did not, with a median of 13,750 copies/mL (range: 500–140,000) versus a median of 1000 copies/mL (range: 500–75,500, $p = 0.001$). At a median follow-up of 19 months (range: 6–33 months), seven (5.3%) EBV-mismatched recipients developed PTLD. All PTLDs were early with a range of 7.5–2.5 months. All cases were positive for EBV by *in situ* hybridization, and 100% were viremic. The effectiveness of sequential EBV PCR monitoring at diagnosis of PTLD at a subclinical stage was only 23%. The positive predictive value of 13% makes this a marginally effective screening tool for subclinical PTLD in the renal transplant population.

12.8   Early and Late PTLD

Posttransplant lymphoproliferative disorder might present early or late (38–41), but the cutoff for these definitions range from 6 to 24 months. Whereas the presence of EBV genome in the tumor has been associated with both early and late PTLD, commonly EBV-negative PTLD occurs later after transplantation, with a median of 50 months, and has a worse prognosis, with an initial reported median survival of 1 month. In contrast, EBV-positive PTLD, which tends to occur earlier following transplantation at a median of 10 months, is associated with an overall survival of 37 months (16, 42). Ghobrial et al. differentiated early versus late PTLD at 12 months (43). For the whole group, the median time to transplantation was 19.5 months (1–208 months) and 49 (46%) patients developed PTLD in less than 12 months and 58 patients developed PTLD beyond 12 months. The patient characteristics in these two groups were similar; however, patients who received pancreas, lung, or multiorgan transplants were more likely to develop PTLD within the first year of transplantation ($p = 0.02$). Early PTLD was also more frequently associated with a positive EBV status ($p \leq 0.0001$) and CD20-positive lymphomas in 36/38 patients versus 34/45 patients ($p = 0.02$). There was no difference in overall survival ($p = 0.2$). This was in contrast to a study of lung transplant patients treated with cyclosporine immunosuppression by Armitage et al. (38). This might be related to a larger cohort of patients, multiple types of transplant, and the use of novel modalities of therapy such as rituximab. The Ghobrial study documented that CD20-positive PTLD occurs early after transplantation (43) and might benefit from rituximab. In contrast to CD20-positive B-cell PTLD, previous studies have documented a poor outcome for T-cell PTLD (44).

12.9   Risk Factors for Developing PTLD

The risk factors for developing PTLD are different than the risk factors for surviving PTLD. Ho et al. first reported that the presence of pretransplantation EBV seronegativity was a significant risk factor for the development of PTLD (26). Other reports followed (45, 46). Swinnen reported that OKT3 was a significant risk factor for PTLD (47). Subsequently, CMV was identified as an independent variable in the development of PTLD (22). Walker et al. reported on the pretransplant assessment of the risk of lymphoproliferative disorders (22). The risk was 0.8% (3/361) in EBV-positive recipients and 50% (9/18) in EBV-negative patients, and four of the EBV-negative cases were fatal. Eight of nine EBV-negative cases occurred in the first 6 months. EBV seronegative recipients had a 24 times higher risk than EBV seropositive patients fordeveloping PTLD. Patients who received OKT3 therapy for rejection had a fourfold to sixfold amplification in their risk. CMV-positive donors to CMV-negative recipients had a fourfold to fivefold amplification. All three synergistically increased the risk of fatal or central nervous system PTLD by 654-fold and all forms by 592-fold versus a low incidence rate (0.458 cases per 100-person years) in patients with none of these factors. Kremers reported that acute fulminant hepatitis in the first 18 months of orthotic liver transplantation put patients at increased risk (HR = 2.6; $p = 0.007$) (9). Rejection therapy was also associated with a risk of developing PTLD in liver transplant patients and included high-dose steroids (HR = 4.5; $p = 0.049$) and OKT3 (HR = 3.9; $p = 0.016$) (9).

The type of organ transplanted is strongly correlated with the incidence of PTLD and is likely related to the immunosuppression program and the extent of lymphoid tissue transplanted. In the Collaborative Transplant Database, 200,000 renal, pancreas, heart, lung, and heart-lung transplant recipients were evaluated (45). The risk of PTLD by organ tranplant in decreasing order was heart-lung, lung, liver, pancreas, and renal, which was consistent with the literature. The incidence in intestinal transplants was particularly high (up to 30%), in large part due to the fact that the recipients were EBV-negative children (46).

12.10   Risk Factors for Surviving PTLD

The risk of surviving PTLD has been complicated by limited data from small series of patients (11, 13, 48–53). Reported prognostic factors in univariate analyses include mulitvisceral disease (five or more sites involved), severe organ dysfunction, presence of "B" symptoms, stage, advanced age, elevated lactate dehydrogenase (LDH), monoclonality, EBV-negative status, late of onset of PTLDs, central nervous system (CNS) PTLDs, and PTLDs associated with allogeneic bone marrow transplantation (11, 13, 48–51). LeBlond reported in a series of 61 patients from 2 institutions that a performance score of 2 or more, the number of extranodal sites (one versus more than one), primary CNS location, T-cell origin, monoclonality, nondetection of EBV, and treatment with chemotherapy were poor prognostic factors for overall survival on univariate analysis (11).

Ghobrial et al. reported on a prognostic analysis for survival in adult organ transplant recipients with PTLD (14). There were 107 patients who were evaluated from 1970 through May 2003. Patients were treated according to a clinicopathologic model. The median age at diagnosis was 48 years. Eighty percent (85) had extranodal disease; 28% (30) had graft involvement; 61% were stage III, IV and 29% performance score of 3–4; 78% were EBV-positive by *in situ* hybridization studies; 86% were CD20-positive. The median survival in this group was 31.5 months (95% confidence interval; 10.7–72.5 months). The median follow-up of the living patients was 51.8 months (5.6–202.6 months). The prognostic model in a multivariate analysis demonstrated that monomorphic disease, graft organ involvement, and a performance score of 3–4 differentiated patients into cohorts with different outcomes. Those patients with a score of 0–1 had a survival that was statistically significantly different from those with a score of 2–3 (HR = 5.31; $p < 0.0001$). The involvement of the graft organ by PTLDs has not been previously reported to correlate with survival. The presence of extranodal disease and high tumor burden has been reported to correlate with poor survival (11, 13, 49). In the Ghobrial series, graft organ involvement was a more meaningful prognostic indicator when adjusted for poor performance score and monomorphic disease. Thus, extranodal disease was not used in the final prognostic model. Other models were assessed in this study, including CD20 status, LDH, EBV status, age, time to PTLD, and the International Prognostic Factor Index (IPI). The IPI is the standard predictive model for NHL survival [54], but previous reports have reported that the IPI was not predictive of survival (11, 43). In the Ghobrial series, the proposed prognostic model performed better than the IPI in separating the survival outcomes of patients.

Posttransplant lymphoproliferative disorder following transplantation does influence overall survival. In a single institution series of liver transplantation patients, Kremers et al. reported that for every 100 deaths, there were roughly 10–15 PTLD patients (9).

12.11   Prophylactic Approaches to PTLD

Retrospective studies have retrospectively reported on the use of prophylactic antiviral therapy (55–59). Darenkov treated 198 patients with prophylactic ganciclovir
or acyclovir (56). The percent of PTLD was 0.5% versus 3.9% in 179 unmatched
institutional controls ($p < 0.03$). Davis et al. reported on 206 patients treated with
high-dose ganciclovir followed by high-dose acyclovir, and 1.5% of prophylaxed
patients versus 8% of retrospective unmatched historical controls developed PTLD
(57). McDiarmid reported on 18 high-risk pediatric patients (donor EBV+ and
recipient EBV−) treated with 100 days of intravenous ganciclovir (60). None who
were prophylaxed developed PTLD, and 10% of unmatched institutional controls
who were not prophylaxed developed PTLD. Thirty-four patients (25 pediatric and
9 adult) were randomized to receive either ganciclovir and placebo or ganciclovir
and immunoglobulin (IG) for 3 months (61). There was no difference in EBV viral
load and 8.8% of patients developed PTLD.

12.12   The Treatment of PTLD

Four major areas of treatment need to be considered: (1) local therapy with surgical
extirpation; (2) reduction of immunosuppression; (3) biological and monoclonal
antibody therapy; (4) immune and cell-based therapies. An International Concensus
Development Meeting on Epstein Barr Virus-Induced Posttransplant Lymphoproliferative Disorders outlined recommendations and future directions in 1999 and
there has been subsequent evolution in management approaches since then (7).

12.12.1   Local Therapy

A small percentage of patients with very limited disease might be managed with
surgical extirpation or localized radiation therapy and minor (e.g., 25%) immunosuppression reduction (7). Localized radiation therapy might be required for patients
emergently or for palliative treatment (62).

12.12.2   Reduction of Immunosuppression in PTLD

The hallmark of the initial treatment of PTLD has been a reduction in immunosuppression with a goal of restoring EBV-specific cellular immunity without inducing
graft rejection. The initial intervention in all patients should be a reduction in
immunosuppression. Regression of monoclonal and polyclonal lesions after reduction
of the dose of immunosuppression been reported to be 20–85% (13, 51, 63–66).

The optimal method for immunosuppression reduction is unclear and adequate prospective trials have not been carried out (67, 68). Consensus guidelines recommended the following (7). In critically ill patients with excessive disease, prednisone should be decreased to a maintenance dose of 7.5–10 mg/day and all other immunosuppressive agents should be stopped. If there is no response (objective reduction in tumor mass within a period of 10–20 days), then further interventions should be considered. In less critically ill patients (who are the majority of patients), the initial management strategy should include reduction of cyclosporine, tacrolimus, prednisone, and related immunosuppressive agents by at least 50%, and azathioprine or Mycophenolate Mofetil (MMF) should be discontinued. After a 14-day trial of decreased immunosuppression, a further decrease of 50% can be considered. This is one of the few times in lymphoproliferative disorders that patients are restaged with scans in such a short time period. It must be emphasized that serial biopsies or other forms of monitoring of the allograft performed during the period of reduced immunosuppression will allow early detection of allograft rejection. This is especially important in the rejection of vital organs such as heart, liver, or lung that might carry the risk of death to the patient. Renal and liver patients are easier to monitor with blood tests than other organ transplants. The consequences of aggressive immunosuppression reduction in heart, liver, and lung patients must always be considered. Clinical improvement occurs within 1.5–4 weeks (51, 69).

Patients with EBV negative disease have been reported to be less likely to respond to immunosuppression reduction(70). The response to immunosuppression reduction in late-onset PTLD is controversial, with experience both supporting and not supporting decreasing immunosuppression (38). Successful management of EBV-negative late-onset disease with immunosuppression reduction has been reported (16, 17, 51).

Tsai et al., in a retrospective analysis of 42 PTLD patients treated with immunosuppression alone or immunosuppression in conjunction with surgical excision, reported a complete response rate of 74% (51). Factors predictive of a poor response included an elevated LDH, organ dysfunction, and multiorgan PTLD involvement. Patients with no risk factors had a response rate of 89%, whereas patients with two or three risk factors had a 0% response.

When comparing the results of the two largest institutional experiences of reduction in immunosuppression in PTLD patients, Ghobrial et al. reported that immunosuppression reduction occurred in 75% of patients, with only 20% of the patients achieving a long-term remission, and Tsai et al. reported long-term remissions in 25% (14, 51).

12.12.3 Rituximab

Rituximab is a chimeric anti-CD20 human immunoglobulin G1 monoclonal antibody that is approved for the treatment of follicular lymphoma as a single agent or as combination therapy with CHOP (cyclophosphamide, doxorubicin, vincristine, and prednisone) in diffuse large B-cell lymphoma (71–73). In contrast to other

NHLs, single-agent rituximab in PTLD is potentially curative. In 1999, Milped and colleagues reported a retrospective analysis of 32 patients treated with rituximab at a dose of 375 mg/m^2 (74, 75). The immunosuppression regimen was reduced in 27 of 32 patients. Rituximab was used as a front-line therapy in 30 patients and as salvage treatment in 2 patients. The overall response rate was 69% (complete remission 20; partial remission, 2). At a median of 10 months, four patients had relapsed. Other reports have followed (21, 76–79). In a retrospective analysis, the major impact was on early response with a significant relapse rate, but in multivariate analysis, rituximab was associated with an improved overall survival ($p = 0.03$) in CD20+ PTLD (78). Phase II data support these observations (80) and show that rituximab therapy after immunosuppression reduction results in overall response rates of 44–75%. Complete response rates have been seen in 35–69% of patients. The variable response rates relate to whether the PTLD was early or late, presence of EBV in the tissue, LDH level, type of organ transplanted, other comorbid conditions, histology variables, retrospective versus prospective studies, and duration of follow-up (78, 80, 81). This is supported by phase II results (80, 81). For example, Choquet et al. reporteda 44% response rate and 35% complete remission rate with few relapses after a CR in a phase II study in which 65% had delayed-onset PTLD, likely accounting for the lower response rate (80).

There are no randomized trials comparing rituximab to chemotherapy. Fifty percent of rituximab failures responded to systemic chemotherapy (75). Retrospective studies report similar response rates, less toxicity, and improved overall survival (77, 79). Monotherapy with rituximab is the standard of care in most patients with PTLD, but rituximab has been utilized with systemic chemotherapy (82). Unique complications with rituximab therapy include transitory neutropenia, reactivation of hepatitis B infection resulting in fulminate hepatic failure, parvo B19 infection resulting in pure red cell aplasia, and disseminated CMV infection in a patient with PTLD on concurrent immunosuppressive medication (73, 83–86).

Currently, rituximab is recommended in the treatment of patients with EBV+ CD20+ PTLD who have not responded to reduction in immunosuppression or as first-line treatment for patients in whom further reduction in immunotherapy is not possible. In EBV– CD20+ PTLD, rituximab should be combined with systemic chemotherapy (72, 73).

Future directions include administering maintenance rituximab following the initial weekly times four schedule of 375 mg/m^2. Maintenance rituximab therapy is now approved for follicular lymphoma and was reported in diffuse large B-cell lymphoma (73, 87). A study treating patients with a partial remission (PR) after the initial dose of rituximab with an additional course of 4 doses of rituximab is underway (77).

Preemptive rituximab has been used (88). Seventeen high-risk patients as manifested by a high EBV viral load consistent with EBV reactivation were treated with a single infusion of rituximab. Two (18%) patients developed PTLD versus 48% of historical controls. The EBV viral load became undetectable in patients who did not develop PTLD. Further studies are needed in this complex area.

12.12.4 Chemotherapy

The respond rates with systemic chemotherapy during the 1980s were reported to be less than 20% (65, 89). Subsequent publications with small numbers of patients treated in noncontrolled studies showed that with anthracycline-based regimens (CHOP and others) a 69% remission rate might be achieved (7, 90–93). In contrast, the reported response rates with CHOP in T-cell PTLD were 0% in series of a small number of patients (94, 95). In a retrospective series of 18 patients with late-onset PTLD treated with systemic chemotherapy, the response rate was 33%, and 50% of patients died of complications of chemotherapy related to end-organ toxicity or infection (96). A review of the Israel Penn International Transplant Tumor Registry reported the outcomes of 193 PTLD patients treated with chemotherapy (97). The 5-year overall survival was 25% in patients treated with R-CHOP, which was similar to other combination chemotherapies that were administered. Single-agent chemotherapy, likely administered to patients with impaired performance status or organ dysfunction, was statistically significantly inferior with a 5-year overall survival of 5% (97). Low-dose chemotherapy regimens have been piloted in children with some success (92, 98).

Indications for the initial treatment with chemotherapy include specific histologies, including Burkitt's lymphoma, Hodgkin's lymphoma, peripheral T-cell lymphoma, other uncommon NHLs, and late-onset CD20+ and EBV– PTLD. Burkitt's lymphoma and Hodgkin's lymphoma must be treated with the standard of care approaches for these specific histologies. Some centers treat late-onset, CD20+/EBV–, advanced stage, and monomorphic PTLD with systemic chemotherapy (16, 96).

12.12.5 Stem Cell Transplantation

Patients who have failed immunosuppression reduction, systemic chemotherapy, and other therapies have been cured with autologous or allogeneic stem cell transplantation (99–101).

12.12.6 Cytokine Therapy

Interleukin-6 (IL-6) promotes the growth of EBV-infected cells (102). Increased levels of IL-6 have been reported in patients with PTLD (103). In a study of 12 patients who failed immune suppression reduction approaches, 8/12 achieved a partial or complete response after treatment with an anti-IL-6 monoclonal antibody, with no increase in graft rejection (104).

12.12.7   Cellular Immunotherapy

The goal of cellular immunotherapy in EBV+ PTLD is to restore EBV-specific
cellular immunity through transfer of selected or unselected EBV-specific cytotoxic T-cells to the patient. Unselected cytotoxic T-cell therapy was initially used
to treat PTLD in the T-cell-depleted allogeneic hematopoietic stem cell transplant
(HSCT) population, as PTLDs in this setting are of donor origin (105). In a series
of 39 patients at high risk of developing PTLD who received prophylactic EBV-
specific cytotoxic T-cells infusions, none of the patients developed PTLD in
comparison to 12% of institutional controls with no increase in graft versus host
disease (106).

Epstein-Barr virus-specific cytotoxic therapy is more complex in solid-organ
transplantation because PTLD is usually of host origin, donors are not routinely
HLA matched, and cytotoxic T-cells are unlikely to recognize the malignant cells
of host origin (107). Various strategies have been tried in this setting. Nonselected
infused autologous lymphocytes cultured with IL-2 were infused into seven
patients with PTLD with four of four completed remissions in EBV+ patients,
none of three responses in EBV− patients, and two graft rejections (108). The
role of autologous EBV-specific cytotoxic T-cells as the preemptive therapy for
the prevention or treatment of EBV+ PTLD in solid-organ transplant patients has
been reported to be safe and effective and resulted in a decreased viral load
(108–114). Strategies to adapt this therapy in EBV− PTLD are ongoing (115,
116). One hundred sixty-four of 568 liver transplant patients received allogeneic
T-cell infusions from HLA-identical donors in a protocol to decrease the side
effects of immunosuppressive therapeutic interventions (117). None of the 164
patients developed PTLD versus 5 of 394 patients in a control group, which was
not statistically significant. Haque and colleagues have developed a bank of 100
EBV-specific T-cell lines of known HLA type from EBV+ donors (118). Five
patients have been treated and three have responded.

12.13   A Clinicopathologic Approach to PTLD

The management of EBV-negative patients is in evolution. One approach is to use
a clinicopathologic model of therapy by initially reducing immunosuppression in
all patients. Then, in those who are CD20-positive and EBV-positive, rituximab
is the next treatment of choice. In those patients who are CD20-positive and
EBV-negative, rituximab-CHOP is the treatment of choice. In patients who are
CD20-negative and EBV-negative, CHOP chemotherapy should be considered. In
those patients with specific histologies such as Hodgkin's lymphoma, peripheral
T-cell lymphoma, and others, disease-specific therapeutic interventions are
required. Where available, cellular immunotherapy should be incorporated into the
management of PTLD.

12.14   Future Directions

Further understanding of the biology of the complex pathology of PTLD will lead to further understanding of this disease, which is different from *de novo* diffuse large B-cell lymphoma. The molecular histogenesis of PTLD is being defined. BCL-6 gene mutations predicted shorter survival and refractoriness to reduced immunosuppression and/or surgical excision (119). Somatic hypermutation of immunoglobulin variable (IgV) genes documented that most monoclonal B-cell PTLDs derive from germinal center-experienced B-cells, but there was remarkable histogenetic diversity (120). Vaccine approaches for EBV could alter the natural history of this disease state.

Discovering new clinical risk factors will lead to different directions in therapy. The recipient of a heart from a hepatitis C virus (HCV)-positive donor is associated with decreased survival in heart transplant recipients (121).

New immunosuppressive drugs are being implemented in solid-organ transplantation. Rapamycin is an immunosuppressive and antineoplastic agent that inhibits the mammalian target of rapamycin (mTOR). The mTOR inhibitors might induce apoptosis in B- and T-lymphocytes. Rapamycin inhibits the growth of human EBV-transformed B-lymphocytes (122). The impact of incorporating rapamycin into solid-organ transplant programs has not been reported to date.

12.15   Outcomes of PTLD

The response rate and survival of patients diagnosed with PTLD remains poor despite the advances in management strategies. Muti et al. reported a cumulative probability of survival at 1 year of 57% (95% confidence interval: 37.6–73.4) in 40 solid-organ transplantation adult patients diagnosed with PTLD, with a median survival that was not reached at 54 months (52). Leblond et al. reported a median survival of 24 months from a two-institution study of 61 patients (11). Ghobrial et al. reported a median survival of 31.5 months (95% confidence interval: 10.7–72.5); 62 patients (58%) had died at the time of this analysis (14). The median follow-up of patients who were alive was 51.8 months (range: 5.6–202.6 months). These series span a significant time frame. Newer approaches to immunosuppression management, risk management, and therapeutic interventions might well lead to improved overall survival.

12.16   Conclusion

Posttransplant lymphoproliferative disorder is related to EBV and immunosuppression. The multiple lymphoma histologic diagnoses make a clinicopathologic approach to management essential. The factors associated with the risk of developing the disease are different than those associated with surviving the disease. PTLD is related to impaired immune reconstitution. Our future understanding and intervention in other EBV disorders, immunosuppression strategies, and T-cell biology infusion strategies will likely lead to new approaches and improved outcomes in this disease.

References

1. Starzl TE. Discussion of Murray JE, Wilson RE, Tilney NL, et al. Five years' experience in renal transplantation with immunosuppressive drugs: survival, function, complications and the role of lymphocyte depletion by thoracic duct fistula. Ann Surg 1968;168:416–435.
2. Penn I. Posttranspantation de novo tumors in liver allograft recipients. Liver Transplant Surg 1996;2:52–59.
3. Penn I. Cancers complicating organ transplantation. N Engl J Med 1990;323:1767–1769.
4. Hanto DW. Classification of Epstein-Barr virus associated post-transplant lymphoprolifera-tive diseases: mplications for understanding their pathogenesis and developing rational treat-ment strategies. Annu Rev Med 1995;46:381–394.
5. Nalesnik MA. Post-transplanation lymphoproliferative disorders (PTLD): current perspectives. Semin Thorac Cardiovasc Surg 1996;8:139–148.
6. Morrison VA, Dunn DL, Manivel LC, et al. Clinical characteristics of post-transplant lym-phoproliferative disorders. Am J Med 1994;97:14–24.
7. Paya CV, Fung JJ, Nalesnik MA, et al. Epstein-Barr virus-induced post-transplant lympho-proliferative disorders. ASTS/ASTP EBV-PTLD Task Force and the Mayo Clinic Organized International Consensus Development Meeting. Transplantation. November 27, 1999; 68(10):1517–1525.
8. Leblond V, Choquet S. Lymphoproliferative disorders after liver transplantation. J Hepatol 2004; 40:728–735.
9. Kremers WK, Devarbhavi HC, Wiesner RH, et al. Post-transplant lymphoproliferative disor-ders following liver transplantation: Incidence, risk factors and survival. Am J Transplant 2006;6:1017–1024.
10. Habermann TM, Steensma DP. Lymphadenopathy. Mayo Clin Proc 2000;75:723–732.
11. Leblond V, Dhedin N, Marnzer Bruneel MF, et al. Identification of prognosticfactors in 61 patients with posttransplant lymphoproliferative disorders. J Clin Oncol 2001;19:772–778.
12. Benkerrou MJJ, Jais JP, Leblond V, et al. Anti-B-cell monoclonal antibody treatment of severe posttransplant B-lymphoproliferative disorder: Prognostic factors and long-term out-come. Blood 1998;92:3137–3147.
13. Nalesnik MA, Jaffe R, Starzl TE, et al. The pathology of posttransplant lymphoproliferative disorders occurring in the setting of cyclosporine A-prednisone immunosuppression. Am J Pathol 1988;133:173–192.
14. Ghobrial IM, Habermann TM, Maurer MJ, et al. Prognostic analysis for survival in adult solid organ transplant recipients with posttransplantation lymphoproliferative disorders. J Clin Oncol 2005;23:7574–7582.
15. Cohen JI. Epstein-Barr virus infection. N Engl J Med 2000;343(7):481–492.
16. Leblond V, Davi F, Charlotte F, et al. Post-transplant lymphoproliferative disorders not associated with Epstein-Barr virus: a distinct entity? J Clin Oncol 1998;16(6):2052–2059.
17. Nelson BP, Nalesnik MA, Bahler DW, et al. Epstein-Barr virus-negative post-transplant lymphoproliferative disorders: a distinct entity? Am J Surg Pathol 2000; 24(3):375–385.
18. Dotti G, Fiocchi R, Motta T, et al. Epstein-Barr virus-negative lymphoproliferative disorders in long-term survivors after heart, kidney, and liver transplant. Transplantation. March 15, 2000; 69(5):827–833.

19. Swerdlow AJ, Higgins CD, Hunt BJ, et al. Risk of lymphoid neoplasia after cardiothoracic transplantation. A cohort study of the relation to Epstein-Barr virus. Transplantation. March 15, 2000; 69(5):897–904.
20. Cohen JI. Epstein-Barr virus infection. N Engl J Med 2000;343:481–492.
21. Glickman JN, Howe JG, Steitz JA. Structural analysis of EBER1 and EBER2 ribonucleoprotein particles present in Epstein-Barr virus-infected cells. J Virol 1988;62:902–911.
22. Walker RC, Marshall WF, Strickler JG, et al. Pretransplantation assessment of the risk of lymphoproliferative disorder. Clin Infec Dis 1995;20(5):1346–1353.
23. Straus SE, Cohen JI, Tosato G, et al. NIH conference. Epstein-Barr virus infections: biology, pathogenesis, and management. Ann Intern Med 1993;118:45–58.
24. Yang J, Tao Q, Flinn IW, et al. Characterization of Epstein-Barr virus-infected B cells in patients with posttransplantation lymphoproliferative disease: disappearance after rituximab therapy does not predict clinical response. Blood 2000;96(13):4055–4063.
25. Spiro IJ, Yandell DW, Li C, et al. Brief report: lymphoma of donor origin occurring in the porta hepatitis of a transplanted liver. N Engl J Med 1993;329(1):27–29.
26. Ho M, Miller G, Atchinson RW, et al. Epstein-Barr virus infection and DNA hybridization studies in posttransplantation lymphoma and lymphoproliferative lesions: the role of primary infection. J Infect Dis 1985;152:876–886.
27. Weissmann DJ, Ferry JA, Harris NL, et al. Posttransplantation lymphoproliferative disorders in solid organ recipients are predominantly aggressive tumors of host origin. Am J Clin Pathol 1995;103:748–755.
28. Chadbum A, Suciu-Foca N, Cesarman E, et al. Post-transplantation lymphoproliferative disorders arising in solid organ transplant recipients are usually of recipient origin. Am J Clin Pathol 1995;1862–1870.
29. Muti G, Veronese S, Poli F, et al. Donor or recipient origin of post-transplant lymphoproliferative disorders in liver transplanted patients: two different, clinically relevant, patterns of disease. Blood 2003;102:629a.
30. Geis WP, Iwatsuki S, Molnar Z, et al. Pseudolymphoma in renal allograft recipients. Arch Surg 1978;113:461–466.
31. Fizzera G, Hanto DW, Gajl-Peczalska RJ, et al. Polymorphic diffuse B-cell hyperplasias and lymphomas in renal transplant recipients. Cancer Res 1981;41:4262–4279.
32. Harris N, Swerdlow S, Frizzera G, Knowles D. Post-transplant lymphoproliferative disorders. In: Jaffe E, Harris N, Stein H, Vardiman J. editors. World Health Organization classification of tumours. Pathology and genetics of hematopoietic and lymphoid tissues. Lyon: IARC Press; 2001. p. 264–269.
33. Nalesnik MA. The diverse pathology of post-transplant lymphoproliferative disorders: The importance of a standardized approach. Transplant Infect Dis 2001;3:88–96.
34. Rae D, Delecluse HJ, Hamilton-Dutoit SJ, et al. Epstein-Barr virus latent and replicative gene expression in post-transplant lymphoproliferative disorders and AIDS-related non-Hodgkin's lymphomas. French Study Group of Pathology for HIV-associated Tumors. Ann Oncol 1994;5(Suppl 1):113–116.
35. Badley AD, Portela DF, Patel R, et al. Development of monoclonal gammopathy precedes the development of Epstein-Barr virus-induced posttransplant lymphoproliferative disorder. Transplant Surg 1996;2:375–382.
36. Wagner HJ, Fischer L, Jabs WJ, et al. Longitudinal analysis of Epstein-Barr load in plasma and peripheral blood mononuclear cells of transplanted patients by real-time polymerase chain reaction. Transplantation 2002;74:656–664.
37. Gera M, Habermann TM, Stegall MD, et al. Viral DNA quantification in EBV-mismatched kidney transplant recipients: utility for early detection of PTLD. The 2006 World Transplant Congress, 2006. p. 416a.
38. Armitage JM, Kormos RL, Stuart RS, et al. Posttransplant lymphoproliferative disease in thoracic organ transplant patients: ten years of cyclosporine-based immunosuppression. J Heart Lung Transplant 1991;10:877–887.

39. Alfrey EJ, Freidman AL, Grossman RA, et al. A recent decrease in the time to development of monomorphous and polymorphous post-transplant lymphoproliferative disorder. Transplantation 1992;54:250–253.
40. Au WY, Lie AK, Lee CK, et al. Late onset post-transplantion lymphoproliferative disease of recipietn origin following cytogenetic relapse and occult autologous heamatopoietic regeneration after allogeneic bone marrow transplantation for acute myelogenous leukemia. Bone Marrow Transplant 2001;28:417–419.
41. Nalesnik MA. Clinicopathologic characteristics of post-transplant lymphoproliferative disorders. Recent Results Cancer Res 2002;159:9–18.
42. Nelson BP, Nalesnik MA, Bahler DW, et al. Epstein-Barr virus negative post-transplant lymphoproliferative disorders: A distinct entity? Am J Surg Pathol 2000;24:375–385.
43. Ghobrial IM, Habermann TM, Macron WR, et al. Differences between early and late post-transplant lymphoproliferative disorders in solid organ transplant patients: Are they two different diseases? Transplantationb 2005;79(2):244–247.
44. Horwitz SM, Ranheim EA, Morgan DS, et al. A unified approach to posttransplant lymphoproliferative disorder (PTLD): improved outcome and analysis of prognostic factors (Abstract 2295). Blood 1999;94(Suppl 1):10.
45. Opelz G, Dohler B. Lymphomas after solid organ transplantation: a collaborative transplant study report. Am J Transplant 2004;4:222–230.
46. Finn L, Reyes J, Bueno J, et al. Epstein-Barr virus infections in children after transplantation of the small intestine. Am J Surg Pathol 1998;22:299–309.
47. Swinnen LJ, Costatanzo-Nordin MR, Fisher SG, et al. Increased incidence of lymphoproliferative disorder after immunosuppression with monoclonal antibody OKT3 in cardiac transplant recipients. N Engl J Med 1990;323:1723–1728.
48. Cockfield SMA, Preiksaitis JK, Jewell LD, et al. Post-transplant lymphoproliferative disorder in renal allograft recipients. Transplantaion 1993;56:88–96.
49. Benkerrou MJJ, Jais JP, Leblond V, et al. Anti-B-cell monoclonal antibody treatment of severe posttransplant B-lymphoproliferative disorder: Prognostic factors and long-term outcome. Blood 1998;92:3137–3147.
50. Choquet S, Marnzer BM, Hermine O, et al. Identification of prognostic factors in post-transplant lymphoproliferative disorders. Recent Results Cancer Res 2002;159:67–80.
51. Tsai DE, Hardy CL, Tomaszewski JE, et al. Reduction in immunosuppression as initial therapy for posttransplant lymphoproliferative disorder: analysis of prognostic variables and long-term follow-up of 42 adult patients. Transplantation 2001;71:1076–1088.
52. Muti G, Cantoni S, Oreste P, et al. Post-transplant lymphoproliferative disorders: improved outcome after clinico-pathologically tailored treatment. Haematologica 2002;87:67–77.
53. Horwitz SM, Ranheim EA, Morgan DS, et al. A unified approach to posttransplant lymphoproliferative disorder (PTLD): improved outcome and analysis of prognostic factors. Blood 1999;94:513a.
54. The International Non-Hodgkin's Lymphoma Prognostic Factor Project. A predictive model for aggressive non-Hodgkin's lymphoma. N Engl J Med 1993;329:987–994.
55. Shapiro RS, McClain K, Frizzera G, et al. Epstein-Barr virus associated B-cell lymphoproliferative disorders following bone marrow transplantation. Blood 1988;71:1234–1243.
56. Darnekov IA, Marcarelli MA, Basadonna GP, et al. Reduced incidence of Epstein-Barr virus-associated posttransplant lymphoproliferative disorder using preemtive antiviral therapy. Transplantation 1997;64:848–852.
57. Davis CL, Harrison KL, McVicar JP, et al. Antiviral prophylaxsis and the Epstein Barr virus-related post-transplant lymphoproliferative disorder. Clin Transplant 1995;9:53–59.
58. Gross TG, Steinbuch M, DeFor T, et al. B-cell lymphoproliferative disorders following hematopoietic stem cell transplantation: risk factors, treatment and outcome. Bone Marrow Transplant 1999;23:251–258.
59. Green M, Bueno J, Rowe D, et al. Predictive negative value of persistent low Epstein-Barr virus viral load after intestinal transplantation in children. Transplantation 2000;70:593–596.

60. McDiarmid SV, Jordan S, Kim GS, et al. Prevention and preemptive therapy of posttransplant lymphoproliferative disease in pediatric liver recipients. Transplantation 1998;66:1604–1611.
61. Humar A, Herbert D, Davies HD, et al. A randomized trial of ganciclovir versus ganciclovir plus immune globulin for prophylaxsis against Epstein-Barr virus related posttransplant lymphoproliferative disorder. Transplantation 2006;81:856–861.
62. Kang SK, Kirkpatrick JP, Halperin EC. Low-dose radiation for posttransplant lymphoproliferative disorder. Am J Clin Oncol 2003;26:210–214.
63. Penn I. Immunosuppression-a contributory factor in lymphoma formation. Clin Transplant 1992;6:214–219.
64. Benkerrow M, Durandy A, Fischer A. Therapy for transplant-related lymphoproliferative diseases. Hematol Oncol Clin North Am 1993;7:467–475.
65. Starzl TE, Porter KA, Iwatsuki S, et al. Reversibility of lymphomas and lymphoproliferative lesions developing under cyclosporine-steroid therapy. Lancer 1984;1:583.
66. Heslop HE, Brenner MK, Rooney C, et al. Administration of neomycin-resistance-gene-marked EBV-specific cytotoxic T lymphocytes to recipients of mismatched-related or phenotypically similar unrelated donor marrow grafts. Hum Gene Ther 1994;5:381–397.
67. Loren AW, Tsai DE. Post-transplant lymphoproliferative disorder. Clin Chest Med 2005;26:631–645.
68. Taylor AL, Marcus R, Bradley JA, et al. Post-transplant lymphoproliferative disorders (PTLD) after solid organ transplantation. Crit Rev Oncol Hematol 2005;56:155–167.
69. Green M. Management of Epstein-Barr virus-induced post-transplant lymphoproliferative disease in recipients of solid organ transplantation. Am J Transplant 2001;1:103–108.
70. Doti G, Fiocchi R, Motta T, et al. Epstein-Barr virus-negative post-transplant lymphoproliferative disorders: a distinct entity? Am J Surg Pathol 2000;24:375–385.
71. McLaughlin P, Grillo-Lopez AJ, Link BK, et al. Rituximab chimeric anti-CD20 monoclonal antibody therapy for relapsed indolent lymphoma: Half of patients respond to a four-dose treatment program. J Clin Oncol 16:2825–2833.
72. Coffier B, Lepage E, Briere J, et al. CHOP chemotherapy plus rituximab compared with CHOP alone in elderly patients with diffuse large B-cell lymphoma. N Engl J Med 2002;346:235–242.
73. Habermann TM, Weller E, Morrison VA, et al. Rituximab-CHOP versus CHOP alone or with maintenance rituximab in older patients with diffuse large B-cell lymphoma. J Clin Oncol 2006;24:3121–3127.
74. Milpied N, Vasseur B, Antoine B, et al. Post-transplant lymphoproliferative disorder. Chimeric anti-CD20 monoclonal antibody (rituximab) in B-post-transplant lymphoproliferative disorders: A retrospective analysis of 32 patients (Abstract 2803). Blood 1999;94:631A.
75. Milpied N, Vasseur B, Parquet, et al. Humanized anti-CD20 monoclonal antibody (rituximab) in post-transplant B-lymphoproliferative disorder: a retrospective analysis of 32 patients. Ann Oncol 2000;11:113–116.
76. Cook R, Connors JM, Gascoyne RD, et al. Treatment of post-transplant lymphoproliferative disease with rituximab monoclonal antibody after lung transplantation. Lancet 1999;354:1698–1699.
77. Gonzalez-Barca E, Domingo-Domenech E, Gomez-Codina J, et al. First-line treatment with rituximab improves survival of patients with post-transplant lymphoproliferative disease (PTLD). Blood 2004;104:394a.
78. Ghobrial IM, Habermann TM, Ristow KM, et al. Prognostic factors in patients with post-transplant lymphoproliferative disorders (PTLD) in the rituximab era. Leuk Lymphoma 2005;46:191–196.
79. Elstrom RI, Andreadis C, Aqui NA, et al. Treatment of PTLD with rituximab or chemotherapy. Am J Transplant 2006;6:569–576.
80. Choquet S, Leblond V, Herbrecht R, et al. Efficacy and safety of rituximab in B-cell post-transplantation lymphoproliferative disorders: results of a prospective multicenter phase 2 study. Blood 2006;107:3053–3057.

81. Oertel SH, Verschuuren E, Reinke P, et al. Effect of anti-CD20 antibody rituximab in patients with post-transplant lymphoproliferative disorder (PTLD). Am J Transplant 2005;5:2901–2906.
82. Orjeula M, Gross TG, Cheung YK, et al. A pilot study of chemoimmunotherapy (cylophosphamide, prednisone, and rituximab) in patients with post-transplant lymphoproliferative disorder following solid organ transplantation. Clin Cancer Res 2003;9:3945S–3952S.
83. Voog E, Morschhauser F, Solal-Celigny P, et al. Neutropenia in patients treated with rituximab. N Engl J Med 2003;348:2691–2694.
84. Dervite I, Hober D, Morel P. Acute hepatitis B in a patient with antibodies to hepatitis B surface antigen who was receiving rituximab. N Engl J Med 2001;344:68–69.
85. Sharma VR, Fleming DR, Slone SP. Pure red cell aplasia due to parvovirus B19 in a patient treated with rituximab. Blood 2000;96:1184–1186.
86. Suzan F, Ammor M, Ribrag V. Fatal reactivation of cytomegalovirus infection after use of rituximab for a post-transplantion lymphoproliferative disorder. N Engl J Med 2001;345:1000.
87. Hochster HS, Weller E, Gascoyne RD, et al. Maintenance rituximab after CVP results in superior clinical outcome in advanced follicular lymphoma (FL): Results of the E1496 phase III trial from the Eastern Cooperative Oncology Group and the Cancer and Leukemia Group B. Blood 2005;106:196a.
88. van Esser JW, Niesters HG, van der Holt B, et al. Prevention of Epstein-Barr virus-lymphoproliferative disease by molecular monitoring and preemptive rituximab in high-risk patients after allogeneic stem cell transplantation. Blood 2002;99:4364–4369.
89. Hanto DW, Frizzera G, Galj-Peczalska, et al. Epstein Barr virus, immunodeficiency, and B-cell lymphoproliferation. Transplantation 1985;39:461–472.
90. Raymond E, Tricottet V, Samuel D, et al. Epstein-Barr virus-related lymphoproliferative disorders treated with cyclophosphamide-doxorubicin-vincristine-prednisone chemotherapy. Cancer 1995;72:1344–1351.
91. Lien Y-H, Schroter GPJ, Weil R III, et al. Complete remission and possible immune tolerance after multidrug combination chemotherapy for cyclosporine-related lymphoma in a renal transplant patient with acute pancreatitis. Transplantation 1991;52:739–742.
92. Garrett TJ, Chadburn A, Barr ML, et al. Posttransplantation lymphoproliferative disorders treated with cyclophosphamide-doxorubicin-vincristine-prednisone chemotherapy. Cancer 1993;72:2782–2785.
93. Swinnen LJ, Mullen GM, Carr TJ, et al. Aggressive treatment for postcardiac transplant lymphoproliferation. Blood 1995;86:3333–3340.
94. VanGorp J, Doornewaard H, Verdonck LF, et al. Post-transplant T-cell lymphoma. Cancer 1994;73:3064–3072.
95. Hanson MN, Morrison VA, Peterson BA, et al. Posttransplant T-cell lymphoproliferative disorders-an aggressive, late complication of solid-organ transplantation. Blood 1996;88:3626–3633.
96. Dotti G, Fiocchi R, Motta T, et al. Lymphomas occurring late after solid-organ transplantaion: influence of treatment on the clinical outcome. Transplantation 2002;74:1095–1102.
97. Buell JF, Gross TG, Hanaway MJ, et al. Chemotherapy for posttransplant lymphoproliferative disorder: the Isreal Penn International Transplant Tumor Registry experience. Transplant Proc 2005;37:956–957.
98. Gross TG, Bucuvalas JC, Park JR, et al. Low-dose chemotherapy for Epstein-Barr virus-positive post-transplantation lymphoptoliferative disease in children after solid organ transplantation. J Clin Oncol 2005;23:6481–6488.
99. Oertel SH, Papp-Vary M, Anagnostopoulos I, et al. Salvage chemotherapy for refractory or relapsed post-transplant lymphoproliferative disorder in patients after solid organ transplantation with a combination of carboplatin and etoposide. Br J Haematol 2003;123:830–835.
100. Komrokji RS, Oliva JL, Zand M, et al. Mini-BEAM and autologous hematopoietic stem-cell transplant for treatment of post-transplant lymphoproliferative disorders. Am J Hematol 2005;79:211–215.
101. Bobey NA, Stewart DA, Woodman RC, et al. Successful treatment of posttransplant lymphoproliferative disorder in a renal transplant patient by autologous peripheral blood stem cell transplantation. Leuk Lymphoma 2002;43:2421–2423.

102. Tosato G, Tanner J, Jones KD, et al. Identification of interleukin-6 as an autocrine growth factor for Epstein-Barr virus-immortalized B cells. J Virol 1990;64:3033–3041.
103. Tosato G, Jones K, Breinig MK, et al. Interleukin-6 production in posttransplant lymphoproliferative disease. J Clin Invest 1003;91:2906–2814.
104. Haddad E, Paszesny S, Leblond V, et al. Treatment of B-lymphoproliferative disorder with a monoclonal anti-interleukin-6 antibody in 12 patients: a multicenter phase 1–2 clinical trial. Blood 2001;97:1590–1597.
105. Papadopoulos EB, Ladanyi M, Emanuel D, et al. Infusions of donor leukocytes to treat Epstein-Barr virus-associated lymphoproliferative disorders after allogeneic bone marrow transplantation. N Engl J Med 1994;330:1165–1191.
106. Rooney CM, Smith CA, Ng CY, et al. Infusion of cytotoxic T cells for the prevention and treatment of Epstein-Barr virus-induced lymphoma in allogeneic transplant recipients. Blood 1998;92:1549–1555.
107. Gulley ML, Swinnen LJ, Plaisance KT, et al. Tumor origin and CD20 expression in posttransplant lymphoproliferative disorder occurring in solid organ transplant recipients: implications for immune-based therapy. Transplantation 2003;76:959–964.
108. Nalesnik MA, Rao AS, Furukawa H, et al. Autologous lymphokine activated killer cell therapy of Epstein-Barr virus-positive and –negative lymphoproliferative disorder in solid organ transplant recipients with evidence of active virus replication. Blood 2002;99:2592–2598.
109. Comoli P, Labirio M, Basso S, et al. Infusion of autologous Epstein-Barr virus (EBV)-specific cytotoxic T cells for prevention of EBV-related lymphoproliferative disorder in solid organ transplant recipients with evidence of active viral replication. Blood 2002;99:2592–2598.
110. Comoli P, Maccario R, Locatelli F, et al. Treatment of EBV-related post-renal transplant lymphoproliferative disease with a tailored regimen including EBV-specific T cells. Am J Transplant 2005;5:1415–1422.
111. Haque T, Amlot PL, Helling N, et al. Reconstitution of EBV-specific T cell immunity in solid organ transplant recipients. J Immunol 1998;160:6204–6209.
112. Khanna R, Bell S, Sherritt M, et al. Activation and adoptive transfer of Epstein-Barr virus-specific cytotoxic T cells in solid organ transplant patients with posttransplant lymphoproliferative disease. Proc Natl Acad Sci USA 1999;96:10,391–10,396.
113. Sherritt MA, Bharadwaj M, Burrows JM, et al. Resconstitution of the latent T-lymphocyte response to Epstein-Barr virus is coincident with long-term recovery from transplant lymphoma after adoptive immunotherapy. Transplantaion 2003;75:1556–1560.
114. Savoldo B, Gross JA, Hammer MM, et al. Treatment of solid organ transplant recipients with autologous Epstein Barr virus-specific cytotoxic T lymphocytes (CTLs). Blood 2006;108:2942–2949.
115. Metes D, Storkus W, Zeevi A, et al. Ex vivo generation of effective Epstein-Barr virus (EBV)-specific CD8+ cytotoxic T lymphocytes from the peripheral blood of immunocompetent Epstein Barr virus-seronegative individuals. Transplantation 2000;70:1507–1515.
116. Popescu I, Macedo C, Zeevi A, et al. Ex vivo priming of naive T cells into EBV-specific Th1/Tc1 effector cells by mature autologous DC loaded with apoptotic/necrotic LCL. Am J Transplant 2003;3:1369–1377.
117. Haque T, Wilkie GM, Taylor C, et al. Treatment of Epstein-Barr-virus-positive posttransplantation lymphoproliferative disease with partly HLA-matched allogeneic cytotoxic T cells. Lancet 2002;360:436–442.
118. Wilkie GM, Taylor C, Jones MM, et al. Establishment and characterization of a bank of cytotoxic T lymphocytes for immunotherapy of Epstein-Barr virus-associated diseases. J Immunother 2004;27:309–316.
119. Cesarman E, Chadburn A, Yi-Fang Liu, et al. BCL-6 gene mutations in posttransplantation lymphoproliferative disorders predict response to therapy and clinical outcomes. Blood 1998;92:2294–2302.
120. Capello D, Cerri M, Muti G, et al. Molecular histgenesis of posttransplantation lymphoproliferative disorders. Blood 2003;102:3775–3785.

121. Gasink LB, Blumberg EA, Lacalio AR, et al. Hepatitis C virus seropositivity in organ donors and survival in heart transplant recipients. JAMA 2006;296:1843–1850.
122. Majewski M, Korecka M, Kossev P, et al. The immunosuppressive macrolide RAD inhibits growth of human Epstein-Barr virus-transformed B lymphocytes in vitro and in vivo; a potential approach to prevention and treatment of posttransplant lymphoproliferative disorders. Proc Natl Acad Sci USA 2000;97:4285–4290.

Chapter 13
Castleman Disease

Angela Dispenzieri

13.1 Introduction

Castleman's disease (CD) was first described in 1954 and further defined in 1956 by Dr. Castleman (1) (Figure 13.1). He reported on patients possessing localized mediastinal lymph node enlargement that was characterized by redundancy of lymphoid follicles with germinal-center involution as well as marked capillary proliferation with endothelial hyperplasia in both follicular and interfollicular regions. Prior cases had been reported, but were anecdotal in nature (2, 3). In 1962, Lattes and Pachter evaluated 12 cases and suggested that these lymph nodes were hamartomatous in nature (4). Lee described refractory anemia associated with CD that responded to surgical resection 5, and by 1967, Tung and McCormack described 5 new cases and reviewed the 62 cases described to that point in the literature (6), highlighting the potential for associated hypochromic anemia, hyper-gammaglobulinemia, and bone marrow plasmacytosis.

In 1969, in a review of his own 13 patients plus a review of the 92 cases reported in the literature, Flendrig described three types of: benign giant lymphoma": the plasma cell variant,the hyalinized variant, and the "intermediate variant" (7, 8). Flendrig noted that those patients with what is now called the plasma cell variant were more likely to have B-symptoms as well as anemia and hypergammaglob-ulinemia. He postulated that the plasma cell variant transitions into the hyaline vascular variant, defining what we now call the "mixed" variant, but which he called an intermediate variant (9). In 1972, Keller et al expanded upon Flendrig's work after performing a clinicopathologic analysis of 81 cases of angiofollicular lymph node hyperplasia (8). He coined the expressions plasma cell type (PCV) and hyaline vascular type (HVV), which have superseded Flendrig's: type I" and "type II" nomenclature. Gaba and associates reported the first case of multicentric Castleman disease in 1978 (10). By the mid-1980s, investigators began describing several of the salient differences between HVV and PCV and their respective associations with unicentric (unifocal or localized) and multicentric (multifocal or generalized) presentations (11, 12) (Table 13.1).

Also during this time frame, there were increasing numbers of cases of CD that were associated with peripheral neuropathy (10, 13–17), highlighting the overlap

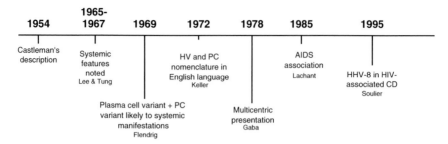

Figure 13.1 Timeline of Castleman disease discoveries.(Compiled from Refs. 1 and 5–10)

Table 13.1 Classification of Castleman disease

	Unicentric	Multicentric
Age	Fourth decade	Sixth decade
Symptoms	Incidental or compressive; occ systemic symptoms	Fever, sweats, weight loss, malaise, autoimmune manifestations; might be associated with peripheral neuropathy and POEMS syndrome
Organomegaly	Rare	Yes
Distribution of lymphadenopathy	Central (mediastinal, abdominal) most common	Peripheral plus central
Laboratory abnormalities	Occasional. Anemia, hypergammaglobulinemia, increased ESR, CRP	Common. Anemia, thrombocytopenia, hypergammaglobulinemia, increased ESR, CRP, abnormal LFTs, low albumin, renal dysfunction
Pathology	HV, occ mixed or PC	PC, mixed, and occ HV
HIV association	No	Some
HHV-8 association	No	Yes (23, 83, 197, 203)
Therapy	Surgery; occ radiation if inoperable	Assorted systemic therapies with variable success (see text)
Clinical course	Benign	Usually aggressive

occ, occasional; POEMS, peripheral neuropathy, organomegaly, endocrinopathy, monoclonal protein, and skin changes; HV, hyaline vascular variant; PC, plasma cell variant; CRP, C-reactive protein, ESR, erythrocyte sedimentation rate; LFTs, liver function tests.
Source: Data compiled from Refs. 12, 19, 21, 24, 28–30, and 85.

between CD and POEMS syndrome (peripheral neuropathy, organomegaly, endocrinopathy, monoclonal protein, skin changes).

Other terminology used historically to describe the entity known as Castleman disease or angiofollicular lymph node hyperplasia included angiofollicular and plasmacytic polyadenopathy, benign giant lymphoma, giant lymph node hyperplasia, follicular lymphoreticuloma, giant hemolymph node, idiopathic plasmacytic lymphadenopathy with polyclonal hypergammaglobulinemia, lymph nodal hamartoma, lymphoid hamartoma or choristoma, multicentric angiofollicular hyperplasia, and tumorlike proliferation of lymphoid tissue (18, 19).

13.2 Epidemiology

As many men as women are affected. The age distribution is bimodal, with unifocal patients being in their fourth decade versus patients with multicentric disease being in their sisxth decade (11, 20, 21). CD occurs not uncommonly in the pediatric population, and there is a suggestion that the pediatric population might have a better prognosis than that of the adult population (22). There are little data of the actual incidence or prevalence of this disorder, but it is considered to be a rare lymphoproliferative disease. With the AIDS epidemic, the incidence has increased (23); but even in this population, it is a rare condition, with CD lymph nodes accounting for fewer than 2% of lymph node biopsies in HIV⁺ patients (24). Nearly all HIV⁺ CD patients are infected with human herpes virus-8 [HHV-8; also known as Kaposi's sarcoma virus (KSV]) (23).

13.3 Pathogenesis/Pathology

The underlying pathogenesis of CD is not understood. Early on, it was thought that the HVV tumors were possibly hamartomas (4). An extraordinary case of identical twins who developed CD in the same location 2 years apart from each other (25) supported this notion. However, most authors including Castleman have speculated that CD is a chronic nonspecific inflammatory process in reaction to an unknown stimulus (1, 8). The differential phenotype (HVV vs. PCV) would then be explained by either a continuum of disease, a differential host-dependent immune response, or reactions to two different but closely related stimuli. Further speculation has revolved around which cell type (stromal cells, endothelial cells, lymphocytes, or plasma cells) drives the process. A number of viral pathogens, like Epstein-Barr virus (EBV), cytomegalovirus (CMV), and HHV-8, have been studied looking for a pathogenic link.

13.3.1 Pathology of Hyaline Vascular Variant

On gross pathology these lesions tend to be large, single, rounded, encapsulated masses—more commonly to be found in central than peripheral lymph node regions. Adjacent lymph nodes might be enlarged and involved with the identical process (8, 11). Most masses are between 5 and 10 cm, although lesions as large as

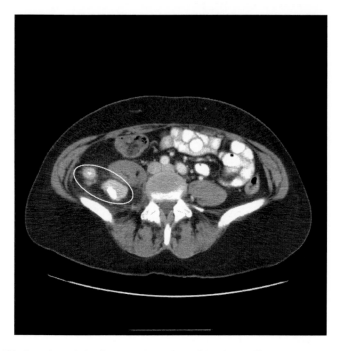

Figure 13.2 CT of a unicentric hyaline vascular variant of Castleman disease displacing the right psoas muscle

Table 13.2 Histology of Castleman disease variants

	Hyaline Vascular Variant (HVV)	Plasma cell variant (PCV)
Follicular size	Small	Normal to large
Capillaries	Increased in number (hyalinized)	No increase
Interfollicular zone	Plasma cells, eosinophils, lymphoblasts	Sheets of plasma cells

Source: Modified from Ref. 87.

25 cm have been described (Figure 13.2). On microscopic examination (Table 13.2), HVV is characterized by the presence of large follicles separated by vascular lymphoid tissue containing lymphocytes (1) (Figure 13.3). There is regressive transformation of the germinal centers, often producing multiple small, burned-out geminal centers within one follicular area. Within and between the follicles there are increased numbers of small vessels with sclerosis and loss of sinuses, which is pathonomic for HVV. The endothelial cells of the capillaries are often plump and mitotic figures might be seen (6, 8). Among the vessels, there is a variable mixture of cells, usually dominated by lymphocytes, but polyclonal plasma cells and eosinophils might also be seen. There is, however, a large variation in the proportions of these components. Large areas of some lesions might be sclerosed, and within such areas, calcification might be present (8). In most cases, there are remnants of lymph node architecture within an affected lymph node. Adjacent lymph nodes

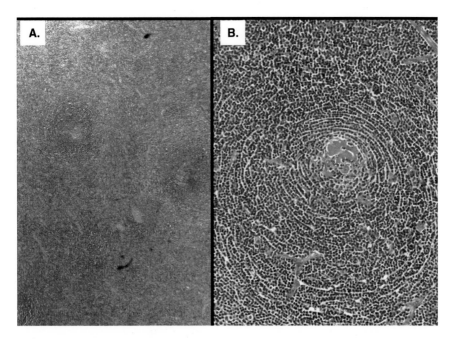

Figure 13.3 Hyaline vacular variant histology. **(A)** Hyaline vascular variant low-power view with reactive follicles and an interfollicular infiltrate of small lymphoid cells and fibrosis as well as increased vascularization of the interfollicular space. **(B)** High-power view showing the B-cell follicle with typical expanded mantle zone showing "onion skin'" pattern and depleted, hyalinized germinal center with increased vascularity. (Courtesy of Dr. Ahmet Dogan)

might be involved, with a spectrum of findings from normal nodal architecture to identical histology to the initial site to somewhere in between (8).

13.3.2   Pathology of Plasma Cell Variant

The gross specimen is that of multiple discrete lymph nodes, comprising the clinically observed "mass." This is distinct from the single rounded mass that is typically seen with HVV (8, 11). Microscopically (Table 13.2), PCV is distinguished by the presence of sheets of plasma cells (PCs) in the interfollicular zone (Figure 13.4) (8). This marked plasmacytosis might be comprised of immunoblastic proliferation along with prominent high endothelial venules, or of mature plasma cells without increased vascularity. Russell bodies are commonly present (8, 26) and binucleated plasma cells might be seen, but mitoses of PCs are rare (26). Some eosinophils and mast cells might also be present (26). There is germinal-center hyperplasia also characterized by sharp borders within the mantle zones and by "polarization" with the light area directed toward the capsular or trabecular sinus (27). Within the follicles, there are mitotic figures, nuclear fragments, histiocytes, and cells resembling lymphoblasts.

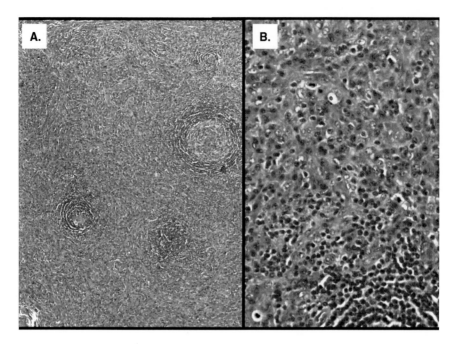

Figure 13.4 Plasma cell variant histology. **(A)** Low-power view with small reactive follicles and an interfollicular infiltrate of plasma cells; lack of vascular proliferation. **(B)** High-power view showing the plasma cell component. Lower left corner contains a small part of a reactive follicle. (Courtesy of Dr. Ahmet Dogan)

13.3.3 Mixed Variant of Castleman Disease

Lymph nodes have characteristics of both HVV and PCV. Focal accumulations of plasma cells next to extensive areas without plasma cells are found in the interfollicular tissue (9). Characteristic lymphoid follicles with normal reaction centers and pseudo-Hassall's corpuscles are found in small areas.

13.3.4 Histologic Differential Diagnosis of CD

The differential diagnoses for CD are broad. Initially, HVV cases were most commonly confused with thymomas because the intrafollicular capillaries with thick hyalinized walls take on a concentric arrangement—the so called "onion skin appearance"—that can be confused for Hassall corpuscle of the thymus (1). More often, HVV might be confused with other conditions in which there is regressive transformation of germinal centers (GCs), like angioimmunoblastic lymphadenopathy, other atypical lymphoproliferative disorders, and advanced phase of HIV-related lymphadenopathy (27–29). In these cases there is a variable degree of condensation of the germinal center. This condensation is due to the progressive disappearance of the lymphoid component of the GC, crowding and sclerosis of the vessels, and increased prominence of the follicular dendritic reticular cell (FDRC) component. The increase in the FDRC can occur, either by concentration or by proliferation.

The PCV "is an overabused diagnosis for a lymph node pattern of germinal center hyperplasia (with or without some regressive transformation) and marked plasmacytosis" (27). This pattern, which might be associated with either immunoblastic proliferation and prominent high endothelial venules or with all mature plasma cells with no increase of the vascularity, might be seen in several other conditions, like autoimmune diseases, primary or acquired immunodeficiencies, or in association with malignancies (27–29). Increased follicular size, mitotic rate, and numbers of intrafollicular tingible body macrophages per follicle can be used to distinguish nonspecific reactive lymph nodes from CD (30).

13.3.5 Histology of Other Tissues

About 75% of patients with multicentric disease have hepatosplenomegaly. Splenic findings might include altered germinal centers, white pulp or marginal zone fibrosis, and prominent plasmacytosis (11, 31). Splenic findings parallel those found in the lymph nodes.

Liver biopsy results are quite varied. Findings might be nonspecific. Peliosis hepatitis, the presence of blood filled cysts in the liver parenchyma secondary to dilated hepatic sinusoids, has been seen (11, 32–34). Micronodular cirrhosis associated with large fibrotic masses resembling hyaline vascular germinal centers of the lymph node has also been described.

13.3.6 Stromal Cells in CD

The stromal background of CD, especially in HVV, is quite striking. How much stroma is present can be variable, and Krishnan et al. have proposed subdividing HVV into a lymphoid variant, in which the lymphoid follicles largely predominate, and a stromal-rich variant, in which the follicles are almost overrun by the proliferation of vessels and/or stromal cells (27). By immunohistochemistry, these whorled centers contain some factor VIII-positive cells suggesting endothelial origin (35). By electron microscopy (EM), the whorled follicle centers are comprised mainly of dendritic reticulum cells (36). Moreover, these FDRCs might be polyploid and have prominent nucleoli, which connotes dysplasia (37). These cells might also aberrantly express adhesion molecules (38). These dysplastic changes are more common in HVV (27, 37, 38) but mightalso be seen in PCV (37). In the majority of PCV cases, the network these FDRCs form is similar to that seen in normal or reactive germinal centers. However, two aberrant phenotypes are commonly seen in HVV: an expanded, disrupted follicular dendritic cell network or multiple tight collections of follicular dendritic cells (39). There are data that suggest that the FDRCs are the primary source of interleukin (IL)-6 in CD (40, 41), which drives the lymphocyte infiltrate seen in PCV (41). Finally, there are four reports of clonal karyotypic abnormalities derived from the stromal elements: (1) 46,XX, t(1;16) (p11;p11), del(7)(q21q22), del(8)(q12q22) (42); (2) 46,XX, add(1)(q21), der(6)t(6;12) (q23;q15), add(7)(p22), -9, inv(9)(p11q13), del(12)(q15),+mar (43); (3) t(1;22)qter;q13 44; and 4) t(7;8)(q37.3;q12) (44).

These observations about the FDRCs are compelling for two reasons. The first is that there is an apparent increased incidence of dendritic sarcoma in patients with CD (45) and other non-KSV vascular neoplasms (46, 47). The second is the association of HHV-8 (aka KSV), CD, Kaposi's sarcoma, and lymphoma in AIDS patients.

13.3.7   The Lymphoplasmacytic Compartment

In addition to FDRCs, there are lymphocytes, plasma cells, and eosinophils within CD lymph nodes. The spectrum of distribution can be broad. Frizzera has divided PCV into proliferative and accumulative patterns based on the number and size of germinal centers, their composition, and the extent of immature lymphoid cells (11). Menke et al have speculated that PCV is a immune disorder characterized by proliferation of an immunophenotypically abnormal population of mantle zone lymphocytes (aberrantly lacking Ki-B3 and/or Ki-B5) (37). These lymphocytes might be of CD5$^+$ B-lymphocyte origin (37, 48)—an autoantibody producing subset—which is sustained by local factors such as IL-6 produced by FDRCs (41). In addition, CD45 RA$^+$ lymphocytes are absent in the mantle zone in CD lymph nodes (37). The T-cell infiltrate are predominantly CD4 cells with a paucity of CD8 cells in PCs (12, 49). T-Cell gene rearrangement studies have been performed by a handful of investigators. The vast majority show no T-cell clones (44, 48, 50, 51).

13.3.8   Is Castleman Disease a Clonal Disorder?

There is contradictory information about whether the interfollicular plasma cells are clonal (Table 13.3) (12, 17, 26, 35, 37, 48–64). The majority of studies are based on immunohistochemical investigations, but some authors have also looked for clonality using molecular techniques. Despite the contradictions, there are a few unifying points. Typically, the PCV cases were more commonly monotypic than the HVV cases. The lymphocytes found in the follicles or the interfollicular regions are not clonal. Plasma cells in the interfollicular zones might sometimes be monotypic—most commonly lambda light-chain restricted—but the majority are not. If plasmablasts

Table 13.3 Defining clonality in Castleman disease

Ref.	Localization	Subtype	Immunohistochemical	Notes
			HIV-negative patients	
17	1 M	1 PCV	Monotypic	
52	1 U	1 PCV	Monotypic	
53	NS	1 Mixed	Monotypic	
54	1 M	1 PCV	Monotypic	No clonal IGH rearrangement
55	1 U; 1 M	2 PCV	1 polytypic; 1 monotypic	
35	9 U	9 PCV	2 monotypic	
12	16 M	3 HVV; 13 PCV	1 PCV monotypic[a]	
48	4 U 1 M	5 PCV	Monotypic × 2; polytypic × 2; Equiv monotypic ×1	First 3 patients had clonal IgH gene rearrangement
26	15 U 3 M	18 PCV	7 monotypic	
56	2 M	2 PCV	1 monotypic; 1 polytypic	1 IgH rearrangement; 1 w/o clonal IGH rearrangement; TCR germline
37	Not stated	9 HVV 21 PCV	1 monotypic 4 monotypic	IgH rearrangements in 4/9 IgH rearrangements in 3/21
57	5 M	5 PCV	2 monotypic All other polytypic	The 2 monotypic cases were only 2 with detectable plasmablasts
51	2 U 3 M 15 U	2 PCV 3 PCV 15 HVV	1 M was monotypic	1 with IgH gene rearrangement
58	4 U 16 M	4 HVV 3 HVV 9 PCV 4 Mixed	Not done	4 w/o clonal IgH rearrangement 2 IgH rearrangement (both NHL) 15 w/o clonal IgH rearrangement 2 IgH rearrangement (1 HD & 1 POEMS)
59	Not stated	4 HVV; 1 mixed; 1 PCV	All polytypic	
60	1 M	1 PCV	All polytypic	
61	1 U	1 PCV	All polytypic	Adjacent monotypic plasmacytoma
62	5 M	5 PC variant	All polytypic	
63	9 M	9 PCV	All polytypic	
50	4 U 4 M	3 HVV; 1 PCV 4 PCV	All polytypic	3/4 multicentric with IgH gene rearrangement
49	1 U	1 mixed	Polytypic	No clonal IgH rearrangement; TCR germline

(continued)

Table 13.3 (continued)

Ref.	Localization	Subtype	Immunohistochemical	Notes
64	25 M	25 PCV[b]	Polytypic	Only the HHV-8+ cases had mantle zone plasmablasts; these cells were monotypic lambda in 4 of 6.
			HIV-positive patients	
58	30 M	1 HVV; 6 PCV; 7 Mixed	Not done	14 w/o clonal IgH rearrangement
57	8 M	8 PCV	8 monotypic (plasmablasts)	2 of 3 had clonal IgH rearrangements

M, multicentric; U, unicentric; HVV, hyaline vascular variant; PCV, plasma cell variant.
[a]Prior LN biopsy 4 years earlier had been polytypic.
[b]Three HIV-positive.

are present in the mantle zone and/or interfollicular regions, these are the cells most likely to express monotypic light chains and/or have clonal immunoglobulin gene rearrangement (57, 64). Plasmablasts are more likely to be present in HHV-8+ cases. It should be noted, however, that not infrequently is there discordance in determining clonality between the immunostains and molecular techniques [polymerase chain reaction (PCR) or Southern blot analyses].

Even in the context of HIV/AIDS, the issue of clonality is contradictory (57, 58). In one study, of eight MCD PC/HIV+ patients studied, all had lambda-restricted plasmablasts, but only two of the three tested by molecular techniques could be confirmed as being clonal (57). However, in another study in which only molecular techniques were used, only 3 of 14 had minor clones identified (58).

Several possible explanations have been postulated. It is possible that a virus (e.g., HHV-8) might infect IgM-positive naïve B-cells and drive them to differentiate into plasmablasts without undergoing the germinal-center reaction (65). Alternatively, HHV-8 or another similar virus, could naturally target both kappa and lambda light-chain-expressing B-cells without bias, but with only lambda cells expanding preferentially due an intrinsic proliferative response to the viral infection (65).

13.3.9 Cytokines

Overproduction of circulating cytokines is implicated in the pathogenesis and symptomotology of CD and its sister syndrome, peripheral neuropathy, organomegaly, endocrinopathy, monoclonal protein, skin changes (POEMS) syndrome (66). Serum levels of IL-6 in CD patients are significantly higher than those found in patients with Hodgkin's disease, diffuse large cell lymphoma, or multiple myeloma. The causative association is based on several observations. The first is that removal of the lymph node masses causes an abrupt drop in IL-6 levels and resolution of symptoms (67). The second is that treatment with IL-6 receptor antibody also relieves the symptoms and signs of the disorder (68). The third is that overexpression of IL-6 in mice produces a phenotype similar to the MCD phenotype (69). High IL-6 levels might contribute to the plasma cell infiltration of lymph nodes, polyclonal hypergammaglobulinemia, increased level of acute-phase proteins, and constitutional symptoms.

Vascular endothelial growth factor (VEGF) is also elevated in CD patients, but less so than in patients with POEMS syndrome (66). Increased VEGF expression has been observed in the interfollicular area of CD lymph nodes and in the supernatant of cultured PCV lymph nodes (70). In one study, five of eight cases of CD, germinal centers containing small vessels expressed VEGF by *in situ* hybridization (71). VEGF, which induces endothelial proliferation and endothelial permeability, could account for the hypervascular skin lesions, the peripheral edema and anasarca.

13.3.10   The Role of Viruses, Especially HHV-8 and HIV

From the initial recognition of CD, it was postulated that a virus might be a driving factor for the disorder. Although there had been initial reports linking EBV to CD (50), this has not been substantiated (56, 72, 73). CMV does not play a role in CD (50). However, HHV-8 and HIV appear to play a significant role in a subset of patients.

In 1985, Lachant et al. reported on two homosexual males with the acquired immunodeficiency syndrome (AIDS) who developed multicentric CD followed by Kaposi's sarcoma (KS) (74). More cases followed. In 1995, Soulier reported on the incidence of HHV-8 in 31 multicentric Castleman disease (MCD) patients based on the three following observations: lymphoma and KS were malignancies that had been described in 10–20% of patients with MCD prior to the AIDS epidemic; similar clinical and pathologic features of MCD had been reported in HIV$^+$ patients with lymph node hyperplasia; and among HIV$^+$ patients, 75% of MCD patients also had KS during the course of their disease (23). All 14 of the HIV$^+$ patients tested had HHV-8 DNA sequences in their CD lymph nodes, whereas, 7 of 17 HIV-negative MCD patients had HHV-8 DNA sequences present.

Other investigators have confirmed that nearly all HIV$^+$ CD cases contain HHV-8$^+$ and that nearly half of HIV$^-$ MCD are HHV-8$^+$ (64, 72, 73, 75, 76) (Table 13.4). This is in stark contrast to the roughly 7% HHV-8$^+$ rate in non-HIV, non-CD, reactive lymph nodes (73). HHV-8 sequences have also been found in the peripheral blood mononuclear cells (PBMC) of some CD patients, more commonly the HIV$^+$ group (23, 77). HHV-8 has also been found in the bone marrow of HIV$^+$/HHV8$^+$ CD patients (78). HHV-8 can be found in intranodal B-lymphocytes, in endothelial cells, and in subcapsular spindle cell proliferations. In one study, the highest copy number was in subcapsular spindle cells (75); in contrast, viral IL-6 (vIL-6) is not expressed in KS spindle cells (72). The HHV-8 gene expression

Table 13.4 HHV-8 infectivity and Castleman disease

Ref.	N	HIV	HHV-8+	Comments
Soulier et al. 1995 (23)	14 M/PCV	+	14	
Gessain et al. 1996 (77)	6 M	+	5/6	All 5 had cutaneous KS
Suda et al. 2001 (76)	3 M	+	3/3	
O'Leary et al. 2000 (75)	1 U 2 M	+	3/3	
Menke et al. 2002 (80)	PCV	Clinically no	9/15	
O'Leary et al. 2000 (75)	9 U 4 M	−	1/9 3/4	
Suda et al. 2001 (76)	79 M	−	0/79	
Soulier et al. 1995 (23)	17 M/PCV	−	7	
Chadburn et al. 1997 (73)	6 U 5 M	−	0/6 3/5	
Luppi et al. 1996 (204)	7 U (HVV) 5 M (PCV)	−	0/12	
Gessain et al. 1996 (77)	3 U 4 M	− −	0/3 1/4	
Parravinci et al. 1997 (72)	3 U HVV 7 M PCV 6 U PCV	−	0/3 6/7 0/6	4 patients developed KS and 2 patients NHL
Belec et al. 1999 (83)	9 M	−	7/9	All had POEMS
Tohuda et al. 2001 (205)	7 M 3 POEMS	—	3/7 0/3	

U, unicentric; M, multicentric; HVV, hyaline vascular variant; PCV, plasma cell variant.

patterns are different in HHV8-associated CD as compared to the two known HHV-8-associated malignancies, KS and primary effusion lymphoma (PEL). In CD, both latent and lytic proteins are expressed; in KS and PEL, predominantly latent genes are expressed (79). One of these lytic phase proteins is vIL-6. vIL-6 expression occurs in the lymphoid cells of 25–100% of HHV8+ CD patients and is associated with an inferior survival (72, 80).

13.3.11 HIV+ Castleman Disease

There are differences between HIV+ CD and HIV− CD. The former is almost always associated with HHV-8 (81), whereas only a minority of HIV− CD case are. In the HIV+ cases, there is a much higher risk of evolution to lymphoma (57) and the MCD course is more fulminant. Morphologically, there are differences as well. HIV+ patients more typically have plasmablasts (CD20+, CD30−) in the mantle zone

(57). These plasmablasts (or immunoblasts) express IgM with lambda immunoglobulin light-chain restriction by immunohistochemistry. These cells also express HHV-8 latent nuclear antigen and are highly proliferative. This type of plasmablast is not commonly observed in HIV⁻ CD, but when present, it is more likely to be present in the context of HHV-8 infection.

The very remarkable feature of these monotypic plasmablasts—and even some of the resultant plasmablastic lymphomas—is that they are usually shown to be polyclonal by molecular techniques (65). Moreover, they are typically germline consistent with being naïve B-cells, despite their mature phenotype (by morphology and by high expression of cytoplasmic Ig and CD27, which is a marker for memory B-cells) (65).

Castleman disease is has long been thought to be related to overproduction of IL-6 and, to some extent, to hyperresponsiveness to IL-6 (41, 82). The viral homologue of IL-6 exhibits many of the biological activities of human IL-6, but the relative importance of vIL-6 and human IL-6 has not yet been clarified. It appears, however, that the sites of expression of these two types of IL-6 are distinct. Human IL-6 expression can be localized to the germinal centers arising form the follicular dendritic cells, which are located outside the sinuses, but in close contact with blood vessels and plasma cells (41, 81), whereas vIL-6 is localized to the mantle zone and interfollicular regions emanating from lymphoid-derived cells (72, 80, 81). In HIV⁺ MCD, clinical symptoms correlate with high levels of plasma human IL-6 and IL-10 accompanied by a 1.7-log increment of HHV-8 copy numbers in peripheral blood mononuclear cells (81).

13.3.12   HIV⁻ CD

There is some suggestion that HIV⁻ MCD patients who are HHV-8⁺ have a different disease both clinically (72, 73) and morphologically (64), as compared to their HHV8⁻ counterparts. In one series, the three HHV-8⁺ patients had a significantly worse clinical course than did the eight HHV-8⁻ patients; however, six of the eight HHV-8⁻ patients had unicentric disease (73), which is known to be associated with a better outcome. In another study of HIV⁻ CD patients, seven out of eight HHV-8⁻ patients had localized and limited disease, whereas all six HHV-8⁺ patients had multicentric PCV with other features of immune dysfunction (72). In yet another study, HHV-8 DNA sequences were present in the tissues of about 88% of HIV⁻, POEMS associated CD, but fewer than 10% of POEMS patients without CD (23, 83).

In addition, HHV⁺ CD might have morphologic characteristics that differentiate it from HHV⁻ CD. After studying the lymph node architecture of HHV-8⁺ ($n = 6$) and HHV-8⁻ ($n = 19$) patients with PCV, Amin et al. concluded that HHV-8⁺ PCV is morphologically distinct because there is an accumulation of infected lymphocytes in the mantle zone, which leads to progressive blurring and dissolution of the germinal center and altered regulation of the surrounding stroma (64). Other

HHV8⁺ cells found in the mantle zone were immunoblasts/plasmablasts, the majority of which expressed lambda light chain. A caveat to this study is that 3 of the 6 HHV-8⁺ patients were also infected with HIV-1.

13.4   Clinical Presentation

Regardless of the classification system used—unicentric versus multicentric, hyaline vascular versus plasma cell variant, or with peripheral neuropathy versus without—there is considerable overlap of signs and symptoms among populations of CD patients. Part of this blurring of boundaries is a function of the spectrum of disease itself; another part is related to limitations of staging, both past and present. The earliest studies were confounded by the limitations of imaging; therefore, the majority of first reported cases were mediastinal masses (8) detected either because of compressive symptomatology or a mass detected on routine chest radiography. This same limitation of technology also delayed the realization that CD could be multicentric. The actual incidence of (and clinical features associated with) unicentric versus multicentric disease is also confounded by the extent of imaging performed and by the lack of consistency in defining multicentric disease. Given the fact that CD changes can be seen in the spleen (10, 31), should the presence of splenomegaly upstage a patient to multicentric disease? In addition, there are reports in which distant lymph nodes contain only "reactive" tissues rather than CD (11, 26, 84) and other reports in which simultaneous but distant lymph nodes have discordant histology (one with HVV and another with PCs) (10, 12).

With these caveats in mind, there are generalizations that can be made about groups of CD patients, as shown in Table 13.1. The median age of presentation is in the fourth decade for the unicentric and the sixth decade for the multicentric presentations. There does not appear to be any sex predilection. The most common symptoms are malaise/weakness, fever, weight loss, night sweats, and anorexia (12, 19, 21, 24, 28–30, 85). Although the earliest reports suggested that unicentric and HVV accounted for close to 80% of cases, a more modern estimate would be approximately 60%. Most masses occur in typical lymph node regions, but gastric, pulmonary (8), muscle (8), and pancreatic lesions (86) have all been described. By imaging, lesions are often vascular appearing (87), might be heavily calcified (Figure 13.4), especially those found in the pelvis (88), and could be flurodeoxyglucose positron emission tomography (FDG PET) avid (89).

13.4.1   Unicentric Disease

Nearly 90% of patients with unicentric disease have the HV form. These patients often present with either compressive symptoms or a large incidental mass; however, nearly 40% of patients with HVV will have associated systemic symptoms that promptly resolve after surgical extirpation of the solitary mass. Unicentric disease occurs most commonly in the mediastinum, cervical regions, and abdominal/pelvic cavity, but nasopharyngeal, orbital, dural, and oral occurrences have been described. Laboratory tests might be completely normal, but anemia, hypergammaglobulinemia, and elevated sedimentation rate and liver function tests might be present, again all of which promptly resolves after successful surgical removal of the mass.

13.4.2 Multicentric Disease

In the case of multicentric disease, the overlap with PCV is about 90%. Approximately 80% of patients with the PCV or the mixed variant have associated protean symptoms. The most common symptoms include fatigue, fevers, night sweats, and weight loss. Hepatomegaly and/or splenomegaly occurs in 75% of patients. Laboratory abnormalities are common, including anemia, low ferritin levels, elevations of the sedimentation rate, antinuclear antibodies, fibrinogen, C-reactive protein, and liver transaminases, and an abnormal urinalysis.

13.4.3 Paraneoplastic Symtpoms and Syndromes

There are a number of paraneoplastic symptoms/syndromes also associated with CD, more commonly with the multicentric form (Table 13.5) (19, 28, 46, 49, 55, 90–116). These include pleural effusions, pericardial effusions, ascites, anasarca, autoimmune hemolytic anemia, immune thrombocytopenic purpura, a multitude of renal disorders, including secondary (AA) amyloidosis or membranoproliferative glomerulonephritis (105, 117, 118), pulmonary abnormalities ranging from infiltrates to restrictive lung disease to lymphoid interstitial pneumonitis (111) to bronchiolitis obliterans (112–114), and skin abnormalities ranging from rash to hyperpigmentation to paraneoplastic pemphigus (99, 100) to Bechet's disease (101) to Kaposi's sarcoma. In one series over the course of the disease, 40% of patients developed central nervous system (CNS) signs, including seizures and aphasia (28). This finding should be tempered by the fact that a number of cases from the 1980s might have been AIDS-associated CD, which is known to have a particularly dismal prognosis (24). Neuropathy occurs in nearly 10% of patients, again more commonly than those with multicentric disease, but it is also possible in patients with unicentric disease. When present, other features of POEMS syndrome (also known as Crow-Fukase and Takatsuki disease) should be sought, including a monoclonal protein and osteosclerotic bone lesions (29, 30) (Figure 13.5).

Table 13.5 Paraneoplastic or autoimmune associations with Castleman disease

Hematologic	Renal
Anemia of chronic disease	Membranoproliferative glomerulonephritis (GN) (93
Pure red cell aplasia (90)	Mesangial proliferative GN (118), mMembranous GN (102, 103)
Autoimmune hemolytic anemia (91)	Interstitial nephritis (104)
Autoimmune thrombocytopenia (92)	Fibrillary glomerulonephritis (105)
Acquired hemophilia (93)	Secondary (AA) amyloidosis (55, 106–109)
Osteosclerotic myeloma (POEMS syndrome) (19, 94)	**Neurologic**
Thrombotic thrombocytopenic purpura (95)	Demyelinating polyneuropathy (POEMS syndrome) (19, 94)
Oncologic	Myasthenia gravis (110)
Non-Hodgkin's lymphoma (96)	**Pulmonary**
Hodgkin disease (96)	Bronchiolitis obliterans (112–114
Follicular dendritric cell sarcoma 97)	Lymphoid interstitial pneumonia (111)
Kaposi's sarcoma98	Pulmonary fibrosis (113)
Mesenchymal spindle-cell neoplasm (46)	**Rheumatologic**
Dermatologic	Systemic lupus erythematosus (115)
Pemphigus (99, 100)	Positive autoantibodies (antinuclear antibodies, antiphospholipid antibodies, Coombs antibodies)
Bechet's disease (101)	**Endocrine**
	Growth failure, delayed puberty (49)
	Adrenal insufficiency (116)

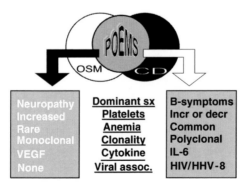

Figure 13.5 Relationship amongn Castleman disease, osteosclerotic myeloma, and POEMS syndrome

13.4.4   CD and POEMS Syndrome

POEMS syndrome is a rare paraneoplastic syndrome most often associated with osteosclerotic myeloma (OSM). The hallmark features of the OSM variant of POEMS are peripheral neuropathy (PN), monoclonal lambda plasmaproliferative disorder, sclerotic bone lesions, as well as the other features shown in Table 13.6, not all of which are required to make a diagnosis. In some cases, the lymph nodes of these patients have Castleman-like (15) or full-fledged CD histology (16, 94, 119). In a series of 30 patients with POEMS syndrome, 19 of 32 biopsied lymph nodes showed angiofollicular hyperplasia typical of CD (16).

Authors have noted that MCD with PN has a different quality to it when compared to MCD without and have even proposed that the presence or absence of PN should be part of the MCD classification system (29, 30). When CD is associated with PN, edema and impaired peripheral circulation are the most common systemic

Table 13.6 Spectrum of multicentric Castleman disease, osteosclerotic myeloma, and POEMS

	MCD	POEMS-MCD variant	POEMS-OSM variant	OSM
Fever/sweats	Defining	+++	+	−
Generalized lymphadenopathy	Defining	+++	++	−
Peripheral neuropathy	−	Defining	Defining	−
Monoclonal PCD	−	+	Defining	Defining
Sclerotic bone lesions	−	+	Defining	Defining
Skin changes[a]	++	++	Defining	−
Papilledema	−	Defining	Defining	−
Edema/ascites/effusions	+	Defining	Defining	−
Endocrinopathy[b]	−	Defining	Defining	−
Interleukin-6 elevation	+++	+++	+	+
VEGF elevation	+	+	+++	+
Weight loss	+++	+++	+++	−
Fatigue	+++	+++	+++	++
Polyclonal hypergammaglobulenima	+++	+++	−	−
Organomegaly	++	++	++	−
Platelets	L or H	L or H	H or N	−
Anemia	+++	+++	−	++
Autoimmune diseases[c]	++	++	−	−
Restrictive lung disease	+	+	++	−
Renal disease	+	+	−	++
Thrombosis	-	+	+	−

MCD, multicentric Castleman's disease; OSM, osteosclerotic myeloma; VEGF, vascular endothelial growth factor; L, low; H, high; N, normal; −: rare or absent; +, occasional; ++, common; +++, very common.

[a]CD-associated skin changes include nonspecific rash, autoimmune pemphigus, and telangectasia; POEMS-associated skin changes include hyperpigmentation, skin thickening, hypertrichosis, cherry angiomata, white nails, clubbing, flushing, and peripheral cyanosis.

[tb]Endocrinopathy should appear to coincide with ongoing illness.[c]See Table 13.5.

abnormalities seen (12, 13, 17, 120–124). In one series, 11 of 12 cases of CD with PN had a monoclonal lambda protein in their serum and/or urine (30). PCV and the mixed HVV/PCV are more like to have associated neuropathy (13, 17, 37, 121–123), but PN has been also seen with HVV (10, 37, 125).

The PN in OSM-POEMS usually has a significant motor component and is one of the dominating features of the syndrome; whereas the PN in CD patients tends to be more subtle and more often sensory. In its most severe form, it is a mixture of demyelination and axonal degeneration, with normal myelin spacing on electron microscopy (121, 123). There might be evidence of abnormal capillary proliferation, similar to that seen in the affected lymph nodes (123).

Table 13.6 presents the spectrum of lymphoproliferative disorder to plasmaproliferative disorder in the context of POEMS. Whereas OSM-POEMS patients have a monoclonal plasma cell disorder, CD is characterized by a brisk polyclonal hypergammaglobulinemia, which, on occasion, also contains a monoclonal protein. Both entities have a proinflammatory cytokine profile, but in the OSM variant of POEMS, VEGF is the most consistently elevated cytokine; in contrast, in CD, IL-6 is the dominant aberrantly overexpressed cytokine. Although renal failure is rare in OSM-POEMS, it is more common when patients have associated CD.

13.4.5   Diagnosis, Classification, and Prognosis

The diagnosis of CD is a pathologic one that can be clouded by discrepant pathology at different sites. It is therefore imperative that more than one biopsy be performed if the clinical level of suspicion is high because of the potential lack of lymph node concordance at distant sites.

Once the diagnosis is made, in addition to a thorough review of systems (B-symptoms, endocrinopathy, peripheral neuropathy) and physical examination (papilledema, skin changes), additional testing is required. Patients should have a complete blood count, erythrocyte sedimentation rate, C-reactive protein, liver function tests, serum creatinine, serum protein electrophoresis with immunofixation, IL-6, VEGF, serology for HHV-8 and HIV, urinalysis, and computed tomography (CT) of the chest abdomen and pelvis. If there are any pulmonary symptoms, the threshold for performing pulmonary function tests should be low. If there is associated neuropathy, imaging of the bones should be done looking for sclerotic bone lesions. If elements of POEMS syndrome are present, then more extensive endocrine testing should also be performed.

The course of CD can be quite variable. Typically, those with localized disease are cured by surgical resection. The multicentric form is more difficult to manage and median survival has been reported to be as short as 26 months (12). Frizzera et al. divided patients' courses into two categories—episodic and persistent (28). Those patients with more extensive disease (systemic symptoms, lymphadenopathy, hepatosplenomegaly, and effusions) were more likely to have the episodic pattern of evolution. These authors also found that male gender, episodic evolution, and predominantly proliferative morphology in involved lymph nodes were associated with worse survival in univariate analysis (28). Weisenberger et al. divided the course for MCD patients into five categories: (1) cure; (2) stable and persistent; (3) relapse and remission; (4) rapidly fatal disease; and (5) evolution to malignant lymphoma (12).

Our group has looked at a prognostic modeling system for survival using the clinical information of 114 patients with CD. We found that after adjusting for age, the multivariable model included organomegaly, respiratory symptoms, and an abnormal platelet count. Depending on whether patients had 0 or 1+ adverse factors, their 10-year survival rates were 80% [95% confidence interval (CI): 65–98%] and 41% (95% CI: 28–59%) (126).

13.4.6 HIV Clinical

Castleman disease in the HIV population distinguishes itself from CD in an HIV-negative population with the following features: (1) more likely to be multicentric; (2) systemic symptoms more common and more intense; (3) adenopathy more likely to be peripheral; (4) pulmonary symptoms more prevalent; (5) leukopenia and thrombocytopenia more common; (6) a much higher incidence of HHV-8 coinfectivity and clinical KS; (7) histologic type most commonly the mixed HV/PC variant; (8) a 15-fold risk of developing malignant lymphoma; and (9) prognosis dismal, with a median survival of 12–22 months (24, 127, 128).

In one series, the duration of known HIV seropositivity before CD diagnosis was less than 2 years in six cases, between 2 and 5 years in eight cases, and more than 5 years in six patients (24). The mean CD4 count was 156×10^6/L. Fifteen of 20 patients had KS: 6 with KS predating the MCD; 6 with concurrent diagnoses; and 3 who went on to develop KS 6–14 months later. This high incidence of KS is mirrored in another smaller series of 11 patients (128). Splenic histology mirrored lymph node histology when evaluated. Bone marrow involvement was observed in 12 of the 15 patients who were tested (24).

The symptoms of MCD might wax and wane for unclear reasons. Often this variability appears to correlate with high HHV8 viral load in peripheral blood mononuclear cells, high level of serum C reactive protein, and high plasma human IL-6 and IL-10 levels (81). The most common symptoms are fevers, sweats, fatigue, fluctuating lymphadenopathy, and hepatosplenomegaly, but patients might also develop pulmonary symptoms (dyspnea and cough) and infiltrates (129). Pulmonary symptoms manifest in approximate 20% of patients (129).

13.4.7 CD in Pediatric Population

Castleman disease is believed to have a more benign course in the pediatric population than in the adult population. Approximately 85% of cases are unicentric (22, 28).

Within the pediatric population, the disease is more common in teenagers, with 72% of cases between ages 10 and 17 years. General symptoms of fever, failure to thrive, weight loss, and fatigue are the presenting complaints in 45% of cases (22).

The distribution of tumor localization is about one-third each in the thorax, the abdomen, and in the periphery (22). Laboratory abnormalities, including anemia, hypergammaglobulinemia, and elevated erythrocyte sedimentation rate, are seen in 23% of the HV cases, in all of the PC cases, and in 82% of the mixed types. Two of the patients with multicentric disease had glomerulonephritis. In a very large review of 83 pediatric cases, patients with localized disease were treated with surgery in all but 4 cases. Two of these patients received radiation and the other two had spontaneous regressions. No relapses were documented in the localized patients. Patients with multicentric disease received various therapies, with half of them achieving a complete response (22).

13.4.8   CD and Lymphoma and Other Secondary Malignancies

Secondary malignancies are not uncommon in CD. This is especially true in the HIV$^+$ population, who are estimated to have a frequency of lymphoma of 15-fold of an HIV$^+$ population without CD (127). However, even in the HIV-negative population, as many as one-third of MCD patients develop malignancies, most notably lymphoma (~15%) (28, 30, 64, 96, 130) and Kaposi sarcoma (28). Both unicentric and multicentric patients appear to be a risk.

13.4.8.1   HIV$^-$ Lymphoma

Larroche et al. reviewed the association between CD lymphoma in the HIV$^-$ population by describing 23 cases of non-Hodgkin's lymphoma (NHL) and 27 cases of Hodgkin's disease (HD) (96). They found that NHL is more often associated with multicentric CD, its diagnosis being concurrent with CD diagnosis or occurring within 2 years. In contrast, HD occurs more commonly in localized CD of the plasma cell type (96), but it also occurs in multicentric disease (64). The spectrum of NHL seen includes diffuse mixed cell lymphoma (12), pleomorphic large-cell lymphoma (12), and peripheral T-cell lymphoma (64). Other secondary B-cell neoplasms have included.: γ-heavy-chain disease (131), multiple myeloma (MM) (132), and small B-lymphocytic lymphoma (133).

13.4.8.2   HIV$^+$ Lymphoma

Within a prospective cohort study on 60 HIV$^+$ patients with MCD and a median follow-up period of 20 months, 14 patients developed HHV-8-associated NHL: 3 with "classic" EBV$^+$ PEL) 5 with EBV$^-$ visceral large-cell NHL with a PEL-like phenotype, and 6 with plasmablastic lymphoma/leukemia (127). All of the plasmablastic cells that were phenotyped expressed IgM lambda on their surface. The estimated 2-year probability of developing NHL after a diagnosis of multicentric Castleman disease (MC) was 24.3%. At the time of NHL diagnosis, the median CD4 count was 248 × 10⁶/L. Those patients with the leukemic phase had a dismal outcome and died within 1 week. The overall median survival from NHL in these patients was 1 month (127).

13.4.8.3   Follicular Dendritic Cell Tumor

Follicular dendritic cell (FDC) sarcoma is an extremely rare neoplasm. However, there have been a number of cases reported in patients with CD (97, 134–138). There are even reports of possible progression from CD to FDC malignancies (97, 134). It appears to occur more frequently in patients with HVV.

13.4.8.4   Kaposi Sarcoma

As mentioned, the association between KS and CD became evident during the AIDS epidemic of the 1980s (12, 24, 28, 139–142). Several of these first cases did not have their HIV status specified (12, 28, 139–141). Over ensuing decades there have been reports of the association in patients who are clearly defined as being HIV⁻ 143. The association has also been in solid-organ transplant recipients (144). Finally, there are sporadic case reports of MCD associated with other carcinomas (145, 146), sarcomas (147) and thymic malignancies. (148).

13.5   Treatment

Treatment options must be considered separately for three different disease presentations: (1) unicentric disease; (2) multicentric disease in patients not infected with HIV; and (3) multicentric disease in HIV-positive patients. Further consideration should be made as to whether patients have coexisting POEMS syndrome.

13.5.1   Treatment of Unicentric Disease

The treatment decision for unicentric disease, regardless of whether it is hyaline vascular, plasma cell variant, or mixed type, is straightforward: surgical removal whenever possible (20, 21, 28, 85, 149). If not possible, irradiation should be considered (Table 13.7) (8, 14, 20, 21, 49, 150–156). For large tumors, embolization of solitary masses prior to surgical removal (157) or neoadjuvant therapy has also

Table 13.7 Role of irradiation in the treatment of Castleman disease

Study	Histology	Response	F/U (months)	Status
		Unicentric Disease		
Fitzpatrick et al. 1968 (150)	—	PR	24+	AWD
Fitzpatrick et al. (1968)	—	CR	72+	NED
Keller et al. 1973 (8)	HVV	Stable disease × 4 patients	—	—
Ernsom et al. 1973 (151)	—	PR	60+	AWD
Nordstrom et al. 1978 (152)	PCV	CR	12+	NED
Weisenburger et al. 1979 (14)	PCV	CR	10+	NED
Stokes et al. 1985 (154)	PCV	Stable	60+	AWD
Massey et al. 1991 (49)	Mixed	CR	26+	NED
Bowne et al. 1999 (20)	HVV	PR	24+	AWD
	HVV	CR	17	DNED
	HVV	CR	12+	NED
Chronowski et al. 2001 (21)	HVV	CR	8	DNED
	HVV	CR	35+	NED
	HVV	Progression	5	DOD
	HVV	CR	23	NED
	HVV	CR	175	NED
Neuhof et al. 2006 (162)	HVV	PR	3	AWD
	Mixed	Stable disease	12	AWD
		Multicentric Disease		
Gaba et al. 1978 (10)	HVV	Mass stable; other symptoms improved	24+	AWD
Nordstrom et al. 1978 (152)	PCV	CR	18+	NED
Marti et al. 1983 (153)	Mixed	CR*	20+	NED
Sethi et al. 1990 (155)	HVV	CR[a]	22+	NED
Veldhuis et al. 1996 (156)	PCV	CR	24+	NED
Bowne et al. 1999 (20)	HVV	CR[b]	—	AWD

HV, hyaline vascular variant; PC, plasma cell variant; CR, complete remission; PR, partial remission; AWD, alive with disease; NED, no evidence of disease.

[a]Local irradiation to dominant mass resulted in shrinkage of distant lymphadenopathy.

[b]Treated with resection followed by irradiation.

been applied. Although there is a low rate of recurrence, these patients appear to have a higher risk of developing HD and NHL. Long-term follow-up should be recommended. A number of patients have seemingly done well with observation alone, but one must be vigilant about subtle development and progression of associated paraneoplastic entities like bronchiolitis obliterans.

If there are associated paraneoplastic or autoimmune conditions associated with CD, these generally resolve within months of the surgery—most notably laboratory abnormalities like anemia, hypergammaglobulinaemia, and high sedimentation rate, C-reactive protein (CRP), and liver function tests. If present, associated pemphigus often (99, 112), but not always (158), improves within the year. NonAA-related

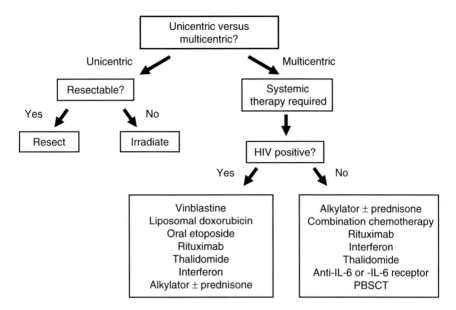

Figure 13.6 Treatment algorithm for patients with Castleman disease

renal disease has also been reported to resolve within 12 months of surgical removal (159). Symptoms from associated AA amyloid typically improves over the ensuing years after removal of unicentric disease (160, 161). Reports of lack of recovery of bronchiolitis obliterans after definitive surgery (112, 113) are difficult to interpret because it is unclear whether earlier intervention (i.e., at a lymphoid interstitial pneumonitis stage or before fibrosis) could reverse pulmonary changes.

Of the 21 patients with unicentric disease treated with irradiation (Table 13.7), 10 had a complete response, 4 had a partial response, 6 had no clinical response, and one had progressive disease (8, 14, 20, 21, 49, 150–155, 162). Even in those patients whose mass does not clearly shrink, the tumors histology changes in that lymphocytes are depleted and nuclear atypicality and hyperchromatism are seen in the plump endothelial cells of the proliferating capillaries (8). Gulati et al. reported on the use of adjuvant radiation therapy in a patient with isolated leptomeningeal disease (163).

13.5.2 Treatment of Multicentric CD in HIV⁻ Patients

For HIV-negative multicentric CD, the best choice of therapy is uncertain because available treatment data are limited to small retrospective series (12, 21, 28, 85, 140) and single case reports. Interpretation of each of these reports is confounded by the absence of uniform response criteria. If B-symptoms abate without shrinkage of lymph node groups, is that a response? If some, but not all, of the autoimmune manifestations abate, is that a response? Is it a meaningful response if it lasts only 2 months? These are just some of the limitations of the available data. With these caveats in mind, therapy to date has been corticosteroid and alkylator based. Small numbers of patients have been treated with alternative therapies like interferon-alpha (IFN-α), thalidomide, rituximab, bortezomib, and anti-IL-6 receptor antibodies (Table 13.8). High-dose chemotherapy with hematopoietic stem cell transplantation has also been used with good effect in a limited number of cases. Exactly where these treatment plans fit into the overall treatment is uncertain.

No prospective studies support the use of corticosteroids in the treatment of CD. Although they have clinical activity (19, 21, 29, 85) and are not infrequently used to maintain clinical improvement, it is unclear whether this strategy is in the best interest of these patients.

Alkylators (cyclophosphamide or chlorambucil) have been used as single-agent therapy, along with low-dose prednisone (85, 164), or as part of combination chemotherapy. Most reports of improvement are from individual or small case studies (19, 21, 29, 85).

Combination chemotherapy (20, 128, 165), including chlorambucil/prednisone, cyclophosphamide/prednisone, cyclophosphamide/vincristine/prednisone (COP) ± doxorubicin (CHOP) or procarbazine (COPP), and rituximab with either COP (166) or CHOP (165) have all been tried in patients with multicentric disease. Some authors suggest that responses are more durable using the high-dose combination chemotherapy (21), but the evidence does not clearly justify this conclusion. Patients with multicentric CD commonly died of infections related to therapy.

Additional anecdotal cases treated with other agents have been reported. An HIV⁻ patient developed MCD and KS associated with active human HHV-8 infection. He was treated initially with sequential antiviral therapy (foscarnet) without clinical benefit or improvement in his HHV-8 viremia (143). Subsequent treatment with chemotherapy and corticosteroids led to clinical improvement. Methotrexate provided benefit in a patient with MCD and rheumatoid arthritis (167). Suramin provided long-lasting response in one patient (20), but it was not effective in another five patients (165).

There is limited experience with anti-CD20 antibodies in patients with CD. There is one report of benefit with single-agent rituximab in a young man with an aggressive form of CD with autoimmune hemolytic anemia and positive outcome (168). A man with orbital CD responded to single-agent rituximab (169). There are two single case reports of treating HIV-negative patients with relapsed CD with rituximab along with cyclophosphamide and prednisone with favorable response (166, 170, 171). Not only did the B-symptoms and lymphadenopathy improve, but the renal failure secondary to CD-related glomerulonephritis in one patient normalized after therapy.

Reports of the use of 2-Chloro-2'-Deoxyadenosine (2-CDA) in patients with CD are limited (172, 173). In a series of three patients with CD (two with multicentric and one with unresectable HV), two patients responded with relapse-free survivals of 24 and 20 months. Both responding patients, however, later devloped NHL (diffuse large B-cell lymphoma and peripheral T-cell NHL, respectively) (172). This

Table 13.8 Novel treatment strategies for MCD

Ref.	Drug	N	Outcomes
Patients Not Infected with HIV			
Jacobs et al. 2006 (167)	MTX	1	HHV8+, rheumatoid arthritis patient—remission × 54+ m
Senanayake et al. 2003 (143)	Antiviral	1	No benefit from antiviral despite HHV-8.
Ide et al. 2003 (169)	Rituximab	1	CR+ 10 m
Ocio et al. 2005 (168)	Rituximab	1 mixed	CR of lymph node, hemolysis, and Raynaud's at 14+ m
Hudnall et al. 2003 (166)	Rituximab, CTX, Pred		CR of lymph nodes and constitutional symptoms; persistant hypergammaglobulinemia at 12+ m
Abdou et al. 2004 (170)	Ritux, CTX, Pred	1	CR of lymph nodes andw acute renal failure at 24+ m
Gholam et al.2003 (171)	Rituximab after chemotherapy	1	PR 2 months, but death secondary to AA amyloidosis
Bordealeau et al. 1995 (173)	2-CDA	2	1 unresectable HV received 2-CDA + XRT resulted in CR 9+ m; 1 MCD had PR
Colleoni et al. 2003 (172)	2-CDA	3	2 MCD patients had response lasting 20–24 m; both patients evolved to NHL (DLBCL; PTCL); 1 unresectable unicentric HVV did not respond
Pavlidis et al. 1992 (174)	Interferon-α	1	CR 11+ m
Tamayo et al. 1995 (175)	Interferon-α	1	CR 32+ m
Strohal et al. 1998 (101)	Interferon-α	1	CR of lymphadenopathy, B-symptoms, and Bechet's disease 25+ m
Simko et al. 2000 (177)	Interferon-α	1	Long-term disease stabilization (8+ years) in 11-year-old with Klinefelter syndrome & HCV.
Andres et al. 2000 (176)	Interferon-α	1	CR 42+ m
Bowne et al. 1999 (20)	Suramin	1	CR 46+ m
Starkey et al. 2006 (179)	Thalidomide	1	Near total resolution of all symptoms and LA 40+ m
Lee et al. 2003 (178)	Thalidomide	1	Improvement of ascites, anemia, albumin, CRP, platelet count, pulmonary hypertension at 13+ m
Hess et al. 2006 (180)	Bortezomib	1	Improved anemia, constitutional symptoms, IL-6, CRP, but stable lymphadenopathy
Beck et al. 1994 (181)	Murine anti-IL-6 monoclonal Ab	1	Response while on therapy, but rapid relapse upon cessation.
Nishimoto et al. 2005 (68)	Humanized anti-IL-6 receptor Ab	28	Improvement of LA and B-symptoms in all for 36+ m
Repetto et al. 1986 (84)	ASCT	1	CR 15+ m

(continued)

Table 13.8 (continued)

Ref.	Drug	N	Outcomes
Advani et al. 1999 (182)	ASCT	1	Failed steroids & chemotherapy, but developed follicular lymphoma. CR 48+ months after ASCT
Dispenzieri et al. 2004 (119)	ASCT	2	Associated POEMS; CR 13+ and 18+ m
Ganti et al. 2005 (124)	ASCT	1	Associated POEMS; response of all manifestations × 24+ m
Lerza et al. 1999 (183)	Splenectomy	1	CR for 12+ m for autoimmune hemolysis, systemic symptoms, and lymphadenopathy
Frizzera et al. 1985 (28)	Splenectomy	1	CR for 78+ m
Patients Infected with HIV			
Lanzafame et al. 2000 (186)	HAART	2	Improvement in both for 12+ m
Aaron et al. 2002 (184)	HAART	7	No response to HAART, but perception that immune reconstitution allowed for better chemotherapy response & overall survival, median 38 m.
Corbellino et al. 2001(188)	Cidofovir	1	No response
Berezne et al. 2004 (189)	Cidofovir	5	No response
Casper et al. 2004 (190)	Ganciclovir	3	Fewer flares of MCD in 2; improvement in acute renal and respiratory failure in one patient who got 12 days of treatment, but who d/c'd Rx due to leucopenia in context of fungal infection–died on day 30.
Nord et al. 2003 (194)	Interferon-α	1	Successful maintenance
Kumari et al. 2000 (193)	Interferon-α	1	Improvement
Jung et al. 2004 (195)	Thalidomide	1	Improvement of hypergammaglobulinemia, thrombocytopenia and constitutional symptoms × 38 weeks
Casquero et al. 2006 (198)	Rituximab	1	CR × 10+ m, but possible aggravation of cutaneous KS
Marcelin et al. 2003 (196)	Rituximab	5	CR × 3 lasting 4+–14+ m, but possible aggravation of cutaneous KS in 2; 2 early deaths
Kofteridis et al.	Rituximab	1	CR 12+ m
Marrache et al. 2003 (206)	Rituximab	1	CR 6+ m
Corbellino et al. 2001(188)	Rituximab	1	CR 14+ m remission of symptoms and HHV-8 viremia

(continued)

Table 13.8 (continued)

Ref.	Drug	N	Outcomes
Newson-Davis et al. 2004 (201)	Rituximab	1	Near CR: HHV-8 viral load, IL-6, and TNF-α levels decreased.
Neuville et al. 2005 (200)	Rituximab	2	No significant response, and exacerbation of KS
Revuelta et al. 1998 (202)	Splenectomy & foscarnet	1	CR of LA, B-symptoms, pulmonary infiltrates, and pancytopenia × 12+ m
Oksenhendler et al. 1996 (24)	Splenectomy	9	Prompt, but transient (1–3 m) improvement in fever and cytopenias.

CR, complete response; KS, Kaposi sarcoma; LA, lymphadenompathy; 2-CDA, 2-chlorodeoxyadenosine; HAART, highly active antiretroviral therapy.

brings into question whether the use of 2-CDA accelerates the transformation of CD to lymphoma (172), reminiscent of the high risk observed in HIV-positive patients (127).

Interferon-α has been reported to control disease in five separate cases (101, 174–177). Novel agents like thalidomide have been used with dramatic success in two patients (178, 179). Bortezomib has been shown to improve the cytokine and biochemical profile in addition to clinical symptoms (180).

Beck et al. demonstrated that an HIV-negative patient with multicentric CD could have his systemic manifestations of multicentric CD alleviated by the use of a monoclonal anti-IL-6 antibody. The patient developed extremely high levels of IL-6, and symptoms of multicentric CD promptly reoccurred after the therapy was discontinued (181). This study demonstrated proof of principle (i.e., that many of the systemic symptoms of multicentric CD are IL-6 mediated). Subsequent studies have focused on blocking the IL-6 receptor. A humanized anti-IL-6 receptor antibody (rhPM-1; aka MRA) was used to treat two patients with multicentric PC or mixed-type CD (82).

These same authors have reported on a prospective multicenter clinical trial employing humanized anti-human IL-6 receptor monoclonal antibody in 28 patients with MCD (68). Within 16 weeks of treatment, fatigue, lymphadenopathy, and all of the inflammatory parameters were alleviated. Hemoglobin, albumin, and total cholesterol levels, high-density lipoprotein cholesterol values, and body mass index all increased significantly. Histopathologic examination revealed reduced follicular hyperplasia and vascularity after treatment (82). Eleven (73.3%) of 15 patients who had received oral corticosteroids before study entry were able to do well on a reduced corticosteroid dose (68). Ninety-six percent of patients remain on therapy for more than 3 years.

High-dose chemotherapy with hematopoietic stem cell transplantation has also been used with good effect in five patients, three of whom had coexisting POEMS syndrome (84, 119, 124, 182).

Somewhat surprisingly, on occasion, localized therapies have provided clinical responses in patients with multicentric disease. There are six reports of using radiation in this setting with dramatic clinical benefit in five (Table 13.8). In two of these cases, radiation of the dominant lymph node group resulted in nodal response at remote locations (153, 155). Even in those patients in whom there was no clear response after irradiation, there was a histologic change [i.e., depletion of lymphocytes, causing nuclear atypia and hyperchromatism in the plump endothelial cells of the proliferated capillaries (8)]. For those patients with POEMS syndrome, radiation to a solitary sclerotic lesion can have resolution of lymphadenopathy (30. In a similar vein, splenectomy has provide durable clinical benefit in two patients with multicentric disease (Table 13.8) (28, 183).

13.5.3 Treatment of Multicentric CD in HIV⁺ Patients

The approaches used for the HIV-positive population are slightly different than the approaches for those not infected with this virus. Because these patients are already severely immunosuppressed, high-dose combination chemotherapy is a riskier prospect. Unlike the dramatic improvements in active KS after the institution of highly active antiretroviral therapy (HAART), MCD does not regress by mere immune reconstitution (184, 185) with only a few exceptions (186). There was one report, which has not been substantiated, that HAART might aggravate the symptoms of MCD (187). The use of HHV-8 directed antivirals, like ganciclovir, foscarnet, and cidofivir in HHV-8-positive patients has yielded conflicting results (188–190), with the majority of cases suggesting no benefit (188, 189).

Singly or in combination, liposomal doxorubicin, oral etoposide, and vinblastine have produced remission—sometimes durable—in HIV-positive patients (24, 128, 184, 191). Vincristine, bleomycin, vinblastine combinations have been used with success (128). Alkylator-based treatment including low-dose chlorambucil have occasionally been helpful (128). More intensive alkylator-based therapies can result in responses, but they should be used with caution because of their extreme immunosuppressive effects (192). Interferon-α has also provided modest benefit (193, 194). There is one case report of the benefit of thalidomide in an HIV-positive patient with multicentric CD (195).

Twelve patients with HIV-associated CD have been treated with rituximab with mixed results (188, 196–201). In the largest series, Marcelin et al. (196) reported on five patients infected with HIV with CD. Two died very quickly after the beginning of rituximab therapy. Three had complete remission with no more clinical symptoms related to CD with a follow-up of 4–14 months. In two of the responders, clinical remission correlated with a dramatic decrease of HHV-8 viral load as well as a transitory but sharp decrease of CD19 cell count and an aggravation of KS (196).

Painful splenomegaly or peripheral cytopenias might trigger splenectomy, which results in a prompt, albeit transient (1–3 months), effect on fever and cytopenia (24), although on occasion the benefit may be durable (202).

13.6   Conclusions

The field of CD has come a long way since it was first described in 1954, but much work is yet to be done. A uniform histologic and clinicopathologic classification system has been the first step. Further advances will come as investigators use the clues imparted from its relationships to AIDS, lymphoma, and the POEMS syndrome. A better understanding of the cytokine networks and the preeminent cell type driving the disease will provide a clearer, more reproducible means to prognosticate, treat, and perhaps even prevent this condition.

References

1. Castleman B, Iverson L, Menendez VP. Localized mediastinal lymph-node hyperplasia resembling thymoma. Cancer 1956;9:822–830.
2. Blades BB. Mediastinal tumous: reports of cases treated at army thoracic surgery centers in the United States. Ann Surg 1946;123:749–765.
3. Symmers D. Primary hemangiolymphoma of the hemal nodes: An unusual variety of malignant tumor. Arch Intern Med 1921;28:467–474.
4. Lattes R, Pachter MR. Benign lymphoid masses of probable hamartomatous nature. Analysis of 12 cases. Cancer 1962;15:197–214.
5. Lee SL, Rosner F, Rivero I, et al. Refractory anemia with abnormal iron metabolism: its remission after resection of hyperplastic mediastinal lymph nodes. N Engl J Med 1965;272:761–766.
6. Tung KS, McCormack LJ. Angiomatous lymphoid hamartoma. Report of five cases with a review of the literature. Cancer 1967;20:525–536.
7. Flendrig JA, Schiillings PHM. Benign giant lymphoma: the clinical signs and symptoms and the morphological aspects. Folia Med 1969;12:119–120.
8. Keller AR, Hocholzer L, Castleman B. Hyaline-vascular and plasma-cell types of giant lymph node hyperplasia of the mediastinum and other locations. Cancer 1972;29:670–683.
9. Flendrig JA. Benign giant lymphoma: cliniccopathologic correlation study. In: Clark RL, Cumley RW, editors. The year book of cancer. Chicago: Year Book Medical; 1970. p. 296–299.
10. Gaba AR, Stein RS, Sweet DL, et al. Multicentric giant lymph node hyperplasia. Am J Clin Pathol 1978;69(1):86–90.
11. Frizzera G, Banks PM, Massarelli G, et al. A systemic lymphoproliferative disorder with morphologic features of Castleman's disease. Pathological findings in 15 patients. Ame J Surg Pathol 1983;7(3):211–231.

12. Weisenburger DD, Nathwani BN, Winberg CD, et al. Multicentric angiofollicular lymph node hyperplasia: a clinicopathologic study of 16 cases. Hum Path 1985;16(2):162–172.

13. Yu GS, Carson JW. Giant lymph-node hyperplasia, plasma-cell type, of the mediastinum, with peripheral neuropathy. Am J Clin Pathol 1976;66(1):46–53.

14. Weisenburger DD, DeGowin RL, Gibson P, et al. Remission of giant lymph node hyperplasia with anemia after radiotherapy. Cancer 1979;44(2):457–462.

15. Bardwick PA, Zvaifler NJ, Gill GN, et al. Plasma cell dyscrasia with polyneuropathy, organomegaly, endocrinopathy, M protein, and skin changes: the POEMS syndrome. Report on two cases and a review of the literature. Medicine (Balt) 1980;59(4):311–322.

16. Nakanishi T, Sobue I, Toyokura Y, et al. The Crow-Fukase syndrome: a study of 102 cases in Japan. Neurology 1984;34(6):712–720.

17. Hineman VL, Phyliky RL, Banks PM. Angiofollicular lymph node hyperplasia and peripheral neuropathy: association with monoclonal gammopathy. Mayo Clin Proc 1982;57(6):379–382.

18. Daley M, Cornog JL Jr. Pelvic retroperitoneal lymphoid hamartoma. J Urol 1967;97(2):235–239.

19. Frizzera G. Castleman's disease and related disorders. Semin Diagn Pathol 1988;5(4):346–364.

20. Bowne WB, Lewis JJ, Filippa DA, et al. The management of unicentric and multicentric Castleman's disease: a report of 16 cases and a review of the literature. Cancer 1999;85(3):706–717.

21. Chronowski GM, Ha CS, Wilder RB, et al. Treatment of unicentric and multicentric Castleman disease and the role of radiotherapy. Cancer 2001;92(3):670–676.

22. Parez N, Bader-Meunier B, Roy CC, et al. Paediatric Castleman disease: report of seven cases and review of the literature. Eur J Pediatr 1999;158(8):631–637.

23. Soulier J, Grollet L, Oksenhendler E, et al. Kaposi's sarcoma-associated herpesvirus-like DNA sequences in multicentric Castleman's disease [see comment]. Blood 1995;86(4):1276–1280.

24. Oksenhendler E, Duarte M, Soulier J, et al. Multicentric Castleman's disease in HIV infection: a clinical and pathological study of 20 patients. AIDS 1996;10(1):61–67.

25. Martin C, Pena ML, Angulo F, et al. Castleman's disease in identical twins. Virchows Arch A: Pathol Anat Histol 1982;395(1):77–85.

26. Radaszkiewicz T, Hansmann ML, Lennert K. Monoclonality and polyclonality of plasma cells in Castleman's disease of the plasma cell variant. Histopathology 1989;14(1):11–24.

27. Krishnan J, Danon AD, Frizzera G. Reactive lymphadenopathies and atypical lymphoproliferative disorders. Am J Clin Pathol 1993;99(4):385–396.

28. Frizzera G, Peterson BA, Bayrd ED, et al. A systemic lymphoproliferative disorder with morphologic features of Castleman's disease: clinical findings and clinicopathologic correlations in 15 patients. J Clin Oncol 1985;3(9):1202–1216.

29. McCarty MJ, Vukelja SJ, Banks PM, et al. Angiofollicular lymph node hyperplasia (Castleman's disease). Cancer Treat Rev 1995;21(4):291–310.

30. Menke DM, Camoriano JK, Banks PM. Angiofollicular lymph node hyperplasia: a comparison of unicentric, multicentric, hyaline vascular, and plasma cell types of disease by morphometric and clinical analysis. Mod Pathol 1992;5(5):525–530.

31. Weisenburger DD. Multicentric angiofollicular lymph node hyperplasia. Pathology of the spleen. Am J Surg Pathol 1988;12(3):176–181.

32. Sherman D, Ramsay B, Theodorou NA, et al. Reversible plane xanthoma, vasculitis, and peliosis hepatis in giant lymph node hyperplasia (Castleman's disease): a case report and review of the cutaneous manifestations of giant lymph node hyperplasia. J Ame Acad Dermatol 1992;26(1):105–109.

33. Molina T, Delmer A, Le Tourneau A, et al. Hepatic lesions of vascular origin in multicentric Castleman's disease, plasma cell type: report of one case with peliosis hepatis and another with perisinusoidal fibrosis and nodular regenerative hyperplasia. Pathol Res Pract 1995;191(11):1159–1164.

34. Saritas U, Ustundag Y, Isitan G, et al. Abdominal Castleman disease with mixed histopathology in a patient with iron deficiency anemia, growth retardation and peliosis hepatis. Am J Med Sci 2006;331(1):51–54.

35. Nagai K, Sato I, Shimoyama N. Pathohistological and immunohistochemical studies on Castleman's disease of the lymph node. Virchows Arch A: Pathol Anat Histopathol 1986;409(2):287–297.

36. Harigaya K, Mikata A, Kageyama K, et al. Histopathological study of six cases of Castleman's tumor. Acta Pathol Jpn 1975;25(3):355–374.

37. Menke DM, Tiemann M, Camoriano JK, et al. Diagnosis of Castleman's disease by identification of an immunophenotypically aberrant population of mantle zone B lymphocytes in paraffin-embedded lymph node biopsies. Am J Clin Pathol 1996;105(3):268–276.

38. Ruco LP, Gearing AJ, Pigott R, et al. Expression of ICAM-1, VCAM-1 and ELAM-1 in angiofollicular lymph node hyperplasia (Castleman's disease): evidence for dysplasia of follicular dendritic reticulum cells. Histopathology 1991;19(6):523–528.

39. Nguyen DT, Diamond LW, Hansmann ML, et al. Castleman's disease. Differences in follicular dendritic network in the hyaline vascular and plasma cell variants. Histopathology 1994;24(5):437–443.

40. Parravicini C, Chandran B, Corbellino M, et al. Differential viral protein expression in Kaposi's sarcoma-associated herpesvirus-infected diseases: Kaposi's sarcoma, primary effusion lymphoma, and multicentric Castleman's disease. Am J Pathol 2000;156(3):743–749.

41. Leger-Ravet MB, Peuchmaur M, Devergne O, et al. Interleukin-6 gene expression in Castleman's disease. Blood 1991;78(11):2923–2930.

42. Pauwels P, Dal Cin P, Vlasveld LT, et al. A chromosomal abnormality in hyaline vascular Castleman's disease: evidence for clonal proliferation of dysplastic stromal cells. Am J Surg Pathol 2000;24(6):882–888.

43. Cokelaere K, Debiec-Rychter M, De Wolf-Peeters C, Hagemeijer A, Sciot R. Hyaline vascular Castleman's disease with HMGIC rearrangement in follicular dendritic cells: molecular evidence of mesenchymal tumorigenesis. American Journal of Surgical Pathology 2002;26(5):662–669.

44. Chen WC, Jones D, Ho CL, et al. Cytogenetic anomalies in hyaline vascular Castleman disease: report of two cases with reappraisal of histogenesis. Cancer Genet Cytogenet 2006;164(2):110–117.

45. Chan JK, Fletcher CD, Nayler SJ, et al. Follicular dendritic cell sarcoma. Clinicopathologic analysis of 17 cases suggesting a malignant potential higher than currently recognized. Cancer 1997;79(2):294–313.

46. Gerald W, Kostianovsky M, Rosai J. Development of vascular neoplasia in Castleman's disease. Report of seven cases. Am J Surg Pathol 1990;14(7):603–614.

47. Lin O, Frizzera G. Angiomyoid and follicular dendritic cell proliferative lesions in Castleman's disease of hyaline-vascular type: a study of 10 cases.[see comment][erratum appears in Am J Surg Pathol 1998 Jan;22(1):139]. Am J Surg Pathol 1997;21(11):1295–1306.

48. Hall PA, Donaghy M, Cotter FE, et al. An immunohistological and genotypic study of the plasma cell form of Castleman's disease. Histopathology 1989;14(4):333–346; discussion 429–432.

49. Massey GV, Kornstein MJ, Wahl D, et al. Angiofollicular lymph node hyperplasia (Castleman's disease) in an adolescent female. Clinical and immunologic findings. Cancer 1991; 68(6):1365–1372.

50. Hanson CA, Frizzera G, Patton DF, et al. Clonal rearrangement for immunoglobulin and T-cell receptor genes in systemic Castleman's disease. Association with Epstein-Barr virus. Am J Pathol 1988;131(1):84–91.

51. Al-Maghrabi J, Kamel-Reid S, Bailey D. Immunoglobulin and T-cell receptor gene rearrangement in Castleman's disease: molecular genetic analysis. Histopathology 2006;48(3):233–238.

52. Kobayashi H, Ii K, Sano T, et al. Plasma-cell dyscrasia with polyneuropathy and endocrine disorders associated with dysfunction of salivary glands. Am J Surg Pathol 1985;9(10):759–763.

53. Chilosi M, Menestrina F, Lestani M, et al. Hyaline-vascular type of Castleman's disease (angiofollicular lymph node hyperplasia) with monotypic plasma cells. An immunohisto-chemical study with monoclonal antibodies. Histol Histopathol 1987;2(1):49–55.
54. Li CF, Ye H, Liu H, et al. Fatal HHV-8-associated hemophagocytic syndrome in an HIV-negative immunocompetent patient with plasmablastic variant of multicentric Castleman disease (plasmablastic microlymphoma). Am J Surg Pathol 2006;30(1):123–127.
55. Chan WC, Hargreaves H, Keller J. Giant lymph node hyperplasia with unusual clinicopatho-logic features. Cancer 1984;53(10):2135–2139.
56. Ohyashiki JH, Ohyashiki K, Kawakubo K, et al. Molecular genetic, cytogenetic, and immu-nophenotypic analyses in Castleman's disease of the plasma cell type. Am J Clin Pathol 1994;101(3):290–295.
57. Dupin N, Diss TL, Kellam P, et al. HHV-8 is associated with a plasmablastic variant of Castleman disease that is linked to HHV-8-positive plasmablastic lymphoma.[see comment]. Blood 2000;95(4):1406–1412.
58. Soulier J, Grollet L, Oksenhendler E, et al. Molecular analysis of clonality in Castleman's disease. Blood 1995;86(3):1131–1138.
59. Dura WT, Mioduszewska O, Porwit-Ksiazek. Cytoplasmic immunoglobulins in giant lymph node hyperplasia (Castlemanans' disease). Virchows Arch 1981;38:239–246.
60. Mufarrij A, Fazzini E, Feiner HD. Giant lymph node hyperplasia. An immunopathologic and ultrastructural study of a case of the multicentric plasma cell variant. Arch Pathol Lab Med 1982;106(2):92–95.
61. Schlosnagle DC, Chan WC, Hargreaves HK, et al. Plasmacytoma arising in giant lymph node hyperplasia. Am J Clin Pathol 1982;78(4):541–544.
62. Tanda F, Massarelli G, Costanzi G. Multicentric giant lymph node hyperplasia: an immuno-histochemical study. Hum Pathol 1983;14(12):1053–1058.
63. Miller RT, Mukai K, Banks PM, et al. Systemic lymphoproliferative disorder with morpho-logic features of Castleman's disease. Immunoperoxidase study of cytoplasmic immunoglob-ulins. Arch Pathol Lab Med 1984;108(8):626–630.
64. Amin HM, Medeiros LJ, Manning JT, et al. Dissolution of the lymphoid follicle is a feature of the HHV8+ variant of plasma cell Castleman's disease. Am J Surg Pathol 2003;27(1):91–100.
65. Du MQ, Liu H, Diss TC, et al. Kaposi sarcoma-associated herpesvirus infects monotypic (IgM lambda) but polyclonal naive B cells in Castleman disease and associated lymphoproliferative disorders.[erratum appears in Blood 2001 Jun 1;97(11):3678]. Blood 2001;97(7):2130–2136.
66. Rieu P, Noel LH, Droz D, et al. Glomerular involvement in lymphoproliferative disorders with hyperproduction of cytokines (Castleman, POEMS). Adva Nephrol Necker Hospital 2000;30:305–331.
67. Yoshizaki K, Matsuda T, Nishimoto N, et al. Pathogenic significance of interleukin-6 (IL-6/BSF-2) in Castleman's disease. Blood 1989;74(4):1360–1307.
68. Nishimoto N, Kanakura Y, Aozasa K, et al. Humanized anti-interleukin-6 receptor antibody treatment of multicentric Castleman disease. Blood 2005;106(8):2627–2632.
69. Brandt SJ, Bodine DM, Dunbar CE, et al. Retroviral-mediated transfer of interleukin-6 into hematopoietic cells of mice results in a syndrome resembling Castleman's disease. Curr Top Microbiol Immunol 1990;166:37–41.
70. Nishi J, Arimura K, Utsunomiya A, et al. Expression of vascular endothelial growth factor in sera and lymph nodes of the plasma cell type of Castleman's disease. Br J Haematol 1999;104(3):482–485.
71. Foss HD, Araujo I, Demel G, et al. Expression of vascular endothelial growth factor in lym-phomas and Castleman's disease. J Pathol 1997;183(1):44–50.
72. Parravinci C, Corbellino M, Paulli M, et al. Expression of a virus-derived cytokine, KSHV vIL-6, in HIV-seronegative Castleman's disease. Am J Pathol 1997;151(6):1517–1522.
73. Chadburn A, Cesarman E, Nador RG, et al. Kaposi's sarcoma-associated herpesvirus sequences in benign lymphoid proliferations not associated with human immunodeficiency virus. Cancer 1997;80(4):788–797.

74. Lachant NA, Sun NC, Leong LA, et al. Multicentric angiofollicular lymph node hyperplasia (Castleman's disease) followed by Kaposi's sarcoma in two homosexual males with the acquired immunodeficiency syndrome (AIDS). Am J Clin Pathol 1985;83(1):27–33.

75. O'Leary J, Kennedy M, Howells D, et al. Cellular localisation of HHV-8 in Castleman's disease: is there a link with lymph node vascularity? Mol Pathol 2000;53(2):69–76.

76. Suda T, Katano H, Delsol G, et al. HHV-8 infection status of AIDS-unrelated and AIDS-associated multicentric Castleman's disease. Pathol Int 2001;51(9):671–679.

77. Gessain A, Sudaka A, Briere J, et al. Kaposi sarcoma-associated herpes-like virus (human herpesvirus type 8) DNA sequences in multicentric Castleman's disease: is there any relevant association in non-human immunodeficiency virus-infected patients? Blood 1996;87(1):414–416.

78. Bacon CM, Miller RF, Noursadeghi M, et al. Pathology of bone marrow in human herpes virus-8 (HHV8)-associated multicentric Castleman disease. Br J Haematol 2004;127(5):585–591.

79. Katano H, Sato Y, Kurata T, et al. Expression and localization of human herpesvirus 8-encoded proteins in primary effusion lymphoma, Kaposi's sarcoma, and multicentric Castleman's disease. Virology 2000;269(2):335–344.

80. Menke DM, Chadbum A, Cesarman E, et al. Analysis of the human herpesvirus 8 (HHV-8) genome and HHV-8 vIL-6 expression in archival cases of castleman disease at low risk for HIV infection. Am J Clinl Pathol 2002;117(2):268–275.

81. Oksenhendler E, Carcelain G, Aoki Y, et al. High levels of human herpesvirus 8 viral load, human interleukin-6, interleukin-10, and C reactive protein correlate with exacerbation of multicentric castleman disease in HIV-infected patients. Blood 2000;96(6):2069–2073.

82. Nishimoto N, Sasai M, Shima Y, et al. Improvement in Castleman's disease by humanized anti-interleukin-6 receptor antibody therapy. Blood 2000;95(1):56–61.

83. Belec L, Mohamed AS, Authier FJ, et al. Human herpesvirus 8 infection in patients with POEMS syndrome-associated multicentric Castleman's disease. Blood 1999;93(11):3643–3653.

84. Repetto L, Jaiprakash MP, Selby PJ, et al. Aggressive angiofollicular lymph node hyperplasia (Castleman's disease) treated with high dose melphalan and autologous bone marrow transplantation. Hematol Oncol 1986;4(3):213–217.

85. Herrada J, Cabanillas F, Rice L, et al. The clinical behavior of localized and multicentric Castleman disease. Ann Intern Med 1998;128(8):657–662.

86. Inoue Y, Nakamura H, Yamazaki K, et al. Retroperitoneal Castleman's tumors of hyaline vascular type: imaging study. Case report. Clin Imaging 1992;16(4):239–242.

87. Spencer TD, Maier RV, Olson HH. Retroperitoneal giant lymph node hyperplasia. A case report and review of the literature. Am Surg 1984;50(9):509–514.

88. Schwartz A, Eid A, Sasson T, et al. Pelvic giant lymph node hyperplasia (Castleman's disease): a surgical and radiological approach. Eur J Surg 1996;162(12):993–996.

89. Reddy MP, Graham MM. FDG positron emission tomographic imaging of thoracic Castleman's disease. Clin Nucl Med 2003;28(4):325–326.

90. Hattori K, Irie S, Isobe Y, et al. Multicentric Castleman's disease associated with renal amyloidosis and pure red cell aplasia. Ann Hematol 1998;77(4):179–181.

91. Liberato NL, Bollati P, Chiofalo F, et al. Autoimmune hemolytic anemia in multicentric Castleman's disease. Haematologica 1996;81(1):40–43.

92. Higashi K, Matsuki Y, Hidaka T, et al. Primary Sjogren's syndrome associated with hyaline-vascular type of Castleman's disease and autoimmune idiopathic thrombocytopenia. Scand J Rheumatol 1997;26(6):482–484.

93. Chan TM, Cheng IK, Wong KL, et al. Resolution of membranoproliferative glomerulonephritis complicating angiofollicular lymph node hyperplasia (Castleman's disease). Nephron 1993;65(4):628–632.

94. Dispenzieri A, Kyle RA, Lacy MQ, et al. POEMS syndrome: definitions and long-term outcome. Blood 2003;101(7):2496–2506.

95. Couch WD. Giant lymph node hyperplasia associated with thrombotic thrombocytopenic purpura. Am J Clin Pathol 1980;74(3):340–344.
96. Larroche C, Cacoub P, Soulier J, et al. Castleman's disease and lymphoma: report of eight cases in HIV-negative patients and literature review. Am J Hematology 2002;69(2):119–126.
97. Chan AC, Chan KW, Chan JK, et al. Development of follicular dendritic cell sarcoma in hyaline-vascular Castleman's disease of the nasopharynx: tracing its evolution by sequential biopsies. Histopathology 2001;38(6):510–518.
98. Rywlin AM, Rosen L, Cabello B. Coexistence of Castleman's disease and Kaposi's sarcoma. Report of a case and a speculation. Am J Dermatopathol 1983;5(3):277–281.
99. Gili A, Ngan BY, Lester R. Castleman's disease associated with pemphigus vulgaris. J Am Acad Dermatol 1991;25(5 Pt 2):955–959.
100. Wang L, Bu D, Yang Y, et al. Castleman's tumours and production of autoantibody in paraneoplastic pemphigus. Lancet 2004;363(9408):525–531.
101. Strohal R, Tschachler E, Breyer S, et al. Reactivation of Behcet's disease in the course of multicentric HHV8-positive Castleman's disease: long-term complete remission by a combined chemo/radiation and interferon-alpha therapy regimen. Br J Haematol 1998;103(3):788–790.
102. Mizutani N, Okada S, Tanaka J, et al. Multicentric giant lymph node hyperplasia with ascites and double cancers, an autopsy case. Tohoku J Exp Med 1989;158(1):1–7.
103. Weisenburger DD. Membranous nephropathy. Its association with multicentric angiofollicular lymph node hyperplasia. Arch Pathol Lab Med 1979;103(11):591–594.
104. Summerfield GP, Taylor W, Bellingham AJ, et al. Hyaline-vascular variant of angiofollicular lymph node hyperplasia with systemic manifestations and response to corticosteroids. J Clin Pathol 1983;36(9):1005–1011.
105. Miadonna A, Salmaso C, Palazzi P, et al. Fibrillary glomerulonephritis in Castleman's disease. Leuk Lymphoma 1998;28(3–4):429–435.
106. Franco V, Aragona F, Rodolico V, et al. Castleman's disease associated with hepatic amyloidosis. An immunohistochemical and ultrastructural study. Haematologica 1984;69(5):556–567.
107. Perfetti V, Bellotti V, Maggi A, et al. Reversal of nephrotic syndrome due to reactive amyloidosis (AA-type) after excision of localized Castleman's disease. Am Journal of Hematol 1994;46(3):189–193.
108. Ordi J, Grau JM, Junque A, et al. Secondary (AA) amyloidosis associated with Castleman's disease. Report of two cases and review of the literature. Am J ClinPathol 1993;100(4):394–397.
109. Pilon VA, Gomez LG, Butler JJ. Systemic amyloidosis associated with a benign mesenteric lymphoid mass. Am J Clin Pathol 1982;78(1):112–116.
110. Day JR, Bew D, Ali M, et al. Castleman's disease associated with myasthenia gravis. Ann Thorac Surg 2003;75(5):1648–1650.
111. Johkoh T, Muller NL, Ichikado K, et al. Intrathoracic multicentric Castleman disease: CT findings in 12 patients. Radiology 1998;209(2):477–481.
112. Fujimoto W, Kanehiro A, Kuwamoto-Hara K, et al. Paraneoplastic pemphigus associated with Castleman's disease and asymptomatic bronchiolitis obliterans. Eur J Dermatol 2002;12(4):355–359.
113. Chin AC, Stich D, White FV, et al. Paraneoplastic pemphigus and bronchiolitis obliterans associated with a mediastinal mass: a rare case of Castleman's disease with respiratory failure requiring lung transplantation. J Pediatr Surg 2001;36(12):E22.
114. Wolff H, Kunte C, Messer G, et al. Paraneoplastic pemphigus with fatal pulmonary involvement in a woman with a mesenteric Castleman tumour.[see comment]. Br J Dermatol 1999;140(2):313–316.
115. Suwannaroj S, Elkins SL, McMurray RW. Systemic lupus erythematosus and Castleman's disease. J Rheumatol 1999;26(6):1400–1403.
116. Crump JA, Beard ME, Angus HB, et al. Acute adrenal insufficiency: a new presentation of Castleman's disease. J Intern Med 1995;238(1):81–84.
117. Seida A, Wada J, Morita Y, et al. Multicentric Castleman's disease associated with glomerular microangiopathy and MPGN-like lesion: does vascular endothelial cell-derived growth factor play causative or protective roles in renal injury? Am J Kidney Dis 2004;43(1):E3–E9.

118. Lui SL, Chan KW, Li FK, et al. Castleman's disease and mesangial proliferative glomerulonephritis: the role of interleukin-6. Nephron 1998;78(3):323–327.
119. Dispenzieri A, Moreno-Aspitia A, Suarez GA, et al. Peripheral blood stem cell transplantation in 16 patients with POEMS syndrome, and a review of the literature. Blood 2004;104(10):3400–3407.
120. Mallory A, Spink WW. Angiomatous lymphoid hamartoma in the retroperitoneum presenting with neurologic signs in the legs. Ann Intern Med 1968;69(2):305–308.
121. Anonymous. Case records of the Massachusetts General Hospital. Weekly clinicopathological exercises. Case 32–1984. N Engl J Med 1984;311:388–398.
122. Anonymous. Case records of the Massachusetts General Hospital. Weekly clinicopathological exercises. Case 10–1987. A 59-year-old woman with progressive polyneuropathy and monoclonal gammopathy. New Engl J Med 1987;316(10):606–618.
123. Donaghy M, Hall P, Gawler J, et al. Peripheral neuropathy associated with Castleman's disease. J Neurol Sci 1989;89(2–3):253–267.
124. Ganti AK, Pipinos I, Culcea E, et al. Successful hematopoietic stem-cell transplantation in multicentric Castleman disease complicated by POEMS syndrome. Am J Hematol 2005;79(3):206–210.
125. Bosco J, Pathmanathan R. POEMS syndrome, osteosclerotic myeloma and Castleman's disease: a case report. Austr NZ J Med 1991;21(4):454–456.
126. Dispenzieri A, Loe MJ, Geyer SM, et al. A prognostic model of 114 patients with Castleman's disease. ASH Annu Meet Abstr 2006;108(11):102.
127. Oksenhendler E, Boulanger E, Galicier L, et al. High incidence of Kaposi sarcoma-associated herpesvirus-related non-Hodgkin lymphoma in patients with HIV infection and multicentric Castleman disease. Blood 2002;99(7):2331–2336.
128. Loi S, Goldstein D, Clezy K, et al. Castleman's disease and HIV infection in Australia. HIV Med 2004;5(3):157–162.
129. Guihot A, Couderc LJ, Agbalika F, et al. Pulmonary manifestations of multicentric Castleman's disease in HIV infection: a clinical, biological and radiological study. Eur Respir J 2005;26(1):118–125.
130. Dickson D, Ben-Ezra JM, Reed J, et al. Multicentric giant lymph node hyperplasia, Kaposi's sarcoma, and lymphoma. Arch Pathol Lab Med 1985;109(11):1013–1018.
131. Okuda K, Himeno Y, Toyama T, et al. Gamma heavy chain disease and giant lymph node hyperplasia in a patient with impaired T cell function. Jpn J Med 1982;21(2):109–114.
132. Artusi T, Bonacorsi G, Saragoni A, et al. Castleman's lymphoadenopathy: twenty years of observation. II. Generalized form. Haematologica 1982;67(1):124–142.
133. Orcioni GF, Mambelli V, Ascani S, et al. Concurrence of localized Castleman's disease and peripheral small B-lymphocytic lymphoma within the same lymph node. Gen Diagn Pathol 1998;143(5-6):327–330.
134. Katano H, Kaneko K, Shimizu S, et al. Follicular dendritic cell sarcoma complicated by hyaline-vascular type Castleman's disease in a schizophrenic patient. Pathol Int 1997;47(10):703–706.
135. Perez-Ordonez B, Rosai J. Follicular dendritic cell tumor: review of the entity. Semin Diagn Pathol 1998;15(2):144–154.
136. Lee IJ, Kim SC, Kim HS, et al. Paraneoplastic pemphigus associated with follicular dendritic cell sarcoma arising from Castleman's tumor. J Am Acad Dermatol 1999;40(2 Pt 2):294–297.
137. Marzano AV, Vezzoli P, Mariotti F, et al. Paraneoplastic pemphigus associated with follicular dendritic cell sarcoma and Castleman disease. Br J Dermatol 2005;153(1):214–215.
138. Kazakov DV, Morrisson C, Plaza JA, et al. Sarcoma arising in hyaline-vascular castleman disease of skin and subcutis. Am J Dermatopathol 2005;27(4):327–332.
139. Chen KT. Multicentric Castleman's disease and Kaposi's sarcoma. Am J Surg Pathol 1984;8(4):287–293.
140. Kessler E. Multicentric giant lymph node hyperplasia. A report of seven cases. Cancer 1985;56(10):2446–2451.
141. De Rosa G, Barra E, Guarino M, et al. Multicentric Castleman's disease in association with Kaposi's sarcoma. Appl Pathol 1989;7(2):105–110.

142. Gironet N, De Muret A, Machet L, et al. [Paraneoplastic pemphigus revealing dendritic cell sarcoma originating from Castleman's disease of the neck]. Ann Dermatol Venereol 2005;132(1):41–44.

143. Senanayake S, Kelly J, Lloyd A, et al. Multicentric Castleman's disease treated with antivirals and immunosuppressants. J Med Virol 2003;71(3):399–403.

144. Mandel C, Silberstein M, Hennessy O. Case report: fatal pulmonary Kaposi's sarcoma and Castleman's disease in a renal transplant recipient. Br J Radiol 1993;66(783):264–265.

145. Baker WJ, Vukelja SJ, Weiss RB, et al. Multicentric angiofollicular lymph node hyperplasia and associated carcinoma. Medi Pediatr Oncol 1994;22(6):384–388.

146. Horio H, Hijima T, Sakaguchi K, et al. Mediastinal Castleman disease associated with pulmonary carcinoma, mimicking N2 stage lung cancer. Jpn J Thorac Cardiovasc Surg 2005;53(5):286–289.

147. Takehara K, Sakai H, Igawa T, et al. Unicentric Castleman's disease with leiomyosarcoma: a rare association. Int J Urol 2003;10(11):619–621.

148. Ulbright TM, Santa Cruz DJ. Kaposi's sarcoma: relationship with hematologic, lymphoid, and thymic neoplasia. Cancer 1981;47(5):963–973.

149. Kasantikul V, Panyavoravut V, Benjavongkulchai S, et al. Castleman's disease: a clinicopathologic study of 12 cases. J Med Assoc Thailand 1997;80(3):195–201.

150. Fitzpatrick PJ, Brown TC. Angiofollicular lymph node hyperplasia. Can Med Assoc J 1968;99(25):1259–1262.

151. Emson HE. Extrathoracic angiofollicular lymphoid hyperplasia with coincidental myasthenia gravis. Cancer 1973;31(1):241–245.

152. Nordstrom DG, Tewfik HH, Latourette HB. Giant lymph node hyperplasia: a review of literature and report of two cases of plasma cell variant responding to radiation therapy. Int J Radiat Oncol Biol Phys 1978;4(11–12):1045–1048.

153. Marti S, Pahissa A, Guardia J, et al. Multicentric giant follicular lymph node hyperplasia. Favorable response to radiotherapy. Cancer 1983;51(5):808–810.

154. Stokes SH, Griffith RC, Thomas PR. Angiofollicular lymph node hyperplasia (Castleman's disease) associated with vertebral destruction. Cancer 1985;56(4):876–879.

155. Sethi T, Joshi K, Sharma SC, et al. Radiation therapy in the management of giant lymph node hyperplasia. Br J Radiol 1990;63(752):648–650.

156. Veldhuis GJ, van der Leest AH, de Wolf JT, et al. A case of localized Castleman's disease with systemic involvement: treatment and pathogenetic aspects. Ann Hematol 1996;73(1):47–50.

157. Safford SD, Lagoo AS, Mahaffey SA. Preoperative embolization as an adjunct to the operative management of mediastinal Castleman disease. J Pediatr Surg 2003;38(9):E21–E23.

158. Caneppele S, Picart N, Bayle-Lebey P, et al. Paraneoplastic pemphigus associated with Castleman's tumour. Clin Exp Dermatol 2000;25(3):219–221.

159. Ruggieri G, Barsotti P, Coppola G, et al. Membranous nephropathy associated with giant lymph node hyperplasia. A case report with histological and ultrastructural studies. Am J Nephrol 1990;10(4):323–328.

160. Mandreoli M, Casanova S, Vianelli N, et al. Remission of nephrotic syndrome due to AA amyloidosis and initiation of glomerular repair after surgical resection of localized Castleman's disease. Nephron 2002;90(3):336–340.

161. Lachmann HJ, Gilbertson JA, Gillmore JD, et al. Unicentric Castleman's disease complicated by systemic AA amyloidosis: a curable disease. Q J Med 2002;95(4):211–218.

162. Neuhof D, Debus J. Outcome and late complications of radiotherapy in patients with unicentric Castleman disease. Acta Oncol 2006;45(8):1126–1131.

163. Gulati P, Sun NC, Herman BK, et al. Isolated leptomeningeal Castleman's disease with viral particles in the follicular dendritic cells. Arch Pathol Lab Med 1998;122(11): 1026–1029.

164. Pavlidis NA, Skopouli FN, Bai MC, et al. A successfully treated case of multicentric angiofollicular hyperplasia with oral chemotherapy (Castleman's disease). Med Ped Oncol 1990;18(4):333–335.

165. van Rhee F, Alikhan M, Munshi N, et al. Anti-IL6 antibody (ab) based strategies improve the management of HIV negative Castleman's disease. Blood 2004;104(11):897a.

166. Hudnall SD, Chen T, Brown K, et al. Human herpesvirus-8-positive microvenular hemangioma in POEMS syndrome. Arch Pathol Lab Med 2003;127(8):1034–1026.
167. Jacobs SA, Vidnovic N, Patel H, et al. Durable remission of HIV-negative, Kaposi's sarcoma herpes virus-associated multicentric Castleman disease in patient with rheumatoid arthritis treated with methotrexate. Clin Rheumatol 2007;26(7):1148–1150.
168. Ocio EM, Sanchez-Guijo FM, Diez-Campelo M, et al. Efficacy of rituximab in an aggressive form of multicentric Castleman disease associated with immune phenomena. Am J Hematol 2005;78(4):302–305.
169. Ide M, Ogawa E, Kasagi K, et al. Successful treatment of multicentric Castleman's disease with bilateral orbital tumour using rituximab. Br J Haematol 2003;121(5):818–819.
170. Abdou S, Salib H. An extra ordinary respone of Castleman's disease to rituximab. Blood 2004;104(11):49b.
171. Gholam D, Vantelon JM, Al-Jijakli A, et al. A case of multicentric Castleman's disease associated with advanced systemic amyloidosis treated with chemotherapy and anti-CD20 monoclonal antibody. Ann Hematol 2003;82(12):766–768.
172. Colleoni GW, Duarte LC, Kerbauy FR, et al. 2-Chloro-deoxyadenosine induces durable complete remission in Castleman's disease but may accelerate its transformation to non-Hodgkin's lymphoma. Acta Oncol 2003;42(7):784–787.
173. Bordeleau L, Bredeson C, Markman S. 2-Chloro-deoxyadenosine therapy for giant lymph node hyperplasia. B J Haematol 1995;91(3):668–670.
174. Pavlidis NA, Briassoulis E, Klouvas G, et al. Is interferon-a an active agent in Castleman's disease? Ann Oncol 1992;3(1):85–86.
175. Tamayo M, Gonzalez C, Majado MJ, et al. Long-term complete remission after interferon treatment in a case of multicentric Castelman's disease. Am J Hematol 1995;49(4):359–360.
176. Andres E, Maloisel F. Interferon-alpha as first-line therapy for treatment of multicentric Castleman's disease. Ann Oncol 2000;11(12):1613–1614.
177. Simko R, Nagy K, Lombay B, et al. Multicentric Castleman disease and systemic lupus erythematosus phenotype in a boy with Klinefelter syndrome: long-term disease stabilization with interferon therapy. J Pediatr Hematolo/Oncol 2000;22(2):180–183.
178. Lee FC, Merchant SH. Alleviation of systemic manifestations of multicentric Castleman's disease by thalidomide. Am J Hematol 2003;73(1):48–53.
179. Starkey CR, Joste NE, Lee FC. Near-total resolution of multicentric Castleman disease by prolonged treatment with thalidomide. Am J Hematol 2006;81(4):303–304.
180. Hess G, Wagner V, Kreft A, et al. Effects of bortezomib on pro-inflammatory cytokine levels and transfusion dependency in a patient with multicentric Castleman disease. Br J Haematol 2006;134(5):544–545.
181. Beck JT, Hsu SM, Wijdenes J, et al. Brief report: alleviation of systemic manifestations of Castleman's disease by monoclonal anti-interleukin-6 antibody. New Engl J Med 1994;330(9):602–605.
182. Advani R, Warnke R, Rosenberg S. Treatment of multicentric Castleman's disease complicated by the development of non-Hodgkin's lymphoma with high-dose chemotherapy and autologous peripheral stem-cell support. Ann Oncol 1999;10(10):1207–1209.
183. Lerza R, Castello G, Truini M, et al. Splenectomy induced complete remission in a patient with multicentric Castleman's disease and autoimmune hemolytic anemia. Ann Hematol 1999;78(4):193–196.
184. Aaron L, Lidove O, Yousry C, et al. Human herpesvirus 8-positive Castleman disease in human immunodeficiency virus-infected patients: the impact of highly active antiretroviral therapy. Clin Infect Dis 2002;35(7):880–882.
185. Bottieau E, Colebunders R, Schroyens W, et al. Multicentric Castleman's disease in 2 patients with HIV infection, unresponsive to antiviral therapy. Acta Clin Belgica 2000; 55(2):97–101.
186. Lanzafame M, Carretta G, Trevenzoli M, et al. Successful treatment of Castleman's disease with HAART in two HIV-infected patients. J Infect 2000;40(1):90–91.

187. Zietz C, Bogner JR, Goebel FD, et al. An unusual cluster of cases of Castleman's disease during highly active antiretroviral therapy for AIDS. N Engl J Med 1999;340(24):1923–1934.
188. Corbellino M, Bestetti G, Scalamogna C, et al. Long-term remission of Kaposi sarcoma-associated herpesvirus-related multicentric Castleman disease with anti-CD20 monoclonal antibody therapy. Blood 2001;98(12):3473–3475.
189. Berezne A, Agbalika F, Oksenhendler E. Failure of cidofovir in HIV-associated multicentric Castleman disease. Blood 2004;103(11):4368–4369.
190. Casper C, Nichols WG, Huang ML, Corey L, Wald A. Remission of HHV-8 and HIV-associated multicentric Castleman disease with ganciclovir treatment.[see comment]. Blood 2004;103(5):1632–1634.
191. Scott D, Cabral L, Harrington WJ Jr. Treatment of HIV-associated multicentric Castleman's disease with oral etoposide. Am J Hematol 2001;66(2):148–150.
192. Liberopoulos E, Tolis C, Bai M, et al. Successful treatment of human immunodeficiency virus-related Castleman's disease: a case report and literature review. Oncology 2003;65(2): 182–186.
193. Kumari P, Schechter GP, Saini N, et al. Successful treatment of human immunodeficiency virus-related Castleman's disease with interferon-alpha. Clin Infect Dis 2000;31(2):602–604.
194. Nord JA, Karter D. Low dose interferon-alpha therapy for HIV-associated multicentric Castleman's disease. Int J STD AIDS 2003;14(1):61–62.
195. Jung CP, Emmerich B, Goebel FD, et al. Successful treatment of a patient with HIV-associated multicentric Castleman disease (MCD) with thalidomide. Am J Hematol 2004;75(3): 176–177.
196. Marcelin AG, Aaron L, Mateus C, et al. Rituximab therapy for HIV-associated Castleman disease. Blood 2003;102(8):2786–2788.
197. Marietta M, Pozzi S, Luppi M, et al. Acquired haemophilia in HIV negative, HHV-8 positive multicentric Castleman's disease: a case report. Eur J Haematol 2003;70(3):181–182.
198. Casquero A, Barroso A, Fernandez Guerrero ML, et al. Use of rituximab as a salvage therapy for HIV-associated multicentric Castleman disease. Ann Hematol 2006;85(3):185–187.
199. Kofteridis DP, Tzagarakis N, Mixaki I, et al. Multicentric Castleman's disease: prolonged remission with anti CD-20 monoclonal antibody in an HIV-infected patient. Aids 2004;18(3): 585–586.
200. Neuville S, Agbalika F, Rabian C, et al. Failure of rituximab in human immunodeficiency virus-associated multicentric Castleman disease. Am J Hematol 2005;79(4):337–339.
201. Newsom-Davis T, Bower M, Wildfire A, et al. Resolution of AIDS-related Castleman's disease with anti-CD20 monoclonal antibodies is associated with declining IL-6 and TNF-alpha levels. Leuk Lymphoma 2004;45(9):1939–1941.
202. Revuelta MP, Nord JA. Successful treatment of multicentric Castleman's disease in a patient with human immunodeficiency virus infection.[see comment]. Clin Infect Diss 1998;26(2):527.
203. Yamasaki S, Iino T, Nakamura M, et al. Detection of human herpesvirus-8 in peripheral blood mononuclear cells from adult Japanese patients with multicentric Castleman's disease. Br J Haematol 2003;120(3):471–477.
204. Luppi M, Barozzi P, Maiorana A, et al. Human herpesvirus-8 DNA sequences in human imunodeficiency virus-negative angioimmunoblastic lymphadenopathy and benign lymphadenopathy with giant germinal center hyperplasia and increased vascularity. Blood 1996;87(9):3903–3909.
205. Tohda S, Murakami N, Nara N. Human herpesvirus 8 DNA in HIV-negative Japanese patients with multicentric Castleman's disease and related diseases. Int J Mol Med 2001;8(5):549–551.
206. Marrache F, Larroche C, Memain N, et al. Prolonged remission of HIV-associated multicentric Castleman's disease with an anti-CD20 monoclonal antibody as primary therapy. Aids 2003;17(9):1409–1410.

Chapter 14
Rare T-Cell Lymphomas

Ana Maria Molina and Steven M. Horwitz

14.1 Introduction

T-Cell lymphomas are a group of rare or, at least uncommon, hematologic malignancies comprising about 10–15% of all non-Hodgkin's lymphomas in North America (6). Overrepresentation of certain subtypes such as natural killer (NK)/T-cell lymphoma makes them relatively more common in Asia (105, 106). As classification systems for lymphoid malignancies become more sophisticated, combining morphology, immunophenotype, molecular, and clinical information, more distinct subtypes of T-cell lymphoma have emerged. In the latest version of the WHO and World Health Organization-European Organisation for Research and Treatment of Cancer (WHO-EORTC) consensus on cutaneous lymphomas, there are at least 13 different subtypes of T-cell lymphoma (83).

Despite this heterogeneity, the T-cell lymphomas do share some common features. They have a predilection for extranodal sites, which makes detection, diagnosis, and management challenging. They are poorly studied and often carry a poor prognosis. The continually evolving classification systems make it difficult to collect rigorous retrospective data and their rarity makes prospective studies almost impossible. Although our understanding of the pathology has grown from detailed studies of tumor tissue, our management strategies for T-cell lymphomas are primarily borrowed from those shown effective for more common aggressive B-cell lymphoma.

In this chapter, we will focus on three of the rarest T-cell lymphomas: enteropathy-associated T-cell lymphoma, hepatosplenic T-cell lymphoma, and subcutaneous panniculitis- like T-cell lymphoma. Each of these lymphomas comprises less than 5% of all the T-cell lymphomas and fewer than 1% of all non-Hodgkin's lymphomas, making them truly rare hematologic malignancies. Each section reviews increasingly well-described clinical and pathologic characteristics of these lymphomas. We also review strategies for management that are collected from case reports, small series, personal experiences, and retrospective reviews. Underlying the treatment discussions must be an awareness on the part of the reader of the inherent biases in case reports and small series and the lack of data available to formulate a preferred management approach.

14.2 Enteropathy-type T-Cell lymphoma

Enteropathy-type T-cell lymphoma (ETL) is a rare, predominantly extranodal non-Hodgkin's lymphoma strongly associated with underlying celiac disease. In the recent international T-cell NHL study, ETL accounts for 4.7% of all T-cell lymphomas (32). Originally termed *malignant histiocytosis of the intestine*, this entity was shown to be of T-cell lineage, arising from intraepithelial cells (IELs) in the gastrointestinal tract (17, 33). In the World Health Organization classification enteropathy-type T-cell lymphoma is categorized under the extranodal grouping of mature T-cell and NK-cell neoplasms (41).

14.2.1 Clinical Features and Diagnosis

Enteropathy-type T-cell lymphoma is strongly associated with celiac disease, with a relative risk ranging from 2.1 to 6.6 (3, 10, 11, 19, 21, 34, 64). It is believed that in many patients, ETL arises from a progressive clonal expansion of IELs in certain at-risk patients with refractory celiac disease and the early changes can be seen long before the manifestations of overt lymphoma. Isaacson and Du have reviewed the multistage development of ETL starting with susceptible individuals with HLA DQA1 and DQB1 to the development of celiac disease (CD), progression to refractory CD, and, finally, the development of ETL (23). ETL has been linked to an HLA type found in northern Europeans consisting of HLA DQA1*0501 and DQB1*0201 genotypes that are characteristic of celiac disease (7). Homozygosity for HLA-DQ2 is associated with refractory celiac disease type II (RCD II) and ETL (66). In patients with refractory sprue, the clonal proliferation of abnormal IELs is an early manifestation of ETL (61). These IELs have normal cytologic appearance but are phenotypically abnormal (CD3€+, CD3−, CD8−, CD4−, and clonal rearrangement of the TCRγ gene) (63). Cellier et al, classified these aberrant populations of IEL as "cryptic enteropathy-associated T-cell lymphoma" (61, 63). Although patients with refractory CD and clonal expansion of IELs have a greatly increased risk of progressing to ETL, not all patients will go on to develop overt lymphoma. In patients with established celiac disease, the absolute rates of non-Hodgkin's lymphoma and small bowel lymphoma are reported to be 1 in 1421 person-years and 1 in 5684 person-years, respectively (34).

Enteropathy-type T-cell lymphoma has an aggressive clinical course. This growth rate coupled with difficulties assessing the bowel by physical exam or radiographic studies results in most patients being diagnosed with advanced disease. ETL commonly occurs in the sixth and seventh decades of life and typically presents in a patient with either a history of childhood celiac disease or during the diagnosis of adult-onset celiac disease. Less often, it presents in patients with no history of celiac disease. At diagnosis, patients complain of abdominal pain, vomiting, and diarrhea. Bowel obstruction and/or perforation are commonly the first signs of disease and subsequent surgery results in the diagnosis. In the two largest series, the presenting features were abdominal pain, diarrhea, vomiting, and up to 23% and 37% of patients presented with small bowel obstruction or perforation, respectively (1, 15). At presentation, B-symptoms, elevated lactate dehydrogenase (LDH), and anemia are also reported (1, 13, 15). Bone marrow involvement is rare, with 2 series reporting 0/9 and 2/24 patients affected (1, 13).

Computed tomography (CT) might show bowel thickening and regional lymphadenopathy but is relatively insensitive at finding sites of bowel involvement. Positron-emission tomography (PET) is reported to assist in staging by identifying sites of bowel involvement not appreciated by CT scan (37, 51, 84). The sensitivity of PET might prove helpful in following patients at high risk of developing ETL. In a retrospective study of a small number of patients, Hoffmann et al. demonstrated that PET findings differ significantly in patients affected by ETL and patients suffering from celiac disease (51). Hadithi et al. demonstrated in a prospective cohort study of 38 patients that 18 Fluorodeoxyglucose-Positron emission tomography (18F-FDG-PET) was more sensitive in detecting ETL in patients with refractory celiac disease than was CT (37). PET scan was 100% sensitive and 90% specific in detecting ETL in patients with refractory celiac disease. The positive likelihood ratio of 10 suggests that PET might be a useful tool in both monitoring and early detection of the development of ETL in patients with RCD by helping to direct biopsy in areas of increased uptake that are suspicious for malignancy. Equivocal PET results in patients can be problematic in the diagnosis of ETL, given the difficulty in assessing the small bowel indirectly or by means other than surgical techniques. Capsule endoscopy, initially used to evaluate obscure gastrointestinal bleeding, is a promising technique that might be useful in directly evaluating the small bowel in patients with ETL and possibly refractory celiac disease. Joyce et al. reported the first use of small bowel capsule endoscopy in a patient with ETL receiving chemotherapy (86). Images revealed erythema, active bleeding, mucosal flattening with villous loss, telangiectasia, and stricturing and nodularity, findings consistent with the presence of persistent lymphoma (86). Early detection has the possibility of improving outcome for these patients, as, at present, due to the lymphoma and underlying celiac disease, many have poor performance status and nutritional status, greatly compromising their ability to receive aggressive therapy. In a prospective, nonrandomized multicenter study of intestinal non-Hodgkin's lymphoma (NHL), 10 out of 35 (29%) of patients with intestinal T-cell lymphoma died within 3 months of diagnosis (15).

14.2.2 Pathology

Characteristic findings on histology include multiple ulcerating and eroding tumors in the mucosa of the small intestine (1, 6). The tumor cells are heterogeneous and pleomorphic, ranging from small to large-sized or anaplastic lymphoid cells. Although these tumors occur most commonly in the jejunum, they are multifocal. The tumor cells represent proliferations of abnormal intraepithelial lymphocytes infiltrating the small bowel wall. The tumor is infiltrated and, at times, is even obscured by a large population of inflammatory cells (1, 23). The tumor cells arise from intraepithelial lymphocytes that usually express the t-cell receptor (TCR) αβ and are TCR γδ-negative (9). They are CD3+, CD4−, CD7+, CD8+/−, CD103+, T-cell-restricted intracellular antigen (TIA-1+) and might also express the cytotoxic protein granzyme B (17, 23, 24). Some anaplastic tumor cells might express CD30 and a subset of monomorphic small to medium-sized cells are CD8- and CD56-positive (6, 9, 24). Epstein-Barr virus (EBV) has been detected in some cases and seems to be epidemiologically dependent (29–67). Quintanilla-Martinez et al. found epidemiological differences in EBV detection in a group of primary intestinal T-cell NHL between Mexican and European populations of 100% and 10%, respectively (67). It is possible that some of the EBV-positive cases are more representative of NK lymphoma-nasal type, which can present in the gastrointestinal tract.

Although genetic abnormalities associated with ETL are largely unknown, common chromosomal abnormalities elucidated in the past years have shed light on the possible evolution of these tumors. Applying comparative genomic hybridization (CGH) and fluorescence *in situ* hybridization (FISH), Zettl et al. investigated genetic alterations in 75 cases of ETL and found recurrent gains and losses of genetic material in 87% of cases (18). Recurrent gains of genetic material involved chromosomes 9q (in 58% of cases), 7q (24%), 5q (18%), and 1q (16%) and recurrent losses involved chromosomes 8p and 13q (24% each) and 9p (18%). Verkarre et al. performed cytogenetic studies in cell lines from clonal abnormal IEL in refractory celiac sprue and found that refractory celiac sprue is strongly associated with partial trisomy of the 1q region, a gain that might be an early event in the development of ETL (36). Obermann et al. also reported that deletions of 9p21, a chromosome that harbors tumor suppressor genes and is associated with the development and progression of lymphomas, is a frequent finding in ETL (25).

14.2.3 Treatment and Prognosis

Due to the rarity and advanced stage at presentation, there are no randomized or large prospective trials for the treatment of ETL. When diagnosed, most patients undergo surgical resection and systemic therapy is initiated. In a retrospective study of 31 patients with ETL, various multiagent chemotherapy regimens were used, including the following: vincristine, doxorubicin, prednisolone, and high-dose methotrexate; cyclophosphamide, doxorubicin, vincristine, and prednisolone (CHOP); alternating 21-day cycles of CHOP with procarbazine, etoposide, and prednisolone orally on days 3–7, and doxorubicin intravenously on day 1; cyclophosphamide, vincristine, doxorubicin and prednisolone; and alternating weekly cycles of prednisolone, doxorubicin, cyclophosphamide, and etoposide with prednisolone, bleomycin, vincristine and methotrexate (PEACE-BOM) (1). Underscoring the difficulty of providing aggressive therapy to these often compromised patients, less than 50% of the patients completed their planned chemotherapy regimens because complications of treatment. Responses seen in 58% of patients [10 complete remission (CR) and 4 partial remission (PR)] were short-lived and 79% of patients relapsed 1–60 months from diagnosis. The 1- and 5-year survival rates were 38.7% and 19.7%, respectively, with 1-and 5-year failure-free survival rates of 19.4% and 3.2%, respectively (1). In a multicenter prospective, nonrandomized study of intestinal NHL, Daum et al. treated 56 patients (28 with ETL) with CHOP and found that patients with intestinal T-cell lymphoma overall had a less favorable response, with an overall 2-year survival rate of only 28% (15). Similarly to other studies, patients frequently could not complete chemotherapy due to complications. Other regimens with success in case series and single case reports include cyclophosphamide, vincristine, doxorubicin, and dexamethasone (hyper-CVAD) with ongoing CR at 34 months; alemtuzumab (CAMPATH) in patients with relapsed or chemotherapy-refractory peripheral T-cell lymphomas; CHOP followed by ProMACE-CytaBOM (consisting of cyclophosphamide, adriamycin, etoposide, cytarabine, bleomycin, vincristine, methotrexate, and prednisolone; and CHOEP (consisting of cyclophos-phamide, doxorubicin, etoposide, vincristine, and prednisone (5, 14, 20, 65, 68, 73, 75). Autologous stem cell transplant (ASCT) also been used successfully in case reports and case series (71, 72). Bishton et al. treated six patients with two cycles of IVE (ifosfamide, etoposide, epirubicin) followed by two cycles of high-dose methotrexate with folinic acid rescue and a BEAM (carmustine, etoposide, cytara-bine, melphalan) autograft, achieving a CR in 4/6 patients at 1.83–4.32 years (72). Overall, the outcome for ETL is very poor, with 1- and 5-year survival rates in the range of 31–39% and 9–20%, respectively (1, 2, 15, 35, 65).

Responding to the dismal results in treating ETL, recently more aggressive approaches consisting of systemic therapy and ASCT have been used to treat patients with refractory celiac disease. Al-toma et al. used ASCT in seven patients with refractory celiac disease with aberrant T-cells (RCD type II) conditioned with fludarabine and melphalan and showed a significant reduction in the aberrant T-cells in duodenal biopsies and a reduction in clinical symptoms (69). In a series of 17 patients with RCD II treated with cladribine, Al-toma et al. again showed a significant decrease in aberrant T-cells, but the development of ETL was not prevented (70).

The improved understanding of the pathobiology of celiac disease and the progression to ETL is paramount in the development of treatment regimens, assess-ment tools, and, possibly, prevention measures. Treatment with a gluten-free diet might reduce the risk of intestinal lymphoma (4).

14.3 Hepatosplenic T-Cell Lymphoma

Hepatosplenic T-cell lymphoma (HSTCL) is an almost exclusively extranodal NHL with infiltration of the spleen, bone marrow, and liver that typically presents with marked hepatosplenomegaly. Originally described as a unique subtype of T-cell lymphomas in 1990, HSCTL was commonly referred to as hepatosplenic γ/δ T-cell lymphoma (12, 37, 56). However, there are now reports of α/β expressing tumors sharing the same clinical and pathologic characteristics and clinical course (60, 65). HSTCL are rare tumors accounting for 1.4% of all T-cell lymphomas in the recent International T-cell NHL study (32). The rarity of this disease results in most of our understanding coming from small series and case reports. There is also significant overlap in these series with many individual cases being reported more than once.

14.3.1 Clinical Features and Diagnosis

Hepatosplenic T-cell lymphoma can occur at any age but is more often seen in teenagers or young adults with a strong male predominance. Patients present with significant hepatosplenomegaly, cytopenias, constitutional symptoms, and an absence of lymphadenopathy. In the two largest series, the presenting features included splenomegaly in all but one case and over 80% had hepatomegaly (28, 57). Splenic rupture is reported (59). Presentation is usually aggressive, with symptoms leading promptly to diagnosis; however, there are reports of more indolent cases with symptoms present for years (28, 57). Cytopenias are very common with thrombocytopenia in over 85% of patients at diagnosis (28, 57). Anemia and leukopenia, often with striking lymphopenia, is also seen in the majority (28, 57). Although most patients have bone marrow involvement and/or splenomegaly to explain the cytopenias, hemophagocytic syndrome is reported (28, 57). Small numbers of circulating tumor cells might be seen on careful review of blood smears (28, 57). Central nervous system involvement is reported but rare (101). Constitutional symptoms including fevers, weight loss, jaundice, drenching night sweats, and infection are frequently seen, whereas autoimmune phenomena such as immune thrombocytopenic purpura and autoimmune hemolytic anemia might precede the diagnosis (28, 58, 59).

Corresponding to liver involvement and an aggressive growth rate, an elevated LDH level, alkaline phosphatase, aspartate aminotransferase, and alanine aminotransferase are the most frequent serum chemistry abnormalities at the time of diagnosis.

Immunocompromised patients are overrepresented, with numerous reports of HSCTL developing years after solid-organ transplantation (28, 57, 102–104). Unlike the more commonly described EBV- associated posttransplantation lymphoproliferative disorders, which often develop soon after transplantation; cases of HSTCL seem to occur many years later. Other reported cases include patients with lupus erythematosus, previous treatment for Hodgkin's disease and acute myelogenous leukemia, malarial infection, and inflammatory bowel disease (55). The importance of immunosuppression as a potential cofactor for the development of HSCTL has recently come to the forefront, with eight cases developing in children or young adults treated with infliximab (a tumor necrosis factor (TFN)-α blocking agent) for inflammatory bowel disease. Previous cases have been reported after azathioprine use and all of the infliximab-treated patients were using concomitant immunosuppression (azathioprine, mercaptopurine, and/or corticosteroids).

Nonetheless, these reports strongly suggest a significant increase in the risk of developing HSTCL in this specific population.

Computed tomography usually shows marked hepatomegaly and splenomegaly with significant lymphadenopathy. Likely due to the absence of lymphadenopathy and diffuse involvement of liver and spleen, PET has not been useful (84). Diagnosis has most commonly been at splenectomy or liver biopsy. Although bone marrow involvement is frequent, the histologic findings often show a hypocellular marrow with subtle infiltration with abnormal lymphocytes. Immunostaining to highlight the T-cells and better define the abnormal lymphocyte population as well as molecular studies demonstrating clonal T-cell receptor rearrangements are often very helpful or essential in confirming the diagnosis.

14.3.2   Pathology

The tumor infiltrate is made up of monomorphic small to medium-sized cells with pale cytoplasms. The cells infiltrate the sinuses of the bone marrow, spleen, and liver with sparing of the portal triads and white pulp.

Pathologic cells of T-cell origin are most often characterized by a specific profile: CD2, CD3, γ/δ TCR positivity, CD7 variable, and CD4, CD5, and CD8 negativity (9, 10). CD8 has been detectable at low levels by flow cytometry on cases described as CD8-negative by immunohistochemistry on paraffin-embedded tissue (54).

Expression of NK markers have frequently been described, including expression of the CD56 and the killer cell immunoglobulinlike receptor (KIR) CD94 (54, 57). T-Cell antigens more commonly expressed on other forms of T-cell lymphoma such as CD30 seem not to be expressed and expression of B-cell markers are not described (57). Most of the tumor cells demonstrate staining for the granule-associated protein TIA-1 but are rarely positive for granzyme B (57). The TCR gamma gene is always clonally rearranged. Reports have described similar presentations with tumor cells expressing an α/β phenotype, usually defined by expression of Beta F-1 (60, 85). In the γ/δ patients investigated, there appears to be preferential use of the Vδ1 chain (53, 57). T-Lymphoblastic lymphomas might be excluded by expression of TdT.

The recurrent abnormality of isochromosome 7q has been recognized and at times found to be associated with other chromosomal abnormalities such as trisomy 8. These chromosomal abnormalities are seen in a number of hematologic malignancies; the combination of both seems most specific to HSTCL (28). There is no association with EBV.

14.3.3   Treatment and Outcome

There are no prospective studies of treatment for HSTCL. In general, patients have been treated with combination chemotherapy such as CHOP or CHOP-like regimens.

The results of this therapy are almost uniformly poor. In the two larger series reporting on 66 patients (although at least 5 cases are included in both series), only 6 patients were alive at the time of the reports. One of these patients is reported with only 3 months of follow-up and four of these patients received some form of high-dose therapy. Thus, only 2 of these 66 patients were in a durable remission after a conventional-dose chemotherapy regimen such as CHOP. There is another case report of a patient with durable remissions after chemotherapy alone (52). Many patients have disease primarily refractory to chemotherapy, with short remission durations in others. Although the course is aggressive in most patients, one series reports several patients who were free from progression for several years after splenectomy or relatively mild chemotherapy, suggesting that there might be rare patients with a more indolent clinical course. Multiple other agents such as pentostatin, alemtuzumab, 2-CDA, and fludarabine are reported to give transient responses.

Somewhat less bleak in the small numbers of reported cases is the use of high-dose therapy and stem cell transplantation. In the larger series, four of the six patients alive in remission at the time of their report had undergone some form of high-dose therapy treatment. Due to publication bias, there is, of course, a high risk of error in drawing conclusions from case series and collections of case reports; however, this is the extent of the data we have for this rare disease. In the report by Belhadj et al. (57) six patients underwent autologous stem cell or bone marrow transplantation with two of these patients alive in remission at 42 and 52 months, respectively. Both of these patients were treated initially with a platinum–cytarabine-based combination as opposed to a CHOP-like regimen, suggesting better activity with these agents. Both of these patients also underwent high-dose therapy as a consolidation phase of their initial treatment program. Long-term remissions are not reported for those undergoing high-dose therapy and ASCT at relapse. Allogeneic stem cell transplantation shows similar results, with 4 of 12 patients alive in remission in a recent review series. All patients reported were treated prior to undergoing allogeneic stem cell transplantation, with four progressing or relapsing and four dying of treatment-related causes in addition to the four who are alive. Details on the conditioning regimen and stem cell source are not provided for most cases, although two of the three patients with total-body irradiation as part of their treatment were alive in remission.

14.4 Subcutaneous Panniculitis-like T-Cell lymphoma and Cutaneous γδ T-Cell Lymphoma

Subcutaneous panniculitis-like T-cell lymphoma (SPTL) and cutaneous γδ T-cell lymphoma (CGD-TCL) are cytotoxic, postthymic T-cell neoplasms that predominantly affect the skin. Both entities express T-cell receptors (TCRs) consisting of either an α/β or a γ/δ heterodimer. The importance of the TCR phenotype has been evaluated, leading to a distinction in these two cutaneous lymphomas. In the

WHO-EORTC classification for cutaneous lymphomas, the term "SPTL" is only used for cases with an α/β+ T-cell phenotype and CGD-TCL classified as a provisional entity and includes cases with a γ/δ T-cell phenotype previously known as SPTL (46, 83). SPTL and CGD-TCL account for 0.9% and 0.1%, respectively, of all T-cell lymphomas in the recent International T-cell NHL study (32).

14.4.1 Clinical Features and Diagnosis

Subcutaneous panniculitis-like T-cell lymphoma and cutaneous γδ T-cell lymphoma predominantly affect young adults and present primarily as skin lesions. The skin lesions consist of solitary or multiple nodules and erythematous plaques predominantly affecting the lower extremities (42, 43, 44, 47, 50). Some of these skin lesions might ulcerate. Extracutaneous involvement and constitutional symptoms are uncommon (50). Although rare, involvement of extracutaneous sites reported in case reports and case reviews include the bone marrow, lymph nodes, liver, spleen, and peripheral blood (13, 43, 44, 50, 79, 82, 88). Elevated LDH, liver dysfunction, and cytopenias are also reported (13, 43, 47, 79, 83). The clinical course is often complicated by a hemophagocytic syndrome with a reported mortality as high as 81% (40, 42, 44, 47, 49, 50, 79, 88, 89, 91).

Overall, two clinical courses have been appreciated, whereby some patients have rapidly progressive disease and others have a more indolent course based on TCR phenotype. Patients with a α/β TCR phenotype have a more indolent course and might experience spontaneous regressions of skin lesions (43, 49, 87, 88). Toro et al. investigated the prognostic value of γ/δ TCR expression in a retrospective study in which the skin biopsy specimens of 104 patients (33/104 γ/δ) were reviewed (43). Patients predominantly presented with plaques, tumors, and subcutaneous nodules, some with ulceration of the lower extremities. Of the patients with γ/δ TCR expression, none had bone marrow involvement, one had lymph node involvement, and four had lymphadenopathy. TCRδ1 expression was associated with decreased survival, with a median survival for individuals with γδ cutaneous T-cell lymphoma of 15 months compared with a median survival of 166 months in individuals with αβ cutaneous T-cell lymphoma (43).

14.4.2 Pathology

Characteristically, atypical lymphoid cells of varying size infiltrate subcutaneous adipose tissue, mimicking panniculitis (42, 47, 49, 50). Rimming of adipocytes with karyorrhexis, tumor necrosis, and angioinvasion are typical findings (42, 50). Although minimal dermal invasion can be observed, the dermis and epidermis are often spared.

Extension into the reticular dermis can be seen with CGD-TCL tumor cells (80, 87). The tumor consists of mature T-cells that express T-cell-associated antigens (CD3, CD45RO, or CD43); cytotoxic proteins [granzyme B, perforin, and (TIA-1)

T-cell intracellular antigen], and T-cell receptors and are EBV-negative (50, 81). SPTL express the α/β T-cell phenotype and are usually CD8-positive (81, 83). CGD-TCL express the γ/δ T-cell phenotype and are typically CD4- and CD 8-negative (80, 83). CD56-positive tumor cells in CGD-TCL have been reported and found to carry a poor prognosis compared to CD56-negative tumors (40, 49, 50, 53, 82, 83, 87). Clonal TCR rearrangements are described in both SPTL and CGD-TCL (53). In contrast to HSTCL, there appears to be preferential use of the Vδ2 chain in γ/δ patients investigated (50, 53). There is no association with EBV.

14.4.3   Treatment and Prognosis

Treatment modalities for indolent disease might include radiotherapy or immuno-suppressive therapy with corticosteroids. In a review of cytotoxic lymphomas, Massone et al. reported that in 10 patients with the α/β T-cell phenotype, the disease could be controlled for long periods with systemic steroid therapy (45). Combination chemotherapy regimens used to treat aggressive NHLs are often used. These regimens frequently consist of anthracylcine-based chemotherapy, other combinations, single agents (fludarabine), FND (fludarabine, mitoxantrone and dexamethasone) and, less frequently, high-dose chemotherapy followed by stem cell transplant (16, 39, 50, 76–79, 87).

In a systematic review of 156 patients with SPTL in the literature, Go and Wester reported overall response rates using different modalities (40). Patients with indolent disease were generally treated initially with modalities that consisted of radiotherapy, prednisone and cyclosporine, and single-agent low-dose chemotherapy (i.e., cyclophosphamide or methotrexate). Patients with more aggressive disease received combination chemotherapy, most of which were anthracycline-based regimens. Examples of overall response (OR) rates reported using the various modalities include the following: 81% in patients treated with radiation; 50% in patients treated with prednisone or a corticosteroid equivalent; and 53% in patients treated with combination-chemotherapy regimens. Overall responses were often short-lived, regardless of the therapy provided, ranging from ≥2 months to ≥72 months and the median survival for the entire group was approximately 27 months.

Additionally, in this review, 13 patients with refractory or recurrent disease received high-dose chemotherapy and stem cell transplantation. Of these patients, 12 (92%) had a CR with a median response duration of ≥14 months at last follow-up (40, 50, 53, 77, 79, 90, 95–100). One out of the 13 patients had an allogeneic transplant and achieved a CR for 70 months (40, 90). Overall, the expression of the γ/δ T-cell phenotype and the presence of hemophagocytic syndrome (HPS) at diagnosis were associated with poor survival (40).

In a retrospective study, Ghobrial et al. looked at 21 patients with unknown TCR phenotype treated with different modalities (82). In this study, 13 patients received systemic therapy including CHOP, CNOP (doxorubicin replaced by mitoxantrone), ProMACE CytaBOM (doxorubicin, vincristine, bleomycin, methotrexate, cyclophosphamide, cytarabine, etoposide, prednisone, leucovorin), vincristine, ICE (ifosfamide, carboplatin, etoposide), CDE (cyclophosphamide, doxorubicin, etoposide), FND (fludarabine, mitoxantrone, dexamethasone), and other interventions, including surgical excision, corticosteroids alone or in combination with either plaquenil, colchicine, hydroxychloroquine, or azathioprine, and bone marrow transplantation. In this group of patients, the OR rate was 43% and was short-lived with subsequent disease progression and a median survival of 7 months from the time of diagnosis. In a small number of patients eligible for autologous bone marrow transplant, median overall survival was 44 months (range 15–90 months).

There are a few case reports that describe treating HPS with cyclosporine A (91, 92). A patient who received methylprednisolone pulse therapy followed by prednisolone and cyclosporine A remained asymptomatic for at least 6 months (91). Another case report described the possibility of graft-versus-lymphoma effect in a patient refractory to conventional chemotherapy who responded after getting total-body irradiation, Ara-C, and cyclophosphamide and then undergoing allogeneic peripheral blood stem cell transplantation (89).

Overall, lasting responses to chemotherapy are rare in SPTL. Biological and immunological therapies such as interferon-α, interleukin-12, retinoids, denileukin difitox (Ontak), and monoclonal antibodies (mAb) such as alemtuzumab (Campath) used in the treatment of cutaneous T-cell lymphoma (CTCL) are promising for the treatment of SPTL (94). Recently, bexarotene, an oral retinoid used to treat mycosis fungoides (48), showed a high response rate in a series of 10 patients with SPTL (93). In this series, 60% of patients responded and the duration of response ranged from 8 to 33 months at last follow-up.

14.5 Summary

The evolving classification systems in lymphoma have been driven by advances in the pathologic characterization of lymphoid malignancies. As evidenced by the detailed pathology descriptions earlier, subdividing heterogenous diseases results in an increasing number of distinct subtypes. This has allowed pathologists to provide more accurate diagnoses and begin to shed light on the molecular mechanisms that underlie these disorders. However, clinical information on these rare subtypes has lagged. Standard staging studies are less useful for these primarily extranodal diseases, although newer technologies such as PET scanning might be useful in detecting and following sites of disease. Optimal management remains undefined. Although these lymphomas are often aggressive, particularly in the case of ETCL, HSTCL, and GD-TCL, standard combination-chemotherapy regimens have only rarely provided durable remissions. Highdose therapy strategies have shown early promise, particularly for HSTCL, although conclusive data to support its routine use is lacking. Other strategies such as biologic therapies as with retinoids for SPTCL have provided durable benefit for some patients with less toxicity. Ultimately, it will take larger series with these rare but increasingly recognized entities to better define a preferred management approach.

References

1. Gale J, Simmonds PD, Mead GM, et al. Enteropathy-type intestinal T-cell lymphoma: clinical features and treatment of 31 patients in a single center. J Clin Oncol 2000;18(4):795–803.
2. Egan LJ, Walsh SV, Stevens FM, et al. Celiac-associated lymphoma: a single institution experience of 30 cases in the combination chemotherapy era. J Clin Gastroenterol 1995;21:123–129.
3. Morton JE, Leyland MJ, Vaughan HG, et al. Primary gastrointestinal non-Hodgkin's lymphoma: a review of 175 British National Lymphoma Investigation cases. Br J Cancer 1993;67:776–782.
4. Holmes GKT, Prior P, Lane MR, et al. Malignancy in celiac disease: effect of a gluten free diet. Gut 1989;30:333–338.
5. Okada M, Maeda K, Suzumiya J, et al. Primary colorectal T-cell lymphoma. J Gastroenterol 2003; 38:376–384.
6. Kluin PM, Feller A, Gaulard P, et al. Peripheral T/NK-cell lymphoma: a report of the IXth Workshop of the European Association for Haematopathology. Histopathology 2001;38:250–270.
7. Jaffe ES, Krenacs L, Raffeld M. Classification of cytotoxic T-cell and natural killer cell lymphomas. Semin Hematol 2003;40(3):175–184.
8. Jaffe ES, Harris NL, Stein H, et al. Pathology and genetics of tumours of haematopoietic and lymphoid tissues. World Health Organization classification of tumours. Lyon: IARC Press; 2001.
9. Chott A, Haedicke W, Mosberger I, et al. Most CD56+ intestinal lymphomas are CD8+ CD5- T-cell lymphomas of monomorphic small to medium size histology. Am J Pathol 1998;153:1483–1490.
10. Isaacson PG, Wright DH. Intestinal lymphoma associated with malabsorption. Lancet 1978; 311(8055):67–70.
11. Holmes GK. Coeliac disease and malignancy. Dig Liver Dis 2002;34:229–337.
12. Cooke CB, Krenacs M, Stetler-Stevenson M, et al. Hepatosplenic gamma/delta T-cell lymphoma: a distinct clinicopathologic entity of cytotoxic gamma/delta T-cell origin. Blood 1996;88:4265–4274.
13. Savage KJ, Chhanabhai M, Gascoyne RD, et al. Characterization of peripheral T-cell lymphomas in a single North American institution by the WHO classification. Ann Oncol 2004;15:1467–1475.
14. Wohrer S, Chott A, Drach J, et al. Chemotherapy with cyclophosphamide, doxorubicin, etoposide, vincristine and prednisone (CHOEP) is not effective in patients with enteropathy-type intestinal T-cell lymphoma. Ann Oncol 2004;15:1680–1683.
15. Daum S, Ullrich R, Heise W et al. Intestinal non-Hodgkin's lymphoma: a multicenter prospective clinical study from the German Study Group on Intestinal non-Hodgkin's Lymphoma. J Clin Oncol 2003; 21:2740–2746.
16. Johnson SA. Use of fludarabine in the treatment of mantle cell lymphoma, Waldenström's macroglobulinemia and other uncommon B- and T-cell lymphoid malignancies. Hematol J 2004;5(Suppl 1):50–61.
17. Isaacson PG, O'Connor NT, Spencer J, et al. Malignant histiocytosis of the intestine: a T-cell lymphoma. Lancet 1985;2:688–691.
18. Zettl A, Ott G, Makulik A, et al. Chromosomal gains at 9q characterize enteropathy-type T-cell lymphoma. Am J Pathol 2002;161:1635–1645.
19. Catassi C, Fabiana E, Corrao G, et al. Risk of non-Hodgkin's lymphoma in celiac disease. JAMA 2002;287:1413–1419.
20. Enblad G, Hagberg H, Erlanson M, et al. A pilot study of alemtuzumab (anti CD52 monoclonal antibody) therapy for patients with relapsed or chemotherapy- refractory peripheral T-cell lymphomas. Blood 2004;103:2920–2924.

21. Halfdanarson TR, Litzow MR, Murray JA. Hematological manifestations of celiac disease. Blood 2007;109:412–421.
22. Anon. A clinical evaluation of the International Lymphoma Study Group classification of non-Hodgkin's lymphoma. The Non-Hodgkin's Lymphoma Classification Project. Blood 1997;89:3909–3918.
23. Isaacson PG, Du M. Gastrointestinal lymphoma: where morphology meets molecular biology. J Pathol 2005;205:255–274.
24. Isaacson PG. Gastrointestinal lymphomas of T- and B-cell types. Mod Pathol 1999; 12(2):151–158.
25. Obermann EC, Diss TC, Hamoudi RA, et al. Loss of heterozygosity at chromosome 9p21 is a frequent finding in enteropathy-type T-cell lymphoma. J Pathol 2004;202:252–262.
26. Wei S, Liu T, Wang D, et al. Hepatosplenic γ/δ T-cell lymphoma. World J Gastroenterol 2005;11(24):3729–3734.
27. Farcet J, Gaulard P, Marolleau J, et al. Hepatosplenic T-cell lymphoma: sinusal/sinusoidal localization of malignant cells expressing the T-cell receptor γδ. Blood 1990;75: 2213–2219.
28. Weidmann E. Hepatosplenic T cell lymphoma. A review of 45 cases since the first report describing the disease as a distinct lymphoma entity in 1990. Leukemia 2000;14:991–997.
29. Pan L, Diss TC, Peng H, et al. Epstein-Barr virus (EBV) in enteropathy-associated T-cell lymphoma (EATL). J Pathol 1993;170:137–143.
30. De Bruin PC, Jiwa NM, Van der Valk P, et al. Detection of Epstein-Barr virus nucleic acid sequences and protein in nodal T-cell lymphomas: relation between latent membrane protein-1 positivity and clinical course. Histopathology 1993;23:509–518.
31. De Bruin PC, Jiwa NM, Oudejans JJ, et al. Epstein-Barr virus in primary gastrointestinal T cell lymphomas. Association with gluten-sensitive enteropathy, pathological features, and immunophenotype. Am J Pathol. 1995;146:861–867.
32. Weisenburger DD, Wilson WH, Vose JM. Peripheral T-cell lymphoma, not otherwise specified: a clinicopathologic study of 340 cases from the International T-Cell Lymphoma Project. Blood (ASH Annual Meeting Abstracts) 2006;108:2458.
33. Fairley NH, Mackie FP. The clinical and biochemical syndrome in lymphoma and allied diseases involving the mesenteric lymph glands. Br Med J 1937;1:375–380.
34. Catassi, C, Bearzi, Holmes G. Association of celiac disease and intestinal lymphomas and other cancers. Gastroenterology 2005;128:S79–S86.
35. Howdle PD, Jalal PK, Holmes GKT, et al. Primary small bowel malignancy in the UK and its association with coeliac disease. Q J Med 2003;96:345–353.
36. Verkarre V, Romana S, Cellier C, et al. Recurrent partial trisomy 1q22–q44 in clonal intraepithelial lymphocytes in refractory celiac sprue. Gastroenterology 2003;125:40–46.
37. Hadithi M, Mallant M, Oudejans J, et al. 18F-FDG PET versus CT for the detection of enteropathy-associated T-cell lymphoma in refractory celiac disease. J Nucl Med 2006;47:1622–1627.
38. Slater DN. The new World Health Organization-European Organization for Research and Treatment of Cancer classification for cutaneous lymphomas: a practical marriage of two giants. Br J Dermatol 2005;153:874–880.
39. Go RS, Gazelka H, Hogan JD, et al. Subcutaneous panniculitis-like T-cell lymphoma: complete remission with fludarabine. Ann Hematol 2003;82:247–250.
40. Go RS, Wester SM. Immunophenotypic and molecular features, clinical outcomes, treatments, and prognostic factors associated with subcutaneous panniculitis-like T-cell lymphoma. A systematic analysis of 156 patients reported in the literature. Cancer 2004;101:1404–1413.
41. Jaffe ES, Ralfkiaer E. Subcutaneous panniculitis-like T-cell lymphoma. In: Jaffe ES, Harris NL, Stein H, et al., editors. World Health Organization classification of tumors: pathology and genetics of tumors of hematopoietic and lymphoid tissues. Lyon: IARC Press; 2001, p. 212–215.
42. Gonzalez CL, Medeiros J, Braziel RM, et al. T-Cell lymphoma involving subcutaneous tissue. A clinicopathologic entity commonly associated with hemophagocytic syndrome. Am J Surg Pathol 1991;15:17–27.

43. Toro JR, Liewehr DJ, Pabby N, et al. Gamma-delta T-cell phenotype is associated with significantly decreased survival in cutaneous T-cell lymphoma. Blood 2003;101: 3407–3412.
44. Toro JR, Beaty M, Sorbara L, et al. Gamma delta T-cell lymphoma of the skin: a clinical, microscopic, and molecular study. Arch Dermatol 2000;136:1024–1032.
45. Massone C, Chott A, Metze D, et al. Subcutaneous, blastic natural killer (NK), NK/T-cell, and other cytotoxic lymphomas of the skin a morphologic, immunophenotypic, and molecular study of 50 patients. Am J Surg Pathol 2004;28:719–735.
46. Willemze R, Kerl H, Sterry W, et al. EORTC classification for primary cutaneous lymphomas: A proposal from the Cutaneous Lymphoma Study Group of the European Organization for the Research and Treatment of Cancer. Blood 1997;90:354–371.
47. Weenig RH, Ng CS, Perniciaro C. Subcutaneous panniculitis-like T-cell lymphoma: an elusive case presenting as lipomembranous panniculitis and a review of 72 cases in the literature. Am J Dermatopathol 2001;23:206–215.
48. Duvic M, Hymes K, Heald P, et al. Bexarotene is effective and safe for treatment of refractory advanced-stage cutaneous T-cell lymphoma: multinational phase II-III trial results. J Clin Oncol 2001;19:2456–2471.
49. Hoque SR, Child FJ, Whittaker SJ, et al. Subcutaneous panniculitis-like T-cell lymphoma: a clinicopathological, immunophenotypic and molecular analysis of six patients. Br J Dermatol 2003;148:516–525.
50. Salhany KE, Macon WR, Choi JK, et al. Subcutaneous panniculitis-like T-cell lymphoma: clinicopathologic, immunophenotypic, and genotypic analysis of alpha/beta and gamma/delta subtypes. Am J Surg Pathol 1998;22:881–893.
51. Hoffmann M, Vogelsang H, Kletter K, et al. 18F-Fluoro-deoxy-glucose positron emission tomography (18F-FDG-PET) for assessment of enteropathy-type T cell lymphoma. Gut 2003;52:347–351.
52. Moleti ML, Testi AM, Giona F, et al. Gamma-delta hepatosplenic T-cell lymphoma. Description of a case with immunophenotypic and molecular follow-up successfully treated with chemotherapy alone. Leuk Lymphoma. 2006;47:333–336.
53. Przybylski GK, Wu H, Macon WR, et al. Hepatosplenic and subcutaneous panniculitis-like γ/δ T cell lymphomas are derived from different Vδ subsets of γ/δ T lymphocytes. J Mol Diagn 2000;2:11–19.
54. Morice WG, Macon WR, Dogan A, et al. NK-Cell-associated receptor expression in hepatosplenic T-cell lymphoma, insights into pathogenesis. Leukemia. 2006;20:883–886.
55. Hassan R, Franco SA, Stefanoff CG, et al. Hepatosplenic gamma delta T-cell lymphoma following seven malaria infections. Pathol Int 2006;56:668–673.
56. Harris NL, Jaffe ES, Stein H, et al. A revised European-American classification of lymphoid neoplasms: a proposal from the International Lymphoma Study Group. Blood 1994;84:1361–1392.
57. Belhadj K, Reyes F, Farcet J, et al. Hepatosplenic γδ T-cell lymphoma is a rare clinicopathologic entity with poor outcome: report on a series of 21 patients. Blood 2003;102:4261–4269.
58. Motta G, Vianello F, Menin C, et al. Hepatosplenic gammadelta T-cell lymphoma presenting with immune-medicated thrombocytopenia and hemolytic anemia (Evan's syndrome). Am J Hematol 2002;69:272–276.
59. Chen JH, Chan DC, Lee HS, et al. Spontaneous splenic rupture associated with hepatosplenic gammadelta T-cell lymphoma. J Formos Med Assoc 2005;104:593–596.
60. Kumar S, Lawlor C, Jaffe ES. Hepatosplenic T-cell lymphoma of alphabeta lineage. Am J Surg Pathol 2001;25:970–971.
61. Cellier C, Patey N, Mauvieux L, et al. Abnormal intestinal intraepithelial lymphocytes in refractory sprue. Gastroenterology 1998;114:471–481.
62. Cellier C, Delabesse E, Helmer C, et al. Refractory sprue, coeliac disease, and enteropathy-associated T-cell lymphoma. Lancet 2000;356:203–208.

63. Daum S, Weiss D, Hummel R, et al. Frequency of clonal intraepithelial T lymphocyte pro-liferations in enteropathy-type intestinal T cell lymphoma, coeliac disease, and refractory sprue. Gut 2001;49:804–812.
64. Smedby KE, Akerman M, Hildebrand H, et al. Malignant lymphomas in coeliac disease: evidence of increased risks for lymphoma types other than enteropathy-type T cell lym-phoma. Gut 2005;54:54–59.
65. Novakovic BJ, Novakovic S, Frkovic-Grazio S. A single-center report on clinical features and treatment response in patients with intestinal T cell non-Hodgkin's lymphomas. Oncol Rep 2006;16:191–195.
66. Al-Toma A, Goerres MS, Meijer JW, et al. Human leukocyte antigen-DQ2 homozygosity and the development of refractory celiac disease and enteropathy-associated T-cell lym-phoma. Clin Gastroenterol Hepatol 2006;4:315–319.
67. Quintanilla-Martinez L, Lome-Maldonado C, Ott G, et al. Primary non-Hodgkin's lym-phoma of the intestine: high prevalence of Epstein-Barr virus in Mexican lymphomas as compared with European cases. Blood 1997;89:644–651.
68. Honemann D, Prince HM, Hicks RJ, et al. Enteropathy-associated T-cell lymphoma without a prior diagnosis of coeliac disease: diagnostic dilemmas and management options. Ann Hematol 2005;84:118–121.
69. Al-toma A, Visser OJ, van Roessel HM, et al. Autologous hematopoietic stem cell transplan-tation in refractory celiac disease with aberrant T-cells. Blood 2007;109(5):2243–2249.
70. Al-toma A, Goerres MS, Meijer JW, et al. Cladribine therapy in refractory celiac disease with aberrant T cells. Clin Gastroenterol Hepatol 2006;11:1322–1327.
71. Rongey C, Micallef I, Smyrk T, et al. Successful treatment of enteropathy-associated T-cell lymphoma with autologous stem cell transplant. Dig Dis Sci 2006;51:1082–1086.
72. Bishton M, Andrew H. Combination chemotherapy followed by autologous stem cell trans-plant for enteropathy-associated T cell lymphoma. Br J Haematol 2006;136:111–113.
73. Vivas S, Ruiz de Morales JM, Ramos F, et al. Alemtuzumab for refractory celiac disease in a patient at risk for enteropathy-associated T-cell lymphoma. N Engl J Med 2006;354:2514–2515.
74. Verbeek W, Mulder C, Zweegman S. Alemtuzumab for refractory celiac disease. N Engl J Med 2006;355:1396–1397.
75. Lundin KE, Farstad IN, Raki M, et al. Alemtuzumab treatment of refractory celiac disease type II (Abstract). Gastroenterol 2006;130(Suppl 2):A-666.
76. Au WY, Ng WM, Choy C, et al. Aggressive subcutaneous panniculitis-like T-cell lym-phoma: complete remission with fludarabine, mitoxantrone and dexamethasone. Br J Dermatol 2000;143:408–410.
77. Reimer P, Rudiger T, Muller J, et al. Subcutaneous panniculitis-like T-cell lymphoma during pregnancy with successful autologous stem cell transplantation. Ann Hematol 2003;82:305–309.
78. Mukai HY, Okoshi Y, Shimizu S, et al. Successful treatment of a patient with subcutaneous panniculitis-like T-cell lymphoma with high-dose chemotherapy and total body irradiation. Eur J Haematol 2003;70:413–416.
79. Ghobrial I, Weenig R, Pittlekow MR, et al. Clinical outcome of patients with subcutaneous panniculitis-like T-cell lymphoma. Leuk Lymphoma 2005;46:703–708.
80. De Wolf-Peeters C, Achten R. γδ T-cell lymphomas: a homogenous entity? Histopathology 2000;36:294–305.
81. Kumar S, Krenac, L, Medeiros J, et al. Subcutaneous pannicultic T-cell lymphoma is a tumor of cytotoxic T lymphocytes. Hum Pathol 1998;29:397–403.
82. Takeshita M, Imayama S, Oshiro Y, et al. Clinicopathologic analysis of 22 cases of subcuta-neous panniculitis-like CD56– or CD56+ lymphoma and review of 44 other reported cases. Am J Clin Pathol 2004;121:408–416.
83. Willemze R, Jaffe E, Burg G, et al. WHO-EORTC classification for cutaneous lymphomas. Blood 2005;105:3768–3785.

84. Horwitz S, Foss F, Goldfarb S, et al. FDG-PET scans as an additional staging study for T-cell lymphomas: high rates of positivity do not result in frequent changes in stage. Blood (ASH Annual Meeting Abstracts) 2006;108:2399.
85. Suarez F, Wlodarska I, Rigal-Huquet F, et al. Hepatosplenic alphabeta T-cell lymphoma: an unusual case with clinical histologic and cytogenetic features of gammadelta hepatosplenic T-cell lymphoma. Am J Surg Pathol 2000;24:1027–1032.
86. Joyce AM, Burns DL, Marcello PW, et al. Capsule endoscopy findings in celiac disease associated enteropathy-type intestinal T-cell lymphoma. endoscopy 2005;37:594–596.
87. Santucci M, Pimpinelli N, Massi D, et al. Cytotoxic/natural killer cell cutaneous lymphomas report of the EORTC Cutaneous Lymphoma Task Force Workshop. Cancer 2003;97:610–627.
88. Bekkenk MW, Jansen PM, Meijer CJLM, et al. CD56+ hematological neoplasms presenting in the skin: a retrospective analysis of 23 new cases and 130 cases from the literature. Ann Oncol 2004;15:1097–1108.
89. Ichii M, Hatanaka K, Imakita M, et al. Successful treatment of refractory subcutaneous panniculitis-like T-cell lymphoma with allogeneic peripheral blood stem cell transplantation from HLA-mismatched sibling donor. Leuk Lymphoma 2006;47:2250–2252.
90. Leo E, Bertz H, Koehler G, et al. Successful treatment of aggressive, recurrent, subcutaneous panniculitis-like T cell lymphoma (SPTCL) with high-dose chemotherapy followed by allogeneic peripheral stem cell transplantation (Abstract). Blood 2001;98:377b.
91. Tsukamato Y, Katsunobu Y, Omura Y, et al. Subcutaneous panniculitis-like T-cell lymphoma: successful initial treatment with prednisolone and cyclosporin A. Intern Med 2006;45:21–24.
92. Al Zolibani AA, Al Robaee AA, Qureshi MG, et al. Subcutaneous panniculitis-like T-cell lymphoma with hemophagocytic syndrome successfully treated with cyclosporin A. Skinmed 2006;5:195–197.
93. Molina A, Advani R, Reddy S, et al. Bexarotene is highly active in the treatment of subcutaneous panniculitis-like T-cell lymphoma. Blood (ASH Annual Meeting Abstracts) 2005 106:3344.
94. McFarlane V, Friedman PS, Illidge TM. What's new in the management of cutaneous T-cell lymphoma? Clin Oncol 2005;17:174–184.
95. Romero LS, Goltz RW, Nagi C, et al. Subcutaneous T-cell lymphoma with associated hemophagocytic syndrome and terminal leukemic transformation. J Am Acad Dermatol. 1996;34:904–910.
96. Munn SE, McGregor JM, Jones A, et al. Clinical and pathological heterogeneity in cutaneous gamma-delta T-cell lymphoma: a report of three cases and a review of the literature. Br J Dermatol. 1996;135:976–981.
97. Haycox CL, Back AL, Raugi GJ, et al. Subcutaneous T-cell lymphoma treated with systemic chemotherapy, autologous stem cell support, and limb amputation. J Am Acad Dermatol 1997;37:832–825.
98. Koizumi K, Sawada K, Nishio M, et al. Effective high-dose chemotherapy followed by autologous peripheral blood stem cell transplantation in a patient with the aggressive form of cytophagic histiocytic panniculitis. Bone Marrow Transplant 1997;20:171–173.
99. Dargent JL, Roufosse C, Delville JP, et al. Subcutaneous panniculitis-like T-cell lymphoma: further evidence for a distinct neoplasm originating from large granular lymphocytes of T/NK phenotype. J Cutan Pathol 1998;25:394–400.
100. Magro CM, Crowson AN, Kovatich AJet al. Lupus profundus, indeterminate lymphocytic lobular panniculitis and subcutaneous T-cell lymphoma: a spectrum of subcuticular T-cell lymphoid dyscrasia. J Cutan Pathol 2001;28:235–247.
101. Ferrari D, Girmenia G, Migliorini L, et al. Hepatosplenic gamma delta T-cell lymphoma with a novel cytogenetic alteration and cerebrospinal fluid infiltration: biological and clinical features. Haematologica 2002;87:ERC11.
102. Khan WA, Yu L, Eisenbrey AB, et al. Hepatosplenic gamma/delta T-cell lymphoma in immunocompromised patients report: Report of two cases and review of literature. Am J Clin Pathol 2001;116:41–50.

103. Francois A, Lesesve JF, Stamatoullas A, et al. Hepatosplenic gamma/delta T-cell lymphoma: a report of two cases in immunocompromised patients, associated with isochromosome 7q. Am J Surg Pathol 1997;21:781–790.
104. Kraus MD, Crawford DF, Kaleem Z, et al. T Gamma/delta hepatosplenic lymphoma in a heart transplant patient after an Epstein-Barr virus positive lymphoproliferative disorder: a case report. Cancer. 1998;82:983–992.
105. Jaffe ES, Chan JK, Su IJ, et al. Report of the Workshop on Nasal and Related Extranodal Angiocentric T/Natural Killer Cell Lymphomas. Definitions, differential diagnosis, and epidemiology. Am J Surg Pathol 1996;20:103–111.
106. Shih LY, Liang DC. Non-Hodgkin's lymphomas in Asia. Hematol Oncol Clin North Am 1991;5:983–1001.

Chapter 15
CD30+ Diseases

Anaplastic Large-Cell Lymphoma and Lymphomatoid Papulosis

Peter Borchmann

15.1 Introduction

The CD30 antigen was first detected in 1982 using a Hodgkin-Reed/Sternberg (H-RS) cell line and it was cloned and characterized as a member of the tumor necrosis factor (TNF) receptor superfamily a decade later in 1992 (1–3). Soon it became clear that, although restricted to hematopoietic cells, it was not only expressed by H-RS cells but also by activated T- and B-cells and some other lymphoid malignancies. In addition to Hodgkin's lymphoma (HL), the following primary systemic lymphomas also express CD30: anaplastic large-cell lymphoma (ALCL) in all cases, the majority of posttransplant lymphoproliferative disorders (PTLDs, see Chapter 12), the primary mediastinal B-cell lymphoma with a comparably weak CD30 expression (see Chapter 10), and the lymphomatoid granulomatosis (Lyg) in some instances (see Chapter 11). In addition, CD30 is expressed in primary cutaneous CD30-positive T-cell lymphoproliferative disorders, to which the primary cutaneous ALCL (C-ALCL), the lymphomatoid papulosis (LyP), and the borderline lesions belong.

This chapter will focus on the systemic ALCL and the primary cutaneous CD30-positive T-cell lymphomas, although CD30 is expressed by many others of the rare lymphoid malignancies. Because CD30 is the red thread for this chapter, this receptor will be described more in detail first.

15.2 The CD30 Antigen

CD30 belongs to the TNF-R superfamily, which consists of 26 receptors and 18 ligands known so far (4). These receptors are characterized by the presence of 40-amino-acid, cysteine-rich repeats in their extracellular domains. CD30 is the largest TNF-R with six of these motifs in its extracellular domain (see Figure 15.1) (5). The whole protein has a molecular weight of 120 kDa and is a type I transmembrane protein. The extracellular part of CD30 can be shed by metalloproteinases and is then released into the plasma. This soluble CD30 (sCD30) is an ~90-kDA

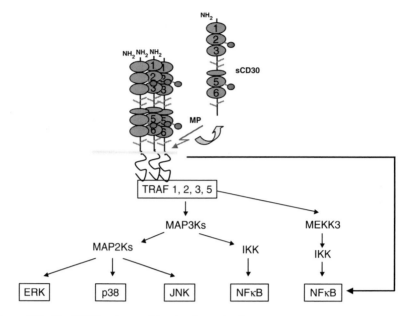

Figure 15.1 The CD30 antigen and its signal transduction

protein that can be found in the sera of patients with CD30-positive lymphoid malignancies, with autoimmune diseases or with acute or chronic viral infections, especially during infection with the Epstein-Barr virus (EBV).

CD30 signaling is induced by its trimerization. Physiologically, aggregation of CD30 is mediated by binding to its counterpart, the CD30 ligand (CD30L, CD153). In contrast to other TNF-Rs, CD30 contains no intracellular death domain (DD), which could cause the cell death upon receptor activation. CD30 acts via so-called TRAFs (TNF receptor-associated factors). So far, six TRAFs are known and the cytoplasmatic tail of CD30 interacts through its binding sites with four of them: TRAF-1, -2, -3, and -5. Trimerisation of CD30 thereby leads to the activation of different pathways, including extracellular signal-regulated kinase (ERK), c-jun amino terminal kinase (JNK), p38 mitogen-activated protein kinase (MAPK), and NF-κB (nuclear factor-κB) (see Figure 15.2). This can then result in the secretion of cytokines, including interleukin (IL)-2, IL-6, IL-8, IL-12, and granulocyte colony-stimulating factor (G-CSF). Based on these diverse possibilities of intracellular signaling, CD30 activation can have pleiotropic and even opposing effects for the cell, ranging from proliferation induction and enhanced cell survival over growth arrest to induction of apoptosis. CD30 deficiency does not result in overt defects in either the T-cell or the B-cell homeostasis. CD30 has been reported to control thymic negative selection, but this could not be confirmed in a more recent study with CD30–/– mice (6). Some studies have shown that CD30L/CD30 might provide proliferation and/or survival signals to allow the generation of high numbers

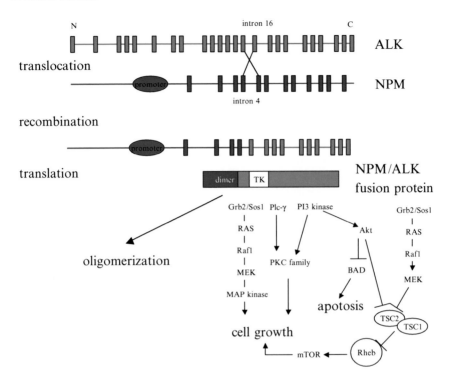

Figure 15.2 The NPM/ALK fusion protein. TSC: tuberous sclerosis complex proteins. (Adapted from Ref. 23)

of antigen-specific T-cells (7, 8). Adoptive transfer of antigen-specific CD8 T-cells into CD30L–/– mice resulted in defective primary and secondary expansion after challenge with antigen. So far, no human diseases have been linked with defects of the CD30 genes (1p36 for CD30 and 9q33 for CD30L), which might be interpreted as a further hint that CD30 is more likely to play a role in the fine-tuning of the immune system, as described earlier.

In malignant cells, the overexpression of CD30 (e.g., by H-RS cells in HL) can lead to self-aggregation, recruitment of TRAF-2 and TRAF-5, NF-κB activation, and strong pro-proliferative signals. Therefore, CD30 was thought to have a critical role in the malignant phenotype of H-RS and ALCL cells. Recent studies suggest that CD30 overexpression is not the driver lesion but is caused by constitutive expression of transcription factors belonging to the AP-1 family, in particular JunB (9). Interestingly, in cases of primary cutaneous CD30-positive LyP showing coexpression of CD30 and CD30L, spontaneous regression has been frequently observed, suggesting a causal relationship (10). This observation suggests pro-apoptotic effects under specific conditions.

15.3   Anaplastic Large-Cell Lymphoma

It is now two decades ago that large-cell lymphomas with anaplastic morphology were first described as an entity by Stein and colleagues (11). This novel lymphoma category was defined by large pleomorphic blasts and the CD30 overexpression on all neoplastic cells. Despite these common features, heterogeneity in the cytology and in the antigen profile of the tumor cells, as well as in the clinical features of patients affected by this condition, was noticed in the original description and led to the distinction of several morphologic, immunophenotypic, and clinical sub-forms of ALCL, as reviewed by Stein et al. recently (12). For practical reasons, in this chapter we will classify the different ALCLs with reference to their origin (T- or B-cell) and clinical presentation (primary systemic vs. primary cutaneous; see Table 15.1). Also for practical reasons, the primary cutaneous ALCL will be described together with the lymphomatoid papulosis under the chapter heading "primary cutaneous CD30 positive T-cell lymphoproliferative disorders", as both are obviously closer related to each other than to the systemic form of CD30 positive T-cell lymphomas.

15.3.1   Primary Systemic ALCL

About 60% of all primary systemic ALCL are positive for the "anaplastic lymphoma kinase" (ALK) (see Table 15.1) (13–15). The remaining cases are either ALK-negative T-cell ALCL or of B-cell origin. Morphologic analysis and immunohistochemical staining can further subclassify systemic ALCL into the *common* (or classic) subtype, the *small cell*, and the *lymphohistiocytic* ALCL. The common type is ALK-positive in about 60–85% of all cases, whereas the small-cell and the lymphohistiocytic ALCL are positive in nearly all cases. The common type is characterized by sheets of large lymphoid cells with chromatin-poor horseshoe-shaped nuclei that contain

Table 15.1 ALCL classification system

ALCL				
B-cell[a]	**T-cell[b]**			
	Primary systemic ALCL		Primary cutaneous CD30-positive T-cell lymphoproliferative disorders	
	ALK-positive[c]	ALK-negative	ALCL-like	Lymphomatoid papulosis

[a]Mostly EBV latent membrane antigen-positive, ALK-negative, often HIV-related lymphoma, accounting for ~15% of all cases.

[b]EBV-negative, sometimes not expressing T-cell antigens (null-cell), but clonally expression of rearranged TCR β and γ genes is detectable in 90% of cases of T-cell and null-type (55). Up to a third of all cases express cytotoxic molecules, indicating NK-cells as possible precursors in some cases.

[c]Representing 60% of all cases.

multiple nucleoli. These are the so-called "hallmark cells," because they can be found in all ALCL variants, including the small-cell and lymphohistiocytic subtypes (16). The small-cell variant is characterized by a mixture of small, medium-sized, and large lymphoid cells (17). Additionally, there are the following rare subtypes: the *giant cell-rich*, and the *Hodgkin-like* ALCL. In both, ALK overexpression is found only in a minority of cases (~40% in giant cell-rich and ~15% in Hodgkin-like ALCL). In the WHO (World Health Organization) classification though, Hodgkin-like ALCL is not considered to be a "real" entity, as ALCL is a T-cell lymphoma and HL is a B-cell lymphoma in almost all cases. This has been confirmed in difficult cases by antigen-receptor gene rearrangement analysis. Due to the expression of cytotoxic molecules in about 30% of all cases, the postulated cell of origin is an activated mature cytotoxic T-cell for the primary systemic ALCL.

15.3.2 The Role of ALK in ALK-Positive ALCL

Soon after the first description of anaplastic large-cell lymphomas as a distinct entity, an association with a balanced (2;5)(p23;q35) chromosomal translocation was reported from different groups (18–21). As a result of this translocation, an 80-kDa fusion protein containing the ALK tyrosine kinase linked to the NPM (nulcleophosmin) N-terminal dimerization domain arises (see Figure 15.2). The fusion gene NPM/ALK is under control of the ubiquitously active NPM promoter, resulting in an overexpression of the NPM/ALK protein.

Anaplastic lymphoma kinase is a member of the insulin receptor superfamily receptor tyrosine kinase and is a 205-kDa type I transmembrane glycoprotein. ALK is physiologically expressed only within the developing and mature nervous system, but not in normal lymphoid cells. As with CD30 (see earlier section), ALK knockout mice develop without major abnormalities, indicating no essential role for this kinase.

Normal NPM is a 37-kDa phosphoprotein that is physiologically highly expressed during embryogenesis. NPM plays a role in ribosome assembly and protein synthesis. Accordingly, the expression of NPM is increased when cell division and growth are stimulated. It is active as a homohexamer that shuttles ribonuclear complexes between the nucleolus and the cytoplasm.

Consequently, the NPM/ALK fusion protein forms oligomers in the nucleus and cytoplasm of NPM/ALK-expressing cells, causing a constitutive activation of the ALK tyrosine kinase, also indicated by its heavily phosphorylated tyrosine residues (22, 23). This constitutive tyrosine kinase activation certainly plays a major role in the malignant phenotype of ALK-positive ALCL. Although not fully understood, activation of phospholipase C (PLC)γ, phosphatidylinositol 3-kinase (PI3K)/protein kinase B (Akt), STAT3, STAT5, and mitogen-induced extracellular kinase (MEK)/ERK have been shown to be involved in the malignant phenotype in NPM/ALK-expressing cell lines (see Figure 15.2). In addition, mTOR (mammalian target of rapamycin) activation might play a major role, as recent research suggests. As shown in Figure 15.2, the NPM/ALK-generated signal is transmitted through the MEK/ERK and, to a much lesser degree, the PI3K/Akt pathways. In addition, mTOR also appears to participate in this signaling cascade. Interestingly, the mTOR inhibitor rapamycin profoundly suppresses proliferation and enhances the apoptotic rate of ALK-positive ALCL cells. Thus, activation of the rapamycin-sensitive mTOR signaling pathway might be a new mechanism by which NPM/ALK promotes malignant transformation (24).

On the other hand, activated ALK is probably not sufficient to transform otherwise normal lymphoid cells, as indicated by several observations. In ALK transgenic mice, tumors occur only in a subset of animals and, in addition, this takes a rather long time (25). In addition, several studies using polymerase chain reaction (PCR) tests have detected ALK fusion genes in reactive lymphoid tissues and peripheral blood of healthy individuals (26). This might explain why ALK rearrangements have been found in various diseases. So far, the secondary events that collaborate with ALK in malignant transformation are not known.

In the meantime, many other translocations involving the ALK gene have been detected; they are listed in Table 15.2. Of these, the TFG and the TPM3 proteins also contain dimerization regions. Thus, they can spontaneously form homodimers of x-ALK proteins to mimic ligand binding. Again, this results in the constitutive activation of the ALK kinase domain and certainly has an oncogneic capacity. Interestingly, these different fusion proteins exhibit different growth kinetics with regard to colony formation in soft agar, invasion, migration through the endothelial barrier, and tumorigenicity, again underscoring the importance of the different ALK-containing fusion proteins for the malignant phenotype (27)

15.3.3 The Role of CD30 in ALK-Positive ALCL

Although these ALCLs all express the CD30 antigen at very high levels, the role of this overexpression for the malignant phenotype remains unclear. Obviously, in

Table 15.2 x-ALK fusion genes

Gene	Chromosomal location	Frequency in ALK-positive ALCL (%)	Size of fusion protein (kDa)	Localization of fusion protein
Nucleophosmin, NPM	5q35	75	80	Cytoplasmic, nuclear, nucleolar
Tropomyosin 3, TPM3	1q21	15	104	Membranous and diffuse cytoplasmic
TRCK fusion gene, TFG	3q21	2	85, 97	Diffuse cytoplasmic
ATIC	2q35	2	96	Cytoplasmic
Clathrin heavy chain, CLTC	17q23	2	250	Punctate cytoplasmic
Moesin, MSN	Xq11-12	1	125	Plasma membrane

ALCL cell lines such as Karpas 299, CD30 trimerization can induce apoptosis. However, under conditions in which new protein synthesis is blocked, the ability of CD30 to trigger cell death in ALCL cell lines is substantially enhanced. Furthermore, CD30-induced cell death in ALCL cells can be inhibited by the pan-caspase inhibitor zVAD-fmk, suggesting that CD30 triggers cell death by an apoptotic pathway. These data suggest that CD30 induces *de novo* synthesis of a survival protein(s) that blocks its cell-death-promoting activity (28). Anti-CD30 antibodies can transduce this signal only if they are hyper-cross-linked, and even then, binding by the natural ligand CD30L is more efficient (29). Taken together, although CD30 can induce apoptosis in ALCL, this does not occur on a regular basis and the factors contributing to these different effects are not yet known. Recent results indicate that this might be due to the activation of the p38 MAP kinase pathway (29) due to the fact that pharmacologic inhibition of p38 MAPK unmasked a CD30-triggered apoptotic pathway involving caspase-8. Additionally, the DD-containing adaptor protein FADD seems to be involved in the signal transduction and might be activated by TNFR1, as CD30 does not contain a DD and therefore cannot activate FADD directly.

15.3.4 Clinical Aspects of Primary Systemic ALCL

15.3.4.1 Clinical Features and Prognosis

There is evidence that the clinical features and prognosis of systemic ALCL differ significantly depending on the presence of x-ALK fusion proteins. ALK-positive ALCL occurs mostly in the first three decades, whereas ALK-negative ALCL shows the highest incidence in the sixth decade. For ALK-positive cases, there is a strong male predominance (male/female ratio: 6.5:1), which is completely missing in ALK-negative patients (see Figure 15.3A). The prognosis for ALK-negative patients is much poorer, with a median overall survival of about 2 years (30). In contrast, long-term survival is seen in ALK-positive patients in almost 75% (see Figure 15.3B). This prognostic difference between ALK-positive and ALK-negative patients was first described by Shiota and colleagues, and then confirmed by two larger series. These studies could also show that the survival difference does not depend on the different age at first diagnosis (14, 31, 32). In these studies, the 5-year overall survival of ALK-positive versus ALK-negative ALCL was 71% versus 15% in one study and 79% versus 46% in the other. New prognostic markers as MUC-1 are also becoming apparent (33). In ALK-positive patients, the 5-year progression-free survival (PFS) rate was 52% in those who were MUC-1 positive versus 100% for those who were MUC-1 negative. On the other hand, the overall survival (OS) was not statistically different. In contrast, MUC-1 expression was predictive in ALK-negative patients for the 5-year PFS (26% in MUC-1-positive vs. 70.8% in MUC-1-negative patients) and OS (55.6% vs. 93.3%). Another useful marker might be survivin, a member of the inhibitor of apoptosis (IAP) family that inhibits cell

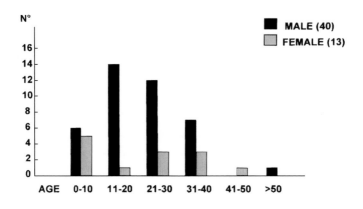

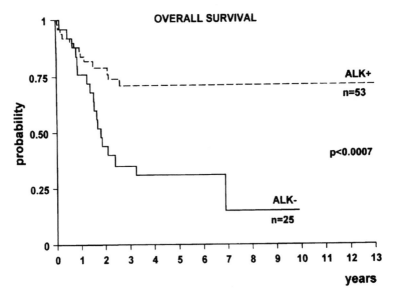

Figure 15.3 (**A**) Age distribution in primary systemic ALCL; (**B**) prognosis in primary systemic ALCL

death via inhibition of apoptotic pathways (34). In patients with ALK-positive tumors, the 5-year failure-free survival (FFS) rate was 34% for patients with sur-vivin-positive tumors versus 100% for patients with survivin-negative tumors. The 5-year OS in ALK-positive patients was 56% for survivin-positive tumors (versus 100% for survivin-negative tumors). Accordingly, in the ALK-negative group, the 5-year OS rate was 60% for survivin-positive tumors (92% for nega-tive tumors) and the 5-year FFS rate was 46% versus 89% for (survivin-positive vs. surviving-negative) (35).

Clinically, ALK-positive ALCL frequently presents as an aggressive stage III–IV disease, usually associated with B-symptoms (75%), especially high fever.

Extranodal involvement is frequent (60%), with ~40% of patients showing two or more extranodal sites of the disease. In a large study, the frequency of extranodal sites of lymphoma involvement was as follows: skin, 21%; bone (solitary or multiple lesions), 17%; soft tissues, 17%; lung, 11%; and liver. 8%, with involvement of the gut and central nervous system only rarely (30). The incidence of bone marrow involvement is ~30% when checked with immunohistochemistry (36). Of course, almost all patients present with disseminated lymphadenopathy, whereas about 40% have lymphadenopathy as their only clinical manifestation. The age-adjusted International Prognostic Index (IPI) is valuable in ALCL regardless of the x-ALK expression. Patients with an IPI of 0 and 1 show a 5-year OS of 94%, whereas for patients with a higher IPI, the OS is only 41%.

Thus, depending on the x-ALK protein expression and the IPI, certainly different initial treatment strategies are necessary for patients with a diagnosis of an ALCL. Whether other predictive markers as MUC-1 or survivin should be incorporated into the treatment algorithm remains unclear to date.

15.3.4.2   First-Line Therapy

The excellent outcome of low-risk ALK-positive lymphoma (age-adjusted IPI 0 and 1) justifies the use of a treatment protocol consisting of alkylating agents, anthracyclines, vinca alkaloids, and corticosteroids (i.e., cyclophosphamide, doxorubicin, vincristine, prednisone—CHOP-like regimens) as first-line therapy. It must be stated though that many other more aggressive polychemotherapy regimens have been reported [as reviewed by Jacobsen recently (37)], including so-called third-generation regimens. Unfortunately, none of them was tested in a prospectively randomized study and the limited numbers of patients and the marked heterogeneity of patient characteristics and schedules used makes it impossible to favor one of them. This situation would warrant a randomized comparison of less versus more intensive conventional polychemotherapy as induction therapy, but if the results of aggressive B-cell lymphomas can be extrapolated to ALCL, this approach is not very promising.

15.3.4.3   High-Dose Chemotherapy and Stem Cell Transplantation

An even more aggressive strategy is represented by upfront high-dose chemotherapy and autologous stem cell transplantation (APBSCT). The largest report on this strategy so far is the EBMT (European Group for Blood and Marrow Transplantation) registry analysis. In this retrospective analysis, only 1 out of 15 patients transplanted in first complete remission relapsed. In contrast, 6 of 15 patients who were transplanted in a second or higher complete remission relapsed. Accordingly, patients with a partial remission prior to transplant or refractory disease showed a much worse outcome (progressive disease in 6/18 and 14/16, respectively). Disease status at transplant, younger age, absence of B-symptoms, and lack of extranodal disease indicated a better prognosis (38). Also, prospective trials have evaluated the use of APBSCT in the first complete remission. All of them are rather small and do not have a comparative arm or a prospectively defined control group, which makes the interpretation of the results difficult. Nevertheless, results of these trials are good for ALK-positive ALCL with an OS of around 90% (39–41). However, APBSCT is not regarded as the standard of care for patients with ALK-positive, IPI low–intermediate-risk ALCL, and the use of APBSCT in first remission warrants further prospective investigation.

For patients with high-risk ALK-positive or ALK-negative lymphoma, the situation is unclear as well and APBSCT has not been shown to improve the outcome so far. ALK-negative patients with relapsed disease are not likely to benefit from APBSCT. Thus, at least, these patients might be enrolled into clinical trials investigating new therapies different from conventional chemotherapy.

Although allogeneic stem cell transplantation has been reported to be successful in single cases, this option still is experimental and might be reserved for younger patients with refractory disease.

15.3.4.4 Experimental Approaches

Experimental approaches in clinical trials include anti-CD30 immunotherapy. Because strong CD30 overexpression is a common feature of ALCL and CD30 is, therefore, an attractive target, evaluation of this approach is ongoing for several years now. So far, two antibodies have entered clinical trials with some encouraging responses in phase I/II studies (SGN-30 and MDX-060) (see Figure 15.4). The SGN-30 antibody is currently being evaluated in an international phase II study. In addition to CD30, ALCL also often expresses the CD25 antigen (IL-2 receptor). Therefore, a recombinant fusion protein of IL-2 and diphtheria toxin (denileukin diftitox) is currently being studied in combination with CHOP in a phase II study.

Another new class of drugs are the histone deacetylase inhibitors (HDACs). HDACs regulate gene expression in a variety of cells and inappropriate deacetylation of antiproliferating genes is thought to be important in the pathogenesis of neoplasias. HDAC inhibitors can induce gene activation, cellular differentiation, cell growth arrest, and apoptosis in cancer cells by restoring the balance between

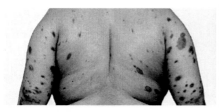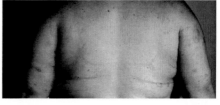

Figure 15.4 Skin lesions due to cutaneous ALCL before **(A)** and after treatment **(B)** with the anti-CD30 antibody MDX-060

the acetylation and deacetylation of genes (42). A variety of HDAC inhibitors are currently in clinical trials [including depsipeptide, SAHA (vorinostat), and PXD101] and should be taken into account for patients with relapsed or refractory ALCL.

Of course, direct targeting of the ALK-containing fusion protein in ALK-positive ALCL would be an ideal therapy. So far, only one preclinical study is available, using a fused pyrrolocarbazole-derived small molecule. This molecule showed ALK-inhibitory activity and induced apoptosis in NPM/ALK-transfected mouse embryonic fibroblasts (43).

In summary, some new therapeutic options are currently available for relapsed or refractory ALCL patients and, thus, these patients should be treated within clinical trials to further improve the knowledge about this rare disease.

15.4 Primary Cutaneous CD30-Positive T-cell Lymphoproliferative Disorders

15.4.1 Introduction

Primary cutaneous CD30-positive lymphoproliferative disorders (LPDs) account for ~30% of cutaueous T-cell lymphomas (CTCL). According to the WHO-EORTC classification system for cutaneous lymphomas, this group includes C-ALCL, LyP, and borderline cases (44). It is now generally accepted that C-ALCL and LyP form a spectrum of disease and that the histology is not sufficient to differentiate between these two ends of this spectrum. LyP, as the starting point of this spectrum, is a rather indolent chronic, recurrent, self-healing papulonecrotic or papulonodular skin disease, whereas C-ALCL is defined by its large anaplastic cells and the rapid growth of the mostly solitary or localized nodules at the end of the spectrum (44). The course of the disease and the clinical appearance must be taken into account to confirm the diagnosis (see Figure 15.5). Accordingly, the term "borderline case" should be used only in cases in which a definite distinction between C-ALCL and LyP cannot be made despite this thorough clinico-pathologic correlation. The course of the disease will usually exhibit the final diagnosis (45).

15.4.2 Clinical Presentation

Lymphomatoid papulosis has been first described in 1968 as recurrent, self-healing, clinically benign disease (46). It occurs mainly in adults (median age: 45 years; male-to-female ratio: 1.5:1) and is characterized by the presence of papular, papulonecrotic, and/or nodular skin lesions at different stages of development. Lesions

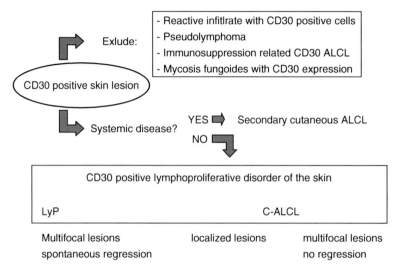

Figure 15.5 Diagnosis of LPD. (Adapted from Refs.45 and 51)

are found predominantly on the trunk and limbs and usually disappear within 3–12 weeks. Coexpression of CD30 and CD30L has been proposed to be responsible for the spontaneous regression often observed in this disease (10). It is a chronic disease that might last from some months to more than 40 years in individual patients. As outlined earlier, LyP is often (20%) associated with other lymphomas, especially HL, mycosis fungoides, or ALCL (45).

Primary cutaneous anaplastic lymphoma also affects mainly adults, with a predominance of the male gender (2–3:1). In contrast to LyP, most patients present with solitary or localized nodules or tumors, with only 20% of all patients showing multifocal lesions. The tumors, which often grow out, commonly ulcerate. Spontaneous regression, as in LyP, occurs, but not as often. After complete resection, relapses are seen frequently in the skin. Extracutaneous dissemination occurs in 10% of the patients and mainly involves the regional lymph nodes.

Importantly, the prognosis for patients with C-ALCL infiltration of regional lymph nodes is not worse than for those with cutaneous disease only. Overall survival is very good, exceeding 90% at 10 years. The prognosis for patients with LyP is even better, with only 2% disease-related mortality at ~6 years.

15.4.3 Therapy

The first choice of therapy for C-ALCL is surgical resection if the patient has only a solitary skin lesion or a few localized nodules. If resection is not possible in patients with few lesions, radiotherapy is also very effective. In cases with disseminated skin involvement, low-dose methotrexate on a weekly schedule often exhibits good clinical results. This is also the first choice of treatment for patients with LyP, who usually present with disseminated disease. Due to the chronic indolent course of the disease, a more aggressive approach is not justified in LyP. However, treatment is indicated in patients with scarring lesions. If low- dose methotrexate cannot achieve clinical improvement, psoralene and ultraviolet A phototherapy (PUVA) or locally administered chemotherapy has been used successfully. In patients with non-carring lesions, a watch-and-wait strategy is justified.

15.4.4 Diagnosis, Histopathological, and Genetic Findings

The histology of LyP is very variable and, in part, correlates with the age of the skin lesion. Three histologic subtypes of LyP (types A, B, and C) represent a spectrum with overlapping features (45). In LyP type A lesions, scattered or small clusters of large, CD30-positive, sometimes multinucleated cells are intermingled with numerous inflammatory cells, such as histiocytes, small lymphocytes, neutrophils, and/or eosinophils. LyP type B amounts to less than 10% of the three subclasses and is characterized by an epidermotropic infiltrate of small atypical cells with cerebriform nuclei similar to that observed in mycosis fungoides. In LyP type C lesions, the large CD30-positive T-cells dominate the picture and demonstrate clusters of cells mixed with relatively few inflammatory cells. For the most common LyP subtypes A and C, immunophenotyping of the neoplastic cells shows an activated CD4-positive T-cell phenotype with variable loss of CD2, CD5, and/or CD3 and frequent expression of cytotoxic proteins (granzyme B, TIA-1, perforin) (47). Only very few cases have a CD8-positive T-cell phenotype. CD30 must be expressed by more than 75% of the malignant cells by definition. In contrast to systemic CD30-positive lymphomas, LPDs express the cutaneous lymphocyte antigen (CLA) but not the epithelial membrane antigen (EMA). Also, x-ALK proteins cannot be found in LPDs (48). CD15 is generally negative. The atypical cells with cerebriform nuclei in the LyP type B lesions stain positive for CD3 and CD4 but negative for CD8 and CD30.

With regard to its genetic features, LyP is a clonal T-cell disorder with rearranged T-cell receptor genes in ~60–70% of all lesions. In C-ALCL, almost all cases show this T-cell receptor rearrangement. In some cases of C-ALCL, polyclonal CD30-positive cells could be detected, suggesting that the malignant CD30-positive clone has emerged from this background population (49). There are no other typical genetic aberrations; especially the t(2;5)(p23;q35) is not found in LPDs in contrast to the primary systemic ALCL. Interestingly, identical rearrangements have been demonstrated in LyP lesions and associated lymphomas (50). This observation has been made for many other cases of LPD and accompanying lymphomas, including mycosis fungoides, HL, and ALCL (49) These cases suggest a common tumor stem cell harboring this rearrangement. Different and distinct lymphomas can arise from this stem cell in one patient, depending on additional genetic events caused by genetic instability.

15.4.5 Differential Diagnosis

Some LPDs express CD30 as well and therefore must be considered in the differential diagnosis. Mycosis fungoides and Sezary syndrome, which have transformed into high-grade lymphomas, might express CD30 as well as Pagetoid reticulosis, systemic T-cell lymphoma, HL, and lymphoma- and leukemia-associated cutaneous atypical T-cell reactions (51). Because CD30-positive lymphocytes can be found in reactive inflammatory disorders, these conditions might mimic LPDs (52, 53). In contrast to LyP, no waxing and waning is found in these so-called pseudolymphomas, which might be infectious or noninfectious. Typically, no clonal T-cell receptor rearrangement can be found in these lesions. All kinds of viral (e.g., herpes simplex or varicella zoster in immunocompromised patients), parasitic (e.g., scabies), and bacterial infections (e.g., tuberculosis) can be accompanied by CD30-positive lymphoid blasts (51). These observations suggest that LyP also might arise from an infection. Viruslike particles have been identified by electron microscopy in LyP lesions (54). Based on this finding, it was hypothesized that endogenous retroviral elements might be involved in the pathogenesis of LyP, although no specific virus could be detected so far.

From a practical point of view, differential diagnosis mostly involves LyP type C, C-ALCL, and mycosis fungoides in transformation. Again, the definite diagnosis cannot be made on the histopathological finding alone, but the clinical presentation must also be considered. However, patients suffering from LyP with large nodules that may last for several months before spontaneous regression might be difficult to differentiate from patients with C-ALCL. These are the so-called borderline lesions, but the term has not been included into the WHO-EORTC classification. Also, histological differentiation of primary and secondary ALCL is often impossible and additional markers as ALK or EMA must be used to distinguish these lymphomas. This differential diagnosis also depends on the staging results (see Figure 15.5). Taken together, the dermatopathologist can provide a list of differential diagnoses in most cases, but the clinical presentation must be considered to get a complete picture and to initiate the appropriate treatment for patients with CD30-positive LPDs.

References

1. Schwab U, Stein H, Gerdes J, et al. Production of a monoclonal antibody specific for Hodgkin and Sternberg-Reed cells of Hodgkin's disease and a subset of normal lymphoid cells. Nature 1982;299:65–67.
2. Durkop H, Latza U, Hummel M, et al. Molecular cloning and expression of a new member of the nerve growth factor receptor family that is characteristic for Hodgkin's disease. Cell 1992;68:421–427.
3. Stein H, Gerdes J, Schwab U, et al. Evidence for the detection of the normal counterpart of Hodgkin and Sternberg-Reed cells. Hematol Oncol 1983;1:21–29.
4. Younes A, Kadin ME. Emerging applications of the tumor necrosis factor family of ligands and receptors in cancer therapy. J Clin Oncol 2003;21:3526–3534.

5. Nagata S, Ise T, Onda M, et al. Cell membrane-specific epitopes on CD30: potentially superior targets for immunotherapy. Proc Natl Acad Sci USA 2005;102:7946–7951.

6. DeYoung AL, Duramad O, Winoto A. The TNF receptor family member CD30 is not essential for negative selection. J Immunol 2000;165:6170–6173.

7. Podack ER, Strbo N, Sotosec V, et al. CD30-governor of memory T cells? Ann NY Acad Sci 2002;975:101–113.

8. Florido M, Borges M, Yagita H, et al. Contribution of CD30/CD153 but not of CD27/CD70, CD134/OX40L, or CD137/4-1BBL to the optimal induction of protective immunity to *Mycobacterium avium*. J Leukoc Biol 2004;76:1039–1046.

9. Al-Shamkhani A. The role of CD30 in the pathogenesis of haematopoietic malignancies. Curr Opin Pharmacol 2004;4:355–359.

10. Mori M, Manuelli C, Pimpinelli N, et al. CD30-CD30 ligand interaction in primary cutaneous CD30(+) T-cell lymphomas: a clue to the pathophysiology of clinical regression. Blood 1999;94:3077–3083.

11. Stein H, Mason DY, Gerdes J, et al. The expression of the Hodgkin's disease associated antigen Ki-1 in reactive and neoplastic lymphoid tissue: evidence that Reed-Sternberg cells and histiocytic malignancies are derived from activated lymphoid cells. Blood 1985;66:848–858.

12. Stein H, Foss HD, Durkop H, et al. CD30(+) anaplastic large cell lymphoma: a review of its histopathologic, genetic, and clinical features. Blood 2000;96:3681–3695.

13. Benharroch D, Meguerian-Bedoyan Z, Lamant L, et al. ALK-positive lymphoma: a single disease with a broad spectrum of morphology. Blood 1998;91:2076–2084.

14. Falini B, Bigerna B, Fizzotti M, et al. ALK expression defines a distinct group of T/null lymphomas ("ALK lymphomas") with a wide morphological spectrum. Am J Pathol 1998;153:875–886.

15. Pulford K, Lamant L, Morris SW, et al. Detection of anaplastic lymphoma kinase (ALK) and nucleolar protein nucleophosmin (NPM)-ALK proteins in normal and neoplastic cells with the monoclonal antibody ALK1. Blood 1997;89:1394–1404.

16. Chan JK, Buchanan R, Fletcher CD. Sarcomatoid variant of anaplastic large-cell Ki-1 lymphoma. Am J Surg Pathol 1990;14:983–988.

17. Kinney MC, Collins RD, Greer JP, et al. A small-cell-predominant variant of primary Ki-1 (CD30)+ T-cell lymphoma. Am J Surg Pathol 1993;17:859–868.

18. Le Beau MM, Bitter MA, Larson RA, et al. The t(2;5)(p23;q35): a recurring chromosomal abnormality in Ki-1-positive anaplastic large cell lymphoma. Leukemia 1989;3:866–870.

19. Kaneko Y, Frizzera G, Edamura S, et al. A novel translocation, t(2;5)(p23;q35), in childhood phagocytic large T-cell lymphoma mimicking malignant histiocytosis. Blood 1989;73:806–813.

20. Rimokh R, Magaud JP, Berger F, et al. A translocation involving a specific breakpoint (q35) on chromosome 5 is characteristic of anaplastic large cell lymphoma ('Ki-1 lymphoma'). Br J Haematol 1989;71:31–36.

21. Mason DY, Bastard C, Rimokh R, et al. CD30-positive large cell lymphomas ('Ki-1 lymphoma') are associated with a chromosomal translocation involving 5q35. Br J Haematol 1990;74:161–168.

22. Bischof D, Pulford K, Mason DY, et al. Role of the nucleophosmin (NPM) portion of the non-Hodgkin's lymphoma-associated NPM-anaplastic lymphoma kinase fusion protein in oncogenesis. Mol Cell Biol 1997;17:2312–2325.

23. Kutok JL, Aster JC. Molecular biology of anaplastic lymphoma kinase-positive anaplastic large-cell lymphoma. J Clin Oncol 2002;20:3691–3702.

24. Marzec M, Kasprzycka M, Liu X, et al. Oncogenic tyrosine kinase NPM/ALK induces activation of the rapamycin-sensitive mTOR signaling pathway. Oncogene 2007. Aug 23; 26(38), 5606–5614.

25. Kuefer MU, Look AT, Pulford K, et al. Retrovirus-mediated gene transfer of NPM-ALK causes lymphoid malignancy in mice. Blood 1997;90:2901–2910.

26. Trumper L, Pfreundschuh M, Bonin FV, et al. Detection of the t(2;5)-associated NPM/ALK fusion cDNA in peripheral blood cells of healthy individuals. Br J Haematol 1998;103:1138–1144.

27. Armstrong F, Duplantier MM, Trempat P, et al. Differential effects of X-ALK fusion proteins on proliferation, transformation, and invasion properties of NIH3T3 cells. Oncogene 2004;23:6071–6082.

28. Mir SS, Richter BW, Duckett CS. Differential effects of CD30 activation in anaplastic large cell lymphoma and Hodgkin disease cells. Blood 2000;96:4307–4312.

29. Krysov SV, Rowley TF, Al-Shamkhani A. Inhibition of p38 mitogen-activated protein kinase unmasks a CD30-triggered apoptotic pathway in anaplastic large cell lymphoma cells. Mol Cancer Ther 2007;6:703–711.

30. Falini B. Anaplastic large cell lymphoma: pathological, molecular and clinical features. Br J Haematol 2001;114:741–760.

31. Gascoyne RD, Aoun P, Wu D, et al. Prognostic significance of anaplastic lymphoma kinase (ALK) protein expression in adults with anaplastic large cell lymphoma. Blood 1999;93:3913–3921.

32. Shiota M, Nakamura S, Ichinohasama R, A. et al. Anaplastic large cell lymphomas expressing the novel chimeric protein p80NPM/ALK: a distinct clinicopathologic entity. Blood 1995;86:1954–1960.

33. Rassidakis GZ, Goy A, Medeiros LJ, et al. Prognostic significance of MUC-1 expression in systemic anaplastic large cell lymphoma. Clin Cancer Res 2003;9:2213–2220.

34. Altieri DC. Validating survivin as a cancer therapeutic target. Nat Rev Cancer 2003;3:46–54.

35. Schlette EJ, Medeiros LJ, Goy A, et al. Survivin expression predicts poorer prognosis in anaplastic large-cell lymphoma. J Clin Oncol 2004;22:1682–1688.

36. Fraga M, Brousset P, Schlaifer D, et al. Bone marrow involvement in anaplastic large cell lymphoma. Immunohistochemical detection of minimal disease and its prognostic significance. Am J Clin Pathol 1995;103:82–89.

37. Jacobsen E. Anaplastic large-cell lymphoma, T-/null-cell type. Oncologist 2006;11:831–840.

38. Fanin R, Ruiz de Elvira MC, Sperotto A, et al. Autologous stem cell transplantation for T and null cell CD30-positive anaplastic large cell lymphoma: analysis of 64 adult and paediatric cases reported to the European Group for Blood and Marrow Transplantation (EBMT). Bone Marrow Transplant 1999;23:437–442.

39. Fanin R, Silvestri F, Geromin A, et al. Primary systemic CD30 (Ki-1)-positive anaplastic large cell lymphoma of the adult: sequential intensive treatment with the F-MACHOP regimen (+/– radiotherapy) and autologous bone marrow transplantation. Blood 1996;87:1243–1248.

40. Fanin R, Sperotto A, Silvestri F, et al. The therapy of primary adult systemic CD30-positive anaplastic large cell lymphoma: results of 40 cases treated in a single center. Leuk Lymphoma 1999;35:159–169.

41. Deconinck E, Lamy T, Foussard C, et al. Autologous stem cell transplantation for anaplastic large-cell lymphomas: results of a prospective trial. Br J Haematol 2000;109:736–742.

42. Marks P, Rifkind RA, Richon VM, et al. Histone deacetylases and cancer: causes and therapies. Nat Rev Cancer 2001;1:194–202.

43. Wan W, Albom MS, Lu L, et al. Anaplastic lymphoma kinase activity is essential for the proliferation and survival of anaplastic large-cell lymphoma cells. Blood 2006;107:1617–1623.

44. Willemze R, Jaffe ES, Burg G, et al. WHO-EORTC classification for cutaneous lymphomas. Blood 2005;105:3768–3785.

45. Bekkenk MW, Geelen FA, van Voorst Vader PC, et al. Primary and secondary cutaneous CD30(+) lymphoproliferative disorders: a report from the Dutch Cutaneous Lymphoma Group on the long-term follow-up data of 219 patients and guidelines for diagnosis and treatment. Blood 2000;95:3653–3661.

46. Macaulay WL. Lymphomatoid papulosis. A continuing self-healing eruption, clinically benign–histologically malignant. Arch Dermatol 1968;97:23–30.

47. Kaudewitz P, Stein H, Dallenbach F, et al. Primary and secondary cutaneous Ki-1+ (CD30+) anaplastic large cell lymphomas. Morphologic, immunohistologic, and clinical-characteristics. Am J Pathol 1989;135:359–367.

48. DeCoteau JF, Butmarc JR, Kinney MC, et al. The t(2;5) chromosomal translocation is not a common feature of primary cutaneous CD30+ lymphoproliferative disorders: comparison with anaplastic large-cell lymphoma of nodal origin. Blood 1996;87:3437–3441.

49. Kadin ME. Pathobiology of CD30+ cutaneous T-cell lymphomas. J Cutan Pathol 2006;33 (Suppl 1):10–17.
50. Davis TH, Morton CC, Miller-Cassman R, et al. Hodgkin's disease, lymphomatoid papulosis, and cutaneous T-cell lymphoma derived from a common T-cell clone. N Engl J Med 1992;326:1115–1122.
51. Kempf W. CD30+ lymphoproliferative disorders: histopathology, differential diagnosis, new variants, and simulators. J Cutan Pathol 2006;33(Suppl 1):58–70.
52. Durkop H, Foss HD, Eitelbach F, et al. Expression of the CD30 antigen in non-lymphoid tissues and cells. J Pathol 2000;190:613–618.
53. Cepeda LT, Pieretti M, Chapman SF, et al. CD30-positive atypical lymphoid cells in common non-neoplastic cutaneous infiltrates rich in neutrophils and eosinophils. Am J Surg Pathol 2003;27:912–918.
54. Kempf W, Kadin ME, Dvorak AM, et al. Endogenous retroviral elements, but not exogenous retroviruses, are detected in CD30-positive lymphoproliferative disorders of the skin. Carcinogenesis 2003;24:301–306.
55. Foss HD, Anagnostopoulos I, Araujo I, et al. Anaplastic large-cell lymphomas of T-cell and null-cell phenotype express cytotoxic molecules. Blood 1996;88:4005–4011.

Chapter 16
Nodular Lymphocyte Predominant Hodgkin's Lymphoma

Michelle A. Fanale and Anas Younes

16.1 Introduction

Whereas it is estimated that 7800 new cases of Hodgkin's lymphoma (HL) will be diagnosed in 2006, nodular lymphocyte predominant Hodgkin lymphoma (NLPHL) will only account for 3–8% of newly diagnosed HL (1, 2). The majority of the incidence is accounted for by the classical Hodgkin lymphoma (cHL) subtypes (nodular sclerosing, lymphocyte rich, lymphocyte depleted, and mixed cellularity). There exists today a large breadth of literature that describes the pathology and epidemiology and provides data that supports the current acceptable standard approaches for both front-line and relapsed/refractory treatment of cHL (3). Given the rarity of the diagnosis of NLPHL, there are significantly fewer publications that are available to establish treatment algorithms and predict both short-term and long-term outcomes. However, as more has become understood about the pathology that underlies the diagnosis of NLPHL, more studies have now come forth that provide the rationale and evidence to support stage-based treatment approaches for the care of patients with this unusual diagnosis.

16.2 Pathology

Previously there were two described classifications of LPHL: nodular and diffuse. These were defined by morphologic appearance and growth pattern. However, the most recent WHO classification system published in 2001 now documents only NLPHL. The pathologic entity that previously was described as diffuse lymphocyte predominant Hodgkin lymphoma is actually now classified as either T-cell-rich large B-cell lymphoma or lymphocyte-rich classical HL (4–6). The principal distinctive cell in NLPHL is the L&H cell (lymphocytic and/or histiocytic of Lukes and Butler), which is often described as a "popcorn" cell, given the characteristic appearance of the nuclei (Figures 16.1 and 16.2). In contrast to classical HL, Reed-Sternberg (RS) cells are not generally seen in NLPHL (7). The cells surrounding the L&H cells are predominantly lymphocytes; however, epithelioid histiocytes, plasma cells, eosinophils, and neutrophils can be seen. Also, occasionally there can be sclerosis in the specimen, which can resemble nodular sclerosing cHL (8).

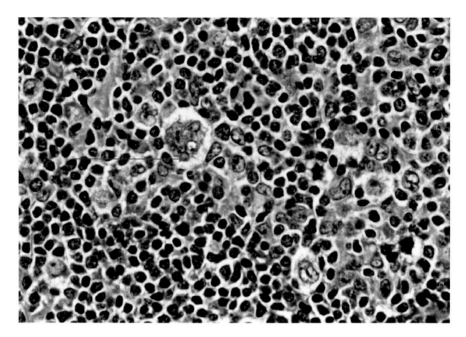

Figure 16.1 Higher-power microscopic view of a nodule of NLPHL showing that the neoplastic L&H cells or "popcorn cells" (red line) generally account for a minority of the cells seen, and there are numerous histiocytes and lymphocytes. Also, no necrosis or granulocytes are visualized. (Courtesy of Dr. Joan Admirand, UT M.D. Anderson Cancer Center, Department of Pathology)

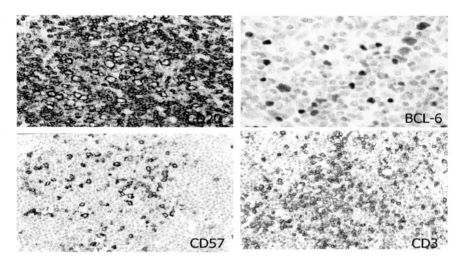

Figure 16.2 Immunophenotyping of NLPHL allows for accurate diagnosis and reveals strong staining for CD20 and BCL-6 positivity of the L&H cells, with surrounding T-cells being positive for CD3 and CD57. (Courtesy of Dr. Joan Admirand, UT M.D. Anderson Cancer Center, Department of Pathology)

A unique aspect of NLPHL that can occur is the progressive transformation of the germinal center. This has been described to occur in 20% of the lymph nodes involved in NLPHL, as well as in other non-NLPHL-positive lymph nodes in these patients (9). This progressive transformation of the germinal center is a distinctive type of follicular lymphoid hyperplasia with follicles that are enlarged and contain many B-cells, which are of mantle zone derivation (IgM- and IgD-positive). The key part of defining a diagnosis of NLPHL is the immunophenotype. Unlike the classical RS cells, L&H cells stain positive for CD45 (leukocyte common antigen) as well as typically B-cell-associated antigens including CD19, CD20, CD22, CD79a, and EMA but lack CD15(Leu-M1) and C30(Ki-1) staining (Table 16.1). Adherence to these immunophenotypic findings is crucial to reliably distinguish NLPHL from lymphocyte-rich cHL and T-cell-rich B-cell lymphomas. It has been shown that prior to the use of these routine markers, the entities of NLPHL, lymphocyte-rich HL, and indolent non-Hodgkin's lymphoma (NHL) often overlapped in classifications (10).

A characteristic finding is that kappa light chain restriction is detected in a majority of cases as shown by *in situ* hybridization (11). Bcl-6, which is a marker of normal B-cell germinal center development, is also expressed, as are CD40 and CD86, which are associated with the B-cell interaction with T-cells. Heavy-chain immunoglobulin (Ig) and bcl-6 juxtapositions with a t(3;14)(q27;q32) have been detected in patients with recurrent NLPHL (12–14). Also, these Bcl-6 rearrangements including t(3;22)(q27;q11), t(3;7)(q27;p12), or t(3;9)(q27;p13) have not been described to occur in cHL (15). Chemokine receptors, which play a key role in the localization of malignant hematopoietic cells, have also been noted to have differential expression in classical HL versus NLPHL, with classical HL showing CCR7 upregulation that was mediated by nuclear factor (NF)-kappa B, whereas NLPHL lacked CCR7 upregulation (16).

A subset of distinct recurrent genomic imbalances have also been described in NLPHL (17). Comparative genomic hybridization (CGH) studies have revealed an average of nearly 11 genomic imbalances per NLPHL tissue sample. All chromosomes were involved except 19, 22, and Y, thus showing a high degree of complexity. Gains of 2q, 4q, 5q, 6, and 11q were noted much more frequently than seen in NHL, thus showing a potential association with NLPHL. In addition, there

Table 16.1 Immunophenotype of NLPHL compared with cHL

CD marker	NLPHL	cHL
CD15	−	+
CD30	−	+
CD20	+	+/−
EMA	+	−
CD57 + T cells	+	−

Source: Adapted from DeVita et al. Cancer. Principles & practice of oncology. Philadelphia: Lippincott Williams and Wilkins; 2000.

was also a frequent overrepresentation seen of chromosome 6q, which is frequently deleted in NHL and rearrangements of Bcl-6 were also observed.

The nodules of NLPHL are made up of altered germinal centers of mantle zone-derived polyclonal B-cells and T-cells that are CD57-positive. These T-cells resemble centrocytes and surround the L&H cells by forming small aggregates, which give NLPHL follicles their irregular contours. Follicular dendritic cells are also present throughout the nodules but are lacking in the diffuse regions (18).

Bcl-2 gene rearrangements have not yet been described, and in contrast to RS cells, L&H cells in NLPHL are generally all Epstein-Barr virus (EBV)-negative. Data describing Ig gene rearrangements is mixed with some studies showing clonal rearrangements, whereas other studies show only polyclonal findings. It is unclear whether these results are dependent on whether tissue sections or single cells are used to perform the tests. For example, using the complementarity-determining region 3 (CDR3) of the Ig heavy chain as an assessment of clonality did yield five out of five positive results when single-cell analysis was used (19). Somatic hypermutation has also been noted, with the most frequent proto-oncogene mutation being PAX-5, which was mutated in seven out of nine NLPHL cases and was also present in cHL and diffuse large B-cell lymphoma cases, supporting a common pathologic root (20). When clonal rearrangements and hypermutations have been found, they have been most consistent with common findings for germinal center cells (21–23). Thus, the L&H cell currently is thought to be most similar to a centroblast within a proliferating germinal cell. A recent study further described that somatic hypermutation in L&H cells remains active throughout malignant proliferation and is not just active in the early stages of lymphoma. This was documented by showing upregulation of the enzyme activation-induced cytidine deaminase (AID) as a surrogate marker for somatic hypermutation (24).

16.3 Epidemiology and Staging

Patients with NLPHL generally have a more favorable prognosis compared to cHL. This is felt to be due to a more indolent presentation, longer time to disease progression, prolonged time to disease recurrence, and higher percent of early-stage disease at time of diagnosis. NLPHL has a high male predominance, with 70% of patients being male, and a median age at diagnosis of 35 years. The disease also tends to present with adenopathy in a peripheral location that is readily detected on exam (10).

A history should be taken to evaluate systemic symptoms such a fever, night sweats, weight loss, as well as performance status, history of prior malignancies, prior treatment with chemotherapy or radiation, history of immunosuppressive diseases, and family history of malignancy. Pruritus and alcohol-induced pain are not as commonly noted in NLPHL as they are in patients with cHL.

A careful physical exam should be performed with attention focused on examination of peripheral nodal sites in addition to the liver and spleen. Similar to cHL, the diagnosis of NLPHL is established by a tissue biopsy. A fine-needle aspirate (FNA) is generally not sufficient for evaluation of architecture and for immunophenotyping. Thus, if a peripheral lymph node is accessible, a surgical excision lymph node biopsy is preferred, although if not feasible, a core-needle biopsy can sometimes suffice.

Staging studies are similar to those performed for the evaluation of cHL. Laboratory studies include a CBC with differential, electrolytes and renal/liver function tests. Radiographic studies should include a chest radiograph and computed tomography (CT) of the neck, chest, and abdomen/pelvis. In addition, a bone marrow biopsy with flow cytometry for B-cell markers and peripheral blood flow cytometry with B-cell markers should also be performed.

Although there is a documented role for whole-body positron-emission tomography (PET scan) for initial staging and follow-up assessment of treatment response for cHL, the role in NLPHL is not established (25, 26). One theoretically useful role of PET scan in NLPHL potentially could be to evaluate the SUV positivity of sites of adenopathy in conjunction with the CT scan, as, typically, patients with NLPHL have SUV values of less than 10 and higher values that this could alert the clinician to do a biopsy to rule out transformation to large B-cell lymphoma.

Staging of both classical HL and NLPHL is based on the Ann Arbor system that was developed in 1971 (27) and subsequent modified in Cotswolds, England in 1988 (28). These staging criteria allow clinicians to define areas of involvement as well as offer appropriate treatment recommendations.

Unlike classical HL, NLPHL patients do not tend to present with bulky (>10 cm) mediastinal masses. In addition, NLPHL patients are less likely to have pulmonary, hepatic, splenic, or bone marrow positivity when compared to their classical HL counterparts.

16.4 Treatment: Front Line

Given the rarity of the diagnosis, there are significantly fewer published clinical trials to support the clinical care of patients with NLPHL as compared to cHL. However, several key publications over the past 2–3 years have served as references and sources of data to begin to develop algorithms for treatment of NLPHL, such as those published in the 2006 NCCN Practice Guidelines.

Often lymphadenopathy is slowly progressive and can be present several years prior to the diagnosis being made. Overall, the general prognosis is favorable. The European Task Force found that, in general, treatment with radiotherapy, chemotherapy, or a combined modality approach can lead to a complete remission (CR) in 95% of patients overall. It was shown that patients with advanced-stage NLPHL do have inferior outcomes compared to their early-stage counterparts with lower rates of survival (OS) and freedom from treatment failure (FFTF). However, data suggest that those with early-stage disease can be treated with less intense treatments and still have excellent outcomes with fewer side effects (2).

16.4.1   Early Stage: Stage I and II

Accepted treatment approaches for early-stage NLPHL range from involved field radiation therapy (IFRT) alone to chemotherapy followed by radiation therapy. The recently updated NCCN guidelines offer potential approaches to treatment (Table 16.2).

Several studies provide the rationale that supports these treatment options. A retrospective German Hodgkin Study Group (GHSG) study examined the outcomes for 131 patients with clinical stage IA disease (29). Cases in the GHSG database from three prior prospective randomized control studies (HD 4, HD7, and HD10) were reviewed. Patients in the HD4 trial were randomized between 40 Gy of extended field radiation (EFRT) and 30 Gy EFRT plus 10 Gy IFRT. Patients in HD7 were randomized between 30 Gy EFRT plus 10 Gy IFRT and two cycles of ABVD (adriamycin, doxorubicin, vinblastine, and dacarbazine) plus 30 Gy EFRT plus 10 Gy IFRT. Patients in HD10 were randomized among four treatment arms consisting of: four cycles of ABVD plus 30 Gy IFRT, four cycles of ABVD plus 20 Gy IFRT, two cycles of ABVD plus 30 Gy IFRT, and two cycles of ABVD plus 20 Gy IFRT. Of the 131 patients analyzed, 45 patients received EFRT, 45 patients received IFRT, and 41 patients received combined modality therapy (CM) with two to four cycles of ABVD plus EFRT or IFRT. The median age ranged from 35 to 41 years for the respective treatment groups, whereas the median follow-up ranged from 17 months in the IFRT group to 78 months in the EFRT group. Responses were excellent in all treatment groups, with 129/131 patients (99%) achieving a CR/CRu (98% with EFRT, 100% with IFRT, and 98% with CM). The FFTF rate was 95% at

Table 16.2 NCCN practice guidelines for NLPHL

Stage IA	Involved-field or regional radiation therapy
Stage IIA	Involved-field or regional radiation therapy
	OR
	Chemotherapy + involved-field radiation therapy
	OR
	Observation if patient can't tolerate radiation
Stage IB or IIB	Chemotherapy + involved-field radiation therapy
Stage IIIA or IVA	Chemotherapy +/− radiation therapy
	OR
	Observation
	OR
	Local radiation therapy for palliation
	OR
	Rituximab in selected patients who are symptomatic but not good candidates for chemotherapy
Stage IIIB or IVB	Chemotherapy ± radiation therapy
	OR
	Rituximab in selected patients who are symptomatic but not good candidates for chemotherapy

Source: Adapted from NCCN Practice Guidelines in Oncology-v.1.2006. www.NCCN.org

43 months, with an OS rate of 99%. Toxicity of CM treatment was comparable to other studies with similar agents, with 48.8% WHO grade 3/4 events and 2.2% WHO grade 3 toxicities for the EFRT and IFRT groups. The secondary malignancy rate was 2% in the EFRT group but 0% in the other treatment groups.

Although the above-described GHSG trial is the largest trial for early-stage NLPHL, other studies provide supporting evidence, including a clinical analysis of 603 HL patients with stage IA and stage IIA HL30. Patients in this study were randomized to receive IFRT or EFRT with either mantle or inverted Y fields. Relapse rates at 25 years after radiation therapy (RT) were 54% for IFRT and 44% for EFRT. Although the IFRT arm had an 11% higher risk of relapse than the EFRT arm, the outcomes for OS and risk of secondary malignancies were limited. Although it was a well-conducted study, the notable limitation was that there was no subset analysis done for the NLPHL patients. Also, it is probable that because these patients were enrolled 25 years ago and given the limitations of immunophenotyping, patients with varying HL subtypes could have been misclassified. Furthermore, because the majority of patients enrolled had classical HL, the relapse rates at 25 years were high given that combined modality and not radiation treatment alone is now the accepted standard of care for this cHL patient population.

Pediatric oncology groups have also published small nonrandomized clinical studies. One such study reviewed the cases of 27 children with predominantly localized stage IA or stage IIA NLPHL who received either four courses of VBVP (vinblastine, bleomycin, etoposide, prednisone) combined with 20 Gy of IFRT after removal of the involved lymph nodes versus another group who received surgical treatment only (31). Notably with a follow-up of 70 months the OS and event-free survival (EFS) was equal between the two groups - 100% and 69% Respectively. However, patients with residual disease after lymphadenectomy did seem to benefit from additional treatment with chemotherapy plus radiation.

Another retrospective trial analyzed 13 consecutive NLPHL children and adolescents seen at a single institution since 1989 (32). Twelve patients had stage I disease and one patient had stage II disease. Six patients received no further treatment after an excisional biopsy. The rest of the patients who had stage I disease with residual disease after excisional biopsy or stage II disease underwent brief chemotherapy with 9 weeks or an estimated three courses of CHOP (cyclophosphamide, adriamycin, vincristine, and prednisone). All patients had a CR and only one patient with stage II disease relapsed 6 years after initial diagnosis and was treated at relapse with radiation.

A separate analysis was conducted on 36 patients with nonbulky stage IA or IIA adult patients who were treated with radiation alone (33). IFRT was given to 28 patients, and 8 patients received EFRT, with a median overall dose of 40 Gy. Treatment for patients who relapsed consisted of MOPP (mechlorethamine, vincristine, prednisone, and procarbazine), CVPP/ABDIC (cyclophosphamide, vinblastine, procarbazine, prednisone/ doxorubicin, bleomycin, lomustine, prednisone) or ABVD chemotherapy, and/or IFRT. Median follow-up was 8.8 years. The 5-year relapse-free survival (RFS) and OS rates for the 20 patients treated for stage IA NLPHL was 95% and 100%, respectively. Also, no cases of secondary malignancies developed in the IFRT group with 11.6 years of follow-up.

The EORTC-GELA (European Organization for Research and Treatment of Cancer–Groupe d'Etude des Lymphomes de l'Adulte) has also published their outcomes for patients treated with early-stage NLPHL (34). Patients in this trial were categorized both by stage and prognostic factors. Patients were grouped by EORTC-GELA criteria that defined either very favorable (women age 16–39, non-bulky stage IA disease, NLPHL or NS subtypes, and an erythrocyte sedimentation rate (ESR) <50 mm/h) or favorable subgroups (age 16–49 years, nonbulky stage I or II disease, and an ESR <50 mm/h if no B-symptoms or an ESR of <30 mm/h if B-symptoms are present). Forty-eight consecutive patients' data were evaluated with stage I (40 patients), stage II (18 patients), very favorable (5 patients), and favorable (43 patients) patients. Thirty-seven patients received radiation alone and 11 patients received chemotherapy followed by radiation, with patients balanced based on the EORTC-GELA criteria between these two treatment groups. A median of three courses of MOPP or NOVP (mitoxantrone, vincristine, vinblastine, and prednisone) were delivered and all patients received 40 Gy of irradiation, although fields varied among IFRT, EFRT, mantle, subtotal lymph node irradiation (STNI), and total lymph node irradiation (TNI). The median follow-up was 9.3 years and the RFS was similar in both arms, with a 10-year RFS of 77% for radiation alone versus 68% for chemotherapy followed by radiation (p = NS). Similarly, the OS rates were 90% versus 100%, respectively (p = NS). In addition, MOPP or NOVP chemotherapy was not found to reduce the rate of distant recurrence outside of the radiation fields.

The rationale to potentially include a brief course of anthracycline-based chemotherapy is supported by a retrospective analysis of the Groupe Quest-Est d'Etude des Leucémies et Autres Maladies du Sang (GOEL-AMS) H81 and H90 clinical trials (35). Of the 500 patients with stage IA or IIA HL treated, 42 were later reclassified to have NLPHL. None of these 42 patients had mediastinal involvement and they were compared to the 458 patients who had cHL, including 144 without mediastinal involvement and 314 with mediastinal involvement. In the H81 trial, patients with peripheral Stage IA were treated with one ABVD cycle plus methylprednisolone, whereas those with nonperipheral stage IA and all stage IIA patients received three ABVD cycles plus methylprednisolone. By comparison, patients in the H90 trial with peripheral stage IA disease received either one ABVD cycle plus methylprednisolone or EBVM (epirubicin, bleomycin, vinblastine, methotrexate) plus methylprednisolone, whereas those with nonperipheral stage IA and all stage IIA patients who had nonbulky disease received three ABVD or three EBVM cycles plus methylprednisolone. All patients in CR or partial remission (PR) received irradiation. Patients with supradiaphragmatic disease received tailored mantle field irradiation to 40 Gy. All patients also received 30–40 Gy of radiation to the spleen and the lumboaortic area to L3. Patients with infradiaphragmatic disease also received unilateral or bilateral pelvic radiation to all involved lymph nodes to 40 Gy.

In this retrospective analysis, it was noted that the male-to-female ratio, first site involved, lymphocyte count, and ESR were similar between the NLPHL and cHL patients without mediastinal involvement. Mortality rates at 15 years secondary to HL were also similarly low in both NLPHL (2.4%) and cHL (0.7%) and OS at 15 years was also similar and ranged from 82% to 86% in all patients and was particularly high in patients less than 40 years of age at time of initial diagnosis ranging from 95–100%. Thus, overall, the findings support the potential inclusion of anthracycline-based chemotherapy for NLPHL followed by radiation. However, the use of mantle plus splenic and lumboaortic radiation paired with chemotherapy did cause a rate of secondary hematologic malignancies of 6.3% at 15 years for the NLPHL patients. In addition, rate of secondary solid tumors was 0.7% for the NLPHL patients and likely secondary to the mantle irradiation field. The risk of cardiac events including myocardial infarction or angina pectoris was highest in those treated at age 40 or younger, with a rate of 18.7% at 15 years.

Thus, the overall findings of the literature published for the treatment of stage I NLPHL supports the rationale for IFRT alone as a reasonable option for these patients. However, the length of follow-up between studies is quite variable, making it difficult to compare long-term outcomes, but, overall, the comparisons between the response rates appear similar across studies. For stage II NLPHL, we believe, based on the above-cited publications, that IFRT alone is a valid choice in the setting of nonbulky disease, although brief chemotherapy followed by IFRT is also an acceptable alternative management strategy.

16.4.2   Advanced Stage: Stage III and IV

Data for the treatment of advanced-stage NLPHL is even more limited than for early-stage NLPHL. There is currently interest in including rituximab with or without chemotherapy for management of this disease. Adriamycin-based chemotherapy is favored, with R-CHOP (rituximab plus CHOP) described as a potential regimen. This is based on data that have documented that patients with advanced-stage NLPHL have similar outcomes to their cHL counterparts (10).

Because the NLPHL L&H cell expresses CD20, the anti-CD20 chimeric antibody rituximab has emerged as a biologically targeted treatment option. There is also much interest in rituximab because it is thought that targeted treatment might offer fewer side effects, including the secondary malignancies described in the above studies that often utilized wide irradiation fields in combination with chemotherapy. Also, it has been described that NLPHL patients, while typically demonstrating high initial CR rates, do continue to relapse over time, with relapses continuing to occur even 10 years out from initial treatment.

Rituximab was first described as a promising agent for the treatment of NLPHL in two case reports that described CR with 4 weekly doses of rituximab for the treatment of advanced and chemotherapy-refractory NLPHL (36, 37). In order to further establish the outcomes of rituximab therapy, a clinical trial was performed that enrolled 22 patients with NLPHL who were confirmed to be CD20+ (38) (Table 16.3). The patient population included 12 untreated patients (5 stage III, 2 with B-symptoms) and 10 relapsed patients. All patients were treated with 4 weekly doses of rituximab at $375\,mg/m^2$. The overall response rate (ORR) was 100%, with a 41%

CR. Median follow-up was 13 months, with 41% of patients having relapsed during follow-up. Thus, median freedom from progression was relatively short at 10.2 months. For patients who relapsed with NLPHL, retreatment with rituximab yielded stable disease or better, with one CR. Interestingly, transformation to large B-cell lymphoma was noted to occur at time of relapse in two or the five patients who were biopsied. Further pathologic review of the two patients who had transformed to large B-cell lymphoma revealed one case of diffuse large B-cell lymphoma and one case of T-cell-rich large B-cell lymphoma. In addition, both of the patients who developed transformation were noted to have an increased number of extranodular L&H cells, which has been described to be associated with a higher rate of progression to large B-cell lymphoma (39). Both of these patients received CHOP ± rituximab chemotherapy and went into CR after four courses of chemotherapy. Furthermore, one case report of a mother and her son who both had a diagnosis of NLPHL provides support for consideration of R-CHOP for advanced-stage NLPHL, with CRs for both lasting 34–40 months after treatment with six cycles of R-CHOP (40).

Thus, the current literature provides evidence for the inclusion of rituximab either alone or with CHOP chemotherapy for the treatment of advanced-stage NLPHL. In general, treatment with CHOP and rituximab is preferred in a patient with otherwise good performance status, whereas rituximab as a single agent is reserved for patients who are believed to not be good candidates for chemotherapy.

16.5   Treatment: Relapsed

Nodular LPHL behaves more similarly to indolent NHL in its clinical course. It is known for late relapses (up to 10 years out from time of initial treatment) compared to the typically more early relapses of cHL. The positive data described earlier for rituximab as a front-line treatment for NLPHL paired with data for indolent relapsed follicular NHL suggest that the disease responds well to rituximab with an ORR of 50% (41) and has spurred interest in examining rituximab as a treatment for relapsed NLPHL.

A multicenter trial was initiated by the GHSG to address the outcomes of treating relapsed NLPHL with rituximab (Table 16.3). Patients were eligible if the NLPHL expressed CD20 on greater than 30% of the malignant cells. Fourteen patients were

Table 16.3 Rituximab as a treatment for NLPHL

Authors (Ref.)	Subjects enrolled	Treatment	Outcomes
Ekstrand et al. 2003 (38)	22 patients (12 untreated & 10 relapsed)	Rituximab 375 mg/m2 × 4 × weekly	ORR: 100%
			CR: 41%
			FFP: 10.2 months
			13 months f/u 41% PD
Rehwald et al., 2003 (42)	14 patients (all relapsed)	Rituximab 375 mg/m2 × 4 × weekly	ORR: 86%
			CR: 57%
			12 months f/u 75% durable ORR

treated with 4 weekly infusions of rituximab (42). All patients had received prior radiation or chemotherapy but no prior rituximab for treatment, with a median time from initial diagnosis of 9 years. Treatment was tolerated well and with an ORR of 86% and 57% CR. After 1 year of follow-up, 75% of the patients who achieved PR+CR still continued to be in remission and the median duration of response was not reached after greater than 20 months.

One reason proposed for the excellent outcomes with rituximab for both follicular NHL and NLPHL is the commonly shared origin as germinal B-cell lymphomas. It is also theorized (but not proven) that rituximab, by preventing the survival of germinal-center-derived lymphoma B-cells, could perhaps decrease the subsequent risk of transformation to large B-cell lymphoma.

16.6 Follow-up Surveillance

Long-term follow-up for NLPHL is based on published guidelines for the management of cHL (28). General recommendation for follow-up include 3–4-month visits during the first 3 years, 6-month intervals during years 4 and 5, and annual follow-up from year 5 onward. A CBC, chemistry profile, and chest X-ray should be performed at each follow-up visit. Controversy exists with regard to the frequency of the need for CT scans although it is commonly done at least every 6 months for the first 5 years following completion of therapy (43). Women who received mantle irradiation are also advised to undergo mammograghy annually beginning 8–10 years after radiation (44). Routine yearly testing of thyroid function is also advised, particularly for patients who have undergone irradiation to the neck.

16.7 Transformation: Pathology, Diagnosis, and Treatment

Overall length of time to relapse of NLPHL is quite long, with a median of 53 months (10). Similar to indolent NHL, which has a risk of transformation of 3% per year, transformation can occur in NLPHL (45). However, given the rarity of the diagnosis, the incidence of transformation in NLPHL is less well defined, as are the outcomes and treatment recommendations for these patients.

Nodular LPHL has been described to typically transform to large B-cell lymphoma (LBCL) with both diffuse LBCL (DLBCL) and a unique entity of T-cell-rich large B cell lymphoma (TCR-LBCL) described. The incidence of this occurrence has been variable in NLPHL papers, with citations of 0% (10) to as high as 9% in one small study (38), with the average being typically described as 2.9% in review publications (2).

A diffuse with a T-cell-rich background pattern and a diffuse with a B-cell-rich pattern have been described as distinct immunoarchitectural patterns of NLPHL. The diffuse with a T-cell-rich background pattern was noted to be more common in patients who had disease recurrence. In addition, it was described that patients who start out with a nodular pattern NLPHL tend to evolve to a diffuse with a T-cell-rich background pattern or a diffuse B-cell-rich pattern with time, thus biologically showing the process of transformation to LBCL of, respectively, the TCR-LBCL and DLBCL subtypes (39).

The WHO criteria (6) provide a pathologic framework by which to subclassify lymphomas as NLPHL versus TCR-LBCL, although this distinction can still be immunphenotypically subtle (Figure 16.3). In NLPHL, small B-cells, follicular dendritic cells, and CD3+CD4+CD57+ T-cell are common, whereas in TCR-LBCL, CD8+ T-cells and histiocytes are predominant (46).

There is a great level of interest in understanding the molecular events that result in the progression and transformation of NLPHL to TCR-LBCL. The B-cell transcription factor PU.1 has been proposed by Delabie, et al. to have a role (47). In a review of 10 cases of composite lymphomas containing NLPHL and TCR-LBCL, it was noted that PU.1 had an elevated level of expression in NLPHL but that this expression was lost in the TCR-LBCL, suggesting that reduced expression of PU.1 might be a marker of transformation. It has also been hypothesized that differential expression of cytokines also could play a key role in transformation by supporting the growth of different cell types (47).

Treatment of NLPHL that has transformed to TCR-LBCL or DLBCL is based on the evidence that supports the treatment of other transformed indolent lymphomas, including follicular or marginal zone lymphomas that have transformed to DLBCL. It is also based on current evidence that supports the front-line and relapsed treatment of DLBCL. Patients who are diagnosed with TCR-LBCL have been described

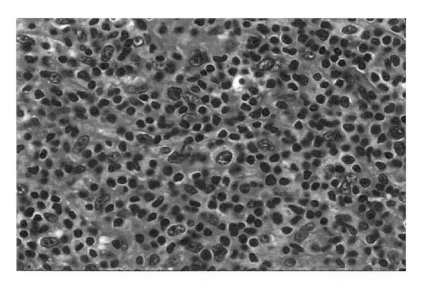

Figure 16.3 Higher-power microscopic view of T-cell-rich large B-cell lymphoma (TCR-LBCL). TCR-LBCL generally is thought to pathologically evolve from NLPHL. A diffuse large B-cell pattern is present and CD8+ T-cells and histiocytes surround these CD20+ large B-cells. This morphologic appearance combined with immunohistochemistry allow for TCR-LBCL to be distinguished from NLPHL or diffuse large B cell lymphoma. (courtesy of Dr. Jeffrey Medeiros, UT M.D. Anderson Cancer Center, Department of Pathology)

to have stage III/IV disease more frequently. Bone marrow positivity was noted in 35% of the patients and splenomegaly in 60% of the patients, and outcomes were similar, as predicted by the International Prognostic Index (IPI), to their classically regarded DLBCL counterparts (47). This evidence provides a rationale for the use of anthracyline-based chemotherapy such as R-CHOP. Consideration is also given for the inclusion of salvage-based chemotherapy followed by autologous peripheral blood stem cell transplantation for those who have previously received anthracy-cline-containing chemotherapy at the time of initial diagnosis of NLPHL; however, this is based on clinical judgment, as there is not a prospective randomized clinical trial that addresses this issue.

16.8 Summary and Conclusions

Nodular LPHL is a pathologic diagnosis distinct from cHL. Its unique pathology contributes to a more indolent clinical behavior than cHL. Although management strategies initially overlapped with therapies recommended for cHL, a growing interest in this unique disease process has led to several prospective clinical trials, particularly in early-stage NLPHL. This has allowed for treatment recommendations for NLPHL to become further defined following an evidence-based approach. Rituximab and radiation therapy have emerged as key components in therapy. Through our study of outcomes of NLPHL patients we have also been able to further define the delayed recurrences that can occur as well as the biologic transformations to TCR-LBCL and DLBCL. Further research is particularly important to increase our understanding of the biological factors that influence transformation as well as the best therapeutic regimens for the treatment of advanced NLPHL as well as NLPHL that has transformed to TCR-LBCL or DLBCL. It is hoped that a continued growth of research in NLPHL will allow us to better stratify treatment approaches and thus improve both short-term and long-term outcomes for the NLPHL patients.

References

1. Jemal A, Siegel R, Ward E, et al. Cancer statistics, 2006. CA Cancer J Clin 2006;56:106–130.
2. Diehl V, Sextro M, Franklin J, et al. Clinical presentation, course, and prognostic factors in lymphocyte-predominant Hodgkin's disease and lymphocyte-rich classical Hodgkin's disease: Report from the European Task Force on Lymphoma Project on Lymphocyte-Predominant Hodgkin's Disease. J Clin Oncol 1999;17:776.
3. Ansell SM, Armitage JO. Management of Hodgkin lymphoma. Mayo Clin Proc 2006;81:419–426.
4. Marafioti T, Hummel M, Anagnostopoulos I, et al. Origin of nodular lymphocyte-predominant Hodgkin's disease from a clonal expansion of highly mutated germinal-center B cells. N Engl J Med 1997;337:453–458.
5. Borg-Grech A, Radford J, Crowther D, et al. A comparative study of the nodular and diffuse variants of lymphocyte- predominant Hodgkin's disease. J Clin Oncol 1989;7:1303–1309.
6. Jaffe ES, Harris, N.L., Stein, H., et al. World Health Organization classification of tumours: Pathology and genetics of tumours of haematopoietic and lymphoid tissues. Lyons: IARC Press; 2001.

7. von Wasielewski R, Wilkens L, Nolte M, et al. Light-chain mRNA in lymphocyte-predominant and mixed-cellularity Hodgkin's disease. Mod Pathol 1996;9:334–338.

8. Falini B, Bigerna B, Pasqualucci L, et al. Distinctive expression pattern of the BCL-6 protein in nodular lymphocyte predominance Hodgkin's disease. Blood 1996;87:465–471.

9. Yatabe Y, Oka K, Asai J, et al. Poor correlation between clonal immunoglobulin gene rearrangement and immunoglobulin gene transcription in Hodgkin's disease. Am J Pathol 1996;149:1351–1361.

10. Bodis S, Kraus M, Pinkus G, et al. Clinical presentation and outcome in lymphocyte-predominant Hodgkin's disease. J Clin Oncol 1997;15:3060–3066.

11. Schmid C, Sargent C, Isaacson PG. L and H cells of nodular lymphocyte predominant Hodgkin's disease show immunoglobulin light-chain restriction. Am J Pathol 1991;139:1281–1289.

12. Renne C, Martin-Subero JI, Hansmann M-L, et al. Molecular cytogenetic analyses of immunoglobulin loci in nodular lymphocyte predominant Hodgkin's lymphoma reveal a recurrent IgH-BCL6 juxtaposition. J Mol Diagn 2005;7:352–356.

13. Kanzler H, Kuppers R, Hansmann ML, et al: Hodgkin and Reed-Sternberg cells in Hodgkin's disease represent the outgrowth of a dominant tumor clone derived from (crippled) germinal center B cells. J Exp Med 1996;184:1495–505, 1996

14. Sextro M, Diehl V, Franklin J, et al. Lymphocyte predominant Hodgkin's disease: a workshop report. European Task Force on Lymphoma. Ann Oncol 1996;7(Suppl 4):61–65.

15. Wlodarska I, Nooyen P, Maes B, et al. Frequent occurrence of BCL6 rearrangements in nodular lymphocyte predominance Hodgkin lymphoma but not in classical Hodgkin lymphoma. Blood 2003;101:706–710.

16. Hopken UE, Foss H-D, Meyer D, et al. Up-regulation of the chemokine receptor CCR7 in classical but not in lymphocyte-predominant Hodgkin disease correlates with distinct dissemination of neoplastic cells in lymphoid organs 10.1182/blood.V99.4.1109. Blood 2002;99:1109–1116.

17. Franke S, Wlodarska I, Maes B, et al. Lymphocyte predominance Hodgkin disease is characterized by recurrent genomic imbalances. Blood 2001;97:1845–1853.

18. Burns BF, Colby TV, Dorfman RF. Differential diagnostic features of nodular L & H Hodgkin's disease, including progressive transformation of germinal centers. Am J Surg Pathol 1984;8:253–261.

19. Ohno T, Stribley JA, Wu G, et al: Clonality in nodular lymphocyte-predominant Hodgkin's disease. N Engl J Med 1997;337:459–466.

20. Liso A, Capello D, Marafioti T, et al. Aberrant somatic hypermutation in tumor cells of nodular-lymphocyte-predominant and classic Hodgkin lymphoma. Blood 2006;108:1013–1020.

21. Said JW, Sassoon AF, Shintaku IP, et al. Absence of bcl-2 major breakpoint region and JH gene rearrangement in lymphocyte predominance Hodgkin's disease. Results of Southern blot analysis and polymerase chain reaction. Am J Pathol 1994;138:261–264.

22. Hansmann ML, Stein H, Dallenbach F, et al. Diffuse lymphocyte-predominant Hodgkin's disease (diffuse paragranuloma). A variant of the B-cell-derived nodular type. Am J Pathol 1994;138:29–36.

23. Inghirami G, Macri L, Rosati S, et al. The Reed-Sternberg cells of Hodgkin disease are clonal. Proc Natl Acad Sci USA 1994;91:9842–9846.

24. Mottok A, Hansmann M-L, Brauninger A. Activation induced cytidine deaminase expression in lymphocyte predominant Hodgkin lymphoma. J Clin Pathol 2005;58:1002–1004.

25. Gallamini A, Rigacci L, Merli F, et al. The predictive value of positron emission tomography scanning performed after two courses of standard therapy on treatment outcome in advanced stage Hodgkin's disease. Haematologica 2006;91:475–481.

26. Hutchings M, Loft A, Hansen M, et al. FDG-PET after two cycles of chemotherapy predicts treatment failure and progression-free survival in Hodgkin lymphoma. Blood 2006;107:52–59.

27. Carbone PP, Kaplan HS, Musshoff K, et al. Report of the Committee on Hodgkin's Disease Staging Classification. Cancer Res 1997;31:1860–1861.

28. Lister TA, Crowther D, Sutcliffe SB, et al. Report of a committee convened to discuss the evaluation and staging of patients with Hodgkin's disease: Cotswolds meeting. J Clin Oncol 19897:1630–1636.

29. Nogova L, Reineke T, Eich HT, et al. Extended field radiotherapy, combined modality treatment or involved field radiotherapy for patients with stage IA lymphocyte-predominant

Hodgkin's lymphoma: a retrospective analysis from the German Hodgkin Study Group (GHSG). Ann Oncol 2005;16:1683–1687.
30. Hoskin P, Smith P, Maughan T, et al. Long-term results of a randomised trial of involved field radiotherapy vs extended field radiotherapy in stage I and II Hodgkin lymphoma. Clin Oncol (R Coll Radiol) 2005;17:47–53.
31. Pellegrino B, Terrier-Lacombe MJ, Oberlin O, et al. Lymphocyte-predominant Hodgkin's lymphoma in children: therapeutic abstention after initial lymph node resection—a study of the French Society of Pediatric Oncology. J Clin Oncol 2003;21:2948–2952.
32. Murphy S, Morgan E, Katzenstein H, et al. Results of little or no treatment for lymphocyte-predominant Hodgkin disease in children and adolescents. J Pediatr Hematol Oncol 2003;25:684–687.
33. Schlembach P, Wilder R, Jones D, et al. Radiotherapy alone for lymphocyte-predominant Hodgkin's disease. Cancer J 2002;8:377–383.
34. Wilder R, Schlembach P, Jones D, et al. European Organization for Research and Treatment of Cancer and Groupe d'Etude des Lymphomes de l'Adulte very favorable and favorable, lymphocyte-predominant Hodgkin disease. Cancer 2002;94:1731–1738.
35. Feugier P, Labouyrie E, Djeridane M, et al. Comparison of initial characteristics and long-term outcome of patients with lymphocyte-predominant Hodgkin lymphoma and classical Hodgkin lymphoma at clinical stages IA and IIA prospectively treated by brief anthracycline-based chemotherapies plus extended high-dose irradiation. Blood 2004;104:2675–2681.
36. Keilholz U, Szelenyi H, Siehl J, et al. Rapid regression of chemotherapy refractory lymphocyte predominant Hodgkin's disease after administration of rituximab (anti CD 20 mono- clonal antibody) and interleukin-2. Leuk Lymphoma 1999;35:641–642.
37. Lush R, Jones S, Haynes A: Advanced-stage, chemorefractory lymphocyte-predominant Hodgkin's disease: long-term follow-up of allografting and monoclonal antibody therapy. Br J Haematol 2001;114:734–735.
38. Ekstrand BC, Lucas JB, Horwitz SM, et al. Rituximab in lymphocyte-predominant Hodgkin disease: results of a phase 2 trial. Blood 2003;101:4285–4289, 2003
39. Fan Z, Natkunam Y, Bair E, et al. Characterization of variant patterns of nodular lymphocyte predominant hodgkin lymphoma with immunohistologic and clinical correlation. Am J Surg Pathol 2003;27:1346–1356.
40. Unal A, Sari I, Deniz K, et al. Familial nodular lymphocyte predominant Hodgkin lymphoma: successful treatment with CHOP plus rituximab. Leuk Lymphoma 2005;46:1613–1617.
41. McLaughlin P, Grillo-Lopez AJ, Link BK, et al. Rituximab chimeric anti-CD20 monoclonal antibody therapy for relapsed indolent lymphoma: half of patients respond to a four-dose treatment program. J Clin Oncol 1998;16:2825–2833.
42. Rehwald U, Schulz H, Reiser M, et al. Treatment of relapsed CD20+ Hodgkin lymphoma with the monoclonal antibody rituximab is effective and well tolerated: results of a phase 2 trial of the German Hodgkin Lymphoma Study Group 10.1182/blood.V101.2.420. Blood 2003101:420–424.
43. Dryver ET, Jernstrom H, Tompkins K, et al. Follow-up of patients with Hodgkin's disease following curative treatment: the routine CT scan is of little value. Br J Cancer 2003;89:482–486.
44. Swerdlow AJ, Douglas AJ, Hudson GV, et al. Risk of second primary cancers after Hodgkin's disease by type of treatment: analysis of 2846 patients in the British National Lymphoma Investigation. Br Med J 1992;304:1137–1143.
45. Bastion Y, Sebban C, Berger F, et al. Incidence, predictive factors, and outcome of lymphoma transformation in follicular lymphoma patients. J Clin Oncol 1997;15:1587–1594.
46. Boudova L, Torlakovic E, Delabie J, et al. Nodular lymphocyte-predominant Hodgkin lymphoma with nodules resembling T-cell/histiocyte-rich B-cell lymphoma: differential diagnosis between nodular lymphocyte-predominant Hodgkin lymphoma and T-cell/histiocyte-rich B-cell lymphoma. Blood 2003;102:3753–3758.
47. Rudiger T, Gascoyne RD, Jaffe ES, et al. Workshop on the relationship between nodular lymphocyte predominant Hodgkin's lymphoma and T cell/histiocyte-rich B cell lymphoma. Ann Oncol 2002;13:44–51.

Chapter 17
Langerhans Cell Histiocytosis

Karen L. Chang and David S. Snyder

17.1 Introduction

Langerhans cell histiocytosis refers to a rare group of diseases that derive from a clonal proliferation and accumulation of Langerhans cells (1). The latter are specialized antigen-presenting cells of dendritic origin present at the dermal/epidermal border of the skin and as a meshwork throughout the epidermis. The Histiocyte Society, an international network of European, North and South American, and Asian groups that conduct cooperative studies of the histiocytoses, has divided histiocytic diseases into three groups: Langerhans cell histiocytosis (class I), non-Langerhans cell histiocytoses (class II), and malignant histiocytoses (class III) (2, 3). Langerhans cell histiocytosis, historically known as histiocytosis X, eosinophilic granuloma, or Langerhans cell granulomatosis, encompasses many different clinical manifestations. The Histiocyte Society classifies Langerhans cell histiocytosis according to the number of sites and types of tissue/organ involved and the presence or absence of involved organ failure. Historically, the disease comprises three main and sometimes overlapping clinical syndromes: unifocal disease (solitary eosinophilic granuloma), multifocal unisystem disease (including cases of Hand-Schüller-Christian syndrome), and multifocal multisystem disease (including cases of Letterer-Siwe syndrome) (1; 4–6). Langerhans cell histiocytosis also encompasses some cases belonging to syndromes previously described as reticuloendotheliosis, Hashimoto-Pritzker syndrome, self-healing histiocytosis, pure cutaneous histiocytosis, Type II histiocytosis, and nonlipid reticuloendotheliosis.

17.2 Epidemiology

Langerhans cell histiocytosis is an extremely rare disease that affects approximately five in a million children and approaches one in a million adults (2, 4, 7–9). Approximately 1200 new cases are reported annually in the United States. These figures may be spuriously low because of the failure to diagnose and report cases with a mild course or spontaneous healing of isolated lesions (10). Males are affected twice as often as females. Patients of northern European descent are more frequently afflicted than patients of Hispanic heritage, and the disease has only rarely been described in patients of African ancestry (11–13). The age at presentation varies with the clinical syndrome, but the disease occurs primarily in the pediatric population. Langerhans cell histiocytosis involving a solitary site (other than the lung) is found predominantly in older children (4, 8, 13). The age of presentation with multifocal unisystem disease is approximately 2–10 years. The median age of presentation with multifocal multisystem disease is less than 3 years (4, 7, 8). Solitary lung involvement is a unique clinical manifestation of Langerhans cell histiocytosis and usually occurs in young adults between 20 and 40 years of age, with a slight female predominance (4, 14). However, all of the clinical syndromes have been reported in all age groups. Early reports describe sibships and kindreds who had what appears to be Letterer-Siwe disease. Although many of the earlier reports were actually describing non-Langerhans cell histiocytosis reticulohistio-cytic disorders, rare well-documented cases of Langerhans cell histiocytosis have appeared in families (15–17).

17.3 Etiology

The etiology of the disease is unknown, but the abnormal cells of Langerhans cell histiocytosis from bone/chronic lesions have been shown to be immature Langerhans-type dendritic cells, thought to arise from blockage in the normal maturational pathway of Langerhans cells (2, 18, 19). However, whether Langerhans cell histio-cytosis is a neoplastic, immunodysregulatory, or reactive disorder has been the sub-ject of considerable debate. Many observations favor a reactive etiology, including the bland cytologic features of the Langerhans cells, the presence of numerous inflammatory cells (including granulomalike lesions), reports of spontaneous remissions, inability of Langerhans cell histiocytosis tissue samples to establish cell lines, and patterns of disease spread in individual patients (19). However, evidence in favor of a Langerhans cell histiocytosis being a neoplastic process includes the infiltrative nature of the atypical cells, the occurrence of bona fide familial cases, and the patterns of X-chromosome inactivation in the X-linked human androgen-receptor gene, which demonstrate that Langerhans cell histiocytosis is a monoclonal proliferation (17, 20, 21). Similar studies using X-linked polymorphic DNA probes have not found clonality in the T-lymphocytes of Langerhans cell histiocytosis. Except for rare reports of HHV6- and Epstein-Barr virus (EBV)-associated cases, most investigators have not found molecular evidence of a viral etiology (22–24). Comparative genomic hybridization, conventional cytogenetics, and loss of heterozygosity analyses have shown some mutational events in Langerhans cells histiocytosis, particularly involving chromosomes 1p and 7 (25–27). Interestingly, some early reports of Langerhans cell histiocytosis concurrent with myelodysplasia in children also involved chromosomes 7 and 1 (28). In fact, certain patients with myelodysplasia or acute myeloid leukemia with monosomy 7 have been reported to develop diabetes insipidus, a common feature of some forms of Langerhans cell histiocytosis (29, 30).

Isolated Langerhans cell histiocytosis of the lung is the only form of the disease known to be associated with an environmental risk factor, namely cigarette smoking. Cessation of smoking often results in tumor regression (14, 31). Lesions from these patients have been found to be nonclonal by HUMARA assay (32) Many investigators consider isolated pulmonary Langerhans cell histiocytosis associated with smoking to be a different disease process from the other forms of Langerhans cell histiocytosis, including those that might involve the lung as part of multisystem involvement.

Malignant diseases such as carcinoma, lymphoma, and leukemia have long been associated with Langerhans cell histiocytosis and may precede, follow, or occur at the same time (33). A focus of Langerhans cell histiocytosis may be seen adjacent to a hematopoietic malignancy, which may include non-Hodgkin or Hodgkin lymphomas, or leukemia (usually acute nonlymphocytic leukemia) (33–36). In cases associated with non-Hodgkin lymphoma, the Langerhans cell histiocytosis lesion is usually small and concurrent, but rarely, Langerhans cell histiocytosis has subsequently developed at other sites in these patients (35, 37). In contrast, in cases of Langerhans cell histiocytosis associated with leukemia, the Langerhans cell histiocytosis typically precedes the diagnosis of malignancy (33, 35). Langerhans cell histiocytosis has also been described in association with a variety of solid tumors. Cigarette smoking is the most likely etiology for the high prevalence of pulmonary and extrapulmonary malignancies in patients with pulmonary Langerhans cell histiocytosis (37) Most cases of malignancy follow Langerhans cell histiocytosis therapy and one cannot state with certainty whether such cases are due to individual predisposition to tumor development, with or without the contribution of potentially mutagenic Langerhans cell histiocytosis therapy.

Immune dysfunction most likely plays a large role in the pathogenesis of Langerhans cell histiocytosis. One hypothesis is that Langerhans cell histiocytosis development may be due to a failure to switch from the innate to adaptive immune response (38). Most investigators accept that the innate immune response in Langerhans cell histiocytosis patients is defective, but no specific immune system defect has been identified. However, there do appear to be defects in interactions between T-cells and macrophages, as well as between T-cells and Langerhans cells, which might result in a cytokine amplification cascade both locally and systemically (39). This cytokine "storm" may explain some of the clinical features of Langerhans cell histiocytosis such as fibrosis, necrosis, osteolysis, wasting, and fever. The cells of Langerhans cell histiocytosis are considered immature and unable to present antigens effectively, which is the usual role of normal Langerhans cells. Rather than an intrinsic defect, this is thought to be heavily influenced by the microenvironment, namely the production of numerous cytokines by the different types of cells, including non-Langerhans cells such as macrophages (18). A possible mechanism for the accumulation of defective Langerhans cells in lesions is related to chemokines of the cell surface. The Langerhans cell histiocytosis cells may aberrantly express chemokines of immature dendritic cells (40). This abnormal expression might help contribute to homing to lymphoid and nonlymphoid organs and might recruit eosinophils and CD4+ T-cells, both of which secrete more cytokines that influence the Langerhans cell histiocytosis cells to remain in an immature state.

17.4 Clinical Features

Langerhans cell histiocytosis is currently classified into localized and disseminated disease, as listed in Table 17.1 (2, 41). Localized disease, a form of "single-system disease," usually includes a single lesion in the bone, skin, or lymph node. As previously discussed, isolated pulmonary involvement probably represents a different disease entity. "Single-system disease" may also involve multiple sites within the same organ system, such as multiple lesions in one bone, multiple lesions in two or more different bones, multiple lymph node involvement, or multiple skin lesions. Lesions that have a tendency to involve the nervous system, usually by direct extension, include those involving the facial bones, sinuses, maxilla, or anterior or middle cranial fossa. These forms of "single-system disease" account for approximately one-third of patients (8). The other two-thirds of patients have a disseminated or multisystemic form of Langerhans cell histiocytosis, which is further divided into two categories ("low risk" and "high risk"), according to clinical course and response to treatment (42). The "risk organs" include the hematopoietic system, lungs, liver, or spleen. The low-risk group comprises patients with Langerhans cell histiocytosis lesions in multiple organs, but not involving the risk organs. The high-risk group comprises patients whose Langerhans cell histiocytosis lesions involve

Table 17.1 Classification of Langerhans cell histiocytosis

Single system disease	
Localized (single site)	Monostotic bone involvement
	Isolated skin involvement
	Solitary lymph node involvement
Multiple site	Polyostotic bone involvement
	Multifocal bone lesions (in two or more different bones)
	Multiple skin lesions
	Multiple lymph node involvement
Multisystem disease	
Low-risk group	Disseminated disease (≥ 2 organs involved), without involvement of lymph nodes, bone marrow, spleen, lungs, or liver
High-risk group	Disseminated disease (≥ 2 organs involved), with involvement of lymph nodes, bone marrow, spleen, lungs, or liver
CNS risk lesions	
	Involvement of facial bones, sinuses, maxilla, or anterior or middle cranial fossa (temporal, mastoid, sphenoidal, ethmoidal, zygomatic, orbital bones) with intracranial tumor extension

Source: Adapted from Ref. 41.

multiple organs, with involvement of one or more of the risk organs. Thus, adults with solitary pulmonary involvement would not be considered to have a high-risk lesion, despite involvement of lung.

The clinical presentation of Langerhans cell histiocytosis depends on the extent of dissemination (4, 8, 27, 43). The most common site of presentation of single site (or unifocal unisystem) disease is the bone. Single site bony disease may be asymptomatic and the incidental finding in the workup of an unrelated disorder. However, pain and tender swelling are common symptoms. The radiograph shows a single, sharply demarcated osteolytic lesion. Patients with single system, multiple site (or multifocal unisystem) disease may have bony defects with exophthalmos (usually due to tumor infiltration of the orbital cavity and the orbital bones), diabetes insipidus (due to involvement of the sella turcica with invasion of the pituitary gland), and loss of teeth (due to mandibular involvement and gum infiltration). Regardless of whether the disease is solitary or multiple, bony lesions usually are found in the long or flat bones: in children, the calvaria and the femur, and in adults, the skull or ribs. The mandible, scapula, ilium, and the anterior portion of the vertebral bodies of the lumbosacral vertebrae may also be affected in both the unifocal and multifocal variants of bony Langerhans cell histiocytosis (3, 4). The bones of the hands, wrists, knees, feet, and cervical vertebrae are uncommonly affected. Spontaneous fractures might result from the Langerhans cell histiocytosis lesions in the long bones, and vertebral collapse may result in spinal cord compression. Neurologic symptoms may occur if the skull lesion extends into the nervous system. Likewise, when Langerhans cell histiocytosis involves the temporal or mastoid bones, purulent external otitis media is common. Diabetes insipidus affects 25–40% of patients who present with unisystemic bone Langerhans cell histiocytosis and involvement of the skull (41, 43, 44). The diabetes insipidus may worsen in patients with Langerhans cell histiocytosis who are pregnant (45). Hypothalamic infiltration and pancreatic and thyroid involvement may result in hyperprolactinemia and hypogonadism (46). Single system Langerhans cell histiocytosis may also present in the skin as noduloulcerative lesions in the oral, perineal, perivulvar, or retroauricular regions. Skin lesions may also manifest as extensive coalescing, scaling, or crusted papules. One-third of patients with the classic multifocal single system form of Langerhans cell histiocytosis have skin mucocutaneous lesions that might present as described earlier, with nodular infiltrates and ulcerated plaques in the mouth, axillae, or anogenital region (47). Patients with lymph node involvement (usually cervical or inguinal region) are usually afebrile but may have painful lymphadenopathy (48). Lymphadenopathy and skin rashes due to Langerhans cell histiocytosis have been reported to transiently regress during pregnancy (49). Other reported sites of isolated disease include the thymus and soft tissue.

Patients with isolated lung involvement usually present with cough, dyspnea, chest pain, fever, hemoptysis, or weight loss. Approximately 20% of patients are asymptomatic (50). The chest radiograph varies from a micronodular and interstitial pattern in the early stages to a "honeycomb lung" appearance (50, 51). Depending on the stage of the lesions, high-resolution computed tomography (CT) scan of the chest shows nodules to cavitated nodules and thick-walled cysts to cysts to confluent cysts (52).

Multisystem disease is the rarest (10% of all cases) and most aggressive form of Langerhans cell histiocytosis and generally involves the skin, lymph nodes, lung, and liver (4, 43). Symptoms include anorexia, failure to thrive, fever, and pulmonary lesions/symptoms, such as cough, dyspnea, tachypnea, hemoptysis, chest pain, and pneumothorax. Chronic otitis media, lymphadenopathy, and hepatosplenomegaly are also common. Skin involvement is present in almost 80% of patients and may be the first sign of disease (47). They usually manifest as a generalized erythematous or weeping eczematoid rash extensively affecting the scalp, ear canals, abdomen, buttocks, intertriginous areas, and face. Ulcerated and denuded skin may serve as a portal for microorganisms and may lead to sepsis. Osteolytic lesions are not common in the multifocal multisystemic form of Langerhans cell histiocytosis, but the mastoid may be affected, resulting in otitis media. Aural discharge, conductive hearing loss, and postauricular swelling have been described. Lung involvement may result in diminished oxygen diffusion and lung capacity. Laboratory abnormalities include anemia in the absence of iron deficiency or significant infection, leukopenia, neutropenia, or thrombocytopenia.

The workup of a patient suspected of having Langerhans cell histiocytosis should include a complete blood cell count (CBC) with differential, a reticulocyte count, an erythrocyte sedimentation rate, a direct and indirect Coombs test, and immunoglobulin levels (2). If the CBC reveals any cytopenia, a bone marrow study should be performed (53). Coagulation studies may be useful. Other laboratory tests may include liver function tests, which, if abnormal, should prompt a liver biopsy, and urine osmolarity, to screen for diabetes insipidus. Imaging studies should include chest radiographs, a skeletal radiograph survey, and CT scan or magnetic resonance imaging (MRI) scans of the hypothalamic–pituitary region. Patients with radiographic evidence of pulmonary involvement, in whom chemotherapy is being considered, should undergo a bronchoalveolar lavage (and biopsy if necessary) to exclude opportunistic infections. Pulmonary function testing may show reduced carbon monoxide diffusing capacity of the lungs in 70–90% of cases (54).

Depending on the clinical situation, workup should also include a small bowel series and biopsy (for cases of unexplained diarrhea, failure to thrive, and malabsorption), hormonal studies (to investigate the hypothalamic–pituitary axis), and visual or neurologic testing. Skin biopsy, lymph node biopsy, or bone marrow or liver biopsy procedures may be warranted.

17.5   Diagnosis and Pathology

The diagnosis of Langerhans cell histiocytosis is made by biopsy of the affected organ. In general, the microscopic features do not allow distinction between the disseminated and localized forms of Langerhans cell histiocytosis. Langerhans cell histiocytosis may affect a portion of the biopsied tissue or might totally replace any normal anatomic structures. Despite the variation in the site, size, and architecture of Langerhans cell histiocytosis lesions, one always sees a proliferation of pathognomonic Langerhans cells in the appropriate cellular milieu. In fact, it is the histologic picture of these unique cells that unifies the protean clinical presentations of Langerhans cell histiocytosis (Figure 17.1) (2, 4).

Normal Langerhans cells are mononuclear cells, approximately 12–15 μm in diameter, with a moderate amount of eosinophilic cytoplasm, and are usually found in the basal layer of the epidermis. The cells of Langerhans cell histiocytosis may be slightly larger, but like their normal counterpart, they usually contain an irregularly shaped nucleus, which may be folded, grooved, or lobulated. Nucleoli are usually inconspicuous. Slight cytologic atypia may be observed. The nuclear membrane is thin, and the chromatin is finely dispersed or vacuolated. In addition to the Langerhans cells, Langerhans cell histiocytosis lesions contain variable numbers of reactive cells, including eosinophils, histiocytes, neutrophils, and small lymphocytes. Eosinophilic microabscesses and granulomas are often seen. Plasma cells usually are not seen. The number of mitoses varies widely from lesion to lesion (4). Bony lesions may contain more necrosis, eosinophils, and multinucleated histiocytes than lesions found in the skin, lung, or lymph node (4, 55). As lesions age, they tend to have more histiocytes and fibrosis and fewer Langerhans cells and eosinophils (55, 56). In very late lesions, fibrosis is markedly increased and the cellular composition may predominantly be foamy histiocytes, lymphocytes and plasma cells, with only rare Langerhans cells.

The Langerhans cells are not morphologically distinctive; thus, ancillary studies are necessary. In fact, Birbeck granules by ultrastructural examination and/or CD1a positivity by immunohistochemistry are required for a definitive diagnosis of

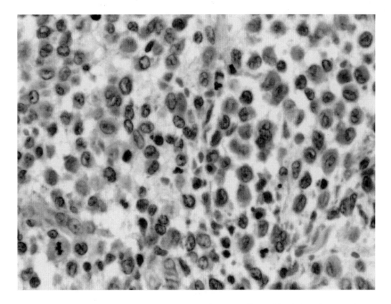

Figure 17.1 Langerhans cell histiocytosis. Langerhans cells, with their characteristic grooved nuclei, are seen admixed with eosinophils and plasma cells

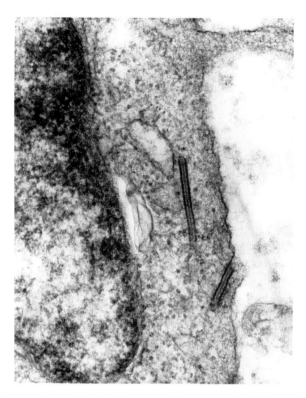

Figure 17.2 Electron micrograph of a Birbeck granule shows two rods, which are 33 nm in diameter, each with a central zipperlike striation. (Courtesy of Dr. Stephen Romansky, Long Beach, CA)

Langerhans cell histiocytosis (2). Ultrastructural examination shows that the cells have numerous lysosomes, small vesicles, multivesicular bodies, and irregular plasma membranes, and the absence of cell junctions, microvilli, desmosomes, tonofilaments, and melanosomes. The Birbeck granule, a pentilaminar "tennis-racket"-shaped intracytoplasmic membranous body with a zipperlike "handle," has remained for years the ultrastructural hallmark of Langerhans cell histiocytosis (Figure 17.2) (57). Formation of Birbeck granules are thought to be induced by a surface protein, which investigators have termed "langerin" (58). Birbeck granules are about 200–400 nm in length and about 33 nm in width, with an osmiophilic core and a double outer sheath. These unique granules are very fragile and are often destroyed in routine processing. Thus, although they are theoretically present in every Langerhans cell histiocytosis lesion, the percentage of cells containing the pathognomonic granules varies from case to case (4, 55).

Paraffin section immunohistochemical studies of Langerhans cell histiocytosis show that the Langerhans cells always express CD1a (Figure 17.3) and almost always express S100 protein (Figure 17.4) (4, 41, 43). The expression of CD1a is virtually pathognomonic and has been accepted as the strongest positive indicator

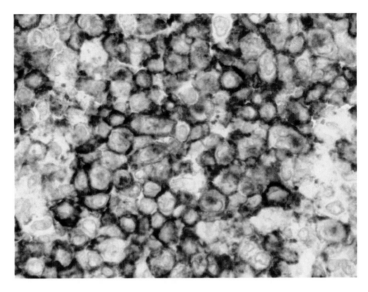

Figure 17.3 Langerhans cell histiocytosis. CD1a immunohistochemistry shows crisp membrane staining of Langerhans cells

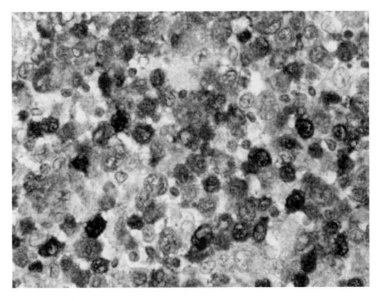

Figure 17.4 Langerhans cell histiocytosis. S100 immunohistochemistry shows variable intensity nuclear and cytoplasmic staining of Langerhans cells

of a Langerhans cell histiocytosis diagnosis, with the exception of Birbeck granules. Other histiocytic and dendritic cells do not express CD1a. In fact, CD1a expression is limited to reactive and lesional Langerhans cells, immature thymocytes, and T-lymphoblastic neoplasms. Langerhans cells also frequently express langerin, peanut agglutinin lectin, vimentin, CD74, the Fc receptor, and HLA-DR, as well as cytoplasmic CD2 and CD3 (59, 60). CD68 and antiplacental alkaline phosphatase may show a granular cytoplasmic pattern of variable intensity in a fraction of Langerhans cell histiocytosis cells (61). They are variably positive for CD45 and lysosome. They do not express CD163, CD35, CD30, CD34, or most B- and T-cell lineage markers (60, 62). The histiocytes, foamy histiocytes, and multinucleated cells often found in the lesions of Langerhans cell histiocytosis mark as ordinary nonneoplastic histiocytes and do not possess the antigenic characteristics of Langerhans cells.

Molecular hybridization studies show a germline configuration for the immunoglobulin heavy chain and α-, β-, and γ-T-cell receptor genes (21, 63). The enzyme histochemical profile of Langerhans cell histiocytosis cells is similar to normal Langerhans cells and other antigen-presenting cells in that they have low levels of lysosomal enzymes, have ATPase activity, and do not have peroxidase activity (64). They strongly express Class II histocompatability proteins and HLA-DR antigen, and they have receptor sites for the Fc portion of the IgG molecule and the third component of complement (18).

17.6   Differential Diagnosis

The clinical differential diagnosis of Langerhans cell histiocytosis includes the seborrheic dermatitides, Wiskott-Aldrich syndrome, mastocytosis, congenital candidiasis, neonatal varicella, and perianal herpes simplex. The patient's age, clinical course, laboratory and microbiology studies, and radiographic films will lead most astute clinicians to obtain a biopsy. However, because the presenting symptoms of Langerhans cell histiocytosis are nonspecific, particularly in single site involvement, the diagnosis is often delayed by a few to several months (44).

The microscopic differential diagnosis of Langerhans cell histiocytosis is quite varied and depends on the site of involvement. As previously stated, the identification of Birbeck granules or the presence of CD1a positivity in the Langerhans cells of Langerhans cell histiocytosis is specific, with the caveat that pertinent negative markers are also examined (2). However, prior to ordering these ancillary studies, the pure histologic differential diagnosis of Langerhans cell histiocytosis may include, in lymph nodes, reactive sinusoidal hyperplasia or dermatopathic lymphadenitis, or, in any other biopsied site, sinus histiocytosis with massive lymphadenopathy, metastatic neoplasms, and sinusoidal malignant lymphoma. In these cases, the distinctive ultrastructural and immunohistochemical profile that characterize the Langerhans cells of Langerhans cell histiocytosis can distinguish it from the other benign and malignant lesions.

17.7 Treatment

In the past, the multifaceted clinical presentations of Langerhans cell histiocytosis seemed to demand a unique approach to the therapy of each patient. Fortunately, data from international cooperative studies of childhood Langerhans cell histiocytosis have been very helpful in assessing the response to therapy, as well as elucidating the clinical features and underlying nature of the disease as previously described (2, 9, 19, 41, 43, 65). The different treatment options for Langerhans cell histiocytosis include watchful waiting, local treatment, immunomodulation, irradiation, chemotherapy, and liver, lung, and allogeneic hematopoietic cell transplantation.

When Langerhans cell histiocytosis is limited to a single skull lesion in the frontal, parietal, and occipital areas or a solitary lesion in a skeletal bone, watchful waiting, surgical curettage, excision, or resection might be sufficient. Painful bone lesions may require intralesional steroid injection. Polyostotic bone lesions may be treated with vinblastine or a short course of systemic steroids. Localized skin disease may be treated with a moderate to potent topical steroid or surgery. Topical nitrogen mustard (20% solution) may be needed for severe cutaneous involvement. PUVA (psoralen plus ultraviolet A) is an excellent treatment for solitary cutaneous disease. Regional lymph node enlargement can be resected or treated with a short course of systemic steroids. Involvement of the jaw bones requires a 6-month course of vincristine and prednisone.

The first clinical trials for Langerhans cell histiocytosis (LCH-I and LCH-II) by the Histiocyte Society were opened for children in the 1990s and resulted in three important observations (19, 42, 66). First, radiation or single-drug administration is not sufficient for patients with multiple bone lesions. Second, etoposide as a treatment agent did not have any additional therapeutic benefit when examining response, survival, or reactivation frequency, either as a single agent or in combination with vinblastine and prednisone. Because of the link between etoposide and an increased risk of therapy-related myelodysplasia or acute myeloid leukemia, vinblastine has remained the preferred treatment for Langerhans cell histiocytosis (67, 68). Third, importantly and unexpectedly, LCH-1 showed that poor response to initial 6-week therapy in children with risk-organ involvement was an adverse prognostic factor. Stratification of children into low-risk and high-risk groups was based on findings from LCH-II. The aim of clinical trial LCH-III, which opened for patient accrual in 2001, is to evaluate the relative efficacies of two multiagent treatment regimens (prednisone, vinblastine, and 6-mercaptopurine (6-MP), with or without methotrexate) in patients with multisystem Langerhans cell histiocytosis considered to be at high risk of disease progression or recurrence (19). This clinical trial will examine whether methotrexate improves the outcome of patients with high-risk Langerhans cell histiocytosis and will define optimal treatment for patients with lower-risk disease, such as multifocal bone disease.

A new international cooperative study of adult Langerhans cell histiocytosis opened in 2004 (LCH-A1) and continues to accrue patients (41). The aims of LCH-A1 include the following: (1) defining a uniform initial evaluation for adults with single-system disease, central nervous system lesions, isolated pulmonary disease, and multisystem Langerhans cell histiocytosis; (2) evaluating the effectiveness of a standard multiagent chemotherapy protocol in adults with multisystem Langerhans cell histiocytosis; and (3) evaluating the effectiveness of smoking cessation and of steroid therapy in adults with isolated pulmonary Langerhans cell histiocytosis. Adults with single system disease who are enrolled in the LCH-A1 clinical trial will receive 6 weeks of prednisone and vinblastine followed by continuation treatment with 6-mercaptopurine, prednisone, and vinblastine for 6 months. Under the LCH-A1 clinical trial, adults with multisystem disease will also receive prednisone and vinblastine for 6 weeks, followed by continuation treatment with 6-MP, prednisone, and vinblastine for 6 or 12 months. Patients with solitary pulmonary disease who stop smoking have a high rate of regression; thus, smoking cessation is essential for patients with lung disease. Those who have persistent lung disease after a trial of smoking cessation (typically 6 weeks) might benefit from a course of steroids. Chemotherapy will be reserved as salvage therapy for patients with progressive lung disease despite not smoking and receiving treatment with steroids.

Radiation therapy has traditionally been reserved for residual disease, disease that recurs following curettage, lesions that increase in size, or lesions in a critical site, such as the orbit, mandible, or vertebral column, and might be needed for lesions that are unusually large and painful or occur in inaccessible areas (69). Radiation therapy is mandatory in patients who develop diabetes insipidus. PUVA has also been used for extensive skin disease or for cutaneous disease in a multisystemic form of Langerhans cell histiocytosis.

Salvage therapy with 2-chloro-2'-deoxyadenosine (2CdA) for patients with recurrent or progressive Langerhans cell histiocytosis following standard therapy is the focus of protocol LCH-S-98, which was recently closed to patient accrual (19, 70). The results are not yet published, but preliminary data evaluation showed that monotherapy with 2CdA does not significantly improve prognosis in patients with severe progressive Langerhans cell histiocytosis. However, 2CdA has shown promise in combination chemotherapy and remains to be studied further.

About 20% of the patients with multisystem Langerhans cell histiocytosis do not respond to the currently available first-line treatment and have extremely poor prognosis. A phase II prospective trial salvage protocol (LCH-S-2005) for patients with severe disease (involvement of liver, spleen, or hematopoietic system) who do not respond to at least 6 weeks of "conventional" therapy will soon be opened for patient accrual (19). This study is expected to assess the efficacy of a potentially more toxic combination therapy (2CdA and cytosine arabinoside) in Langerhans cell histiocytosis patients with extremely poor prognosis.

Patients with resistant multisystem disease have been reported to undergo allogeneic hematopoietic cell transplantation or chemotherapy followed by transplantation of affected organ (kidney, lung, or liver), but the true efficacy of these transplants is not yet known, as no widely disseminated clinical trials have been conducted (71–73). Other emerging therapies include the use of immunomodulatory agents such as thalidomide or monoclonal antibodies directed against the CD1a or CD52 epitopes found on Langerhans cells (74,75). Specific therapies directed against the cytokines that are apparently critical to the abnormal proliferation have not yet been defined. Cooperative trials examining the efficacy and optimal treatment plan for these therapeutic options would be important to develop.

17.8 Clinical Course

The clinical course of the disease is greatly influenced by the number of affected organs at presentation, especially if involvement is accompanied by organ dysfunction (2, 4, 8, 10). Also, as previously stated, response to therapy at 6 weeks is an important prognostic variable (41–43). Age and histologic features such as nuclear atypia and mitotic rate are not independent prognostic indicators (41–43).

In one large study, those children who responded at 6 weeks to multiagent chemotherapy had a 3-year survival of 94%; that dropped to 34% in children who did not have a favorable 6-week response to chemotherapy (42). A recent study of adults with Langerhans cell histiocytosis showed that patients with "single-system disease" have a 5-year event-free survival of 100%, patients with solitary lung involvement have a 5-year event-free survival of 87.8%, and patients with multisystem disease have a 5-year event-free survival of 91.7% (10). The annual death rate in adults is estimated at 1.1% and a 5-year survival rate of >90% has been calculated (10). Disease recurrence in children varies, but it is approximately 50% in multifocal bony disease treated with single-agent chemotherapy, radiotherapy, or observation (43, 66).

Approximately 70% of patients with multisystem involvement develop late effects of Langerhans cell histiocytosis compared to approximately 24% of single system patients (43, 76). Diabetes insipidus, orthopedic abnormalities, and hearing loss are the most common problems. Neurologic problems, particularly cerebellar symptoms, might not manifest until 10 years or more after initial diagnosis. Endocrine abnormalities other than diabetes insipidis, such as growth hormone deficiency, may appear later in the course, possibly secondary to disease infiltration and secondary physical pressure by a growing tumor. Impaired liver function and therapy-related second neoplasms are other long-term adverse sequelae (33).

References

1. Coppes-Zantinga A, Egeler RM. The Langerhans cell histiocytosis X files revealed. Br J Haematol 2002;116:3–9.
2. Favara BE, Feller AC, Paulli M, et al. A contemporary classification of histiocytic disorders. The WHO Committee on Histiocytic/Reticulum Cell Proliferations. Reclassfication Working Group of the Histiocyte Society. Med Pediatr Oncol 1997;29:157–166.
3. Writing Group of the Histiocyte Society. Histiocytosis syndromes in children. Lancet 1987;i:209.
4. Lieberman PH, Jones CR, Steinman RM, et al. Langerhans cell (eosinophilic) granulomatosis: a clinicopathologic study encompassing 50 years. Am J Surg Pathol 1996;20:519–552.
5. Nezelof C, Basset F. Langerhans cell histiocytosis research; past, present, and future. Hematol Oncol Clin North Am 1998;12:385–406.

6. Lichtenstein L. Lichtenstein L. Histiocytosis X: integration of eosinophilic granuloma of bone, Letterer-Siwe disease and Schüller-Christian disease as related manifestations of a single nosologic entity. Arch Pathol 1953;56:84–102.
7. Baumgartner I, vonHochstetter A, Baumert B, et al. Langerhans'-cell histiocytosis in adults. Med Pediatr Oncol 1997;28:9–14.
8. Nicholson HS, Egeler RM, Nesbit ME. The epidemiology of Langerhans cell histiocytosis. Hematol Oncol Clin North Am 1998;12:379–384.
9. Howarth DM, Gilchrist GS, Mullan BP, et al. Langerhans cell histiocytosis: diagnosis, natural history, management, and outcome. Cancer 1999;85:2278 –2290.
10. Arico M, Girschikofsky M, Genereau T, et al. Langerhans cell histiocytosis in adults. Report from the International Registry of the Histiocyte Society. Eur J Cancer 2003;39:2341–2348.
11. Mickelson MR, Bonfiglio M. Eosinophilic granuloma and its variations. Orthop Clin North Am 1997;8:933–945.
12. Winkelmann RK. The skin in histiocytosis X. Mayo Clin Proc 1969;44:535–548.
13. Alessi DM, Maceri D. Histiocytosis X of the head and neck in a pediatric population. Arch Otolaryngol Head Neck Surg 1992;118:945–948.
14. Colby TV, Lombard C. Histiocytosis X in the lung. Hum Pathol 1983;14:847–856.
15. Katz AM, Rosenthal SD, Jakubovic HR, et al. Langerhans cell histiocytosis in monozygotic twins. J Amer Acad Dermatol 1991;24:32–37.
16. Hanapiah F, Yaacob H, Ghani KS, et al. Histiocytosis X: evidence for a genetic etiology. J Nihon Univ Sch Dent 1993;35:171–174.
17. Arico M, Nichols K, Whitlock JA, et al. Familial clustering of Langerhans cell histiocytosis. Br J Haematol 1999;107:883–888.
18. Geissmann F, Lepelletier Y, Fraitag S, et al. Differentiation of Langerhans cells in Langerhans cell histiocytosis. Blood 2001;97:1241–1248.
19. McClain KL. Langerhans cell histiocytosis: what is the orphan telling us? Am Soc Hematol Educ Program Book 2004;xx:284–295.
20. Willman CL, Busque L, Griffith BB, et al. Langerhans'-cell histiocytosis (Histiocytosis X): a clonal proliferative disease. N Engl J Med 1994;331:154–160.
21. Yu RC, Chu C, Buluwela L, et al. Clonal proliferation of Langerhans cells in Langerhans cell histiocytosis. Lancet 1994;343:767–768.
22. Leahy MA, Krejci SM, Friedmash M, et al. Human herpsvirus 6 is present in lesions of Langerhans cell histiocytosis. J Invest Dermatol 1993;101:642–645.
23. Chen C-J, Ho TY, Lu JJ, et al. Identical twin brothers concordant for Langerhans' cell histiocytosis and discordant for Epstein-Barr virus-associated haemophagocytic syndrome. Eur J Pediatr 2004;163:539.
24. McClain K, Jin H, Gresik V, et al. Langerhans cell histiocytosis: lack of a viral etiology. Am J Hematol 1994;47:16–20.
25. Murakami I, Gogusev J, Fournet JC, et al. Detection of molecular cytogenetic aberrations in Langerhans cell histiocytosis of bone. Hum Pathol 2002;33:555–560.
26. Betts DR, Leibundgut KE, Feldges A, et al. Cytogenetic abnormalities in Langerhans cell histiocytosis. Br J Cancer 1998;77:552–555.
27. Scappaticci S, Danesino C, Rossi E, et al. Cytogenetic abnormalities in PHA-stimulated lymphocytes from patients with Langerhans cell histiocytosis. Br J Haematol 2000;111:258–262.
28. Surico G, Muggeo P, Rigillo N, et al. Concurrent Langerhans cell histiocytosis and myelodysplasia in children. Med Pediatr Oncol 2000;35:434–438.
29. Lavabre-Bertrand T, Bourquard P, Chiesa J, et al. Diabetes insipidus revealing acute myelogenous leukaemia with a high platelet count, monosomy 7 and abnormalities of chromosome 3: a new entity? Eur J Haematol 2006;66:66–69.
30. Brescia M, Petti MC, Ottaviani E, et al. Diabetes insipidus as first manifestation of acute myeloid leukaemia with EVI-1-positive, 3q21q26 syndrome and T cell-line antigen expression: what is the EVI-1 gene role? Br J Haematol 2001;118:438–441.
31. Vassalo R, Ryu JH, Colby TV, et al. Pulmonary Langerhan's-cell histiocytosis. N Eng J Med 2000;342:1969–1978.

32. Yousem SA, Colby TV, Chen YY, et al. Pulmonary Langerhans' cell histiocytosis: molecular analysis of clonality. Am J Surg Pathol 2001;25:630–636.
33. Egeler RM, Neglia JP, Arico M, et.al. The relation of Langerhans cell histiocytosis to acute leukemia, lymphomas, and other solid tumors. The LCH-Malignancy Study Group of the Histiocyte Society. Hematol Oncol Clin North Am 1998;12:369–378.
34. Burns BF, Colby TV, Dorfman RF. Langerhans' cell granulomatosis (histiocytosis X) associated with malignant lymphomas. Am J Surg Pathol 1983;7:529–533.
35. Egeler RA, Neglia JP, Puccetti DM, et al. Association of Langerhans cell histiocytosis with malignant neoplasms. Cancer 1993;71:865–873.
36. Egeler RM, Neglia JP, Arico M, et al. Acute leukemia in association with Langerhans cell histiocytosis. Med Pediatr Oncol 1994;23:81–85.
37. Neuman MP, Frizzera G. The coexistence of Langerhans' cell granulomatosis and malignant lymphoma may take different forms: Report of seven cases with a review of the literature. Hum Pathol 1986;17:1060–1065.
38. Nezelof C, Basset F. An hypothesis Langerhans cell histiocytosis: the failure of the immune system to switch from an innate to an adaptive mode. Pediatr Blood Cancer 2004;42:398–400.
39. Egeler RM, Favara BE, vanMeurs M, et al. Differential in situ cytokine profiles of Langerhans-like cells and T cells in Langerhans cell histiocytosis: abundant expression of cytokines relevant to disease and treatment. Blood 1999;94:4195–4201.
40. Annels NE, daCosta CE, Prins FA, et al. Aberrant chemokine receptor expression and chemokine production by Langerhans cells underlies the pathogenesis of Langerhans cell histiocytosis. J Exp Med 2003;197:1385–1390.
41. Stockschlaeder M, Sucker C. Adult Langerhans cell histiocytosis. Eur J Haematol 2006;76:363–368.
42. Gadner H, Grois N, Arico M, et al. A randomized trial of treatment for multisystem Langerhans' cell histiocytosis. J Pediatr 2001;138:734.
43. Savasan S. An enigmatic disease: childhood Langerhans cell histiocytosis in 2005. Int J Dermatol 2006;45:182–188.
44. Maghie M, Cosi G, Genovese E, et al. Central diabetes insipidus in children and young adults. N Eng J Med 2000;343:998–1007.
45. DiMaggio LA, Lippes HA, Lee RV. Histiocytosis X and pregnancy. Obstet Gynecol 1995;85:806–809.
46. Braunstein GD, Kohler PO. Endocrine manifestations of histiocytosis. Am J Pediatr Hematol Oncol 1981;3:67–75.
47. Munn S, Chu AC. Langerhans cell histiocytosis of the skin. Hematol Oncol Clin North Am 1998;12:269–286.
48. Motoi M, Helbron D, Kaiserling E, et al. Eosinophilic granuloma of lymph nodes: a variant of histiocytosis X. Histopathology 1980;4:585–606.
49. Scherbaum WA, Seif FJ. Spontaneous transient remission of disseminated histiocytosis X during pregnancy. J Cancer Res Clin Oncol 1995;121:57–60.
50. Vassallo R, Ryu JH, Schroeder DR, et al. Pulmonary Langerhans'-cell histiocytosis. N Eng J Med 2002;346:484–490.
51. Travis W, Borok Z, Roum JH, et al. Pulmonary Langerhans' cell granulomatosis (Histiocytosis X). A clinicopathologic study of 48 cases. Am J Surg Pathol 1993;17:971–986.
52. Brauner MW, Greiner P, Mouelhi MM, et al. Pulmonary histiocytosis X: evaluation with high-resolution CT. Radiology 1989;172:255–258.
53. Chang KL, Gaal KK, Huang Q, et al. Histiocytic lesions involving the bone marrow. Semin Diagn Pathol 2003;20:226–236.
54. Crausman RS, Jennings CA, Tuder RM, et al. Pulmonary histiocytosis X: Pulmonary function and exercise pathophysiology. Am J Respir Crit Care Med 1996;153:426–435.
55. Nezelof C, Frileux-Herbet F, Cronier-Sachot J. Disseminated histiocytosis X. Analysis of prognostic factors based on a retrospective study of 50 cases. Cancer 1979;44:1824–1838.
56. Favara BE, Jaffe R. Pathology of Langerhans cell histiocytosis. Hematol Oncol Clin North Am 1987;1:75–97.

57. Birbeck M, Breahnach A. An electron microscopy study of basal melanocytes and high-level clear cells (Langerhans Cells) in vitiligo. J Invest Dermatol 1961;37:51–63.
58. Valladeau J, Dezutter-Dambuyant C, Saeland S. Langerin/CD207 sheds light on formation of birbeck granules and their possible function in Langerhans cells. Immunol Res 2003;28:93–107.
59. Chikwava K, Jaffe R. Langerin (CD207) staining in normal pediatric tissues, reactive lymph nodes, and childhood histiocytic disorders. Pediatr Dev Pathol 2004;7:607–614.
60. Chu PG, Chang KL, Arber DA, Weiss LM. Practical applications of immunohistochemistry for hematolymphoid disorders: an updated review. Ann Diagn Pathol 1999;3:104–133.
61. Ruco LP, Pulford KAF, Mason D. Expression of macrophage-associated antigens in tissues involved by Langerhans' cell histiocytosis (histiocytosis X). Am J Clin Pathol 1989;92:273–279.
62. Lau SK, Chu PG, Weiss LM. CD163: a specific marker of macrophages in paraffin-embedded tissue samples. Am J Clin Pathol 2004;122:794–801.
63. Yu RC, Chu AC. Lack of T-cell receptor gene rearrangements in cells involved in Langerhans cell histiocytosis. Cancer 1995;75:1162–1166.
64. Foucar K, Foucar E. The mononuclear phagocyte and immunoregulatory effector (M-PIRE) system: evolving concepts. Semin Diagn Pathol 1990;7:4–18.
65. Ceci A, deTerlizzi M, Collela R, et al. Langerhans cell histiocytosis in childhood: results from the Italian Cooperative AIEOP-CNR-H.X 83 study. Med Pediatr Oncol 1993;21:259–264.
66. Titgemeyer C, Grois N, Minkov M, et al. Pattern and course of single-system disease in Langerhans cell histiocytosis. Data from the DAL-HX83- and 90- study. Med Pediatr Oncol 2001;37:108–114.
67. Smith MA, Rubenstein L, Anderson JR, et al. Secondary leukemia or myelodysplastic syndrome after treatment with epipodophyllotoxins. J Clin Oncol 1999;17:569–577.
68. Krishnan A, Bhatia S, Slovak ML, et al. Predictors of therapy-related leukemia and myelodysplasia following autologous transplantation for lymphoma: an assessment of risk factors. Blood 2000;95:1588–1593.
69. Seegenschmiedt HM, Micke O, Olschewski T, et al. Radiotherapy is effective in symptomatic Langerhans cell hsitiocytosis (LCH): long-term results of a multicenter study in 63 patients. Int J Radiat Oncol Biol Phys 2003;57(Suppl. 2):S251.
70. Stine KC, Saylors RL, Saccente S, et al. Efficacy of continuous infusion 2-CDA (Cladribine) in pediatric patients with Langerhans cell histiocytosis. Pediatr Blood Cancer 2004;43:81–84.
71. Kinugawa N, Imashuku S, Hirota Y, et al. Hematopoietic stem cell transplantation (HSCT) for Langerhans cell histiocytosis (LCH) in Japan. Bone Marrow Transplant 1999;24:935–938.
72. Akkari V, Donadieu J, Piguet C, et al. Hematopoietic stem cell transplantation in patients with severe Langerhans cell histiocytosis and hematological dysfunction: experience of the French Langerhans Cell Study Group. Bone Marrow Transplant 2003;31:1097–1103.
73. Steiner M, Matthes-Martin S, Attarbaschi A, et al. Improved outcome of treatment-resistant high-risk Langerhans cell histiocytosis after allogeneic stem cell transplantation with reduced-intensity conditioning. Bone Marrow Transplant 2005;36:215–225.
74. Kelly KM, Beverley PC, Chu AC, et al. Successful in vivo immunolocalization of Langerhans cell histiocytosis with use of a monoclonal antibody, NA1/34. J Pediatr 1994;125:717–722.
75. Jordan MB, McClain KL, Yan X, et al. Anti-CD52 antibody, alemtuzumab, binds to Langerhans cells in Langerhans cell histiocytosis. Pediatr Blood Cancer 2005;44:251–254.
76. Haupt R, Nanduri V, Calevo MG, et al. Permanent consequences in Langerhans cell histiocytosis patients: a pilot study from the Histiocyte Society-Late Effects Study Group. Pediatr Blood Cancer 2004;42:438–444.

Chapter 18
Systemic Mastocytosis

Peter Valent

18.1   Introduction

Mastocytosis is a term used for a group of disorders defined by an abnormal accumulation of mast cells (MCs) in one or more organ systems. Clinical symptoms result from MC-derived mediators and/or from infiltration of MCs in the tissues. Cutaneous mastocytosis (CM) is a benign disease of the skin and often regresses spontaneously. Systemic mastocytosis (SM) is a persistent clonal disease of MCs with a variable clinical picture and a variable prognosis. Notably, the clinical course in SM ranges from asymptomatic and indolent over many years to highly aggressive with a short survival. The WHO classification discriminates four categories of SM: indolent SM (ISM), aggressive SM (ASM), SM with an associated clonal hematologic non-MC-lineage disease (SM-AHNMD), and mast cell leukemia (MCL). The genetic hallmark of SM is the somatic *KIT* mutation D816V. In SM-AHNMD, additional or alternative molecular defects might be detected, such as the *FIP1L1/PDGFRA* fusion gene in associated chronic eosinophilic leukemia (SM-CEL) or *AML1/ETO* in SM with acute myeloid leukaemia (AML) and t(8;21). Patients with ISM are treated with 'mediator-targeting' drugs, whereas patients with ASM or MCL are candidates for cytoreductive therapy. The use of 'KIT-targeting' tyrosine kinase (TK) inhibitors has also been suggested. Unfortunately, the D816V *KIT* mutation is associated with resistance against imatinib. However, several second-generation TK inhibitors, such as PKC412 (midostaurin), AMN107 (nilotinib), or BMS354825 (dasatinib) are available and reportedly inhibit growth of MCs carrying KIT D816V. These drugs might be useful for therapy of ASM or MCL in the future.

18.2   Biology of Mast Cells

Mast cells are hematopoietic cells with unique functional properties and a distinct composition of mediators and antigens (1, 2). In contrast to basophils and other leukocytes, MCs are long-lived cells with an estimated life span of at least several

S.M. Ansell (ed.), *Rare Hematological Malignancies.*
© Springer 2008

months. MCs reside in vascularized tissues in diverse organs, often in the vicinity of smaller or larger blood vessels or nerve fibers (1, 2). In routinely processed tissue sections, these cells can usually be identified by their typical metachromatic granules (1, 2). Within their granules, MCs store vasoactive and immunoregulatory mediators, including histamine, heparin, PGD2, and cytokines (1–3). These compounds are released from MCs in response to aggregation of the high-affinity IgE receptor, activation through complement receptors, or activation by cytokines (1–3). Other mediators, such as tryptase, are constitutively secreted from MCs and are rapidly released after MC activation. Baseline tryptase levels can be measured in the serum as a MC-related marker and correlate with the total burden of MC in healthy subjects as well as in patients with MC proliferative disorders (4–6).

Mast cells reportedly are derived from hematopoietic progenitor cells which are detectable in the bone marrow and in the peripheral blood (7–11). It is assumed that pre-committed and MC-committed progenitors are circulating cells that undergo transmigration, and after trafficking into the tissues, they undergo differentiation and maturation (12). Several cytokines and microenvironmental factors are considered to contribute to growth and differentiation of MCs. The most important MC growth factor is stem cell factor (SCF), also termed KIT-ligand. This stromal cell-derived cytokine induces the development of MCs from uncommitted and MC-committed progenitors (8–15). These MC progenitor cells express a specific receptor for SCF, a TK-type receptor encoded by the *KIT* proto-oncogene (10, 12, 16). The respective oncoprotein, KIT, and SCF are considered essential for the development of MCs. Defects in *KIT* or *SCF* genes in mice lead to MC deficiency (17, 18). By contrast, 'gain-of-function mutations' in *KIT* are associated with enhanced survival and growth of MCs (progenitors) (19, 20). Such mutations, particularly *KIT* D816V, are frequently detected in patients with SM (21–26).

18.3   Pathogenesis of Mastocytosis

The common histopathologic feature of mastocytosis, shared by all disease variants, is the focal accumulation (clustering) of MCs in the tissues (27–30). Depending on the disease variant, MCs and their progenitors also show increased proliferative capacity (27–30). However, little is known concerning pathogenetic factors that contribute to the development of disease variants and progression. Likewise, so far, no clear pathogenetic concept has been presented for CM, an indolent disorder confined to the skin. It remains unclear whether all patients with CM suffer from a monoclonal MC disease, as only a subset of them exhibit *KIT* mutations. Interestingly, in those with a *KIT* D816V mutation, the disease process might be programmed to become SM and to persist (23, 24, 31).

In SM, monoclonality of the disease is well established, and several pathogenetic concepts have been developed (32–34). The most important concept relates to the *KIT* mutation D816V, which is detectable in the vast majority (>80%) of all patients (20–26, 35). The D816V *KIT* mutation is considered to represent an important "hit" contributing to MC differentiation and abnormal clustering of neoplastic progenitors (19, 20). In contrast, this mutation alone might be unable to act as a proliferation-enhancing oncogene (36). However, KIT D816V may well play a causative role in indolent SM, for which the pathologic hallmark is MC differentiation and MC-clustering without proliferation. In contrast, in advanced MC neoplasms (i.e., ASM or MCL) in which KIT D816V can also be detected, MC and MC progenitors show increased proliferative capacity (27–30, 32, 33). In these patients, additional (genetic) defects and features, which remain to be identified, are likely to cooperate with KIT D816V and thereby contribute to the uncontrolled growth of MCs.

It has also been suggested that, apart from D816V, other *KIT* mutations might play a role in the development of SM (37–39). Several of these *KIT* mutations are shown in Table 18.1. In addition, various chromosomal defects, other gene defects, and genetic polymorphisms have been discussed to contribute to the pathogenesis of SM (40–44). Some of these defects might play a particular role in patients who

Table 18.1 Cyto/genetic defects and gene polymorphisms described in mastocytosis

Cyto/genetic defect	Reported in patients with	Estimated frequency in patients with SM
KIT D816V	All variants of SM (some with CM)	>80%
KIT D816Y	CM, SM, SM-AHNMD	<5%
KIT D816F	CM, SM	<5%
KIT D816H	SM, SM-AHNMD	<5%
KIT R815K	CM	<5%
KIT I817V	SM	<5%
KIT D820G	ASM	<5%
KIT E839K	CM	<5%
KIT V533D	CM	<5%
KIT V559A	CM	<5%
KIT V560G	SM	<5%
KIT F522C[a]	SM	<5%
KIT V530I	SM-AML	<5%
KIT K509I[a]	SM	<5%
KIT A533D[a]	CM	<5%
FIPL1/PDGFRA[b]	SM-CEL	<5%
IL-4Rα Q576R	CM, indolent SM (ISM)	n.k.
del 20(q12)[b]	SM, SM-AHNMD	<5%
+9[b]	SM, SM-AHNMD	<5%
AML1/ETO[b]	with t(8;21)[b]	

CM, cutaneous mastocytosis; SM, systemic mastocytosis; SM-AHNMD, SM with an associated hematologic clonal non-mast-cell lineage disease. n.k., not known.

[a]Described as germline mutation.

[b]These cyto/genetic defects are indicative of an AHNMD.

have an additional myeloid neoplasm apart from SM (i.e. an AHNMD (Table 18.1). Many of these defects have recently been linked to distinct myeloid neoplasms. A good example is the *FIP1L1/PDGFRA* fusion gene, that has recently been associated with chronic eosinophilic leukemia (CEL), which can also develop in patients with SM. Table 18.1 provides a summary of chromosomal and gene defects that have been identified in patients with SM.

Another important pathogenetic aspect in SM is abnormal expression of cell surface adhesion antigens on neoplastic MCs (45–47). Several of these surface antigens are specifically expressed on neoplastic MCs in SM, but not on normal MCs or MCs in reactive disease states. An intriguing example is CD2 (LFA-2). Because MCs also express CD58 (LFA-3), the natural ligand of CD2, an attractive hypothesis is that CD2–CD58-dependent aggregation of MCs occurs in patients with SM and then contributes to abnormal cluster formation (46). MCs in SM also express other cell–cell adhesion molecules such as CD9 (motilin), CD29 (ß-chain of ß1 integrins), CD54 (ICAM-1), CD63 (LAMP3), or CD172a (SIRPalpha) (48–50). However, these antigens are also detectable on normal MCs, whereas CD2 is only detected on MCs in patients with SM (45–47). Whether these molecules, especially CD2, indeed play a pathogenetic role in SM remains at present unknown. It is also unknown whether *KIT* D816V, or another defect, is responsible for abnormal expression of adhesion-related molecules on MCs in SM. Whatever the relationship is, it is assumed that increased MC differentiation and MC clustering are important aspects in the development of SM in all SM variants, whereas disease progression with enhanced proliferation of MCs might be associated with other gene defects.

18.4 Diagnostic Criteria and WHO Classification

Traditionally, mastocytosis is split into cutaneous mastocytosis and systemic mastocytosis (27–30). Localized MC tumors (mastocytomas, MC sarcoma) are extremely rare entities (27, 28). Whereas CM has its usual onset before puberty (51), most patients presenting in adulthood are diagnosed as having SM. In these patients, the diagnosis is commonly established by bone marrow examination (52, 53). However, apart from the bone marrow, other organs such as the liver or the gastrointestinal tract, might also be affected (54–58). A remarkable aspect is that CM shows spontaneous regression in a significant number of cases (59).

Systemic mastocytosis is a persistent disease in which the *KIT* mutation D816V is commonly detected (20–26). In some of these patients, the mutation is not only found in MCs but also in non-MC-lineage hematopoietic cells (25, 26, 60–64). Based on such data, SM is now accepted to be a myeloproliferative disorder (32–34). This concept is consistent with the notion that MCs derive from myelopoietic progenitor cells (7–11) and is also consistent with the relatively high incidence of AHNMDs, including secondary AML, that occur in these patients (65–68).

During the past two decades, substantial progress has been made in the genetic, molecular, and phenotypic characterization of neoplastic MC (32–35). Based on these advances, a consensus classification for mastocytosis has been developed (69, 70). This World Health Organization (WHO) classification is based on specific criteria that help in the differentiation between SM and CM, between SM and other myeloid neoplasms, and between SM and a reactive increase in MCs or MC activation (69, 70). Respective criteria have been termed SM criteria and are divided into major SM criteria and minor SM criteria (Table 18.2). If at least one major and one minor criteria or at least three minor SM criteria are fulfilled, the diagnosis SM can be established (Table 18.2).

18.5 Histology and Immunohistochemistry (Major Criterion)

The most important step in the diagnostic workup of adult patients is a thorough examination of the bone marrow biopsy and bone marrow aspirate (27–30, 52, 53, 71). The major SM criterion is the presence of dense, compact, multifocal MC infiltrates within a bone marrow biopsy section. The most suitable marker for MC detection in such biopsies is tryptase immunohistochemistry (71–74). Thus, antibodies against tryptase detect even small-sized compact or diffuse MC infiltrates (71–74). Additional markers that can be used to detect MCs in SM by immunohistochemistry are the tetraspan molecule motolin (CD9), LAMP-3 (CD63), and KIT (CD117). Compact MC infiltrates might not only be detected in the bone marrow in SM but may also be detected in extramedullary visceral organs in these patients (53–58).

Apart from compact, sharply demarcated MC infiltrates, other types of MC infiltrates might also be detected in the bone marrow and may correlate with the

Table 18.2 Criteria defining systemic mastocytosis: SM criteria

Major[a]:	Multifocal dense infiltrates of MCs in bone marrow or other extracutaneous organ(s) (>15 MCs in aggregate) detected by immunohistochemistry (tryptase stain)
Minor[a]:	- MC in bone marrow or other extracutaneous organ(s) show an abnormal morphology [i.e., type I MC (>25%) (usually recorded in bone marrow smears)]
	- *KIT* mutation at codon 816[b] in extracutaneous organ(s) (usually, bone marrow cells should be examined)
	- MC in bone marrow express CD2 and/or CD25 (by immunohistochemistry or flow cytometry)
	- Serum tryptase >20 ng/mL (does not count in patients who have AHNMD-type disease)

[a]If at least one major and one minor or at least three minor criteria are fulfilled, the diagnosis SM can be established (69, 70).
[b]Activating mutations at codon 816, in most cases *KIT* D816V.

subtype of SM (52, 53). Notably, in more advanced MC disorders (ASM, MCL), MC infiltrates often are diffuse or mixed (compact plus diffuse component) (52, 53). In patients with ASM or MCL, the remaining bone marrow architecture is usually altered (distorted) by the MC infiltrate, whereas this is not the case in typical ISM. Here, MC infiltration does not lead to an alteration in the architecture of the remaining (surrounding) normal bone marrow even if some of the MCs are diffusely spread in these areas (52, 53).

18.6   Minor Diagnostic Criteria for SM

Minor SM criteria relate to the morphology of MCs (spindle-shaped, atypical MC type I), their phenotype (CD2, CD25), elevated serum tryptase, and demonstration of codon 816 mutations in the *KIT* gene (69, 70). The application of such criteria is often crucial in the diagnostic workup, as MCs might also be increased and form focal infiltrates in reactive MC hyperplasia or in myelomastocytic disorders. For example, advanced myeloid neoplasms might exhibit an increase in diffusely spread MC in the bone marrow without cytological or biochemical evidence of SM (75–78). If the percentage of MCs in these patients exceeds 10% in the bone marrow smear or peripheral blood smear, the final diagnosis is myelomastocytic leukemia (76, 78). Major and minor SM criteria are listed in Table 18.2. Table 18.3 shows differential diagnoses to be considered in suspected SM.

18.6.1   Morphology of Mast Cells: The Bone Marrow Smear

The bone marrow smear in suspected SM might show an increase in MCs, abnormal morphology of MCs, or cytomorphological abnormalities in other cell lineages, such as myelodysplasia, eosinophilia, or an increase in blasts, which raises the suspicion of an AHNMD (69, 70, 79). In the normal bone marrow, the percentage of MCs is low (<0.1%). In patients with SM, the percentage is usually higher (79). A percentage of MC of >10% in bone marrow smears is associated with a poor prognosis and is indicative of aggressive disease (79). If the percentage of MCs exceeds 20%, the diagnosis is MCL, provided that SM criteria are met (79). Four distinct stages of MC maturation have been described: the nongranulated blast, the metachromatic blast, the promastocyte (atypical MC type II = MC with bilobed or multilobed nuclei), and the mature (mononuclear) MC (69, 70, 79). Immature MCs are frequently recorded in patients with ASM or MCL (79). In ISM, bone marrow MCs are more mature, albeit they usually do show characteristic morphological abnormalities, including cytoplasmic extensions, oval nuclei, and a hypogranulated cytoplasm (79). Such MCs are termed "atypical MC type I" and are detected in a majority of cases with ISM (79).

Table 18.3 Systemic mastocytosis: differential diagnosis[a]

a. Systemic disorders mimicking MC mediator effects
Vascular diseases (with hypotension and shock)
Endocrinologic disorders (diabetes, adrenal tumors, VIPoma, etc.)
Neurologic and psychiatric disorders (encephalopathy, neuritis, etc.)
Gastrointestinal disorders (Crohn's disease, ulcerative colitis, etc.)
Infectious diseases (parasitic infections, hepatitis, others)
b. Benign disorders associated with MC activation
Allergies, atopic disorders
Benign cutaneous flushing,
Idiopathic anaphylaxis
Chronic urticaria
Drug effects on MC
MC activation syndrome, monoclonal MC activation syndrome
c. Local (reactive) MC hyperplasia
Immunocytoma or other NHLs with reactive focal increase in MCs
Cutaneous tumors (melanomas, basal cell carcinoma, others)
Chronic inflammation (autoimmune disorders, intestinal ulcer, etc.)
Treatment with recombinant stem cell factor (SCF)
Thromboembolic disorders
d. Other myeloid neoplasms
Myelomastocytic leukemia: myeloid neoplasm with increase in MCs but criteria to diagnose SM are not fulfilled
Tryptase-positive acute myeloid leukemia (AML)
KIT+ AML with blast cells expressing CD2 (FAB AML-M4eo, some M3)
AML with *KIT* mutations at codon 816 (but without detectable occult SM)
Chronic myeloid leukemia with accumulation of tryptase+ cells
Idiopathic myelofibrosis with focal accumulation of MC
Acute or chronic basophilic leukemia

SM, systemic mastocytosis; MC, mast cell, [a]SM criteria are sufficient to discriminate SM from these differential diagnoses.

18.6.2 Abnormal Immunophenotype of Mast Cells in Mastocytosis

Mast cells exhibit a characteristic cell surface antigen phenotype in normal tissues as well as in mastocytosis (32,45–50). In patients with SM, a number of CD antigens are overexpressed on bone marrow MCs (45–47). Likewise, MCs in SM commonly express CD2 and CD25, two surface antigens that are not found on MCs in healthy controls (45–47). Abnormal expression of at least one of these two antigens on MCs is employed as minor SM criterion (69, 70). Expression of these antigens in MCs can be investigated by flow cytometry (45–47) or immunohistochemistry (80, 81). In both instances, CD25 is the more sensitive marker. For flow cytometry, it is thus recommended that a sensitive fluorochrome label is used for detection of CD2 on MCs.

18.6.3   Serum Tryptase Measurement

Tryptase is a well-established disease-related marker enzyme that should be determined in all patients with (suspected) mastocytosis (4–6). In healthy controls, total serum tryptase levels range between <1 and 15 ng/mL (4–6). In those with CM (no systemic involvement), tryptase levels are normal to slightly elevated (4–6). The same holds true for most cases with "isolated" bone marrow mastocytosis without multiorgan disease (6). Higher tryptase values are found in SM patients with multiorgan involvement (seen in most cases of SM). Thus, in most patients with SM, tryptase levels exceed 20 ng/mL (4–6). Moreover, tryptase levels in SM correlate with the burden of neoplastic MCs (5, 6). However, elevated tryptase is not only detected in SM but also in other myeloid neoplasms, especially acute and chronic myeloid leukemias, even in the absence of SM (82–85). Moreover, tryptase levels transiently increase during a severe allergic reaction (85, 86). Therefore, tryptase alone cannot be regarded as a disease-specific and diagnostic marker of SM. Based on these limitations, a persistently elevated serum tryptase level of >20 ng/mL is employed as a minor criterion of SM, provided that an AHNMD has been excluded. In other words, in the presence of an AHNMD, serum tryptase does not count as a criterion of SM (69). All in all, a first important (preinvasive) diagnostic step in suspected mastocytosis is determination of serum tryptase levels, with recognition of potential limitations of the test (4–6, 87).

18.6.4   Recommended Molecular and Cytogenetic Tests

The examination of the bone marrow in suspected SM includes the analysis of *KIT* for codon 816 mutations. The most sensitive (recommended) assays are allele-specific polymerase chain reaction (PCR), PCR plus restriction fragment length polymorphism RFLP, and peptidic nucleic acid PNA-mediated PCR (31, 35). Using these techniques, bone marrow cells (not blood or skin) should be examined for the existence of a codon 816 *KIT* mutation in suspected SM. If the test is negative in a bone marrow sample, sequence analysis to screen for other *KIT* mutations can be considered. However, sequence analysis might yield false-negative results because of a relatively low level of sensitivity (35). By contrast, a false-negative PCR result is unusual even if unfractionated cells are examined or the MC infiltrates are small. Nevertheless, in some cases, the mutation might only be detectable when highly enriched (sorted or microdissected) MCs are analyzed.

In patients with (suspected) AHNMD, bone marrow cells should not only be examined for the presence of mutations in *KIT* but also be subjected to appropriate molecular analyses seeking specific fusion genes or chromosomal defects indicative of specific myeloid neoplasm (34). Likewise, in patients with coexisting eosinophilia, bone marrow and/or blood cells should be examined for the presence of several molecular defects, including BCR/ABL and the FIP1L1/PDGFRA fusion gene (33). In SM-AML, the t(8;21) is often detected (Table 18.1). Apart from molecular markers and chromosomes, it might sometimes be appropriate to measure the numbers of colony-forming progenitor cells in patients with suspected SM-AHNMD (34, 88).

18.7 Categories and Subvariants of Mastocytosis and Current Therapy Options

The delineation of subcategories of CM is based on macroscopic inspection and biopsy of lesional skin (51, 89–91). Based on these aspects, three major variants have been defined: maculopapular CM-urticaria pigmentosa (UP), diffuse CM, and solitary mastocytoma of skin (51, 69, 70, 89–91).

In patients with SM, a number of staging investigations are required to define the exact subtype of disease. Aggressive SM is characterized by progressive infiltration of various organs by MCs with a consecutive impairment of organ function. Respective clinical features have been designated 'C-Findings' (69, 70, 92). Note that MC infiltration with associated organomegaly is not regarded as organopathy (C-Finding) unless accompanied by signs of impaired organ function (69, 92). Thus, organomegaly is also found in patients with an indolent or an uncertain (smouldering) course (60–64), and then is regarded as a B-Finding (69). B- and C-Findings are listed in Table 18.4. In patients with suspected AHNMD (65–68),

Table 18.4 B-Findings and C-Findings

B-Findings = Indication of high burden of MCs, and expansion of the genetic defect into various myeloid lineages
1. Infiltration grade (MCs) in bone marrow >30% in histology *and* serum total tryptase levels >200 ng/mL
2. Hypercellular marrow with loss of fat cells, discrete signs of dysmyelopoiesis without substantial cytopenias or WHO criteria for an MDS or MPD
3. Organomegaly: palpable hepatomegaly, splenomegaly, or lymphadenopathy (on CT or US: >2 cm) without impaired organ function
C-Findings = Indication of impaired organ function due to MC infiltration (has to be confirmed by biopsy in most cases)
1. Cytopenia(s): ANC < 1000/μL or Hb < 10 g/dL or Plt < 100,000/μL
2. Hepatomegaly with ascites and impaired liver function
3. Palpable splenomegaly with hypersplenism
4. Malabsorption with hypalbuminemia and weight loss
5. Skeletal lesions: large-sized osteolyses or/and severe osteoporosis causing pathologic fractures
6. Life-threatening organopathy in other organ systems that is definitively caused by an infiltration of the tissue by neoplastic MCs

Standard - Memorizer: B = B̲orderline B̲enign—B̲e watchful; C = C̲onsider C̲ytoreductive therapy.

WHO criteria (for SM and for AHNMD) are employed to define subvariants (Table 18.1) (69). Sometimes it might be difficult to discriminate among SM-AML, true MCL, and myelomastocytic leukemia (75, 76, 78). MCL is a rare subentity of SM for which SM criteria are fulfilled and there is a diffuse leukemic infiltration of hematopoietic tissues by immature neoplastic MCs (27–30, 69, 70, 92–94). In contrast to ISM, patients with MCL (and also many with ASM) lack UP-like skin lesions [27–30, 69, 70, 92–94). Table 18.5 provides a summary of variants of mastocytosis recognized by the WHO.

An important aspect of mastocytosis is the frequent occurrence of mediator-related symptoms. These symptoms might be mild but might also be severe or even life-threatening (95–97). It is important to be aware that such severe symptoms can occur in any subvariant of mastocytosis (CM or SM variants) and that the symptoms are not, by themselves, diagnostic of aggressive disease (not regarded as C-Findings).

The following subsections give a brief overview of distinct variants of mastocytosis recognized by the WHO, with special reference to diagnostic criteria and available treatment options.

18.7.1   Cutaneous Mastocytosis

True CM usually develops in (early) childhood (51, 90). By definition, MC infiltration in CM is confined to the skin (51, 69). A characteristic maculopapular exanthema is recorded in most patients (51, 89, 90). In a smaller group of patients, skin lesions are diffuse or nodular (51). A positive Darier's sign is a typical clinical feature. Blistering (rare) and flushing might also be observed. The diagnosis CM is based on typical skin lesions, histologic demonstration of MC infiltrates, and lack of diagnostic SM criteria (one or two minor SM criteria are sometimes found in CM) (51, 69). Serum tryptase levels in CM are usually <20 ng/mL (4–6, 69).

Three major variants of CM are described by the WHO: (1) UP, also termed maculopapular cutaneous mastocytosis (MPCM); (2) diffuse CH (DCM; and (3) mastocytoma of the skin (51, 69, 70). MPCM/UP is the most frequent form of CM (89, 90). Apart from the classical form of UP, a number of (rare) subvariants have been described, including a plaque form, a nodular form, and a telangiectatic subvariant (51, 90, 98, 99). The prognosis of UP is good. In many children, skin lesions regress during or shortly after puberty. In some patients, skin lesions are extensive and/or accompanied by mediator-related symptoms requiring therapy. A reasonable approach in adults is to offer mediator-targeting drugs or psoralene with ultraviolet light PUVA (51, 90, 100). In severe cases, glucocorticoids might be necessary. DCM is less frequently diagnosed than UP (51, 90, 91, 101, 102). The prognosis in DCM is reasonable, but the disease might persist into adulthood. Mastocytoma of the skin is rarely diagnosed (51, 90, 103). Histologically, the lesions consist of densely packed MCs without cellular atypia. In most cases, the mastocytoma resolves spontaneously. If this does not occur, excision should be considered (103).

Table 18.5 Classification of mastocytosis according to WHO

Disease variant	Standard abbreviation	Subvariant(s)
Cutaneous mastocytosis	CM	- Urticaria Pigmentosa (UP) = Maculopapular CM (MPCM)
		- Diffuse CM (DCM)
		- Mastocytoma of Skin
Indolent systemic mastocytosis	ISM	- Typical ISM
		- Smouldering SM
		- Isolated bone marrow mastocytosis
Systemic mastocytosis with an associated clonal hematologic non-mast cell lineage disease	SM-AHNMD	- SM-AML
		- SM-MDS
		- SM-MPD
		- SM-CEL; SM-HES
		- SM-CMML
		- SM-NHL
Aggressive systemic mastocytosis	ASM	
		- Lymphadenopathic SM with eosinophilia
Mast cell leukemia	MCL	- Typical MCL
		- Aleukemic MCL
Mast cell sarcoma	MCS	
Extracutaneous mastocytoma	—	

Note: For details of the WHO classification of mastocytosis, see Refs, 69 and 70.

18.7.2 Indolent Systemic Mastocytosis

Indolent systemic mastocytosis is the most frequently diagnosed variant of SM. ISM is defined by SM criteria, involvement of the skin (UP-like lesions), and an indolent clinical course. Progression is rarely seen and the prognosis is good (69, 70, 95). Mediator-related symptoms are reported in a subgroup of patients and might represent the predominant medical problem (95, 96). The bone marrow is almost invariably affected, with multifocal dense infiltrates of MCs (52, 53). In typical ISM, the infiltration grade is rather low, and the infiltrates are sharply demarcated from normal marrow (52, 53). Typically, MCs in bone marrow smears are atypical MC type I (79). Apart from the marrow, MC infiltrates might also be detected in other organs, including the liver, spleen, and the gastrointestinal tract (53–58). In most patients, MCs express CD2 and CD25 and contain the *KIT* mutation D816V (20–23, 45, 69). Serum tryptase levels exceed >20 ng/mL in most cases (4–6, 85, 86). Patients with ISM are treated with 'mediator-targeting' drugs including histamine receptor antagonists but not with cytoreductive agents (Table 18.6) (29, 30, 34, 95, 97, 104). Skin lesions in ISM might also require treatment. In most cases, transient responses are seen with PUVA (105).

Isolated bone marrow mastocytosis is a rare subentity of ISM characterized by the absence of skin lesions and lack of multiorgan involvement (27, 28, 69). It is important to differentiate bone marrow mastocytosis from ASM or MCL, where skin lesions are also absent. In contrast to ASM and MCL, the serum tryptase level in isolated bone marrow mastocytosis usually is low (6). In most patients, no therapy is required.

Smouldering systemic mastocytosis (SSM) is another subentity of ISM (60–64, 69). In contrast to typical ISM, B-Findings (≥ 2) are noted (Table 18.4). These B-Findings reflect a high burden of MCs and extension of the clonal disease into several myeloid non-MClineages (64, 69). Clinically, the smouldering state has an uncertain prognosis and a variable clinical course. In some cases, the clinical course is long-lasting and silent. In other patients, AHNMD or ASM develops with time. Typically, patients with SSM have a bone marrow infiltration grade of >30% (dense infiltrates), serum tryptase levels >200 ng/mL, discrete signs of myelodysplasia or myeloproliferation, and organomegaly (hepatomegaly, splenomegaly, or lymphadenopathy) (64, 69). These B-Findings are due to organ infiltration by MCs or other myeloid cells. However, impairment of organ function (C-Findings) is not observed. The bone marrow in SSM typically contains mixed infiltrates (dense and diffuse component) of MCs (52, 53). These MCs might be quite immature. The *KIT* mutation D816V is detectable in most patients (60–64). In most instances, the mutation is also detected in other myeloid lineages, including unfractionated blood leukocytes (60–64). The treatment of SSM is identical to that in patients with ISM. However, SSM patients should be observed closely for signs of progression or occurrence of an AHNMD.

18.7.3   SM with Associated Clonal Hematologic Non-Mast-Cell Lineage Disease

In a group of patients with SM WHO criteria to diagnose on AHNMD as well as a SM are met (65–70). Patients with SM-AHNMD are categorized according to the AHNMD and the type of SM. In most cases, a myeloid neoplasm such as a myeloproliferative disorder [e.g., idiopathic myelofibrosis (IMF) or the hypereosinophilic syndrome (HES)] or a myeloid leukemia develops (65–70). Myelodysplastic syndromes might also be found. Less frequently, a lymphoid neoplasm is diagnosed. In AHNMD patients, separate treatment plans for the SM component and the AHNMD component of the disease should be established. Notably, in these patients, SM should be treated as if no AHNMD is present, and AHNMD should be treated as if no SM was diagnosed (Table 18.6). Likewise, in patients with SM and an associated CEL with *FIP1L1/PDGFRA* fusion gene,

Table 18.6 Cytoreductive treatment for patients with systemic mastocytosis

Disease variant	Treatment options (recommended)
Typical indolent systemic mastocytosis (ISM)	No cytoreductive treatment required. (exception: consider IFN-α for severe osteoporosis resistant to bisphosphonate therapy).
Smouldering systemic mastocytosis (SSM)	Watch and wait in most cases. However, in select cases (rapidly progressive B-Findings) IFN-α ± glucocorticoids can be considered.
SM-AHNMD	Treat AHNMD as if no SM is present and also treat SM as if no AHNMD is found.
Aggressive systemic mastocytosis (ASM) with slow progression	IFN-α ± glucocorticoids
	If splenomegaly and hypersplenism prohibit therapy, consider splenectomy. In patients without detectable KIT D816V, imatinib might be considered. In those with SM and KIT D816V, novel TK inhibitors are applied in clinical trials.
ASM - rapid progression and patients who do not respond to IFN-α	Polychemotherapy (± IFN-α); consider stem cell transplantation in select cases in whom chemotherapy induces remission.
	For select cases, cladribine (2CdA) or other cytoreductive drugs and novel TK inhibitors (in clinical trials) can be considered.
	Consider hydroxyurea as palliative drug.
Mast cell leukemia (MCL)	Polychemotherapy (± 2CDA; ± IFN-α).
	Consider stem cell transplantation for those in whom chemotherapy can induce remission.
	Consider novel TK inhibitors (clinical trials).
	Consider hydroxyurea as palliative drug.

IFN, interferon; SM-AHNMD, systemic mastocytosis with an associated hematologic clonal non-mast-cell lineage disease.

imatinib induces reasonable responses and, thus, is the recommended drug (106, 107). In patients with SM-AML, polychemotherapy (which would be given in patients with AML without SM) might induce complete hematologic remission of the AML component of the disease (67, 108). An important aspect in SM-AHNMD is that the SM component might present as ISM or ASM, which, in turn, has implications for determining the treatment plan. In some patients, cytoreductive drugs might show beneficial effects for both ASM and the AHNMD component.

18.7.4 Aggressive Systemic Mastocytosis

This rare aggressive subvariant of SM (ASM) is characterized by organopathy caused by pathologic infiltration of diverse organs by neoplastic MCs with consecutive impairment of organ function (27–30, 69, 70,9 2). In contrast to MCL, the bone marrow smear shows less than 20% MCs (69, 92). In contrast to ISM or SSM,

C-Findings are detectable (Table 18.4). In particular, patients show one of the following: (1) significant cytopenia(s); (2) impairment of liver function due to MC infiltration, often with ascites; (3) osteolyses with pathologic fractures; (4) malabsorption with weight loss; (5) splenomegaly with hypersplenism; or (6) significant impairment of organ function in other organ systems (69, 70, 92). The most commonly affected organs are the liver, bone marrow, and the skeletal system. UP-like skin lesions are often absent (69, 70, 92). The histology of the bone marrow shows a variable degree of infiltration, often with mixed (dense focal + diffuse) MC infiltration (52, 53). The bone marrow cytology might disclose major MC atypia, with the occurrence of promastocytes and metachromatic blasts (69, 79). Serum tryptase levels are elevated and often are quite high. Patients with ASM are candidates for treatment with cytoreductive drugs (Table 18.6). Patients with a relatively slow progression are usually treated with glucocorticoids (prednisone) and interferon-alpha (IFN-α) (92, 109–113). Prednisone (50–75 mg p.o. daily) is initiated a few days before IFN-α is administered (3 million IU s.c. three times a week) (34, 92, 97, 113). During the first days of treatment, the patient should be carefully monitored. After a few weeks, the interferon dosage can usually be escalated to 3–5 million units per day and prednisone tapered to a low maintenance dose (92, 97). In case of osteoporosis or osteolysis, the use of biphosphonates is recommended. Patients with ASM with rapid disease progression (e.g., to MCL) or failure to respond to IFN-α are candidates for 2-chlorodeoxy odenoside 2CdA or polychemotherapy (Table 18.6) (34, 92, 94, 114–116). The use of targeted drugs in ASM has also been considered. Imatinib (STI571) has been described to be effective in some of these patients. In fact, several SM patients with wild-type KIT or *KIT* mutations other than D816V appear to respond to imatinib −38, 107). However, most patients with ASM have the D816V *KIT* mutation, which appears to confer (relative) resistance against imatinib (117–119). Therefore, currently, new TK inhibitors such as PKC412 (midostaurin), AHN107 (nilotinib), or BMS354825 (dasatinib) have been tested and used to treat patients with ASM or MCL in clinical trials. In fact, these agents also act on MCs expressing the D816V-mutated vairant of KIT (120–125).

18.7.5 Mast Cell Leukemia and Mast Cell Sarcoma

Mast cell leukemia is a rare aggressive MC neoplasm defined by an increase in atypical immature MCs in bone marrow smears ($\geq$20%) (27–30, 92–94). In typical cases, circulating MCs are detected in the peripheral blood smear (27–30, 92–94). MCL patients typically suffer from rapidly progressive organopathy involving the liver, bone marrow and other organs. The bone marrow typically shows a diffuse plus dense infiltration with MCs (69, 70, 79, 92–94). MCs are often immature, show a blastlike morphology or/and have polylobed nuclei (promastocytes) (69, 79). In many cases, MCs account for more than 10% of blood leukocytes (typical MCL) (69, 79, 94). In other patients, however, MCs account for less than 10% (aleukemic variant) (69, 79, 94). MCs in MCL usually express CD2 and CD25. The

KIT mutation D816V is detected in most patients. The prognosis in MCL is poor. Most patients survive less than 1 year and respond poorly to cytoreductive drugs or chemotherapy (69, 79, 92, 94). A curative therapy is not available for these patients. Chemotherapy regimens employing substances otherwise used in AML patients might be considered (Table 18.6) (94). Another experimental option is stem cell transplantation, although no experience exists concerning responses and outcome.

Mast cell sarcoma (MCS) is an extremely rare form of mastocytosis. To date, the author is aware of only three well-documented cases (126–128). The disease is defined by local destructive sarcomalike growth of a tumor consisting of highly atypical immature MCs (126–128). At diagnosis, systemic involvement is usually not found. However, secondary generalization with involvement of multiple visceral organs and hematopoietic tissues has been described in most cases (126–128) and the terminal phase might be indistinguishable from MCL (126, 128). The prognosis in patients with MC sarcoma is grave. MC sarcoma should not be confused with extracutaneous mastocytoma, a rare benign MC tumor without destructive growth.

18.8   Concluding Remarks

During the past two decades, major advances in mastocytosis research have been made, including the identification of molecular markers and potential drug targets in neoplastic MCs and the formulation of diagnostic criteria. An important aim for the future will be to standardize diagnostic techniques and evaluations, in order to establish a useful basis for the design of clinical trials. There is also hope that the use of novel *KIT* TK inhibitors alone or in combination with other drugs will improve therapy in patients with ASM and MCL in the future.

References

1. Galli SJ. Biology of disease: new insights into "the riddle of the mast cells": microenvironmental regulation of mast cell development and phenotypic heterogeneity. Lab Invest 1990;62:5–33.
2. Valent P, Sillaber C, Bettelheim P. The growth and differentiation of mast cells. Prog Growth Factor Res 1991;3:27–41.
3. Schwartz LB. The mast cell. In: Kaplan AP, editor. Allergy, Volume 1. Edinburgh: Churchill Livingston; 1985. p. 53–92.
4. Schwartz LB, Sakai K, Bradford TR, et al. The alpha form of human tryptase is the predominant type present in blood at baseline in normal subjects and is elevated in those with systemic mastocytosis. J Clin Invest 1995;96:2702–2710.
5. Akin C, Metcalfe DD. Surrogate markers of disease in mastocytosis. Int Arch Allergy Immunol 2002;127:133–136.
6. Sperr WR, Jordan JH, Fiegl M, et al. Serum tryptase levels in patients with mastocytosis: correlation with mast cell burden and implication for defining the category of disease. Int Arch Allergy Immunol 2002;128:136–141.
7. Kitamura Y, Yokoyama M, Matsuda H, et al. Spleen colony forming cell as common precursor for tissue mast cells and granulocytes. Nature 1981;291:159–160.

8. Kirshenbaum AS, Goff JP, Kessler SW, et al. Effects of IL-3 and stem cell factor on the appearance of human basophils and mast cells from CD34+ pluripotent progenitor cells. J Immunol 1992;148:772–777.

9. Kirshenbaum AS, Goff JP, Semere T, et al. Demonstration that human mast cells arise from a progenitor cell population that is CD34+, c-kit+, and expresses aminopeptidase N (CD13). Blood 1999;94:2333–2342.

10. Agis H, Willheim M, Sperr WR, et al. Monocytes do not make mast cells when cultured in the presence of SCF. Characterization of the circulating mast cell progenitor as a c-kit+, CD34+, Ly-, CD14-, CD17-, colony forming cell. J Immunol 1993;151:4221–4227.

11. Rottem M, Okada T, Goff JP, et al. Mast cells cultured from peripheral blood of normal donors and patients with mastocytosis originate from a CD34$^+$/FceRI$^-$ cell population. Blood 1994;84:2489-2496.

12. Valent P. The riddle of the mast cell: c-kit ligand as missing link ? Immunol Today 1994;15:111–114.

13. Mitsui H, Furitsu T, Dvorak AM, et al. Development of human mast cells from umbilical cord blood cells by recombinant human and murine c-kit ligand. Proc Natl Acad Sci USA 1990;90:735–739.

14. Irani AM, Nilsson G, Miettinen U, et al. Recombinant human stem cell factor stimulates differentiation of human mast cells from dispersed fetal liver cells. Blood 1992;80:3009–3016.

15. Valent P, Spanblöchl E, Sperr WR, et al. Induction of differentiation of human mast cells from bone marrow and peripheral blood mononuclear cells by recombinant human stem cell factor (SCF)/kit ligand (KL) in long term culture. Blood 1992;80:2237–2245.

16. Galli SJ, Tsai M, Wershil BK. The c-kit receptor, stem cell factor, and mast cells. What each is teaching us about the others. Am J Pathol 1993;142:965–974.

17. Kitamura Y, Go S, Hatanaka S. Decrease of mast cells in W/W^v mice and their increase by bone marrow transplantation. Blood 1978;52:447–452.

18. Kitamura Y, Go S. Decreased production of mast cells in Sl/Sl^d mice. Blood 1979;53:492–497.

19. Furitsu T, Tsujimura T, Tono T, et al. Identification of mutations in the coding sequence of the proto-oncogene c-kit in a human mast cell leukemia cell line causing ligand-independent activation of the c-kit product. J Clin Invest 1993;92:1736–1744.

20. Feger F, Ribadeau Dumas A, Leriche L, et al. Kit and c-kit mutations in mastocytosis: a short overview with special reference to novel molecular and diagnostic concepts. Int Arch Allergy Immunol 2002;127:110–114.

21. Nagata H, Worobec AS, Oh CK, et al. Identification of a point mutation in the catalytic domain of the protooncogene c-kit in peripheral blood mononuclear cells of patients who have mastocytosis with an associated hematologic disorder. Proc Natl Acad Sci USA 1995;92:10,560–10,564.

22. Longley BJ, Tyrrell L, Lu SZ, et al. Somatic c-kit activating mutation in urticaria pigmentosa and aggressive mastocytosis: establishment of clonality in a human mast cell neoplasm. Nat Genet 1996;12:312–314.

23. Longley BJ, Metcalfe DD, Tharp M, et al. Activating and dominant inactivating c-kit catalytic domain mutations in distinct forms of human mastocytosis. Proc Natl Acad Sci USA 1999;96:1609–1614.

24. Büttner C, Henz BM, Welker P, et al.Identification of activating c-kit mutations in adult-, but not childhood-onset indolent mastocytosis: a possible explanation for divergent clinical behaviour. J Invest Dermatol 1998;111:1227–1231.

25. Akin C, Kirschenbaum AS, Semere T, et al.Analysis of the surface expression of c-kit and occurrence of the c-kit Asp816Val activating mutation in T cells, B cells, and myelomonocytic cells in patients with mastocytosis. Exp Hematol 2000;28:140–147.

26. Yavuz AS, Lipsky PE, Yavuz S, et al. Evidence for the involvement of a hematopoietic progenitor cell in systemic mastocytosis from single cell analysis of mutations in the c-kit gene. Blood 2002;100:661–665.

27. Lennert K, Parwaresch MR. Mast cells and mast cell neoplasia: a review. Histopathology 1979;3:349–365.
28. Parwaresch MR, Horny H-P, Lennert K. Tissue mast cells in health and disease. Pathol Res Pract 1985;179:439–461.
29. Metcalfe DD. Classification and diagnosis of mastocytosis: current status. J Invest Dermatol 1991;96:2S–4S.
30. Valent P. Biology, classification and treatment of human mastocytosis. Wien Klin Wschr 1996;108:385–397.
31. Sotlar K, Escribano L, Landt O, et al. One-step detection of *c-kit* point mutations using peptide nucleic acid-mediated polymerase chain reaction clamping and hybridization probes. Am J Pathol 2003;162:737–746.
32. Valent P, Escribano L, Parwaresch MR, et al. Recent advances in mastocytosis research. Int Arch Allergy Immunol 1999;120:1–7.
33. Tefferi A, Pardanani A. Clinical, genetic, and therapeutic insights into systemic mast cell disease. Curr Opin Hematol 2004;11:58–64.
34. Valent P, Akin C, Sperr WR, et al. Diagnosis and treatment of systemic mastocytosis: state of the art. Br J Haematol 2003;122:695–717.
35. Fritsche-Polanz R, Jordan JH, Feix A, et al. Mutation analysis of *C-KIT* in patients with myelodysplastic syndromes without mastocytosis and cases of systemic mastocytosis. Br J Haematol 2001;113:357–364.
36. Ferrao PT, Gonda TJ, Ashman LK. Constitutively active mutant D816VKit induces megakayocyte and mast cell differentiation of early haemopoietic cells from murine foetal liver. Leuk Res 2003;27:547–555.
37. Pignon JM, Giraudier S, Duquesnoy P, et al. A new c-kit mutation in a case of aggressive mast cell disease. Br J Haematol 1997;96:374–376.
38. Akin C, Fumo G, Yavuz AS, et al. A novel form of mastocytosis associated with a transmembrane *c-Kit* mutation and response to imatinib. Blood 2003;103:3222–3225.
39. Pullarkat VA, Pullarkat ST, Calverley DC, et al. Mast cell disease associated with acute myeloid leukemia: detection of a new *c-kit* mutation Asp816His. Am J Hematol 2000;65:307–309.
40. Pardanani A, Ketterling RP, Brockman SR, et al. CHIC2 deletion, a surrogate for FIP1L1-PDGFRA fusion, occurs in systemic mastocytosis associated with eosinophilia and predicts response to imatinib mesylate therapy. Blood 2003;102:3093–3096.
41. Swolin B, Rodjer S, Roupe G. Cytogenetic studies and in vitro colony growth in patients with mastocytosis. Blood 1987;70:1928–1932.
42. Swolin B, Rodjer S, Roupe G. Cytogenetic studies in patients with mastocytosis. Cancer Genet Cytogenet 2000;120:131–135.
43. Lishner M, Confino-Cohen R, Mekori YA, et al. Trisomies 9 and 8 detected by fluorescence in situ hybridization in patients with systemic mastocytosis. J Allergy Clin Immunol 1996;98:199–204.
44. Daley T, Metcalfe DD, Akin C. Association of the Q576R polymorphism in the interleukin-4 receptor alpha chain with indolent mastocytosis limited to the skin. Blood 2001;98: 880–882.
45. Escribano L, Orfao A, Diaz-Agustin B, et al. Indolent systemic mast cell disease in adults: immunophenotypic characterization of bone marrow mast cells and its diagnostic implication. Blood 1998;91:2731–2736.
46. Schernthaner GH, Jordan JH, Ghannadan M, et al. Expression, epitope analysis, and functional role of the LFA-2 antigen detectable on neoplastic mast cells. Blood 2001;98: 3784–3792.
47. Escribano L, Díaz-Agustín B, Bellas C, et al. Utility of flow cytometric analysis of mast cells in the diagnosis and classification of adult mastocytosis. Leuk Res 2001;25:563–570.
48. Valent P, Bettelheim P. Cell surface structures on human basophils and mast cells: biochemical and functional characterization. Adv Immunol 1992;52:333–423.
49. Valent P, Schernthaner GH, Sperr WR, et al. Variable expression of activation-linked surface antigens on human mast cells in health and disease. Immunol Rev 2001;179:74–81.

50. Ghannadan M, Hauswirth A, Schernthaner G-H, et al. Detection of novel CD antigens on the surface of human mast cells and basophils. Int Arch Allergy Immunol 2002;127:299–307.
51. Wolff K, Komar M, Petzelbauer P. Clinical and histopathological aspects of cutaneous mastocytosis. Leuk Res 2001;25:519–528.
52. Horny H-P, Parwaresch MR, Lennert K. Bone marrow findings in systemic mastocytosis. Human Pathology 1985;16:808–814.
53. Horny H-P, Valent P. Diagnosis of mastocytosis: general histopathological aspects, morphological criteria, and immunohistochemical findings. Leuk Res 2001;25:543–551.
54. Horny H-P, Kaiserling E, Parwaresch MR, et al. Lymph node findings in generalized mastocytosis. Histopathology 1992;21:439–446.
55. Horny H-P, Ruck M, Kaiserling E: Spleen findings in generalized mastocytosis. A clinicopathologic study. Cancer 1992;70:459–468.
56. Horny H-P, Kaiserling E, Campbell M, et al. Liver findings in generalized mastocytosis. A clinicopathologic study. Cancer 1989;63:532–538.
57. Metcalfe DD. The liver, spleen, and lymph nodes in mastocytosis. J Invest Dermatol 1991;96:45S–46S.
58. Travis WD, Li CY. Pathology of the lymph node and spleen in systemic mast cell disease. Mod Pathol 1988;1:4–14.
59. Caplan RM. The natural course of urticaria pigmentosa. Arch Dermatol 1963;87:146–157.
60. Jordan JH, Fritsche-Polanz R, Sperr WR, et al. A case of smouldering mastocytosis with high mast cell burden, monoclonal myeloid cells, and *C-KIT* mutation Asp-816-Val. Leuk Res 2001;25:627–634.
61. Akin C, Scott LM, Metcalfe DD. Slowly progressing mastocytosis with high mast cell burden and no evidence of a non-mast cell hematologic disorder: an example of a smoldering case? Leuk Res 2001;25:635–638.
62. Hauswirth A, Sperr WR, Ghannadan M, et al. A case of smouldering mastocytosis with peripheral blood eosinophilia and lymphadenopathy. Leuk Res 2002;26:601–606.
63. Sotlar K, Marafioti T, Griesser H, et al. Detection of *c-kit* mutation Asp-816-Val in microdissected bone marrow infiltrates in a case of systemic mastocytosis associated with chronic myelomonocytic leukemia. Mol Pathol 2000;53:188–193.
64. Valent P, Akin C, Sperr WR, et al. Smouldering mastocytosis: a new type of systemic mastocytosis with slow progression. Int Arch Allergy Immunol 2002;127:137–139.
65. Horny H-P, Ruck M, Wehrmann M, et al. Blood findings in generalized mastocytosis: evidence of frequent simultaneous occurrence of myeloproliferative disorders. Br J Haematol 1990;76:186–193.
66. Lawrence JB, Friedman BS, Travis WD, et al. Hematologic manifestation of systemic mast cell disease: a prospective study of laboratory and morphologic features and their relation to prognosis. Am J Med 1991;91:612–624.
67. Sperr WR, Horny H-P, Lechner K, et al. Clinical and biologic diversity of leukemias occuring in patients with mastocytosis. Leuk Lymphoma 2000;37:473–486.
68. Travis WD, Li CY, Yam LT, et al. Significance of systemic mast cell disease with associated hematologic disorders. Cancer 1988;62:965–972.
69. Valent P, Horny H-P, Escribano L, et al. Diagnostic criteria and classification of mastocytosis: a consensus proposal. Conference Report of "Year 2000 Working Conference on Mastocytosis". Leuk Res 2001;25:603–625.
70. Valent P, Horny H-P, Li CY, et al. Mastocytosis (mast cell disease). World Health Organization (WHO) classification of tumours. Pathology & genetics. Tumours of haematopoietic and lymphoid tissues. Volume 1. Jaffe ES, Harris NL, Stein H, et al., editors. IARC Press, Lyon, France 2001, p. 291–302.
71. Horny H-P, Sillaber C, Menke D, et al. Diagnostic utility of staining for tryptase in patients with mastocytosis. Am J Surg Pathol 1998;22:1132–1140.
72. Fukuda T, Kamashima T, Tsuura Y, et al. Expression of the c-kit gene product in normal and neoplastic mast cells but not in neoplastic basophil/mast cell precursors from chronic myelogenous leukaemia. J Pathol 1995;177:139–146.

73. Li WV, Kapadia SB, Sonmez-Alpan E, et al. Immunohistochemical characterization of mast cell disease in paraffin sections using tryptase, CD68, myeloperoxidase, lysozym, and CD20 antibodies. Mod Pathol 1996;9:982–988.

74. Li C-Y. Diagnosis of mastocytosis: value of cytochemistry and immunohistochemistry. Leuk Res 2001;25:537–541.

75. Prokocimer M, Polliack A. Increased bone marrow mast cells in preleukemic syndromes, acute leukemia, and lymphoproliferative disorders. Am J Clin Pathol 1981;75:34–38.

76. Valent P, Sperr WR, Samorapoompichit P, et al. Myelomastocytic overlap syndromes: biology, criteria, and relationship to mastocytosis. Leuk Res 2001;25:595–602.

77. Jordan JH, Sperr WR, Lechner K, et al. Stem cell factor-induced bone marrow mast cell hyperplasia mimicking systemic mastocytosis (SM): histopathologic and morphologic evaluation with special reference to novel SM-criteria. Leuk Lymphoma 2002;43:575–582.

78. Valent P, Samorapoompichit P, Sperr WR, et al. Myelomastocytic leukemia: myeloid neoplasm characterized by partial differentiation of mast cell-lineage cells. Hematol J 2002;3:90–94.

79. Sperr WR, Escribano L, Jordan JH, et al. Morphologic properties of neoplastic mast cells: delineation of stages of maturation and implication for cytological grading of mastocytosis. Leuk Res 2001;25:529–536.

80. Jordan JH, Walchshofer S, Jurecka W, et al. Immunohistochemical properties of bone marrow mast cells in systemic mastocytosis: evidence for expression of CD2, CD117/Kit, and bcl-x_L. Hum Pathol 2001;32:545–552.

81. Sotlar K, Horny HP, Simonitsch I, et al. CD25 indicates the neoplastic phenotype of mast cells: a novel immunohistochemical marker for the diagnosis of systemic mastocytosis (SM) on routinely processed bone marrow biopsy specimens. Am J Surg Pathol 2004;28:1319–1325.

82. Sperr WR, Stehberger B, Wimazal F, et al. Serum tryptase measurements in patients with myelodysplastic syndromes. Leuk Lymphoma 2002;43:1097–1105.

83. Sperr WR, Jordan JH, Baghestanian M, et al. Expression of mast cell tryptase by myeloblasts in a group of patients with acute myeloid leukemia. Blood 2001;98:2200–2209.

84. Sperr WR, Hauswirth AW, Valent P. Tryptase a novel biochemical marker of acute myeloid leukemia. Leuk Lymphoma 2002;43:2257–2261.

85. Schwartz LB. Clinical utility of tryptase levels in systemic mastocytosis and associated hematologic disorders. Leuk Res 2001;25:553–562.

86. Schwartz LB, Metcalfe DD, Miller JS, et al. Tryptase levels as an indicator of mast-cell activation in systemic anaphylaxis and mastocytosis. N Engl J Med 1987;316:1622–1626.

87. Valent P, Sperr WR, Schwartz LB, et al. Classification of systemic mast cell disorders: delineation from immunologic diseases and non mast cell lineage hematopoietic neoplasms. J Allergy Clin Immunol 2004;114:3–11.

88. Jordan JH, Jäger E, Sperr WR, et al. Numbers of colony-forming progenitors in patients with systemic mastocytosis: potential diagnostic implications and comparison with myeloproliferative disorders. Eur J Clin Invest 2003;33:611–618.

89. Topar G, Staudacher C, Geisen F, et al. Urticaria pigmentosa: a clinical, hematopathologic, and serologic study of 30 adults. Am J Clin Pathol 1998;109:279–285.

90. Hartmann K, Henz BM. Cutaneous mastocytosis: clinical heterogeneity. Int Arch Allergy Immunol 2002;127:143–146.

91. Willemze R, Ruiter DJ, Scheffer E, et al. Diffuse cutaneous mastocytosis with multiple cutaneous mastocytomas. Report of a case with clinical, histopathological and ultrastructural aspects. Br J Dermatol 1980;102:601–607.

92. Valent P, Akin C, Sperr WR, et al. Aggressive systemic mastocytosis and related mast cell disorders: current treament options and proposed response criteria. Leuk Res 2003;27:635–641.

93. Dalton R, Chan L, Batten E, et al. Mast cell leukemia: evidence for bone marrow origin of the pathological clone. Br J Haematol 1986;64:397–406.

94. Travis WD, Li CY, Hogaland HC, et al. Mast cell leukemia: Report of a case and review of the literature. Mayo Clin Proc 1986;61:957–966.

95. Austen KF. Systemic mastocytosis. N Engl J Med 1992;326:639–640.
96. Castells M, Austen KF. Mastocytosis: mediator-related signs and symptoms. Int Arch Allergy Immunol 2002;127:147–152.
97. Escribano L, Akin C, Castells M, et al. Mastocytosis: current concepts in diagnosis and treatment. Ann Hematol. 2002;81:677–690.
98. Beltrani G, Carlesimo OA. Telangiectasia macularis eruptiva perstans with mastocytosis. Minerva Dermatol 1966;41:436–442.
99. Cohn MS, Mahon MJ. Telangiectasia macularis eruptiva perstans. J Am Osteopath Assoc 1994;94:246–248.
100. Wolff K. Treatment of cutaneous mastocytosis. Int Arch Allergy Immunol 2002;127: 156–159.
101. Verbov JL, Borrie PF. Diffuse cutaneous mastocytosis. Br J Dermatol 1971;84:190–191.
102. Requena L. Erythrodermic mastocytosis. Cutis 1992;49:189–192.
103. McDermott WV, Topol BM. Systemic mastocytosis with extensive large cutaneous mastocytomas: surgical management. J Surg Oncol 1985;30:221–225.
104. Worobec AS. Treatment of systemic mast cell disorders. Hematol Oncol North Am 2000;14:659–687.
105. Godt O, Proksch E, Streit V, Christophers E. Short- and long-term effectiveness of oral and bath PUVA therapy in urticaria pigmentosa and systemic mastocytosis. Dermatology 1997; 195:35–39.
106. Pardanani A, Elliott M, Reeder T, et al. Imatinib for systemic mast-cell disease. Lancet 2003; 362:535–536.
107. Tefferi A, Pardanani A. Imatinib therapy in clonal eosinophilic disorders, including systemic mastocytosis. Int J Hematol 2004;79:441–447.
108. Sperr WR, Walchshofer S, Horny HP, et al. Systemic mastocytosis associated with acute myeloid leukaemia: report of two cases and detection of the c-kit mutation Asp-816 to Val. Br J Haematol. 1998;103:740–749.
109. Kluin-Nelemans HC, Jansen JH, Breukelman H, et al. Response to interferon alfa-2b in a patient with systemic mastocytosis. N Engl J Med 1992;326:619–623.
110. Delaporte E, Pierard E, Wolters BG, et al. Interferon-alpha in combination with corticosteroids improves systemic mast cell disease. Br J Dermatol 1995;132:479–482.
111. Worobec AS, Kirshenbaum AS, Schwartz LB, et al. Treatment of three patients with systemic mastocytosis with interferon alpha-2b. Leuk Lymphoma. 1996;22:501–508.
112. Weide R, Ehlenz K, Lorenz W, et al. Successful treatment of osteoporosis in systemic mastocytosis with interferon alpha-2b. Ann Hematol 1996;72:41–43.
113. Hauswirth AW, Simonitsch-Klupp I, Uffmann M, et al. Response to therapy with interferon alpha-2b and prednisolone in aggressive systemic mastocytosis: report of five cases and review of the literature. Leuk Res 2004;28:249–257.
114. Tefferi A, Li CY, Butterfield JH, et al. Treatment of systemic mast-cell disease with cladribine. N Engl J Med. 2001;344:307–309.
115. Kluin-Nelemans HC, Oldhoff JM, Van Doormaal JJ, et al. Cladribine therapy for systemic mastocytosis. Blood 2003;102:4270–4276.
116. Pardanani A, Hoffbrand AV, Butterfield JH, et al.Treatment of systemic mast cell disease with 2-chlorodeoxyadenosine. Leuk Res 2004;28:127–131.
117. Akin C, Brockow K, D'Ambrosio C, et al. Effects of tyrosine kinase inhibitor STI571 on human mast cells bearing wild-type or mutated forms of c-kit. Exp Hematol 2003;31: 686–692.
118. Ma Y, Zeng S, Metcalfe DD, Akin C, et al. The c-KIT mutation causing human mastocytosis is resistant to STI571 and other KIT kinase inhibitors; kinases with enzymatic site mutations show different inhibitor sensitivity profiles than wild-type kinases and those with regulatory type mutations. Blood 2002;99:1741–1744.
119. Frost MJ, Ferrao PT, Hughes TP, et al. Juxtamembrane mutant V560GKit is more sensitive to Imatinib (STI571) compared with wild-type c-kit whereas the kinase domain mutant D816VKit is resistant. Mol Cancer Ther 2002;1:1115–1124.

120. Growney JD, Clark JJ, Adelsperger J, et al. Activation mutations of human c-KIT resistant to imatinib mesylate are sensitive to the tyrosine kinase inhibitor PKC412. Blood 2005;106: 721–724.
121. Gleixner K, Mayerhofer M, Aichberger K, et al. PKC412 inhibits in vitro growth of neoplastic human mast cells expressing the D816V-mutated variant of KIT: comparison with AMN107, imatinib, and cladribine (2CdA), and evaluation of cooperative drug effects. Blood 2005;107:752–759.
122. Gotlib J, Berube C, Growney JD, et al. Activity of the tyrosine kinase inhibitor PKC412 in a patient with mast cell leukemia with the D816V KIT mutation. Blood 2005;106:2865–2870.
123. Schittenhelm MM, Shiraga S, Schroeder A, et al. Dasatinib (BMS-354825), a dual SRC/ABL kinase inhibitor, inhibits the kinase activity of wild-type, juxtamembrane, and activation loop mutant KIT isoforms associated with human malignancies. Cancer Res 2006;66:473–481.
124. Shah NP, Lee FY, Luo R, Jiang Y, et al. Dasatinib (BMS-354825) inhibits KITD816V, an imatinib-resistant activating mutation that triggers neoplastic growth in most patients with systemic mastocytosis. Blood 2006;108:286–291.
125. Quintas-Cardama A, Aribi A, Cortes J, et al. Novel approaches in the treatment of systemic mastocytosis. Cancer 2006;107:1429–1439.
126. Horny H-P, Parwaresch MR, Kaiserling E, et al. Mast cell sarcoma of the larynx. J Clin Pathol 1986;39:596–602.
127. Kojima M, Nakamura S, Itoh H, et al. Mast cell sarcoma with tissue eosinophilia arising in the ascending colon. Mod Pathol 1999;12:739–743.
128. Guenther PP, Huebner A, Sobottka SB, et al.. Temporary response of localized intracranial mast cell sarcoma to combination chemotherapy. J Pediatr Hematol Oncol 2001;23:134–138.

Index

Cancer Treatment and Research

Steven T. Rosen, M.D., Series Editor

Continued from Pg. ii

Balducci, L., Extermann, M. (eds): *Biological Basis of Geriatric Oncology.* 2004. ISBN

Abrey, L.E., Chamberlain, M.C., Engelhard, H.H. (eds): *Leptomeningeal Metastases.* 2005. ISBN 0-387-24198-1

Platanias, L.C. (ed.): *Cytokines and Cancer.* 2005. ISBN 0-387-24360-7.

Leong, S.P.L., Kitagawa, Y., Kitajima, M. (eds): *Selective Sentinel Lymphadenectomy for Human Solid Cancer.* 2005. ISBN 0-387-23603-1.

Small, Jr. W., Woloschak, G. (eds): *Radiation Toxicity: A Practical Guide.* 2005. ISBN 1-4020-8053-0.

Haefner, B., Dalgleish, A. (eds): *The Link Between Inflammation and Cancer.* 2006. ISBN 0-387-26282-2.

Leonard, J.P., Coleman, M. (eds): *Hodgkin's and Non-Hodgkin's Lymphoma.* 2006. ISBN 0-387-29345.

Leong, S.P.L. (ed): *Cancer Clinical Trials: Proactive Strategies.* 2006. ISBN 0-387-33224-3.

Meyers, C. (ed): *Aids-Associated Viral Oncogenesis.* 2007. ISBN 978-0-387-46804-4.

Ceelen, W.P. (ed): *Peritoneal Carcinomatosis: A Multidisciplinary Approach.* 2007. ISBN 978-0-387-48991-9.

Leong, S.P.L. (ed): *Cancer Metastasis and the Lymphovascular System: Basis for rational therapy.* 2007. ISBN 978-0-387-69218-0.

Raizer, J., Abrey, L.E. (eds): *Brain Metastases.* 2007. ISBN 978-0-387-69221-0.

Woodruff, T., Snyder, K.A. (eds): *Oncofertility.* 2007. ISBN 978-0-387-72292-4.

Angelos, P. (ed): *Ethical Issues in Cancer Patient Care, 2nd edition.* 2008. ISBN 978-0-387-73638-9.

Ansell, S. (ed): *Rare Hematological Malignancies.* 2008. ISBN 978-0-387-73743-0.